DRUG INTERACTIONS

Drug Interactions

Clinical Significance of Drug-Drug Interactions

Philip D. Hansten, *Pharm. D.*

Professor of Clinical Pharmacy
College of Pharmacy
Washington State University
Pullman, Washington

FIFTH EDITION

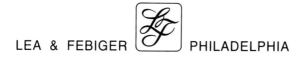

LEA & FEBIGER   PHILADELPHIA

LEA & FEBIGER
600 Washington Square
Philadelphia, Pa. 19106 USA
(215) 922-1330

First edition 1971
Second edition 1973
Third edition 1975
    Reprinted 1976
Fourth edition 1979
Fifth edition 1985

Library of Congress Cataloging in Publication Data

Hansten, Philip D.
    Drug interactions.

    Includes bibliographies and index.
    1. Drug interactions. I. Title. [DNLM: 1. Drug
Interactions. QV 38 H251d]
RM302.H36 1984   615'.7045   84-19397
ISBN 0-8121-0944-9

Printed in the United States of America
Print Number   4   3

PREFACE

The fifth edition of *Drug Interactions* has undergone some substantial changes. Part II (Drug Effects on Clinical Laboratory Results) has been deleted from the book; due to the steadily increasing volume of information, it has become impossible to do justice to both drug interactions and drug effects on laboratory tests. It is planned that the laboratory material will be published separately, with the help of persons who have a special interest in clinical laboratory medicine.

A great deal of information has been published on drug interactions since the last edition, and about 200 interacting pairs have been added. The concise format of previous editions has been maintained to allow rapid access of information and to keep the size of the book within reason. In an effort to maintain clinical relevance, nearly all works cited deal with studies in humans, and all statements refer to humans unless specifically stated otherwise. A basic understanding of pharmacologic and physiologic principles has been assumed in order to keep the discussions as concise as possible.

The continued acceptance of this book has been most gratifying. It has now been translated into Japanese, German, Spanish, and Portuguese. I would also like to acknowledge those persons who helped with the preparation of this edition. The bulging files of journal articles were tamed by Debbie Emrich, Margaret Fanning, Denise Hansten, and Michelle Hansten. Ms. Fanning also prepared the initial material on the smoking-drug interactions included in this edition. Dr. Edward Hartshorn provided both encouragement and invaluable updates of the drug interaction literature; Drs. Leslie Hendeles, Timothey Self, and many others contributed useful information on specific interactions.

PHILIP D. HANSTEN
Pullman, Washington

CONTENTS

INSTRUCTIONS TO USERS

INDEX

The index is the key to the effective use of this book. The drug-drug interactions are arranged as much as possible by drug or drug class, but interactions for a given drug may appear in several locations in the book. For this reason, the index *must* be consulted to ensure finding the desired drug-drug interaction.

CLINICAL SIGNIFICANCE RATING:

All of the drug-drug interactions in this book have been assigned to one of three categories of clinical significance, and these are indicated by differing type faces used both in the index and in the text of the book.

Bold type—Major Clinical Significance: includes those interactions which are relatively well documented and which have the potential of being harmful to the patient.

Italic—Moderate Clinical Significance: includes those interactions for which more documentation is needed and/or the potential harm to the patient is less.

Roman—Minor Clinical Significance: includes those interactions which may occur but which are least significant because of one or more of the following factors:
1) documentation is poor.
2) potential harm to the patient is slight.
3) incidence of the interaction is quite low.

The decision as to the best category for a given drug-drug interaction was based on the severity of the potential interaction, the predictability of the adverse consequences, the amount and quality of literature documenting the existence of the interaction, and finally, the author's own opinions based on personal experience and theoretical considerations. It is important to remember that because of differences in diseases, doses of drugs, routes and duration of administration, renal and hepatic status, etc., an interaction in the "major" category may produce no ill effects, whereas an interaction assigned a "minor" classification may produce a severe adverse drug interaction. Thus, the unique conditions of the individual patient must always be kept in mind when evaluating the clinical significance of drug interactions.

It is important to note that the presence of an interaction in this text (especially if assigned a "minor" rating) should not necessarily be interpreted to mean that it is felt to be of potential clinical significance. Some interactions have been included specifically to demonstrate the tenuous nature of the documentation.

CHAPTER 1

Antiarrhythmic Drug Interactions

AMIODARONE INTERACTIONS

DRUGS	DISCUSSION

Anticoagulants, Oral[373-377]

MECHANISM: Not established. Amiodarone may reduce oral anticoagulant metabolism. Also, since hyperthyroidism enhances the hypoprothrombinemic response to oral anticoagulants, patients who develop amiodarone-induced hyperthyroidism may develop an increased anticoagulant effect.

CLINICAL SIGNIFICANCE: Patients on chronic warfarin therapy have developed excessive hypoprothrombinemia following initiation of amiodarone therapy.[373-377] Several of these patients developed bleeding.[373,376,377] In nine patients on chronic warfarin therapy, the addition of amiodarone resulted in a mean increase in the prothrombin time of approximately 100%.[376] A mean decrease in the warfarin dose of one-third was necessary to maintain the prothrombin time within the therapeutic range. In ten other patients, amiodarone consistently increased the hypoprothrombinemic response to warfarin.[377] In this study the warfarin dose had to be reduced by about one-third to one-half to achieve the desired prothrombin time following the initiation of amiodarone. The increase in hypoprothrombinemic response to warfarin may last long after the amiodarone is discontinued. In four patients on warfarin, the potentiating effect of amiodarone continued for a period of 1.5 to 4 months.[376] The onset of the increased warfarin effect following initiation of amiodarone therapy has not been well studied, but available evidence indicates that enhanced hypoprothrombinemia becomes apparent within 2 to 4 days of concomitant therapy. The hypoprothrombinemia may continue to increase for several more days.[373,374] Bleeding episodes secondary to this interaction usually occur 1 to 4 weeks following the initiation of amiodarone, although bleeding could appear sooner or later.

MANAGEMENT: In patients receiving oral anticoagulants, it would be preferable to avoid the use of amiodarone. If amiodarone is used, the hypoprothrombinemic response to oral anticoagulants should be monitored carefully. Because the onset of the interaction is delayed in some patients, the prothrombin time should be monitored for several weeks following initiation of amiodarone therapy. Because the inter-

DRUGS	DISCUSSION

action may have a long duration, warfarin dosage may need to be adjusted for months following discontinuation of amiodarone.

Aprindine (Fibocil)[372]

MECHANISM: Not established.

CLINICAL SIGNIFICANCE: Two patients on chronic aprindine therapy developed increased serum aprindine levels and symptoms such as nausea, ataxia, and lightheadedness following initiation of amiodarone therapy (1200 mg daily, then 400 to 600 mg daily.)[372] The authors reported that in general patients receiving both drugs tend to require less aprindine than those receiving aprindine alone. More data are needed to establish the incidence and magnitude of this purported interaction.

MANAGEMENT: One should be alert for evidence of altered aprindine response if amiodarone therapy is initiated or discontinued.

Digitalis Glycosides[368-371]

MECHANISM: Not established. Both pharmacokinetic and pharmacodynamic interactions may be involved.

CLINICAL SIGNIFICANCE: Following the observation of unexpectedly high plasma digoxin levels and neurotoxicity in several patients who were receiving amiodarone concurrently, seven patients stabilized on chronic digoxin therapy were given amiodarone (600 mg daily).[368] The plasma digoxin concentrations were increased during the next 4 days by an average of approximately 70%. Although the plasma digoxin concentrations increased in all of the patients, only four developed symptoms consistent with digoxin toxicity. In two other patients on chronic digoxin therapy, a 0.4 and 0.7 ng/ml increase in serum digoxin occurred when the dose of amiodarone was raised from 200 mg to 600 mg daily. A control group of six similar patients receiving digoxin alone did not experience increased plasma digoxin concentrations. However, in a subsequent study of five patients receiving chronic digoxin, the administration of amiodarone (800 mg daily for 5 days, then 400 mg daily) did not affect the serum digoxin concentration.[369] The reason for the disparate results in these two studies is not clear. Nevertheless, until more conclusive data are available one should assume that amiodarone can increase serum digoxin levels. Others have noted sinus arrest in three patients receiving combined therapy with amiodarone and digoxin.[370,371] Although the sinus arrest could have been due to a pharmacodynamic and/or pharmacokinetic interaction between amiodarone and digoxin, this possibility remains largely speculative at present. In summary, the bulk of the evidence indicates that amiodarone is capable of increasing plasma digoxin concentrations.

MANAGEMENT: One should be alert for evidence of altered digoxin response if amiodarone is initiated or discontinued. Plasma digoxin determinations would be useful in following this interaction.

AMIODARONE INTERACTIONS (CONT.)

DRUGS	DISCUSSION

Disopyramide (Norpace), Mexiletine[121]

MECHANISM: Not established. Combined pharmacologic effects may be involved.

CLINICAL SIGNIFICANCE: Isolated cases of prolongation of the QT interval and ventricular arrhythmias have been reported in patients receiving amiodarone plus other antiarrhythmic drugs such as disopyramide and mexiletine.[121] The incidence and magnitude of this potential interaction is not known.

MANAGEMENT: Carefully monitor the cardiac status of patients receiving combined therapy with amiodarone and other agents such as disopyramide or mexiletine (especially at the beginning of combined therapy).

Lidocaine[141]

MECHANISM: Combined depression of the sinus node.

CLINICAL SIGNIFICANCE: A 64-year-old man with sick sinus syndrome developed severe sinus bradycardia following local anesthesia with 15 ml of 2% lidocaine while on amiodarone therapy (600 mg/day).[141] He responded to cardiac massage, atropine, and isoproterenol. The authors proposed that the reaction resulted from the combined effects of amiodarone and lidocaine. More study is needed.

MANAGEMENT: Until more is known about this purported interaction, cardiac status be monitored closely if lidocaine is administered systemically or locally to patients receiving amiodarone.

Quinidine[121]

MECHANISM: Not established. Both pharmacodynamic and pharmacokinetic interactions may be involved.

CLINICAL SIGNIFICANCE: A patient on long-term quinidine therapy (1200 mg daily) developed atypical ventricular tachycardia ("torsades de pointes") and a prolonged QT interval shortly after an injection of amiodarone (150 mg in pulmonary artery).[121] These effects did not recur when quinidine was subsequently administered alone. Another patient receiving quinidine (1200 mg/day) and amiodarone (200 mg/day) developed atypical ventricular tachycardia following routine bicycle ergometry. In addition, a healthy subject was given quinidine (1200 mg daily) and 6 days later amiodarone (600 mg daily) was added. After 3 days of amiodarone administration, the plasma quinidine level was increased by about twofold, and the QT interval was prolonged in comparison to that seen the quinidine alone. In summary, preliminary evidence indicates that amiodarone may interact with quinindine on both a pharmacodynamic and pharmacokinetic basis.

MANAGEMENT: When amiodarone is added to quinidine therapy, one should monitor the cardiac status (e.g., QT interval prolongation) and, if possible, serum quinidine levels.

DISOPYRAMIDE (NORPACE) INTERACTIONS

DRUGS	DISCUSSION

Anticoagulants, Oral[104,125,126]

MECHANISM: Not established.

CLINICAL SIGNIFICANCE: A patient stabilized on warfarin (3 mg/daily) and disopyramide developed a twofold increase in warfarin requirements when the disopyramide was stopped.[104] Other causes for the increased warfarin requirements could not be found. However, disopyramide had little effect on the hypoprothrombinemic response to warfarin in three other patients.[125] It has been proposed that disopyramide-induced hemodynamic changes could affect hepatic clotting factor synthesis,[125,126] thus affecting the prothrombin time. In summary, there is little evidence to support an effect of disopyramide on warfarin response, but one should be aware of the possibility.

MANAGEMENT: Until more information is available, monitor patients for altered anticoagulant response if disopyramide is started or stopped.

Antidiabetics[127,128,389]

MECHANISM: Not established.

CLINICAL SIGNIFICANCE: Isolated cases of hypoglycemia associated with disopyamide therapy have been reported,[127,128,389] but the incidence of this finding is not established. It has been suggested that predisposing factors for disopyramide-induced hypoglycemia may be old age, and serious impairment of renal or hepatic function.[389]

MANAGEMENT: One should be alert for evidence of enhanced hypoglycemic response to antidiabetic drugs if disopyramide is given concurrently.

Beta-Adrenergic Blockers[122–124,140]

MECHANISM: Not established. Combined pharmacologic effects may be involved.

CLINICAL SIGNIFICANCE: Two patients with supraventricular tachycardia developed severe bradycardia after receiving intravenous practolol and then intravenous disopyramide.[122] One of the patients progressed to asystole and died. In studies of healthy subjects, no pharmacodynamic interactions on left ventricular function were noted when the use of propranolol (Inderal) and disopyramide in combination was compared to either drug alone.[123,140] Further, concurrent administration of disopyramide and propranolol does not appear to affect the pharmacokinetics of either drug.[124] In summary, there is only limited clinical information indicating an interaction between disopyramide and practolol. However, the severity of the possible interaction is such (one patient died), that it cannot be ignored.

4

DISOPYRAMIDE (NORPACE) INTERACTIONS (CONT.)

DRUGS	DISCUSSION

MANAGEMENT: Until more clinical information is available, one should administer disopyramide (especially if given intravenously) only with caution and careful monitoring to patients receiving practolol or other beta-adrenergic blockers.

Diazepam (Valium)[124]

MECHANISM: None.

CLINICAL SIGNIFICANCE: Studies in healthy subjects indicate that concurrent use of disopyramide and diazepam does not alter the disposition of either drug.

MANAGEMENT: No special precautions appear necessary.

Digitalis Glycosides[129–131,384]

MECHANISM: None.

CLINICAL SIGNIFICANCE: Three studies involving a total of 24 patients indicated that disopyramide does not affect the disposition of digoxin.[129–131] A subsequent study found a reduction in digoxin half-life in five healthy men given 600 mg/day of disopyramide.[384] However, this was balanced by a reduction in digoxin volume of distribution resulting in no change in the steady-state serum digoxin concentration.

MANAGEMENT: No special precautions appear necessary.

Lidocaine[132]

MECHANISM: Combined cardiodepressant effects.

CLINICAL SIGNIFICANCE: Isolated cases have been reported of impaired intraventricular conduction and ventricular asystole in predisposed patients receiving combined therapy with disopyramide and lidocaine.

MANAGEMENT: Patients receiving combined therapy with disopyramide and lidocaine should be monitored closely, especially in the presence of preexisting impairment of myocardial function of conduction disturbances.

Phenytoin (Dilantin)[132–135]

MECHANISM: The hepatic metabolism of disopyramide may be enhanced by phenytoin-induced enzyme stimulation. Also, disopyramide and phenytoin may exert additive cardiodepressant effects.

CLINICAL SIGNIFICANCE: Data from several patients indicate that phenytoin increases the elimination of disopyramide.[133–135] The magni-

DRUGS	DISCUSSION

tude of the reductions in serum disopyramide appear large enough to reduce the response to disopyramide. However, serum levels of the major metabolite of disopyramide (mono-N-dealkyldisopyramide) are increased, and there is some evidence that this product may have antiarrhythmic activity.[133-134] Thus, it is not yet clear whether the therapeutic response to disopyramide would be reduced by concurrent use of enzyme inducers such as phenytoin. A pharmacodnamic interaction between disopyramide and phenytoin has also been proposed based on a patient who developed an idioventricular rhythm and atrial standstill while receiving both drugs.[132] It should be noted that any pharmacodynamic interaction between phenytoin and disopyramide would occur as soon as sufficient serum levels of both drugs are achieved, while the stimulation of disopyramide metabolism by phenytoin would occur gradually over a period of about 7 to 10 days.

MANAGEMENT: One should be alert for evidence of altered disopyramide response if phenytoin is given concurrently.

Potassium Salts[136]

MECHANISM: The cardiovascular toxicity of disopyramide may be increased by elevated potassium levels.

CLINICAL SIGNIFICANCE: A patient developed conduction disturbances and hypotension which was attributed to the combined effects of disopyramide and potassium supplementation.[136] The serum disopyramide level was 10.8 μg/ml (about twice the upper limit of the therapeutic range), and the serum potassium was 6.9 mEg/L. The degree to which elevated serum potassium levels would predispose to disopyramide toxicity in patients with therapeutic serum levels of disopyramide is not established. The likelihood of elevated serum levels of both disopyramide and potassium would increase in a patient with serious renal impairment, and such patients may be at greater risk of this interaction.

MANAGEMENT: One should be alert for electrocardiographic evidence of disopyramide toxicity (e.g., QRS widening) if potassium supplementation is also given, especially if large doses of disopyramide and potassium are used or if renal function is impaired.

Quinidine[124,137]

MECHANISM: The mechanism for the small changes in serum levels of disopyramide and quinidine is not established. Combined cardiodepressant effects may occur since both drugs are type I antiarrhythmic agents.

CLINICAL SIGNIFICANCE: In healthy subjects quinidine administration has been shown to produce small increases in serum disopyramide levels, while disopyramide produces small decreases in serum quinidine levels.[124,137] Also, anticholinergic effects such as dry mouth,

DISOPYRAMIDE (NORPACE) INTERACTIONS (CONT.)

DRUGS	DISCUSSION

blurred vision, and urinary retention were more common with concurrent therapy with both drugs than with either drug alone.[137] It seems unlikely that the degree of increase in serum disopyramide following quinidine would be sufficient to produce toxicity unless the preexisting disopyramide level was at the upper end of the therapeutic range. Significant additive electrocardiographic effects from disopyramide and quinidine were not noted in healthy subjects,[137] but this does not rule out such effects in patients with cardiac disease.

MANAGEMENT: One should be alert for evidence of enhanced disopyramide effect and anticholinergic side effects if quinidine is given concurrently.

Rifampin (Rimactane, Rifadin)[134]

MECHANISM: Rifampin stimulates the hepatic metabolism of disopyramide.

CLINICAL SIGNIFICANCE: Twelve patients with recently diagnosed tuberculosis were given disopyramide (200 to 300 mg as a single dose) before and 2 weeks after starting therapy with rifampin.[134] Serum disopyramide levels were reduced to about 50% in the presence of rifampin, and the amount of disopyramide excreted unchanged in the urine (% of dose) fell to about one-fourth of that seen without rifampin. The study was complicated by the fact that some of the patients were given isoniazid in addition to the rifampin. In summary, it appears that rifampin is capable of lowering serum disopyramide to subtherapeutic levels in at least some patients.

MANAGEMENT: One should be alert for evidence of altered disopyramide effect if rifampin is started or stopped. Serum disopyramide levels would be useful in monitoring this interaction.

LIDOCAINE INTERACTIONS

DRUGS	DISCUSSION

Ajmaline[2]

MECHANISM: Lidocaine and other antiarrhythmic agents such as ajmaline can exert a combined cardiac depressant effect.

CLINICAL SIGNIFICANCE: One case has been briefly reported in which a 67-year-old woman developed a worsening of her cardiac failure following combined therapy with ajmaline and intravenous lidocaine.[2]

MANAGEMENT: Combined therapy with antiarrhythmic drugs is sometimes necessary but should be accompanied by increased vigilance toward detection of adverse effects.

Aminoglycosides, Polymyxin B[159]

MECHANISM: Enhanced neuromuscular blockade.

7

DRUGS	DISCUSSION

CLINICAL SIGNIFICANCE: In-vitro studies indicate that neomycin and polymyxin B enhance the neuromuscular blocking activity of lidocaine, but the clinical significance of these findings are not clear.

MANAGEMENT: Until clinical information is available one should be alert for evidence of neuromuscular blockade (e.g., impaired respirations) in patients receiving systemic lidocaine plus aminoglycosides or polymyxin B.

Barbiturates[4,5,143–145]

MECHANISM: Barbiturates appear to enhance the disposition of lidocaine. Although this has been assumed to be due to induction of hepatic microsomal enzymes, hepatic blood flow is probably the primary determinant of lidocaine disposition. Thus, the observed effect might be related to barbiturate-induced increases in hepatic blood flow.

CLINICAL SIGNIFICANCE: Barbiturates markedly reduce the bioavailability of oral lidocaine,[143,144] but lidocaine is seldom given by that route. Studies of intravenous lidocaine administration in man[4,143] and dogs[5] have indicated that lidocaine disposition is slightly enhanced by pretreatment with phenobarbital. Thus, it has been proposed that patients receiving barbiturates might be more tolerant to the effects of lidocaine. However, since lidocaine is usually titrated to achieve the desired response, it does not seem likely that patients would frequently be adversely affected. Administration of pentobarbital (30 mg/kg I.V. over 1 minute) to six dogs which had received lidocaine infusions resulted in apnea in all six, and four of them died.[145] The author proposed that the two drugs had additive effects on the respiratory center. However, large doses of pentobarbital were used, and the clinical importance of these findings is not clear.

MANAGEMENT: Until more information is available, patients receiving lidocaine and intravenous barbiturates should be monitored for excessive respiratory depression.

Beta-adrenergic blockers[80,96,146–151]

MECHANISM: Beta-blockers tend to reduce cardiac output and hepatic blood flow, which would in turn reduce hepatic lidocaine metabolism.[146,148] There is also evidence that beta-blockers may inhibit the activity of hepatic microsomal drug metabolizing enzymes.[80,149,151] This effect may be greater for the more lipid-soluble beta-blockers such as propranolol, labetalol, oxprenolol, timolol, and metoprolol than for those which are more polar, such as atenolol, nadolol, and sotalol.[149] Finally, lidocaine may enhance the negative inotropic effect of propranolol (and possibly other beta-blockers).[150]

CLINICAL SIGNIFICANCE: In 11 healthy volunteers, pretreatment with propranolol (80 mg tid for 3 days) substantially reduced the plasma clearance of intravenous lidocaine, resulting in a 30% increase in

DRUGS	DISCUSSION

steady-state serum lidocaine levels during continuous lidocaine infusions.[146] In another study, six healthy subjects were given three single doses of lidocaine (2.5 to 3.0 mg/kg IV over 10 minutes): one alone, one following 1 day of pretreatment with propranolol (40 mg orally every 6 hours), and one following 1 day of pretreatment with metoprolol (50 mg orally every 6 hours).[148] Propranolol reduced lidocaine clearance by 47%, and metroprolol reduced lidocaine clearance by 31%. The magnitude of the changes in lidocaine disposition found in these studies appear sufficient to increase the danger of lidocaine toxicity. Two cases of toxicity which may have been due to this interaction have been reported.[147] The clinical importance of the additive negative inotropic effect of lidocaine and beta-blockers[150] is not yet established.

MANAGEMENT: One should be alert for the need to lower lidocaine dosage in patients who receive concurrent therapy with beta-blockers. The magnitude of the reduction in lidocaine elimination appears to be less with metoprolol than with propranolol, but still may be clinically important.

Cephalosporins[152]

MECHANISM: None.

CLINICAL SIGNIFICANCE: Reconstitution of cefoxitin with 0.5% or 1.0% lidocaine does not appear to affect the disposition of cefoxitin.[152]

MANAGEMENT: No special precautions appear necessary.

Cimetidine (Tagamet)[153–157,380]

MECHANISM: Cimetidine is known to inhibit hepatic microsomal drug metabolism, and there is some evidence that it may reduce hepatic blood flow.[155] Also, cimetidine may alter the distribution and protein binding of lidocaine.[153] Combined effects of cimetidine and lidocaine on cardiac function and mental status are also possible, but little is known about such mechanisms.

CLINICAL SIGNIFICANCE: Six healthy subjects received lidocaine (1 mg/kg body weight I.V. over 10 minutes) with and without pretreatment with cimetidine (300 mg qid for 1 day).[153] Lidocaine clearance was reduced by about 25%, and peak serum lidocaine levels were increased by 50%. Five of the six subjects developed symptoms of lidocaine toxicity (light-headedness, intoxication, paresthesias) during the lidocaine infusions when pretreated with cimetidine. Similar results were found in a subsequent study of 21 patients receiving lidocaine infusions.[154] Cimetidine (300 mg every 6 hours) given to 15 of the 21 patients produced substantial increases in serum lidocaine levels: six had lidocaine levels in the toxic range and two had symptoms of lidocaine toxicity (confusion, lethargy). Lidocaine serum levels did not increase in the six controls who did not receive cimetidine. However, another study in seven patients did not find an effect of intrave-

DRUGS	DISCUSSION

nous cimetidine (2 mg/kg body weight then 0.75 mg/kg body weight/hour) on the disposition of lidocaine given as a continuous intravenous infusion.[380]

MANAGEMENT: One should be alert for evidence of excessive lidocaine effect if cimetidine is given concurrently; reductions in lidocaine dose may be necessary. Ranitidine may be a good alternative to cimetidine since it does not appear to affect lidocaine disposition.[156,157] It also seems unlikely that antacids or sucralfate would affect lidocaine disposition.

Diazepam (Valium)[6,158]

MECHANISM: None.

CLINICAL SIGNIFICANCE: Since diazepam appeared to antagonize the central nervous system toxicity of lidocaine, it was feared that the antiarrhythmic effect of lidocaine might also be antagonized by diazepam. However, studies in dogs indicated that diazepam actually *enhanced* the antiarrhythmic effect of lidocaine.[6] In another study of cats given large doses of lidocaine, diazepam protected against lidocaine-induced seizures but did not enhance the cardiovascular toxicity of lidocaine.[158]

MANAGEMENT: No special precautions appear necessary.

Digitalis glycosides[158]

MECHANISM: None.

CLINICAL SIGNIFICANCE: In three patients receiving digoxin, the mean serum digoxin was 0.60 ng/ml before and 0.83 ng/ml during lidocaine administration.[158] The increase was not statistically significant, but too few patients were studied to determine whether an interaction occurs.

MANAGEMENT: No special precautions appear necessary at this point.

Diphenhydramine (Benadryl)[142]

MECHANISM: None.

CLINICAL SIGNIFICANCE: Diphenhydramine (dose not stated) did not affect serum lidocaine levels in three patients.

MANAGEMENT: No special precautions appear necessary.

Isoproterenol (Isuprel)[85]

MECHANISM: It is proposed that isoproterenol may increase hepatic blood flow, thus enhancing lidocaine disposition.

CLINICAL SIGNIFICANCE: Studies in monkeys have demonstrated enhanced lidocaine disposition when an isoproterenol infusion is given.[85] The significance to human therapy remains speculative.

LIDOCAINE INTERACTIONS (CONT.)

DRUGS	DISCUSSION

MANAGEMENT: Until human data are available, one should be alert for evidence of reduced lidocaine response in the presence of isoproterenol.

Levarterenol (norepinephrine, Leveophed)[85]

MECHANISM: It is proposed that levarterenol may decrease hepatic blood flow, thus slowing lidocaine disposition.

CLINICAL SIGNIFICANCE: Studies in monkeys have demonstrated slowed lidocaine disposition when a levarterenol infusion is given.[85] The significance of these findings to human therapy remains speculative.

MANAGEMENT: Until human data are available, one should be alert for evidence of enhanced lidocaine response in the presence of levarterenol.

Neuromuscular Blocking Agents[3,7,78,159]

MECHANISM: Not established. Lidocaine and other antiarrhythmics may enhance the neuromuscular blockade of skeletal muscle relaxants by impairing transmission of impulses at the motor nerve terminals.[3] It has also been proposed that lidocaine may displace succinylcholine from plasma protein binding.[7]

CLINICAL SIGNIFICANCE: Bolus intravenous doses of lidocaine (from 1.0 to 16.5 mg/kg) have been shown to prolong the duration of succinylcholine (0.7 mg/kg)-induced apnea in humans. Lidocaine doses of 3.3 mg/kg and below produced only a mild increase in duration of apnea. At a dose of 5.0 mg/kg of lidocaine the duration of succinylcholine apnea was approximately doubled, and at 16.5 mg/kg of lidocaine it was about three times that of control.[7] Thus, doses of lidocaine commonly used clinically are not likely to have a major effect on the duration of succinylcholine apnea. In another study intravenous lidocaine (6 mg/kg bolus) prevented succinylcholine-induced increases in intragastric pressure.[78] Studies in cats have shown that the intensity and duration of neuromuscular block from tubocurarine can be enhanced by administration of lidocaine.[3]

MANAGEMENT: Some caution should be observed in the concomitant use intravenous lidocaine and neuromuscular blocking agents such as succinylcholine and tubocurarine, especially if large doses of lidocaine are used.

Phenytoin (Dilantin)[1,4,143]

MECHANISM:
1. Diphenylhydantoin may enhance the diposition of lidocaine.[4]
2. Diphenylhydantoin and lidocaine may have additive cardiac depressant effects.[1]

11

DRUGS	DISCUSSION

CLINICAL SIGNIFICANCE: Phenytoin appears to substantially reduce the bioavailability of oral lidocaine,[143] but lidocaine is seldom given by that route. Patients with epilepsy receiving diphenylhydantoin and other anticonvulsants have shown an increased rate of disappearance of lidocaine administered intravenously.[4] In another similar study, patients on anticonvulsants tended to have a higher clearance of intravenously administered lidocaine than healthy volunteers, but the differences were not clinically significant.[143] The significance of this effect on the antiarrhythmic response to lidocaine is not known, but it probably is not large. The additive depressant effect of lidocaine and intravenous diphenylhydantoin on cardiac pacemaker tissue (Mechanism #2) may have resulted in sinoatrial arrest in one patient.[1]

MANAGEMENT: Combined therapy with intravenous diphenylhydantoin and intravenous lidocaine should be undertaken with the realization that excessive cardiac depression might occur. In the case cited, intravenous isoproterenol reversed the severe ventricular bradycardia seen following combined use of lidocaine and diphenylhydantoin.

Procainamide (Pronestyl)[46]

MECHANISM: Not established. It is possible that additive psychiatric side effects may be seen with concomitant use of lidocaine and procainamide.

CLINICAL SIGNIFICANCE: Not established. A single case has been reported in which delirium occurred in a patient receiving both lidocaine and procainamide.[46] It was proposed that procainamide could have precipitated the delirium by adding to the effects of lidocaine.

MANAGEMENT: The possibility of additive neurologic effects should be realized, but too little information is available to make a statement on management.

Ranitidine (Zantac)[156,157]

MECHANISM: None.

CLINICAL SIGNIFICANCE: In six healthy subjects, the disposition of lidocaine (1 mg/kg body weight IV) was not altered by pretreatment with ranitidine (300 mg/day for 1 day).[156] Similarly, ranitidine (400 mg/day) did not affect lidocaine disposition in a preliminary report of a study in six healthy subjects.[157]

MANAGEMENT: No special precautions appear necessary.

Smoking[160]

MECHANISM: Smoking appears to stimulate the hepatic microsomal enzymes responsible for the metabolism of lidocaine, but smoking also tends to reduce hepatic blood flow.[160]

CLINICAL SIGNIFICANCE: The bioavailability of oral lidocaine is markedly reduced in smokers. However, the enzyme induction caused by

LIDOCAINE INTERACTIONS (CONT.)

DRUGS	DISCUSSION

smoking has relatively little effect on the disposition of intravenous lidocaine, since lidocaine is highly extracted by the liver. In addition, the ability of smoking to reduce hepatic blood flow somewhat would probably more than offset any effect of enzyme induction on lidocaine given intravenously. In summary, it appears that intravenous lidocaine will have similar disposition in smokers and nonsmokers. However, it is possible that in an occasional patient, smoking would have sufficient effect so that lidocaine response would be altered.

MANAGEMENT: No special precautions appear necessary at this point.

PROCAINAMIDE (PRONESTYL) INTERACTIONS

DRUGS	DISCUSSION

Acetazolamide (Diamox)[56,84,100]

MECHANISM: See Clinical Significance.

CLINICAL SIGNIFICANCE: Acetazolamide is a urinary alkalinizer. Although it had been suspected that procainamide might undergo pH dependent urinary excretion, several studies have failed to document such an effect.[56,84,100] Preliminary information indicates that the active metabolite of procainamide (N-acetylprocainamide) is also unaffected by urinary pH changes.[100]

MANAGEMENT: Current evidence indicates that urine pH need not be considered as a significant cause of variation in plasma procainamide levels.

Ammonium Chloride[56,84,100]

MECHANISM: See Clinical Significance.

CLINICAL SIGNIFICANCE: Although it had been suspected that procainamide might undergo pH dependent urinary excretion, neither urinary acidification with ammonium chloride administration nor alkalinization with sodium bicarbonate administration appears to affect renal excretion.[56,84] Preliminary information indicates that the active metabolite of procainamide (N-acetylprocainamide) is also unaffected by urinary pH changes.[100]

MANAGEMENT: Current evidence indicates that urine pH need not be considered as a significant cause of variation in plasma procainamide levels.

Antacids[161]

MECHANISM: Aluminum hydroxide suspension may delay procainamide absorption in dogs.

CLINICAL SIGNIFICANCE: Procainamide (300 mg orally) was administered to six dogs with and without suspensions of aluminum hydrox-

DRUGS	DISCUSSION

ide (1 g/10 ml) or magnesium oxide (1 g/10 ml).[161] Aluminum hydroxide lowered the maximal plasma procainamide concentration by about 20% but the reduction in the area under the procainamide plasma level time curve was not statistically significant. Magnesium hydroxide did not affect procainamide. Antacids appear to have minimal effects on procainamide absorption in dogs, but studies in humans are lacking.

MANAGEMENT: No special precautions appear necessary at this point.

Beta-adrenergic Blockers[213,386]

MECHANISM: Not established.

CLINICAL SIGNIFICANCE: In a preliminary report, six healthy subjects received procainamide with and without long-term propranolol pretreatment.[213] Procainamide elimination half-life increased by about 50%, and procainamide plasma clearance decreased by 16% in the presence of procainamide. However, in a subsequent study of eight subjects neither propranolol (240 mg/day) nor metoprolol (200 mg/day) affected the pharmacokinetics of a single dose of procainamide (500 mg intravenously).[386]

MANAGEMENT: Until more is known about this potential interaction, one should be alert for evidence of altered procainamide response if propranolol therapy is initiated or discontinued.

Cholinergic Agents [57,79]

MECHANISM: Procainamide has neuromuscular blocking properties and may antagonize the effect of cholinergic drugs on skeletal muscle.

CLINICAL SIGNIFICANCE: The therapeutic response of cholinergic drugs used in the treatment of myasthenia gravis may be antagonized by procainamide. Isolated cases have been reported or worsening of myasthenic symptoms several days after starting procainamide therapy.[79] Also edrophonium tests may be unreliable in procainamide-treated patients.[79]

MANAGEMENT: If possible, avoid procainamide in myasthenic patients. Unfortunately, quinidine cannot be used as a substitute since it can produce similar deterioration of myasthenia. Although lidocaine and propranolol might also be expected to worsen myasthenia,[57] limited use of lidocaine in two myasthenic patients did not result in aggravation of symptoms.[79]

Cimetidine (Tagamet)[162-164]

MECHANISM: Preliminary evidence indicates that cimetidine reduces the renal excretion of procainamide and its major metabolite acetylprocainamide.

CLINICAL SIGNIFICANCE: Six healthy subjects were given procainamide (1 g orally) with and without cimetidine pretreatment (1 g/day

DRUGS	DISCUSSION

for 1 day).[162] All six subjects developed an increase in the procainamide plasma concentration time curve (mean increase, 35%) and the procainamide half-life increased from 2.9 to 3.8 hours. Renal procainamide clearance decreased by almost 50% following treatment with cimetidine. Acetylprocainamide was similarly affected by cimetidine treatment. The magnitude of these changes indicate that some patients may develop excessive levels of procainamide and acetylprocainamide in the presence of cimetidine. Patients with marked renal impairment and the elderly are probably more at risk, since they may have reduced renal clearance of all three drugs.[162-164]

MANAGEMENT: One should be alert for evidence of enhanced procainamide and acetylprocainamide response in the presence of cimetidine therapy. A reduction in procainamide dose may be necessary.

Ethanol[99]

MECHANISM: Ethanol appears to enhance the acetylation of procainamide in the liver.

CLINICAL SIGNIFICANCE: Procainamide (10 mg/kg orally) was given to 11 healthy subjects with and without ethanol (0.73 g/kg body weight/ 1.5 hour after procainamide, then 0.11 g/kg body weight hourly for six doses).[99] In eight other subjects ethanol administration was started 2 hours before procainamide. In both experiments ethanol administration was associated with an increase in procainamide clearance and a reduction in procainamide half-life. Accordingly, ethanol was associated with an increase in serum levels of the active procainamide metabolite, acetylprocainamide. The clinical consequences of these changes are not clear since the reduction in serum procainamide levels may be offset by the increase in serum acetylprocainamide.

MANAGEMENT: No special precautions appear necessary at this point.

Isoniazid (INH)[81]

MECHANISM: Procainamide may slightly reduce isoniazid metabolism (acetylation).

CLINICAL SIGNIFICANCE: In a preliminary report of a study in four normal subjects, isoniazid half-life was slightly prolonged by concomitant ingestion of procainamide (6 mg/kg body weight every 4 hours).[81] However, procainamide acetylation rate, as measured by the half-life, did not appear to be affected by isoniazid. The clinical effect of the prolongation of isoniazid half-life is not clear from the data given but probably is not large.

MANAGEMENT: No special precautions appear necessary.

Neuromuscular Blocking Agent[3,44]

MECHANISM: Procainamide is said to potentiate the neuromuscular blocking action of skeletal muscle relaxants.

DRUGS	DISCUSSION

CLINICAL SIGNIFICANCE: No clinical studies could be found to establish the clinical significance of these interactions. Animal studies indicate that large doses of procainamide can increase sensitivity to tubocurarine[3] and succinylcholine.[44]

MANAGEMENT: Procainamide-treated patients should be watched for enhanced or prolonged response to neuromuscular blocking agents.

Sodium Bicarbonate[56,84,100]

MECHANISM: See Clinical Significance.

CLINICAL SIGNIFICANCE: It has been proposed that urinary alkalinization with sodium bicarbonate would reduce urinary excretion of procainamide, thus increasing serum levels. However, several studies have failed to document such as effect.[56,84,100] Preliminary information indicates that the active metabolite of procainamide (N-acetylprocainamide) is also unaffected by urinary pH changes.[100]

MANAGEMENT: Current evidence indicates that urine pH need not be considered as a significant cause of variation in plasma procainamide levels.

QUINIDINE INTERACTIONS

DRUGS	DISCUSSION

Acetazolamide (Diamox)[30,32]

MECHANISM: Acetazolamide tends to render the urine alkaline, resulting in an increased proportion of un-ionized quinidine. Thus, renal tubular reabsorption of quinidine is increased and serum levels may be increased.

CLINICAL SIGNIFICANCE: In one preliminary study of four subjects,[32] average quinidine excretion was 115 mg ± 48 mg/L when urine pH was below 6 while the average excretion was 13 ± 8 mg/L when urine pH was greater than 7.5. It appears likely that quinidine toxicity may result from quinidine and agents which increase urine pH.

MANAGEMENT: Initiation, discontinuation, or a change in dose of acetazolamide in a patient receiving quinidine may necessitate a change in quinidine dosage.

Antacids, Oral[54,55,161,165]

MECHANISM: Some oral antacids can increase urinary pH,[55] which in turn increases the proportion of un-ionized quinidine, resulting in increased renal tubular reabsorption.

CLINICAL SIGNIFICANCE: Gibaldi and co-workers[55] studied the effect of five antacids on urinary pH in 11 subjects. They found that aluminum hydroxide suspension (Amphojel) and dihydroxyaluminum glycinate (Robalate) had no effect on urine pH. Magnesium hydroxide (Phillips

DRUGS	DISCUSSION

Milk of Magnesia) and calcium carbonate-glycine (Titralac) increased urinary pH about one-half unit, which aluminum and magnesium hydroxide suspension (Maalox) increased urinary pH by almost one unit. Zinn[54] also found an increase in urine pH in subjects receiving an aluminum and magnesium hydroxide-containing tablet (Mylanta). He also reported that a patient developed quinidine intoxication following the use of Mylanta Tablets (about eight a day for 1 week) in addition to large quantities of citrus fruit juice. Studies in humans and dogs indicate that aluminum hydroxide does not reduce the extent of quinidine absorption,[161,165] but magnesium oxide did reduce the amount of quinidine absorbed in dogs.[161] In summary, antacids capable of increasing urine pH (e.g., magnesium-aluminum hydroxides) may increase serum quinidine levels. Aluminum hydroxide probably does not impair gastrointestinal quinidine absorption significantly, but the effect of other antacids on quinidine absorption is not established.

MANAGEMENT: In a patient receiving quinidine, antacids which increase urinary pH should be administered with caution. Monitoring quinidine blood levels may allow early detection of the interaction.

Anticoagulants, Oral[25–27,39,48,49]

MECHANISM: Quinidine may produce additive hypoprothrombinemic effects with coumarin anticoagulants. Theoretically, the same effect would be seen with the indandione oral anticoagulants.

CLINICAL SIGNIFICANCE: Quinidine administration appears to have resulted in hemorrhages in a few patients taking warfarin.[25,26] Another patient receiving both quinidine and warfarin developed corpus luteum hemorrhage, although the authors did not mention the possibility of drug interaction.[48] However, in ten patients on chronic warfarin therapy, quinidine (800 mg/day) did not alter the hypoprothrombinemic response.[49] Further, I have carefully observed a number of patients who have received warfarin and then quinidine with no evidence of enhanced warfarin effect. Thus, it appears that quinidine may enhance warfarin hypoprothrombinemia, but only in occasional predisposed patients.

MANAGEMENT: Patients on oral anticoagulants who subsequently receive quinidine should be observed closely for excessive hypoprothrombinemia.

Barbiturates[75,166,171]

MECHANISM: Phenobarbital appears to enhance the hepatic metabolism of quinidine.

CLINICAL SIGNIFICANCE: Several cases have been described wherein barbiturate or phenytoin therapy was associated with low plasma quinidine levers.[75,166,171] Additional study in normal subjects confirmed that phenobarbital can considerably enhance the disposition of quinidine.[75]

QUINIDINE INTERACTIONS (CONT.)

MANAGEMENT: Initiation or discontinuation of barbiturate therapy in patients receiving quinidine may necessitate a change in quinidine dosage. In patients receiving barbiturates initiation of quinidine therapy should be undertaken with the realization that larger than normal quinidine doses may be required.

Cholinergic Drugs[57,79,167]

MECHANISM: Quinidine has anticholinergic properties and may antagonize the effects of cholinergic drugs.

CLINICAL SIGNIFICANCE: Quinidine tends to prevent the cardiac slowing produced by cholinergic drugs. Thus, in patients receiving quinidine, cholinergic drugs may fail to terminate paroxysmal supraventricular tachycardia. Also, quinidine may antagonize the effects of neostagmine (Prostigmin) and edrophonium (Tensilon) in the treatment of myasthenia gravis. This interaction has been used to advantage by using a cholinergic drug (physostigmine) to counteract delirium caused by the combination of quinidine and other anticholinergic agents.[167]

MANAGEMENT: Precribers should remember that the anticholinergic effect of quinidine may antagonize the vagal-stimulating effect of cholinergic drugs. Quinidine should be used with caution in patients with myasthenia gravis who are being treated with cholinergic drugs.

Cimetidine (Tagamet)[168,169,387]

MECHANISM: Cimetidine appears to inhibit the hepatic metabolism of quinidine.

CLINICAL SIGNIFICANCE: A 60-year-old woman developed an elevated plasma quinidine level (9.4 μg/ml) while receiving large doses of cimetidine (600 mg orally qid). The high serum quinidine level was probably caused in part by the cimetidine, but another factor was the increase in quinidine dose (to 300 mg qid) prior to detection of the elevated level. In a preliminary report of a study in nine subjects, quinidine (400 mg orally) was given with and without cimetidine pretreatment (300 mg qid).[169] Cimetidine was associated with a 23% increase in the plasma half-life of quinidine. In another study of six normal subjects, cimetidine (1.2 g/day for 7 days) increased quinidine half-life by 55% and reduced quinidine clearance from 26 L/hour to 16 L/hour.[387] In summary, available evidence indicates that cimetidine inhibits the metabolism and elevates plasma levels of quinidine. The evidence is consistent with the known properties of both drugs.

MANAGEMENT: One should be alert for evidence of altered quinidine response if cimetidine is started or stopped. Changes in quinidine dosage may be necessary in some patients. When available, plasma quinidine determinations would be useful when it is suspected that the interaction is occurring.

DRUGS	DISCUSSION

Digitalis Glycosides[119,120,175-212]

MECHANISM: Quinidine reduces the renal and nonrenal clearance of digoxin, and also appears to displace digoxin from tissue binding sites. Quinidine may also increase the rate (and possibly extent) of gastrointestinal digoxin absorption, but the clinical importance of this mechanism is not clear.

CLINICAL SIGNIFICANCE: Almost all (90% or more) patients who receive digoxin and quinidine will develop a substantial increase in serum digoxin concentration. The increases are usually two- to three-fold, but sometimes patients will manifest a larger or smaller effect. In a patient on chronic digoxin, the serum digoxin level will begin to increase within hours of initiation of quinidine therapy, but a new steady state serum digoxin level will usually take 5 to 7 days (or sometimes longer) to achieve. In patients with chronic renal failure, one would expect a longer period (perhaps weeks) to achieve a new steady-state serum digoxin level, since the digoxin elimination half-life may be increased to a week or more.[175] The magnitude of the increase in serum digoxin is affected by the serum quinidine concentration. Quinidine doses of 400 to 500 mg/day may increase serum digoxin levels, but the degree of increase is generally one-half or less of that seen with larger therapeutic quinidine doses (e.g., 1000 to 1200 mg/day). Although some clinicians contend that quinidine protects the patient against the adverse effects of the elevated serum digoxin levels, the clinical evidence clearly shows that gastrointestinal, cardiac, and other digoxin toxicity may be induced by quinidine administration. The effect of quinidine on *digitoxin* disposition has been disputed, but the bulk of the evidence indicates that quinidine does increase serium digitoxin levels to a clinically significant degree. Quinidine appears to reduce digitoxin renal and nonrenal clearance, but does not affect the volume of distribution of digitoxin.

MANAGEMENT: A 50% reduction in digoxin dose when quinidine is started may reduce the likelihood of digoxin toxicity. However, because the magnitude of the interaction varies considerably from patient to patient, further adjustments in digoxin dose are likely to be necessary. During the first 7 to 10 days of combined therapy, the patient should be observed carefully by symptoms and ECG evidence of digoxin toxicity, and serum digoxin levels should be monitored. In a patient stabilized on both quinidine and digoxin, one should be alert for evidence of reduced digoxin response if the quinidine is discontinued. When digoxin administration is started in a patient on chronic quinidine therapy, one should be aware that the digoxin dose needed to produce the desired serum digoxin concentration may be smaller than expected. In general, all of the above precautions would also apply to the concurrent use of quinidine and digitoxin, although it may take longer to achieve a new steady-state serum digitoxin level after starting quinidine therapy. One way of avoiding the potential adverse effects of the quinidine-digoxin interaction would be to use an

QUINIDINE INTERACTIONS (CONT.)

alternative to quinidine which does not interact with digoxin (e.g., procainamide, disopyramide, mexilitine, and possibly lidocaine).

Docusate (Colace, Doxinate, Surfak)[109–111]

MECHANISM: It has been proposed that docusate might increase the likelihood of quinidine hepatoxicity by increasing the intrahepatic concentration of quinidine.

CLINICAL SIGNIFICANCE: Not established. A case of quinidine hepatotoxicity was reported,[109] and it was subsequently suggested that the hepatotoxicity could have been enhanced by concomitant administration of docusate.[110,111] There is some evidence that surfactants such as docusate might enhance hepatotoxicity of other drugs but effects on quinidine have not been studied.

MANAGEMENT: No special precautions appear necessary at this point.

Food[54,108]

MECHANISM: Foods which alkalinize the urine result in an increased proportion of un-ionized quinidine, thus enhancing tubular reabsorption of the drug.

CLINICAL SIGNIFICANCE: In one patient on chronic quinidine therapy, quinidine intoxication occurred after about 1 week of ingestion of citrus juice (1 quart of orange-grapefruit juice/day) and antacid (eight tablets of magnesium-aluminum hydroxide/day).[54] In six normal subjects the same antacid plus 1 quart of orange-grapefruit juice produced a persistently alkaline urine in five of the subjects.[54] Consumption of 1500 ml per day of orange juice in a study of seven male subjects led to an increase in urinary pH by an average of one pH unit, while 300 ml of orange juice daily did not significantly alter urine pH.[108]

MANAGEMENT: Patients receiving quinidine should be cautioned to avoid excessive intake of foods such as citrus juices which may alkalinize their urine.

Neuromuscular Blocking Agents[28,29,43,44]

MECHANISM: Quinidine appears to potentiate both nondepolarizing and depolarizing muscle relaxants. This effect is mediated by (a) a curare-like action on the myoneural junction and (b) depression of the muscle action potential.

CLINICAL SIGNIFICANCE: Quinidine administration to patients who are recovering from the effects of tubocurarine may result in recurarization leading to unresponsiveness and apnea.[28] A similar effect might be seen with quinine administration. Neostigmine did not appear to reverse the effects of this interaction.

MANAGEMENT: If possible, the use of quinidine should be avoided in the immediate postoperative period when the effects of muscle relax-

DRUGS	DISCUSSION

ants may still be present. If quinidine must be used, the need for respiratory support should be anticipated.

Nifedipine (Procardia)[170,383]

MECHANISM: Not established.

CLINICAL SIGNIFICANCE: A report describes a patient whose serum quinidine levels appeared to be lowered by nifedipine.[170,383] Serum quinidine levels rose when nifedipine was stopped, and fell when nifedipine therapy was reinstituted. It appears that nifedipine may have reduced serum quinidine levels in this patient, but it is not known how often or to what extent this effect would be seen in other patients.

MANAGEMENT: Until more information is available, one should be alert for evidence of reduced quinidine response in the presence of nifedipine.

Phenytoin (Dilantin)[75,171,172,218]

MECHANISM: Phenytoin appears to enhance the hepatic metabolism of quinidine. A study in dogs indicates that other mechanisms may also be involved.[172]

CLINICAL SIGNIFICANCE: A few cases have been described where in phenytoin or phenobarbital therapy was associated with low plasma quinidine levels.[75] Additional study in normal subjects confirmed that phenytoin can considerably enhance the disposition of quinidine.[75] A study in dogs showed that the half-life of quinidine was shortened by phenytoin, but peak quinidine plasma levels were increased about threefold, possibly due to a reduction in the volume of distribution of quinidine.[172] In summary, available evidence indicates that some patients receiving phenytoin and quinidine manifest subtherapeutic quinidine plasma levels. It is not established whether the higher peak plasma quinidine levels found in phenytoin-treated dogs would apply to the clinical situation.

MANAGEMENT: Initiation of discontinuation of phenytoin therapy in patients receiving quinidine may necessitate a change in quinidine dosage. In patients receiving phenytoin initiation of quinidine therapy should be undertaken with the realization that larger than normal quinidine doses may be required.

Rifampin (Rifadin, Rimactane)[173,174,388]

MECHANISM: Rifampin is an enzyme inducer that stimulates the hepatic metabolism of quinidine.

CLINICAL SIGNIFICANCE: A patient whose ventricular arrhythmia responded to quinidine developed a recurrence after rifampin therapy was added.[174] In a subsequent study, eight healthy subjects were

DRUGS	DISCUSSION

given oral or intravenous quinidine (6 mg/kg body weight as a single dose) with and without rifampin pretreatment (600 mg/day for 7 days).[173] Rifampin reduced the elimination half-life of oral quinidine-time curve almost sixfold. The disposition of intravenous quinidine was similarly affected by rifampin pretreatment. A preliminary report describes two additional patients who developed low serum quinidine levels in the presence of rifampin.[388] The magnitude of these changes indicate that rifampin is likely to reduce quinidine plasma concentrations to subtherapeutic levels in a majority of patients.

MANAGEMENT: One should be alert for evidence of reduced quinidine response in patients receiving rifampin. A substantial increase in quinidine dose may be necessary in some patients. Plasma quinidine determinations would be useful in achieving the optimal dose of quinidine in the presence of rifampin.

Sodium Bicarbonate[30-32]

MECHANISM: Sodium bicarbonate tends to render the urine alkaline, resulting in an increased proportion of un-ionized quinidine. Thus, renal tubular reabsorption of quinidine is increased and serum levels may be increased.

CLINICAL SIGNIFICANCE: In one preliminary study of four subjects,[32] average quinidine excretion was 115 mg ± 48 mg/L when urine pH was below 6 while the average excretion was 13 mg ± 8 mg/L when urine pH was greater than 7.5. It appears likely that quinidine toxicity may result from concomitant administration of quinidine and agents which increase urine pH.

MANAGEMENT: Attention should be given to the possible necessity of decreasing quinidine dosage with initiation of therapy with a urinary alkalizer such as sodium bicarbonate.

BETA-ADRENERGIC BLOCKER INTERACTIONS

DRUGS	DISCUSSION

Acetaminophen (Overdose)[95,214]

MECHANISM: It is proposed that beta-blockers may reduce hepatic blood flow, thus decreasing the formation of toxic acetaminophen metabolites in patients with acetaminophen overdose.

CLINICAL SIGNIFICANCE: This interaction is based primarily on animal studies and theoretical considerations with little clinical information available. In one animal study, propranolol and alprenolol protected mice against acetaminophen overdoses, while pindolol did not.[214]

MANAGEMENT: None required (favorable interaction).

DRUGS	DISCUSSION

Allopurinol (Zyloprim)[222]

MECHANISM: None.

CLINICAL SIGNIFICANCE: In six healthy subjects allopurinol (300 mg/day) did not affect the disposition of atenolol (100 mg/day).[222]

MANAGEMENT: No special precautions appear necessary.

Aminoglycosides[385]

MECHANISM: Not established.

CLINICAL SIGNIFICANCE: In eight healthy subjects oral erythromycin (0.5 g qid) and oral neomycin (0.5 g qid) for 2 days more than doubled mean peak plasma nadolol concentration following a single oral dose of nadolol (80 mg).[385] However, nadolol half-life was reduced from 17.3 hours to 11.6 hours in the presence of the antibiotics. The clinical importance of these findings is not established.

MANAGEMENT: Until more information is available, one should be alert for altered nadolol response if antibiotics with effects on bowel flora are given concurrently.

Ampicillin[222]

MECHANISM: Not established.

CLINICAL SIGNIFICANCE: In six healthy subjects, atenolol (100 mg orally) was given with and without ampicillin (1 g orally) in both single-dose and 6-day studies.[222] The bioavailability of atenolol was 60% when given alone, 36% with a single dose of ampicillin, and 24% with combined therapy for 6 days. The possibility that ampicillin may have interfered with the atenolol assay was apparently not addressed. However, the fact that ampicillin reduced atenolol-induced inhibition of exercise tachycardia lends support to the authors' contention that atenolol plasma concentration were actually reduced. The magnitude of the reductions in atenolol bioavailability seems large enough to inhibit the therapeutic response to atenolol, but additional study is needed to confirm such a possibility. One would guess that ampicillin-like agents (e.g., amoxicillin, hetacillin, bacampicillin, cyclacillin) might also affect atenolol, but the effect ampicillin on beta-blockers other than atenolol is not established.

MANAGEMENT: Until more data are available, one should be alert for evidence of altered atenolol response if ampicillin therapy is started or stopped.

Anesthetics, Local[223,224,381]

MECHANISM: See Clinical Significance.

CLINICAL SIGNIFICANCE: If their beta-blocker was discontinued prior to spinal anesthesia with tetracaine, patients on long-term beta-blocker therapy had a higher incidence of adverse effects (e.g., tachycardia, arrhythmias, angina) than patients in whom the beta-blocker was continued.[223] Similar results were obtained in patients receiving bupivacaine for intercostal nerve blockade, although in one patient with heart failure bupivacaine in the presence of beta-blockade may have resulted in slight cardiodepression.[224] However, infiltration of lidocaine plus epinephrine in plastic surgery patients on propranolol has resulted in severe hypertensive reactions, probably as a result of propranolol-induced blockade of the beta-adrenergic stimulatory effect of epinephrine.[381] Cardioselective beta-blockers are probably less likely to predispose patients to epinephrine-induced hypertension.

MANAGEMENT: These studies indicate that chronic beta-blocker therapy should not be discontinued prior to the use of local anesthetics such as tetracaine or bupivacaine, although one should be alert for evidence of cardiodepression. If possible, epinephrine-containing local anesthetics should be avoided in patients receiving propranolol or other nonselective beta-blockers such as nadolol, pindolol, or timolol.

Antacids, Oral[101,102,161,225–227]

MECHANISM: Antacids may inhibit the gastrointestinal absorption of some beta-blockers.

CLINICAL SIGNIFICANCE: In a study involving five normal subjects oral administration of 30 ml of aluminum hydroxide gel with propranolol (80 mg orally) produced a mean decrease in maximum plasma concentration of 57% as compared to propranolol alone in the same subjects.[101] Thus, it appears that propranolol absorption is at least *delayed* by aluminum hydroxide administration, which is consistent with the ability of aluminum hydroxide gel to delay gastric emptying.[102] The area under the plasma concentration time curve was reduced by 58% with aluminum hydroxide, indicating a decrease in total bioavailability. A similar reduction in the propranolol plasma level time curve was found in dogs given concurrent aluminum hydroxide or magnesium oxide.[161] Two studies in healthy subjects indicate that magnesium-aluminum or aluminum antacids may reduce the bioavailability of atenolol.[225,226] Calcium salts also appear to reduce atenolol bioavailability, but that effect is somewhat offset by an increase in the elimination half-life of atenolol.[226] The bioavailability of metoprolol may actually *increase* slightly with concurrent administration of a magnesium-aluminum antacid.[225] In summary, the gastro-intestinal absorption of propranolol and atenolol may be reduced by concurrent administration of aluminum or magnesium antacids, while metoprolol absorption does not appear to be reduced. The impact of these findings on the therapeutic response to beta-blockers has not been assessed.

MANAGEMENT: Until the clinical importance of these findings is determined, it would be prudent to separate the doses of beta-blockers and

DRUGS	DISCUSSION

antacids by an hour or more. One should also be alert for evidence of altered response to beta-blockers if antacids are started or stopped.

Anticholinergics[225,228]

MECHANISM:
1. Anticholinergics may attenuate beta-blocker-induced bradycardia.
2. Anticholinergics may increase the bioavailability of atenolol, probably by slowing gut motility.
3. Propranolol may enhance the likelihood of atropine-delirium (animal study).

CLINICAL SIGNIFICANCE: Atropine has been used to counteract propranolol-induced bradycardia, a favorable use of the interaction. In six healthy subjects, atenolol (100 mg orally) was given with and without propantheline (30 mg orally, 1.5 hours before the atenolol).[225] Propantheline slowed the absorption *rate* of atenolol, but atenolol bioavailability increased by 36%. If this effect is found to be sustained under conditions of multiple dosing, one would expect atenolol response to be enhanced. However, this has not been studied. Dogs given large doses of propranolol (2 mg/kg body weight) and atropine (0.4 mg/kg body weight) during anesthesia developed emergence delirium, whereas either propranolol or atropine alone did not produce this effect.[228] The implications of these findings to humans receiving conventional doses of propranolol and atropine are not established.

MANAGEMENT: In patients receiving beta-blockers and anticholinergics, one should be alert for evidence of altered response to either drug.

Antidiabetic Agents[17–20,33,34,40,58–61,73,89,90,229–262]

MECHANISM:
1. Beta-blocker-induced delayed glucose recovery from insulin-induced hypoglycemia is probably related to inhibition of the hyperglycemic effect of the epinephrine released in response to the hypoglycemia.[230,231]
2. Beta-blocker-induced hypertension during hypoglycemia is related to blockade of the beta-2 (vasodilator) effects of the epinephrine released in response to hypoglycemia, leaving unopposed alpha (vasoconstrictor) effects which increase the blood pressure.
3. Beta-blocker-induced inhibition of the tachycardia during hypoglycemia is related to inhibition of the cardiac stimulatory effect of the epinephrine released in response to the hypoglycemia.
4. Beta-blockers may inhibit insulin secretion, leading to a hyperglycemic effect under certain conditions.
5. Beta-blockers may impair peripheral circulation, and diabetics may already have such impairment.

CLINICAL SIGNIFICANCE:
1. Delayed glucose recovery during hypoglycemia: Propranolol inhibits glucose recovery following insulin-induced hypogly-

25

DRUGS	DISCUSSION

cemia,[229] and may also increase the likelihood of hypoglycemia in predisposed patients not receiving insulin. Predisposing factors include fasting, prolonged exercise, large propranolol doses, and possibly youth (many patients were children), liver dysfunction, and hemodialysis.[229,232–237] Metoprolol may prolong insulin-induced hypoglycemia somewhat,[238] but in at least one study the effect was only slight.[239] Atenolol, penbutolol, and practolol do not appear to affect the magnitude or duration of insulin-induced hypoglycemia,[240–243] while acebutolol may increase slightly the magnitude but not duration of insulin-induced hypoglycemia.[238,240] Timolol eye drops purportedly contributed to hypoglycemic episodes in one patient,[261] but the significance of this is not yet clear.

2. Hypertension during hypoglycemia: A number of case reports and clinical studies have appeared describing increased blood pressure and bradycardia during hypoglycemia in the presence of propranolol treatment.[229,244] Other nonselective beta-blockers such as alprenolol,[245] nadolol, oxprenolol, sotalol, and timolol would be expected to produce a similar effect. Cardiovascular beta-blockers such as metoprolol and atenolol are probably less likely to produce hypertension during hypoglycemia because they have less inhibitory effect on vasodilatory beta-2 receptors.[229,245] However, large doses of metoprolol produce more beta-2 blockade and would be expected to increase blood pressure during hypoglycemia. Hypoglycemia-induced hypertension has occurred in a patient on metoprolol (100 mg bid),[246] but the serum metoprolol levels may have been higher than expected due to concurrent drug therapy.

3. Inhibition of the symptoms of hypoglycemia: Propranolol inhibits the tachycardia that normally accompanies hypoglycemia.[229] In fact, reflex bradycardia may occur as a result of the increased blood pressure when hypoglycemia occurs in the presence of propranolol. Metoprolol also tends to inhibit the tachycardia of hypoglycemia,[259] but is less likely to produce reflex bradycardia since blood pressure usually does not change appreciably; however, large doses of metoprolol may act more like propranolol. Other beta-blockers which have been shown to inhibit hypoglycemia-induced tachycardia include atenolol,[241] acebutolol,[238,240] penbutolol,[242] and alprenolol[245]; other beta-blockers probably act similarly. Sweating as a sign of hypoglycemia is not inhibited by beta-blockers and may actually be prolonged.[229,258]

4. Inhibition of insulin secretion: Propranolol has been shown to inhibit insulin response to glucose[247] or tolbutamide,[248] and has also been used to inhibit insulin secretion in patients with insulinoma.[249,250] Further, long-term propranolol therapy (especially when combined with thiazides) has been associated with reduced glucose tolerance.[229,251–253] Metoprolol appears to be less likely than propranolol to impair glucose tolerance, perhaps because metoprolol is less likely to inhibit insulin secretion.[253–255,260] Because stimulation of beta-2 receptors in the

DRUGS	DISCUSSION

pancreas tends to stimulate insulin secretion,[257] one would expect cardioselective beta-blockers to have less inhibitory effect on insulin secretion than nonselective beta blockers.
5. Impaired peripheral circulation: Propranolol has been associated with reduced circulation to the extremities, leading to gangrene in some extreme cases.[229] This property of propranolol may be a particular problem in the diabetic, who may already have impaired peripheral circulation. Cardioselective beta-blockers would theoretically be less likely to compromise peripheral circulation since they have less effect on beta-2 receptors in peripheral arterioles.

MANAGEMENT: Cardioselective beta-blockers such as metoprolol and atenolol are probably less likely to produce the unwanted effects listed above (although inhibition of hypoglycemic tachycardia should be anticipated from any beta-blocker). Thus, cardioselective agents are preferable in diabetic patients, especially if the patient is prone to hypoglycemic episodes. However, the increased safety of cardioselective agents is only relative, and they may exhibit nonselective beta-blockade (especially if large doses are used). Diabetic patients receiving beta-blockers should be aware that hypoglycemic episodes may not result in the expected tachycardia, but hypoglycemic sweating does not appear to be affected (or may even be increased).

Antipyrine[80]

MECHANISM: It is proposed that propranolol reduces the hepatic clearance of antipyrine.

CLINICAL SIGNIFICANCE: In a preliminary report of a study in six healthy volunteers acting as their own controls, propranolol increased antipyrine half-life from 10.8 hours to 14.9 hours and reduced clearance from 0.71 ml/minute/kg body weight to 0.49 ml/minute/kg body weight.[80] Since antipyrine is seldom used, the primary significance of these findings relates to possible effects of propranolol on the disposition of other drugs.

MANAGEMENT: None appears required at this point.

Barbiturates[106,263-265]

MECHANISM: Barbiturates appear to stimulate the metabolism of beta-blockers that are extensively metabolized (e.g., propranolol, metoprolol, alprenolol).

CLINICAL SIGNIFICANCE: In six healthy subjects pretreatment with pentobarbital (0.1 g/day for 10 days) reduced plasma levels of alprenolol (0.2 g orally) and its active metabolite (4-hydroxy-alprenolol) by about 40%.[263] Similarly, in eight healthy subjects pretreatment with pentobarbital (0.1 g/day for 10 days) reduced the area under the plasma concentration/time curve for metoprolol (0.1 g orally) by 32%.[264] In 68 patients receiving propranolol or sotalol, the three pa-

DRUGS	DISCUSSION

tients on enzyme inducers (phenobarbital or phenytoin) had a higher plasma clearance of propranolol than those not on enzyme inducers.[265] Enzyme inducers did not seem to affect the plasma clearance of sotalol, a drug which undergoes little hepatic metabolism. The degree to which barbiturates would alter the therapeutic response to beta-blockers such as propranolol, metoprolol that undergo hepatic metabolism is not established. However, the magnitude and range of the observed changes suggest that some patients would develop reduced beta-blocker effect.

MANAGEMENT: One should be alert for evidence of altered response to beta-blockers metabolized by the liver (e.g., propranolol, metoprolol, alprenolol) if barbiturate therapy is initiated or discontinued. Beta-blockers excreted primarily unchanged by the kidneys (e.g., atenolol, nadolol, sotalol) are not likely to interact with barbiturates and thus could be used to avoid the interaction.

Caffeine[268,382]

MECHANISM: See Clinical Significance.

CLINICAL SIGNIFICANCE: In 16 healthy subjects caffeine (250 mg orally) did not affect the plasma binding of propranolol (added in vitro to plasma samples). The caffeine did increase urinary excretion of epinephrine and dopamine, reflecting an increase in circulating catecholamines. However, it seems unlikely that the magnitude of the increase in catecholamines would be sufficient to cause difficulties due to a propranolol-catecholamine interaction. Indeed, the effect of coffee on blood pressure and forearm blood flow was not altered by pretreatment with propranolol or metoprolol in 12 healthy subjects, although the coffee-induced fall in heart rate was somewhat greater during treatment with propranolol.[382]

MANAGEMENT: No special precautions appear necessary.

Carbamazepine (Tegretol)[267]

MECHANISM: Carbamazepine therapy tends to increase serum levels of $alpha_1$-acid glycoprotein, a protein to which propranolol is bound in the serum. It is also possible that carbamazepine-induced stimulation of hepatic drug-metabolizing enzymes could increase propranolol metabolism.

CLINICAL SIGNIFICANCE: Serum levels of $alpha_1$-acid glycoprotein were found to be 23% higher in 17 patients receiving carbamazepine than in 21 controls. Propranolol binding was not determined in this study. The ability of carbamazepine to increase the metabolism of beta-blockers metabolized by the liver (e.g., propranolol, metoprolol) is not established but theoretically should occur. In summary, the interactions of carbamazepine and beta-blockers are largely theoretical, and the clinical significance is not yet established.

BETA-ADRENERGIC BLOCKER INTERACTIONS (CONT.)

DRUGS	DISCUSSION

MANAGEMENT: Until the clinical significance of this interaction is established, one should be alert for evidence of altered propranolol response in patients also receiving carbamazepine.

Cholestyramine (Questran)[266]

MECHANISM: None.

CLINICAL SIGNIFICANCE: In five patients with hyperlipidemia, cholestyramine did not affect the blood levels of propranolol administered simultaneously.

MANAGEMENT: No special precautions appear necessary.

Cimetidine (Tagamet)[269-276]

MECHANISM: Cimetidine reduces the activity of the hepatic microsomal enzymes that metabolize propranolol and some other beta-adrenergic blockers. It has been proposed that cimetidine reduces propranolol metabolism by decreasing blood flow, but the contribution of this mechanism to the interaction is not established. The ability of beta-blockers to reduce the pulse rate may also be enhanced by cimetidine.

CLINICAL SIGNIFICANCE: Several studies have shown that cimetidine consistently and substantially increases plasma propranolol levels.[269-274] The studies were performed primarily in healthy subjects and involved both single doses and chronic use of propranolol. Peak and steady state plasma propranolol levels generally increase by about 50% to 100% in the presence of cimetidine, but the degree to which this increases the pharmacologic and toxic effects of propranolol is not well established. As one would expect, the resting pulse rates were considerably lower with cimetidine plus propranolol than with propranolol alone in one study.[269] However, in another report, cimetidine did not alter exercise-induced tachycardia in patients receiving propranolol or metoprolol.[270] One patient on cimetidine and an unspecified beta-blocker developed severe bradycardia (36 beats/minute) and hypotension, effects attributed to combined effects of the drugs. Metoprolol disposition (100 mg orally as a single dose) was not affected by cimetidine in one study,[275] but in another study cimetidine substantially increased plasma levels of metoprolol (given 100 mg bid for 7 days).[270] The reason for this discrepancy is not immediately apparent, but the study that found increased metoprolol levels was more like the clinical situation since it involved multiple doses rather than a single dose. In a preliminary report, the bioavailability of labetolol was increased by about 80% in the presence of cimetidine (1.6 g/day for 3 days).[276] Atenolol disposition appears to be minimally affected by cimetidine therapy,[270,275] and it seems likely that other beta-blockers excreted extensively by the kidneys (e.g., nadolol, sotalol) would not be much affected by cimetidine. Although little clinical information is available, one would expect that plasma levels

DRUGS	DISCUSSION

of beta-blockers that undergo significant hepatic metabolism (e.g., alprenolol, oxprenolol, penbutolol, timolol) would be increased by cimetidine therapy.

MANAGEMENT: One should be alert for evidence of altered response to propranolol, labetalol, and possibly other beta-blockers if cimetidine therapy is initiated or discontinued. Ranitidine may be preferable to cimetidine in this case since it does not appear to interact with propranolol, and probably does not interact with other beta-blockers. Antacids or sucralfate may also be suitable alternatives to cimetidine, although beta-blocker doses should probably be separated from antacids or sucralfate to minimize the possibility of impaired absorption of the beta-blocker.

Clonidine (Catapres)[71,112,118,277–285]

MECHANISM: The hypertension that may accompany rapid clonidine withdrawal is thought to result from increased circulating catecholamine levels. If the patient is receiving a beta-blocker during withdrawal from clonidine, the beta (vasodilating) response of epinephrine would be blocked, resulting in an exaggerated alpha (vasoconstrictor) response and possibly hypertension.

CLINICAL SIGNIFICANCE: In several patients, beta-blockers have seemed to enhance the hypertensive response following clonidine withdrawal.[71,112,118,277–280] The interaction may have contributed to a fatal cerebellar hemorrhage in one case.[280] Even gradual withdrawal of clonidine has been associated with hypertensive reactions in the presence of beta-blockade.[112,278] It seems likely that patients on large doses of clonidine would be more at risk. Also, a paradoxical hypertensive response has also been reported in patients on continued clonidine therapy who also receive propranolol[281] or sotalol.[285] Propranolol has also been shown to inhibit clonidine-induced hypotensive effect in animals.[282] However, neither propranolol nor sotalol increased blood pressure in 12 clonidine-treated patients,[283] and the significance of the hypertensive effect of *continued* clonidine plus beta-blockade remains to be established.

MANAGEMENT: It has been proposed that in patients receiving propranolol and clonidine withdrawing the propranolol before the clonidine may reduce the danger of rebound hypertension.[71] The use of labetalol (which has both alpha- and beta-blocking activity) may prove useful in preventing rebound hypertension following clonidine withdrawal.[284] If clonidine is withdrawn while the patient remains on a beta-adrenergic blocker, the patient should be very carefully monitored for a hypertensive response.

Contraceptives, Oral[286]

MECHANISM: Not established. Oral contraceptives may inhibit the metabolism of metoprolol (Lopressor).

CLINICAL SIGNIFICANCE: A single 100 mg oral dose of metoprolol (Lopressor) was given to 23 healthy women, 12 of whom were taking a

DRUGS	DISCUSSION

low-dose oral contraceptive.[286] Women on the oral contraceptives had a 70% higher area under the plasma concentration-time curve. If a similar effect is seen with chronic metoprolol use, one might expect to see increased metoprolol response. The effect of oral contraceptives on other beta-blockers is not established, but one would expect a similar interaction with beta-blockers extensively metabolized by the liver such as propranolol (Inderal) and timolol (Blocadren).

MANAGEMENT: Although the clinical importance of this interaction is not established, one should be alert for evidence of increased metoprolol response in women taking oral contraceptives.

Digitalis Glycosides[8,37,62,74,91,287]

MECHANISM: Bradycardia due to digitalis may be potentiated by propranolol.

CLINICAL SIGNIFICANCE: Excessive bradycardia has been reported in patients with digitalis intoxication who received propranolol.[37] The adverse effect was felt to represent increased sensitivity to the action of propranolol. Also, some workers have discouraged, on theoretical grounds the concomitant use of propranolol and digitalis in the treatment of patients with angina pectoris but without heart failure.[8] However, another group subsequently presented data to indicate that the combination may actually be beneficial in patients with angina who have abnormal ventricular function or enlarged hearts.[62] Further, the combination of digoxin and propranolol has proved useful in some patients with atrioventricular reentrant tachycardia.[287]

MANAGEMENT: The combination of digitalis and propranolol may be used to advantage in some patients. (See Clinical Significance.)

Dopamine (Intropin)[288]

MECHANISM: Propranolol inhibits dopamine-induced increase in the pulse rate by blocking the beta-stimulatory effect of dopamine on the heart.

CLINICAL SIGNIFICANCE: In 12 healthy subjects, propranolol inhibited the increased pulse rate following dopamine, but did not inhibit the dopamine-induced rise in plasma glucagon and serum insulin.

MANAGEMENT: No special precautions appear necessary.

Doxapram (Dopram)[289]

MECHANISM: Not established. Propranolol may inhibit the beta-stimulatory effects of epinephrine released in response to doxapram.

CLINICAL SIGNIFICANCE: In 12 healthy subjects, propranolol enhanced the pressor response to doxapram (especially diastolic), but inhibited the doxapram-induced increase in pulse rate. The clinical importance of these findings remains to be established.

DRUGS	DISCUSSION

MANAGEMENT: No special precautions appear to be necessary at this time.

Epinephrine (Adrenalin)[17,21,69,77,93,290–299,381]

MECHANISM: Epinephrine alone exerts both alpha effects (vasoconstriction) and beta effects (vasodilation and cardiac stimulation). These effects usually result in a mild increase in heart rate and minimal changes in mean arterial pressure. However, with blockade of the beta effects of epinephrine using propranolol, the alpha (vasoconstrictor) effects predominate, resulting in hypertension and a reflex increase in vagal tone resulting in bradycardia.

CLINICAL SIGNIFICANCE: There is convincing evidence from studies in hypertensive patients, patients with angina, and healthy subjects that propranolol enhances the pressor response to epinephrine, usually with accompanying bradycardia.[21,69,93,293–296] The effect is marked in some people; the hypertensive response resulted in an intracerebral hemorrhage in one patient,[297] and the bradycardia may be associated with atrioventricular block or other cardiac arrhythmias.[21,298] Severe hypertensive reactions have also been noted following infiltration of lidocaine with epinephrine in plastic surgery patients on chronic propranolol therapy.[381] One would expect that nonspecific beta-blockers other than propranolol (e.g., alprenolol, nadolol, pindolol, timolol) would produce a similar effect. Labetalol (which is a nonspecific beta-blocker as well as an alpha-2 blocker) has been shown to increase the diastolic pressure and slow the heart rate during epinephrine infusions.[299] However, metoprolol (Lopressor) has minimal effects on the pressor response to epinephrine even at metoprolol doses of 200 to 300 mg/day.[293–295] Other cardioselective beta-blockers (e.g., acebutolol, atenolol) would be expected to behave as metoprolol, but little clinical information is available. Propranolol has been shown to *inhibit* the pressor and bronchodilation response of epinephrine in patients with anaphylaxis.[290–291] Thus, patients receiving propranolol who develop anaphylaxis may respond poorly to epinephrine injections. Large amounts of intravenous fluids have been required for stabilization in several patients. It has also been noted in five normal subjects that propranolol pretreatment (15 mg intravenously) prevents the decrease in serum potassium that normally follows an epinephrine infusion (10 μg/minute for 30 minutes).[77]

MANAGEMENT: In patients receiving propranolol, or other nonselective beta-blockers, epinephrine should be administered with caution. Blood pressure should be monitored carefully. If the epinephrine is used to treat anaphylaxis, one should be aware that the response to epinephrine may be poor, and vigorous supportive care (e.g., volume replacement) may be needed. Selective beta₁ blockers may be less likely than propranolol to result in hypertension and bradycardia with epinephrine administration or endogenous epinephrine release.

BETA-ADRENERGIC BLOCKER INTERACTIONS (CONT.)

DRUGS	DISCUSSION

Ergot Alkaloids[9,10,11]

MECHANISM: It has been proposed that propranolol blocks the natural pathway for vasodilation in patients receiving vasoconstrictors such as ergotamine.[9] The potential adverse result of this combination would be excessive vasoconstriction.

CLINICAL SIGNIFICANCE: A case report has appeared describing a patient with migraine headaches on ergotamine-caffeine (Cafergot) suppositories who, after being placed on propranolol (30 mg daily), developed "purple and painful" feet which worsened with each Cafergot suppository.[9] However, a number of patients have received ergotamine plus propranolol with no obvious ill effects.[9,10] Further the preceding case may represent ergotism from excessive ergotamine use rather than a drug interaction. One additional report has appeared describing a patient with migraine, controlled with Cafergot, who developed an exacerbation of migraine attacks (refractory to Cafergot) when put on propranolol for a cardiac disorder.[11] The attacks cleared when propranolol was stopped and recurred when it was started again, thus supporting the authors' contention that propranolol was involved. It seems clear from available evidence that if an interaction does exist, it occurs rarely in patients treated with both drugs and may well require a certain set of (as yet undefined) conditions in the patient.

MANAGEMENT: Although many patients can apparently take propranolol and ergot alkaloids without ill effects, there is enough evidence of an interaction to dictate closer surveillance of patients so treated.

Erythromycin[385]

MECHANISM: Not established.

CLINICAL SIGNIFICANCE: In eight healthy subjects oral erythromycin (0.5 g qid) and oral neomycin (0.5 g qid) for 2 days more than doubled the mean peak plasma nadolol concentration following a single oral dose of nadolol 80 mg.[385] However, nadolol half-life was reduced from 17.3 hours to 11.6 hours in the presence of the antibiotics. The clinical importance of these findings is not established.

MANAGEMENT: Until more information is available, one should be alert for altered nadolol response if antibiotics with effects on bowel flora are given concurrently.

Ethanol (Alcohol, ethyl)[300–303]

MECHANISM: Not established. Ethanol-induced increases in hepatic blood flow might be involved.

CLINICAL SIGNIFICANCE: Short-term studies in normal subjects indicate that ethanol increases both the elimination rate and bioavailability of propranolol, but slightly reduces the elimination rate of sotalol.[300–302] However, the changes in beta-blocker pharmacokinetics were not large, and the studies did not typify the clinical situation. In cats, a bolus intravenous injection of propranolol reduced the blood alcohol concentration.[303] More study is needed to assess the clinical significance of these effects.

MANAGEMENT: Pending further clinical information, one should be alert for alteration in the response to propranolol if alcohol is ingested. At this point it would not appear necessary for patients on beta-blockers to abstain from alcohol.

Food[97,98]

MECHANISM: Not established. Gastrointestinal absorption of metoprolol and propranolol appears to be complete. Enhancement of bioavailability may be attributed to changes in the metabolism of the drug during first passage through the liver.[97]

CLINICAL SIGNIFICANCE: A study involving 13 healthy volunteers has shown that food enhances the bioavailability of metoprolol and propranolol as indicated by increased peak serum concentrations and larger areas under the curve when the drug was taken with food as compared to administration of the drug in the fasting state.[97] However, Shand[98] reported that food delayed absorption of propranolol without change in the peak concentrations of the drug.

MANAGEMENT: Each patient should probably take propranolol and metoprolol in a consistent manner with regard to meals so that any variation in absorption may be minimized.

Furosemide (Lasix)[105,226,304]

MECHANISM: Not established.

CLINICAL SIGNIFICANCE: In ten subjects propranolol (40 mg orally) was given with and without furosemide (25 mg orally).[304] Furosemide was associated with a considerable increase in plasma propranolol levels, and study in six additional subjects indicated that the increased plasma propranolol levels were accompanied by increased beta-blockade. Another study in healthy subjects showed reduced renal clearance of practolol due to furosemide,[105] but atenolol does not appear to be affected by concurrent furosemide treatment.[226]

MANAGEMENT: In a patient receiving propranolol one should be alert for altered effect if furosemide is initiated or discontinued.

Glucagon[82,103,111]

MECHANISM: Propranolol partially inhibits the hyperglycemic effect of glucagon. The mechanism for this effect is not established, but those proposed[111] include (a) propranolol inhibition of the hyperglycemic response to catecholamines released by the glucagon and (b) propranolol-induced decrease in hepatic gluconeogenesis.

DRUGS	DISCUSSION

CLINICAL SIGNIFICANCE: In a study of five normal subjects given glucagon with and without propranolol, the hyperglycemic response to glucagon was partially inhibited by the propranolol.[82] Propranolol did not reduce the large increases in plasma cyclic AMP seen following administration of glucagon, leading the authors to conclude that glucagon and beta agonists such as isoproterenol act on independent receptor sites. This proposal is consistent with previously reported animal and clinical data indicating that glucagon may be effective in reversing the adverse myocardial depressant effects of propranolol.[103]

MANAGEMENT: If glucagon is being used for its hyperglycemic effect, one should expect a reduced response in propranolol-treated patients. Glucagon may prove to be of value in the treatment of excessive myocardial effects of propranolol.

Halofenate[70]

MECHANISM: Not established.

CLINICAL SIGNIFICANCE: In a crossover study in four normal subjects, halofenate (1.0 g/day for 21 days) produced marked decreases in steady state plasma propranolol levels as compared to placebo.[70] The propranolol was given during the last 2 days of halofenate or placebo administration, with each subject receiving propranolol doses of 80 mg/day and 160 mg/day in separate experiments. In addition to the reduced propranolol plasma levels, there was a corresponding decrease in beta-blocking activity as measured by the heart rate response to isoproterenol. If these findings are confirmed by further clinical study, one might expect a reduction in the therapeutic response to propranolol in patients receiving halofenate. It has also been proposed that adding halofenate to a patient stabilized on propranolol therapy for angina could result in the propranolol-withdrawal rebound phenomenon,[94] thus increasing anginal morbidity and mortality.

MANAGEMENT: Although evidence does not seem sufficient to avoid concomitant use, patients receiving propranolol and halofenate should be observed for impaired therapeutic response to propranolol. Initiation of halofenate therapy in patients receiving propranolol for angina pectoris should be undertaken with careful monitoring for signs of exacerbation of angina due to the propranolol-withdrawal rebound phenomenon.

Heparin[305–308]

MECHANISM: See Clinical Significance.

CLINICAL SIGNIFICANCE: Heparin administration has been shown to increase free plasma levels of propranolol,[305,306] although the observed effects may be an artifact of the testing method.[307] In any case, preliminary evidence from a study in five healthy subjects indicates that heparin administration does not affect the degree of beta-blockade due to propranolol.

DRUGS	DISCUSSION

MANAGEMENT: No special precautions appear necessary.

Hydralazine (Apresoline)[309-312]

MECHANISM: Hydralazine might reduce the first pass metabolism of propranolol (Inderal) and other highly extracted beta-blockers.

CLINICAL SIGNIFICANCE: In seven healthy subjects propranolol (1 mg/kg body weight orally) was given with and without oral hydralazine in doses of 25, 50, or 100 mg.[309] Propranolol bioavailability was increased by about 75%. In a similar study, hydralazine increased the bioavailability of metoprolol (Lopressor) by 30% but did not affect the bioavailability of nadolol (Corgard) or acebutolol.[310] Hydralazine may not affect propranolol bioavailability under nonfasting conditions,[312] possibly because the food has already increased propranolol bioavailability (see section on Beta-adrenergic Blockers and Food above). Although many patients have received concurrent propranolol and hydralazine with no apparent ill effects, the combination may occasionally result in excessive propranolol response. A possible clinical example has been reported.[311]

MANAGEMENT: One should be alert for altered response to propranolol or metoprolol if hydralazine therapy is initiated or discontinued.

Indomethacin (Indocin)[116,313-315]

MECHANISM: Not established. It is proposed that the antihypertensive action of beta-blockers may involve prostaglandins, and related substances which are in turn affected by prostaglandin inhibitors such as indomethacin.

CLINICAL SIGNIFICANCE: In seven hypertensive patients given beta-adrenergic blockers (three on propranolol; four on pindolol), administration of indomethacin (100 mg/day) was associated with inhibition of the antihypertensive response.[116] In a subsequent double-blind study of eight hypertensive patients on propranolol, indomethacin (100 mg/day for 3 weeks) increased the blood pressure by about 15/7 mm Hg.[313] In another study the antihypertensive response to oxprenolol was reduced by about 50% by indomethacin (100 mg/day).[314] In nine patients with coronary artery disease, indomethacin (0.5 mg/kg body weight IV) reduced coronary blood flow.[315] It is not known whether this property of indomethacin would adversely affect patients receiving beta-blockers for angina, but it certainly seems possible.

MANAGEMENT: Monitor for altered antihypertensive or antianginal to beta-blockers if indomethacin is initiated or discontinued. Adjustments in beta-blocker dosage may be required. Other proglandin inhibitors (e.g., other nonsteroidal anti-inflammatory drugs) probably produce a similar effect, but there may well be differences in the magnitude. Using an antihypertensive other than a beta-blocker may not circumvent the interaction since indomethacin tends to inhibit the effect of antihypertensives in general.

DRUGS	DISCUSSION

Isoproterenol (Isuprel)[45,63,82,83,316]

MECHANISM: Beta-adrenergic blockers can inhibit the actions of isoproternol, which is a beta-adrenergic stimulant.

CLINICAL SIGNIFICANCE: Asthmatic patients pretreated with propranolol are resistant to the bronchodilating effects of isoproterenol as measured by the forced expiratory volume in 1 second (FEV_1).[63,83] The selective $beta_1$-receptor blocking agents such as metoprolol (Lopressor) and practolol (Eraldin) do not appear to inhibit isoproterenol-induced increases in FEV_1.[63,83] Propranolol and other beta-blockers have also been shown (in normal subjects) to inhibit isoproterenol-induced increases in pulse rate, decreases in diastolic blood pressure, and increases in plasma cyclic AMP.[82,316] Contrary to expectations, the concomitant use of isoproterenol and small doses of propranolol in cardiogenic shock has not offered any advantage over isoproterenol alone.[45]

MANAGEMENT: The mutually antagonistic effects of propranolol and isoproterenol indicate that their concomitant use would seldom be justified. If the isoproterenol is being used in treatment of asthma, propranolol should probably be avoided. Cardioselective beta-adrenergic blockers such as metoprolol appear to be preferable to propranolol in asthmatic patients since the bronchodilation from isoproterenol is less likely to be reduced.

Levodopa (L-DOPA)[12,13,51,52,64,65,76]

MECHANISM:
1. Propranolol may antagonize the beta-adrenergic properties of dopamine formed as a result of levodopa administration.
2. Propranolol may enhance the therapeutic effect of levodopa in patients with parkinsonism with tremor.
3. Propranolol may enhance levodopa-induced stimulation of growth hormone secretion.

CLINICAL SIGNIFICANCE: Limited clinical observations indicate that propranolol may antagonize both the hypotensive[52] and positive inotropic[51] effects of levodopa. Antagonism of the hypotensive effect of levodopa would be considered a favorable interaction in most cases. Further, in one study of 25 patients with parkinsonism with tremor, propranolol plus levodopa produced better therapeutic results than either drug used alone,[12] but others have failed to detect additional improvement when a beta blocker is added to levodopa therapy.[76] Propranolol produces a marked enhancement of the elevated plasma growth hormone levels seen following levodopa. The levels of growth hormone were reportedly close to those seen in acromegaly.[13] This combined effect on growth hormone has been used to advantage as a provocative test in children with short stature.[64]

MANAGEMENT: Most of the consequences of this interaction appear to be favorable. However, until more is known concerning the magni-

DRUGS	DISCUSSION

tude and clinical significance of the elevated growth hormone levels, patients on combined therapy for prolonged periods should be monitored more closely (possibly including occasional plasma growth hormone assays).

Marijuana[92,94]

MECHANISM: Not established. It is proposed that propranolol blocks beta-adrenergic stimulation produced by marijuana.

CLINICAL SIGNIFICANCE: Study in six healthy experienced marijuana smokers showed that propranolol (120 mg orally) inhibits the increase in heart rate and systolic blood pressure which normally follows smoking of a marijuana cigarette (10 mg of delta-9-tetrahydrocannabinol).[92] Propranolol also seemed to prevent marijuana impairment on a learning task and reduced marijuana-induced reddening of the eyes.

MANAGEMENT: No special precautions appear necessary.

Methyldopa (Aldomet)[22,66,317]

MECHANISM: The following mechanism has been proposed.[22] Methyldopa results in accumulation of alpha-methyl-norepinephrine in storage sites of the adrenergic neuron. Since alpha-methyl-norepinephrine has greater beta-adrenergic (vasodilating) activity than norepinephrine, it is less potent than norepinephrine as a pressor agent. However, if propranolol is administered, the beta-adrenergic stimulation of alpha-methyl-norepinephrine is inhibited, resulting in unopposed alpha-adrenergic stimulation and increased pressor response.

CLINICAL SIGNIFICANCE: A case report has appeared describing a 36-year-old hypertensive man on methyldopa and hydralazine who, following a cerebrovascular accident, developed an increasing blood pressure following propranolol (5 mg by slow IV injection).[22] However, two subsequent patients on methyldopa did not manifest a hypertensive reaction following propranolol. Subsequent studies in dogs by the same group showed that administration of alpha-methyl-norepinephrine with propranolol pretreatment resulted in a pressor response similar to that of norepinephrine.[22] A similar case was subsequently described wherein administration of neostigmine to a patient who had received methyldopa, atropine, and practolol was followed by a hypertensive reaction (260/140 mm Hg).[66] In this case it was proposed that stimulation of nicotinic receptors in the ganglia by neostigmine resulted in release of alpha-methyl-norepinephrine and/or norepinephrine from nerve endings and possibly some epinephrine from the adrenals. Any beta blockade remaining in this patient would thus result in an overbalance of alpha (vasoconstrictor) activity. In summary, evidence is accumulating that patients receiving a beta-blocker and methyldopa may develop hypertension when there is re-

DRUGS	DISCUSSION

lease of catecholamines. It may be that this interaction is significant only in the patient under stress (e.g., a cerebrovascular accident) in whom there is mobilization of endogenous catecholamines. It should also be noted that paradoxical hypertension following methyldopa has also been noted in the absence of beta-blockers.[317]

MANAGEMENT: Patients receiving methyldopa and a beta-adrenergic blocker should be monitored for hypertensive episodes if there is a likelihood of catecholamine release (e.g., severe physiologic stress, cholinesterase inhibitors, indirect sympathomimetics). Based on one case report,[22] hypertensive reactions to propranolol in methyldopa-treated patients can be treated with phentolamine (Regitine).

Metoclopramide (Reglan)[318]

MECHANISM: None.

CLINICAL SIGNIFICANCE: In 12 healthy subjects, pretreatment with metoclopramide (20 mg orally) did not affect the serum levels of long-acting propranolol (160 mg orally).[318]

MANAGEMENT: No special precautions appear to be necessary.

Monoamine Oxidase Inhibitors (MAOI)[23,35,41,42,50]

MECHANISM:
1. The mechanism which is the basis for the caution against concomitant use of propranolol and MAOI is not stated by those expressing the caution.[35,41]
2. The beta-blocker sotalol (Sotacor) appears to inhibit tranylcypromine (Parnate)-induced insulin secretion, but the effect of propranolol on tranylcypromine was not studied.[23]

CLINICAL SIGNIFICANCE: Propranolol has been stated to be contraindicated in patients receiving MAOI and patients who may still be affected by previous MAOI administration (e.g., within 2 weeks).[35,41] Personal communication with the manufacturer indicates that the caution about interaction between propranolol and MAOI in their literature is based on theoretical considerations.[50] Further, animal studies indicate that interaction probably does not occur.[42] Determining the actual clinical manifestations of concomitant MAOI and propranolol administration must await additional study.

MANAGEMENT: Although there is little clinical evidence to support the existence of this interaction, the combination of MAOI and propranolol should probably be avoided when possible. Medicolegal considerations would also dictate against their concomitant use.

Narcotic Analgesics [319-321]

MECHANISM: Not established.

CLINICAL SIGNIFICANCE: Propranolol markedly enhances the lethality of toxic doses of morphine (and other opiates) in animals.[319-321] The

DRUGS	DISCUSSION

degree to which this applies to humans in the clinical situation is not established.

MANAGEMENT: Until the clinical importance of this potential interaction is established, one should use this combination with caution, especially if large doses of one or both drugs is being used.

Neuromuscular Blockers[3,14,68]

MECHANISM: Propranolol may enhance the neuromuscular blockade of tubocurarine by impairing transmission of impulses at the motor nerve terminals.

CLINICAL SIGNIFICANCE: In one report,[14] two patients with thyrotoxicosis who received propranolol (120 mg/day) prior to surgery appeared to manifest an increase in the duration of action of tubocurarine. Animal studies have shown a similar effect.[3] Beta-adrenergic blockers have also been associated with symptoms of myasthenia gravis,[68] which is further evidence of a neuromuscular blocking action.

MANAGEMENT: One should be alert to a prolonged action of tubocurarine if the patient has been receiving propranolol (especially in high doses).

Nifedipine (Procardia)[326,329-344]

MECHANISM: Nifedipine has intrinsic depressant effects on myocardial contractility, but this tends to be offset by a reflex increase in heart rate resulting from peripheral vasodilation produced by the nifedipine. However, in the presence of beta-blockers the reflex increase in heart rate is reduced, thus allowing the negative inotropic effect of nifedipine to remain unopposed.

CLINICAL SIGNIFICANCE: Numerous studies have indicated that the combination of nifedipine and beta-blocking agents may produce positive clinical responses in patients with angina pectoris or hypertension.[329-338] However, several case reports have appeared describing severe hypotension or cardiac failure associated with the combined use of nifedipine and beta-adrenergic blockers.[340-344] Also, in a study of 12 patients who were given nifedipine (10 mg sublingually) in the presence of beta blockade (atenolol, 100 mg every 6 hours for four doses), a negative intropic response to nifedipine was observed.[339] Factors which may predispose to adverse effects from this interaction include preexisting left ventricular dysfunction and large doses of the beta-blocker.

MANAGEMENT: Although the results of this interaction are usually positive, one should be alert for evidence of excessive cardiodepressant effects and hypotension.

Nylidrin (Arlidin)[24]

MECHANISM: Propranolol inhibits nylidrin-induced increases in gastric acid secretion and volume.[24]

CLINICAL SIGNIFICANCE: In a study of 20 healthy volunteers, nylidrin (10 mg) alone produced increases in the volume of gastric juice and acid secretion. When propranolol (10 mg intravenously) was administered prior to the nylidrin, these effects of nylidrin on gastric secretion were inhibited.[24] Whether propranolol inhibits other effects of nylidrin remains to be determined. However, if the therapeutic effect of nylidrin (such as it is) is due to beta-adrenergic stimulation, it would not be surprising to find that propranolol inhibits its effect. Since there is some question about the efficacy of nylidrin, adding a drug which may inhibit its effect is of questionable clinical significance.

MANAGEMENT: No special precautions appear necessary.

Phenothiazines[40,53,349-351]

MECHANISM:
1. Propranolol (Inderal) and chlorpromazine (Thorazine) appear to mutually inhibit the hepatic metabolism of the other drug.
2. Phenothiazines and beta-blockers both have hypotensive effects which may be additive.
3. Propranolol can reverse some of the electrocardiographic abnormalities induced by phenothiazines.[53]

CLINICAL SIGNIFICANCE: Chlorpromazine (150 mg/day) increased propranolol plasma levels and degree of beta-blockade in five subjects.[349] Further, propranolol (average dose, 8.1 mg/kg body weight) markedly increased plasma chlorpromazine levels in ten schizophrenic patients in a 15-week randomized crossover study.[350] A schizophrenic patient on chlorpromazine and thiothixene developed delirium and grand mal seizures after addition of large doses of propranolol (up to 1200 mg daily).[351] In another case, chlorpromazine and sotalol appeared to produce additive hypotensive effects.[40] In summary, combined use of propranolol and chlorpromazine may result in elevated plasma levels of both drugs, and the magnitude of the changes appear large enough to increase drug response. It seems likely that other phenothiazines would behave similarly, but the interaction might not occur with beta-blockers excreted primarily by the kidneys such as atenolol (Tenormin), nadolol (Corgard), or sotalol.

MANAGEMENT: Patients receiving both phenothiazines and beta-blockers should be monitored for enhanced effects of both drugs. Dosage of one or both drugs should be reduced as necessary.

Phenylephrine (Neo-Synephrine)[345-348]

MECHANISM: Beta-blockers may enhance the pressor response to phenylephrine.

CLINICAL SIGNIFICANCE: A fatal intracerebral hemorrhage occurred in a 55-year-old woman on chronic propranolol (160 mg/day) after she received one drop of 10% phenylephrine in each eye.[345] Presumably, the hemorrhage resulted from an acute hypertensive episode; previ-

DRUGS	DISCUSSION

ous administration of phenylephrine eye drops to this patient in the absence of propranolol produced no apparent ill effects. However, phenylephrine 10% eye drops have occasionally produced acute hypertensive episodes in the absence of propranolol.[346,347] Thus, the role of drug interaction in this case is not established. Intranasal phenylephrine in 14 hypertensive patients on metoprolol (Lopressor) did not increase the blood pressure,[348] but these findings may well not apply to nonselective beta-blockers such as propranolol. In summary, there is very limited evidence which suggests that propranolol may predispose to acute hypertensive episodes when phenylephrine is administered. If the interaction is real, it is likely to be more important with nonselective beta-blockers such as propranolol, nadolol (Corgard), timolol (Blocadren), or pindolol (Visken).

MANAGEMENT: Until this potential interaction is substantiated or disproved, one should carefully monitor the blood pressure if phenylephrine is administered to patients receiving beta-blocking agents.

Phenylpropanolamine (Propadrine)[107,113]

MECHANISM: Not established. Since the patient was receiving both methyldopa an oxprenolol (a beta-blocker) when the phenylpropanolamine was given, it is possible that the following sequence occurred. The methyldopa increased alpha-methylnorepinephrine in storage sites in the adrenergic neuron which were released by the indirect acting sympathomimetic, phenylpropanolamine. The beta effects of the alpha-methyl-norepinephrine were blocked by the oxprenolol, resulting in an overbalance of alpha stimulation and thus hypertension. It should also be noted that patients receiving methyldopa may be more sensitive to the pressor effects of norepinephrine.[113] Thus, any norepinephrine released by the phenylpropanolamine may have produced a larger than usual pressor response.

CLINICAL SIGNIFICANCE: A patient with hypertension well controlled on methyldopa and oxprenolol developed a severe hypertensive reaction (200/150 mm Hg) detected 2 days after beginning therapy with a "cold tablet" containing phenylpropanolamine and acetaminophen.[107] The day after the cold preparation was stopped his blood pressure decreased to 140/110 mm Hg and later to 140/90 mm Hg. It seems likely that, in this case, the phenylpropanolamine was responsible for the hypertensive episode.

MANAGEMENT: The usual warning that hypertensive patients should avoid sympathomimetics may be more important if the patient is receiving both a beta-blocking agent and methyldopa.

Phenytoin (Dilantin)[1]

MECHANISM: It is proposed that propranolol and diphenylhydantoin may have additive cardiac depressant effects.[1]

CLINICAL SIGNIFICANCE: This interaction is based primarily on theoretical considerations.

DRUGS	DISCUSSION

MANAGEMENT: It has been proposed that intravenous diphenylhydantoin be given with "great caution" to a patient who is already receiving a beta-adrenergic blocker such as propranolol.[1]

Prazosin (Minipress)[352-355]

MECHANISM: Not established. Beta-blockers may inhibit the compensatory cardiovascular responses that would normally follow prazosin-induced hypotension. Neither propranolol nor aprenolol appear to affect prazosin pharmacokinetics.[354-355]

CLINICAL SIGNIFICANCE: When hypertensive patients taking propranolol were given prazosin (2 mg orally), the acute postural hypotension that often occurs following the first dose of prazosin appeared to be enhanced.[352] This potentiating effect of beta-adrenergic blockers was confirmed in normal subjects who were given 1 mg of prazosin orally with or without propranolol or primidolol, a cardioselective beta-blocker.[353] A similar increase in the "first dose" hypotensive reaction was observed with combined use of prazosin and alprenolol in hypertensive patients.[354] Other factors that may predispose patients to first does hypotension from prazosin include diuretic therapy and/or low sodium diets.

MANAGEMENT: In patients receiving beta-blockers, initiation of prazosin therapy should be undertaken with caution and with conservative doses. Taking the initial dose at bedtime may be prudent.

Propoxyphene (Darvon, Darvocet-N)[356]

MECHANISM: Propoxyphene may inhibit the metabolism of beta-blockers such as propranolol (Inderal) and metoprolol (Lopressor) that undergo hepatic elimination.

CLINICAL SIGNIFICANCE: Preliminary results from a study in healthy subjects indicates that propoxyphene produces about a threefold increase in the bioavailability of metoprolol (100 mg orally) and reduces metoprolol total body clearance by about 20%.[356] The bioavailabilty of propranolol (40 mg orally) was increased by about 70%, but this effect may have been greater if a larger propranolol does had been used. It does not seem likely that beta-blockers excreted primarily by the kidneys such as atenolol (Tenormin), nadolol (Corgard), and sotalol would be affected by propoxyphene. Although the results of this study indicate that propoxyphene may increase the effect of propranolol and metoprolol, not enough data were presented to fully evaluate the validity of the results.

MANAGEMENT: Until more information is available one should be alert for evidence of altered response to metoprolol and propranolol if propoxyphene is initiated or discontinued.

BETA-ADRENERGIC BLOCKER INTERACTIONS (CONT.)

DRUGS	DISCUSSION

Quinidine[36,38,47,67,357-361]

MECHANISM: Both quinidine and propranolol exert a negative inotropic action on the heart.

CLINICAL SIGNIFICANCE: Due to the possibility of combined cardiac depressant effects, caution has been recommended in concurrent use of quinidine and propranolol.[36,357] However, recent studies in animals have indicated that the negative inotropic effect of these two drugs, when used together, is less than one would expect on an additive basis.[47] Combination therapy with both drugs has been used to advantage in various cardiac arrhythmias.[359] Although one study found that patients on propranolol had a lower quinidine clearance than patients not on propranolol,[360] subsequent crossover studies indicated that propranolol does not affect the pharmacokinetic behavior of quinidine.[358,361] Diarrhea was found in a majority of patients receiving propranolol plus quinidine,[359] but the incidence of diarrhea was not compared to that seen following either drug alone.

MANAGEMENT: Concomitant use should not cause difficulties in experienced hands.

Ranitidine (Zantac)[362-367]

MECHANISM: None.

CLINICAL SIGNIFICANCE: Ranitidine (300 mg/day for 1 or 6 days) did not affect steady state plasma propranolol levels in five healthy subjects receiving oral propranolol (160 mg daily).[362] Similarly, ranitidine pretreatment (300 mg/day for 14 days) did not affect blood propranolol levels following a single oral 80-mg dose of propranolol in six subjects, while cimetidine (1000 mg/day for 14 days) resulted in substantial increases in blood levels of propranolol.[363] In other studies cimetidine, but not ranitidine, reduced propranolol elimination.[364,365] Little information is available on the effect of ranitidine on other beta-blockers.[364,365] Preliminary information from a study in healthy subjects indicates that ranitidine (300 mg/day) substantially increases plasma levels of metoprolol given 200 mg/day for 1 week[366,367]; however, such an effect does not appear consistent with the lack of ranitidine interaction with propranolol. The disposition of atenolol (100 mg/day orally) does not appear to be affected by ranitidine (300 mg/day) in healthy subjects. In summary, ranitidine does not appear to affect propranolol or atenolol disposition, and probably has little effect on other beta-blockers. There is some evidence that metoprolol metabolism may be reduced by ranitidine, but confirmation of this unexpected effect is needed.

MANAGEMENT: No special precautions appear necessary at this point.

Reserpine[35]

MECHANISM: It has been proposed that catecholamine-depleting drugs such as reserpine may add to the beta-adrenergic blocking action of propranolol. Excessive sympathetic blockade may result.

DRUGS	DISCUSSION

CLINICAL SIGNIFICANCE: This interaction is based largely on theoretical considerations rather than clinical studies using the two drugs concomitantly.

MANAGEMENT: It would be prudent to closely observe patients who are receiving both reserpine and propranolol.

Rifampin (Rifadin, Rimactane)[378]

MECHANISM: Rifampin appears to enhance the hepatic metabolism of metoprolol.

CLINICAL SIGNIFICANCE: In 12 healthy subjects, pretreatment with rifampin (600 mg/day for 15 days) resulted in a 33% reduction in the bioavailability of metoprolol (Lopressor) given as 100 mg orally.[378] It seems likely that other highly metabolized beta-blockers such as propranolol (Inderal) would be similarly affected. The degree to which rifampin inhibits the therapeutic response to metoprolol or other beta-blockers is not established.

MANAGEMENT: One should be alert for evidence of altered metoprolol response if rifampin therapy is initiated or discontinued.

Terbutaline (Brethine, Bricanyl)[72]

MECHANISM: A nonspecific beta-adrenergic blocker such as propranolol would be expected to antagonize the bronchodilation produced by terbutaline. However, cardioselective beta-adrenergic blockers would be expected to have little effect on bronchoselective beta agonists such as terbutaline.

CLINICAL SIGNIFICANCE: In a group of 29 patients with chronic bronchial asthma, practolol did not appear to impair the bronchodilator activity of terbutaline.[72] It appears that practolol can be used safely in asthmatics if a beta$_2$-stimulating drug is given concurrently. Nonspecific beta-blockers such as propranolol would appear more likely to antagonize bronchodilators such as terbutaline.

MANAGEMENT: Any beta-adrenergic blocker should be used with caution in asthmatics, but the combination of practolol and terbutaline appears to be reasonably safe.

Theophylline[15,16,80,149,215-217,219-221]

MECHANISM: Beta-blockers have been shown to inhibit hepatic microsomal drug metabolism,[80,149,219-221] and this may be responsible for the reduction in theophylline clearance seen following treatment with propranolol or metoprolol. Also, theophylline and beta-blockers have some antagonistic pharmacologic effects.[15,16]

CLINICAL SIGNIFICANCE: In nine healthy subjects, propranolol (40 mg q 6 hours) and, to a lesser extent, metoprolol (50 mg q 6 hours)

DRUGS	DISCUSSION

reduced the clearance of theophylline.[216] The effect was most pronounced in subjects shows theophylline metabolism was enhanced by cigarette smoking. Propranolol has also been shown to inhibit aminophylline-induced increases in plasma-free fatty acids and insulin and to inhibit aminophylline-induced decreases in growth hormone levels.[15] The inhibition is isoproterenol-induced positive inotropic and chronotropic effects by beta-adrenergic blocking agents can be partially reversed by theophylline administration,[16] while the mild inotropic effect of theophylline in healthy subjects is blocked by pretreatment with propranolol or metoprolol.[217] In summary, theophylline and beta-blockers may have antagonistic pharmacodynamic effects, while pharmacokinetic interactions would tend to increase the effects of theophylline. However, in the absence of reports of adverse effects due to this interaction, its clinical importance remains speculative.

MANAGEMENT: Concomitant use of beta-blockers and aminophylline should be undertaken with some caution, and attention should be given to detecting inhibition of the effect of either drug. If the aminophylline is being used in the treatment of asthma, propranolol should probably not be used because of the possibility of propranolol-induced bronchoconstriction.

Verapamil (Calan, Isoptin)[322-328]

MECHANISM: Verapamil has intrinsic depressant effects on myocardial contractility, but this tends to be offset by a reflex increase in heart rate resulting from peripheral vasodilation produced by the verapamil. In the presence of beta-blockers, the reflex increase in heart rate is reduced, thus allowing the negative inotropic effect of the verapamil to remain unopposed. Also, the intrinsic cardiodepressant effect of the beta-blocker may be additive with that of verapamil. The combined inhibitory effects of verapamil and beta-blockers on the atriorventricular node represent another potential site of adverse interaction.

CLINICAL SIGNIFICANCE: Both theoretical considerations and clinical evidence indicate that the combination of verapamil and beta-blockade can result in additive cardiodepressant effects.[322-326] In many patients (e.g. those with refractory angina pectoris) the positive effects of the combination outweigh the risk of adverse effects.[328] However, some patients have developed marked bradycardia, cardiac failure, and severe hypotension.[323,327] Patients with reasonably good left ventricular function on low to moderate doses of a beta-blocker appear much less likely to experience adverse effects than those with reduced left ventricular performance on large doses of a beta-blocker. Other factors which may predispose to an adverse interaction include cardiac conduction disturbances, aortic stenosis, large does of verapamil (especially if given intravenously), presence of other drugs with negative inotropic effect (e.g., disopyramide), and possibly the presence of drugs that inhibit alpha-adrenergic response (e.g., methyldopa, quinidine).

BETA-ADRENERGIC BLOCKER INTERACTIONS (CONT.)

DRUGS	DISCUSSION

MANAGEMENT: Concurrent use of verapamil and beta-blockers may be used to advantage in cases of refractory angina pectoris. However, one should be alert for evidence of excessive cardiodepressant effects in patients receiving this combination, especially if large beta-blocker doses are used and/or the patient has compromised left ventricular function. Nifedipine produces less myocardial depression than verapamil and may thus be less likely to interact adversely with beta-blockers.[326]

NITROGLYCERIN INTERACTIONS

DRUGS	DISCUSSION

Ergot alkaloids[379]

MECHANISM: Ergot alkaloids may precipitate angina, and thus work against the anti-anginal effects of nitroglycerin. Also, nitroglycerin may reduce the first-pass hepatic metabolism of dihydroergotamine.

CLINICAL SIGNIFICANCE: Ergot alkaloids are known to precipitate angina pectoris, and are even used as a provocative agents in angina studies. Also, nitroglycerin has been shown to markedly enhance the bioavailability of dihydroergotamine in a study of six patients with orthostatic hypotension.[379]

MANAGEMENT: Patients receiving nitroglycerin for angina pectoris should avoid ergot alkaloids if at all possible. If the combination is used, monitor for enhanced ergot alkaloid effect and lower ergot dosage as needed.

Ethanol (Alcohol, ethyl)[114,115]

MECHANISM: Hypotension reportedly may occur following the combined use of ethanol and nitroglycerin.[114] This is presumably due to the vasodilation which both agents may produce.[115]

CLINICAL SIGNIFICANCE: Although clinical reports are lacking, Shafer[114] warns that cardiovascular collapse may result from this combination. Unless the clinician is cognizant of this interaction, he may attribute the collapse to coronary insufficiency or occlusion.

MANAGEMENT: Pending accumulation of further information, patients receiving nitroglycerin should take ethanol cautiously.

Nitrates (long-acting)[86,87,88,117]

MECHANISM: The chronic administration of long-acting nitrates had been reported to produce tolerance, thus decreasing the therapeutic effect of subsequently administered nitroglycerin.

CLINICAL SIGNIFICANCE: Some patients with angina pectoris reportedly have noted decreased effectiveness of nitroglycerin while they

DRUGS	DISCUSSION

were taking long-acting nitrates. A pharmacologic study of ten patients demonstrated that a partial tolerance to nitroglycerin developed after as little as 1 week of pentaerythritol tetranitrate therapy.[86] Study in normal volunteers[88] indicates that isosorbide dinitrate (120 mg/day for 6 to 8 weeks) attenuates the venodilation of nitroglycerin (0.9 mg sublingually) but does not appear to affect the arteriolar dilation. Another study in 17 patients with angina failed to note an impaired response to nitroglycerin due to isosorbide dinitrate.[87] Most recently, a study in 28 patients with coronary artery disease showed that isosorbide dinitrate (120 mg/day for a month) did not alter nitroglycerin-induced improvement in exercise testing.[117] Thus, although there is some evidence of interaction, the preponderance of evidence of actual patients with angina indicates that it has little clinical importance.

MANAGEMENT: The available evidence does not appear sufficient to warrant avoiding the concomitant use of nitroglycerin and long-acting nitrates. However, in patients with suboptimal response to sublingual nitroglycerin, large doses of long-acting nitrates should be considered a potential cause.

References

1. WOOD RA: Sinoatrial arrest: an interaction between phenytoin and lignocaine. Br Med J 1:645, 1971.
2. BLEIFELD W: Side effects of antiarrhythmic drugs. Nauyn Schmiedebergs Arch Pharmacol 267:282, 1971.
3. HARRAH MD et al: The interaction of d-tubocurarine with antiarrhythmic drugs. Anesthesiology 33:406, 1970.
4. HEINONEN J, et al: Plasma lidocaine levels in patients treated with potential inducers of microsomal enzymes. Acta Anaesthesiol Scand 14:89, 1970.
5. DIFAZIO CA, BROWN RE: Lidocaine metabolism in normal and phenobarbital-pretreated dogs. Anesthesiology 36:238, 1972.
6. DUNBAR RW, et al: The effect of diazepam on the antiarrhythmic response to lidocaine. Anesth Analg 50:685, 1971.
7. USUBIAGA JE, et al: Interaction of intravenously administered procaine, lidocaine and succinylcholine in anesthetized subjects. Anesth Analg 46:39, 1967.
8. O'REILLY M, et al: Propranolol and digitalis (Letter). Lancet 1:138, 1974.
9. BAUMRUCKER JF: Drug-interaction—propranolol and cafergot (Letter). N Engl J Med 288:916, 1973.
10. DIAMOND S: Propranolol and ergotamine tartrate (cont.) (Letter). N Engl J Med 289:159, 1973.
11. BLANK NK, REIDER MJ: Paradoxical response to propranolol in migraine (Letter). Lancet 2:1336, 1973.
12. KISSEL P, et al: Levodopa-propranolol therapy in parkinsonian tremor (Letter). Lancet 1:403, 1974.

References (CONT.)

13. CAMANNI F, MASSARA F: Enhancement of levodopa-induced growth-hormone stimulation by propranolol (Letter). Lancet 1:942, 1974.
14. ROZEN MS, WHAN FM: Prolonged curarization associated with propranolol. Med J Aust 1:467, 1972.
15. ENSINCK, JW, et al: Effect of aminophylline on the secretion of insulin, glucagon, luteinizing hormone and growth hormone in humans. J Clin Endocrinol Metab 31:153, 170.
16. STAUCH M, et al: Effets hemodynamiques de la stimulation des beta-recepteurs apres blocage beta-adrenergique et theophylline. Ann Cardiol Angeiol 20:71, 1971.
17. BERCHTOLD P, BESSMAN AN: Propranolol (Letter). Ann Intern Med 80:119, 1974.
18. McMURTRY RJ: Propranolol, hypoglycemia, and hypertensive crisis (Letter). Ann Intern Med 80:669, 1974.
19. MOLNAR GW, et al: Propranolol enhancement of hypoglycemic sweating. Clin Pharmacol Ther 15:490, 1974.
20. ABRAMSON EA, et al: Effects of propranolol on the hormonal and metabolic responses to insulin-induced hypoglycemia. Lancet 2:1386, 1966.
21. KRAM J, et al: Propranolol (Letter). Ann Intern Med 80:282, 1974.
22. NIES AS, SHAND DG: Hypertensive response to propranolol in a patient treated with methyldopa—a proposed mechanism. Clin Pharmacol Ther 14:823, 1973.
23. BRESSLER R, et al: Tranlycypromine: a potent insulin secretagogue and hypoglycemic agent. Diabetes 17:617, 1968.
24. GEUMEI A, et al: Beta-adrenergic receptors and gastric acid secretion. Surgery 66:663, 1967.
25. KOCH-WESER J: Quinidine-induced hypoprothrombinemic hemorrhage in patients on chronic warfarin therapy. Ann Intern Med 68:511, 1968.
26. GAZZANIGA AB, STEWART DR: Possible quinindine-induced hemorrhage in a patient on warfarin sodium. N Engl J Med 280:711, 1969.
27. UDALL, JA: Drug interference with warfarin therapy (Abstract). Am J Cardiol 23:143, 1969.
28. WAY WL, et al: Recurarization with quinindine. JAMA 200:153, 1967.
29. SCHMIDT JL, et al: The effect of quinidine on the action of muscle relaxants. JAMA 183:669, 1963.
30. KNOUSS RF, et al: Variation in quinidine excretion with changing urine pH (Abstract). Ann Intern Med 68:1157, 1968.
31. MILNE MD: Influence of acid-base balance on the efficacy and toxicity of drugs. Proc R Soc Med 58:961, 1965.
32. GERHARDT RE, et al: Quinidine excretion in aciduria and alkaluria. Ann Intern Med 71:927, 1969.
33. KOTLER MN, et al: Hypoglycaemia precipitated by propranolol. Lancet 2:1389, 1966.
34. ABRAMSON EA, ARKY RA: Role of beta-adrenergic receptors in counterregulation to insulin-induced hypoglycemia. Diabetes 17:141, 1968.
35. Inderal. Product Information, Ayerst Laboratories, 1981.
36. DREIFUS LS, et al: Propranolol and quinidine in the management of ventricular tachycardia. JAMA 204:736, 1968.
37. WATT DAL: Sensitivity to propranolol after digoxin intoxication. Br Med J 3:413, 1968.

References (CONT.)

38. STERN S: Synergistic action of propranolol with quinidine. Am Heart J 72:569, 1966.
39. UDALL JA: Quinidine and hypoprothrombinemia (Letter). Ann Intern Med 69:403, 1968.
40. BAKER L, et al: Beta adrenergic blockade and juvenile diabetes: acute studies and long-term therapeutic trial. J Pediatr 75:19, 1969.
41. FRIEDEN J: Propranolol as an antiarrhythmic agent. Am Heart J 74:283, 1967.
42. BARRETT AM, CULLUM VA: Lack of interaction between propranolol and mebanazinc. J Pharm Pharmacol 20:911, 1968.
43. Quelicin® Product Information, Abbott Laboratories, 1969.
44. CUTHBERT MF: The effect of quinidine and procainamide on the neuromuscular blocking action of suxamethonium. Br J Anaesth 38:775, 1966.
45. STUBBS D, et al: Combined use of isoproterenol and propranolol in cardiogenic shock. Clin Pharmacol Ther 11:244, 1970.
46. ILYAS M, et al: Delirium induced by a combination of anti-arrhythmic drugs (Letter). Lancet 2:1368, 1969.
47. STERN S: Haemodynamic change following separate and combined administration of beta-blocking drugs and quinidine. Eur J Clin Invest 1:432, 1971.
48. SOPHER IM, MING SC: Fatal corpus luteum hemorrhage during anticoagulant therapy. Obstet Gynecol 37:695, 1971.
49. UDALL JA: Drug interference with warfarin therapy. Clin Med 77:20, 1970.
50. TRENT J: Personal communication. November 19, 1970.
51. WHITSETT TL, et al: Propranolol blockade of positive inotropic effects of L-dopa in dog and man. The Pharmacologist 12:213, 1970 (Abstract 089).
52. DUVOISIN RC: Hypotension caused by L-dopa (Letter). Br Med J 3:47, 1970.
53. ARITA M, MASHIBA H: Effects of phenothiazine and propranolol on ECG. The effects of propranolol on the electrocardiographic abnormalities induced by phenothiazine derivatives. Jpn Circ J 34:391, 1970.
54. ZINN MB: Quinidine intoxication from alkali ingestion. Texas Med 66:64, 1970.
55. GIBALDI M, et al: Effect of antacids on pH of urine. Clin Pharmacol Ther 16:520, 1974.
56. GALEAZZI RL, et al: The renal elimination of procainamide. Clin Pharmacol Ther 19:55, 1976.
57. FLACKE W: Treatment of myasthenia gravis. N Engl J Med 288:27, 1973.
58. EISALO A, et al: The effect of alprenolol in elderly patients with raised blood pressure. Acta Med Scand (Supplement 554):23, 1974.
59. DEDIVITHS O, et al: Tolbutamide and propranolol (Letter). Lancet 1:749, 1968.
60. SKINNER DJ: Uses of propranolol (Letter). N Engl J Med 293:1205, 1975.
61. LLOYD-MOSTEN RH, ORAM S: Modification by propranolol of cardiovascular effects of induced hypoglycemia. Lancet 1:1213, 1975.
62. CRAWFORD MH, et al: Combined propranolol and digoxin therapy in angina pectoris. Ann Intern Med 83:449, 1975.

References (CONT.)

63. JOHNSON G, et al: Effects of intravenous propranolol and metoprolol and their interaction with isoprenaline on pulmonary function, heart rate, and blood pressure in asthmatics. Eur J Clin Pharmacol 8:175, 1975.
64. COLLU R, et al: Stimulation of growth hormone secretion by levodopapropranolol in children and adolescents. Pediatrics 56:262, 1975.
65. LOTTI G, et al: Enhancement of levodopa-induced growth hormone stimulation by practolol (Letter). Lancet 2:1329, 1974.
66. PALMER RF: Pharmacological autopsy of anesthetic death after aortography for aortic dissection (Question and Answer). JAMA 232:1281, 1975.
67. VISIOLI O, et al: Effects of interaction of quinidine and beta-blocking agents on some cardiodynamic and hemodynamic parameters of normal individuals. Am Heart J 2:217, 1969.
68. HERISHANU Y, ROSENBERG P: Beta-blockers and myasthenia gravis. Ann Intern Med 83:834, 1975.
69. VARMA DR, et al: Response to adrenaline and propranolol in hyperthyroidism (Letter). Lancet 1:260, 1976.
70. HUFFMAN DH, et al: The interaction between halofenate and propranolol. Clin Pharmacol Ther 19:807, 1976.
71. HARRIS AL: Clonidine withdrawal and blockade. Lancet 1:596, 1976.
72. FORMGREN H, ERIKSSON NE: Effects of practolol in combination with terbutaline in the treatment of hypertension and arrhythmias in asthmatic patients. Scand J Resp Dis 56:217, 1975.
73. KAESS H, et al: The influence of propranolol on serum gastrin concentration and hydrochloric acid secretion in response to hypoglycemia in normal subjects. Digestion 13:193, 1975.
74. BINNION PF, DASGUPTA R: Tritiated digoxin metabolism after prior treatment with propranolol or diphenylhydantoin sodium. Int J Clin Pharmacol 12:96, 1975.
75. DATA JL, et al: Interaction of quinidine with anticonvulsant drugs. N Engl J Med 294:699, 1976.
76. SANDLER M, et al: Oxpernolol and levodopa in parkinsonian patients (Letter). Lancet 1:168, 1975.
77. MASSARA F, et al: Propranolol block of epinephrine-induced hypokalaemia in man. Eur J Pharmacol 10:404, 1970.
78. MILLER TD, WAY WL: Inhibition of succinylcholine-induced increased intragastric pressure by nondepolarizing muscle relaxants and lidocaine. Anesthesiology 34:185, 1971.
79. KORNFELD P, et al: Myasthenia gravis unmasked by antiarrhythmic agents. Mt Sinai J Med 43:10, 1976.
80. GREENBLATT DJ: Impairment of antipyrine clearance in humans by propranolol (Abstract). Clin Pharmacol Ther 21:104, 1977.
81. SCHNECK D, et al: Effect of procainamide and isoniazid on each other's acetylation pathway in normal subjects (Abstract). Clin Pharmacol Ther 21:116, 1977.
82. MESSERLI FH, et al: Effects of β-adrenergic blockade on plasma cyclic AMP and blood sugar responses to glucagon and isoproterenol in man. Int J Clin Pharmacol 14:189, 1976.
83. THIRINGER G, SVEDMYR N: Interaction of orally administered metoprolol, practolol and propranolol in asthmatics. Eur J Clin Pharmacol 10:163, 1976.

References (CONT.)

84. MEYER N, et al: A study of the influence of pH on the buccal absorption and renal excretion of procainamide. Eur J Clin Pharmacol 7:287, 1974.
85. BENOWITZ N, et al: Lidocaine disposition kinetics in monkey and man II. Effects of hemorrhage and sympathomimetic drug administration. Clin Pharmacol Ther 16:99, 1974.
86. SCHELLING, JL, LASAGNA L: A study of cross-tolerance to circulatory effects of organic nitrates. Clin Pharmacol Ther 8:256, 1967.
87. ARONOW WS, CHELSUK HM: Evaluation of nitroglycerin in angina in patients on isosorbide dinitrate. Circulation 42:61, 1970.
88. ZELIS R, MASON DT: Isosorbide dinitrate. Effect on the vasodilator response to nitroglycerin. JAMA 234:166, 1975.
89. ANON: Beta blockers for diabetics (Editorial). Lancet 1:843, 1977.
90. FEELY J: Beta blockers for diabetics (Letter). Lancet 1:950, 1977.
91. LeWINTER MM, et al: The effects of oral propranolol, digoxin and combination therapy on the resting and exercise electrocardiogram. Am Heart J 93:202, 1977.
92. SULKOWSKI A, et al: Propranolol effects on acute marijuana intoxication in man. Psychopharmacology 52:47, 1977.
93. VanHERWAARDEN CLA, et al: Effects of adrenalin during treatment with propranolol and metoprolol (Letter). Br Med J 2:1029, 1977.
94. BENOWITZ NL, JONES RT: Prolonged delta-9-tetrahydrocannabinol ingestion effects of sympathomimetic amines and autonomic blockades. Clin Pharmacol Ther 21:336, 1977.
95. AUTY RM, BRANCH RA: Paracetamol toxicity and propranolol (Letter). Lancet 2:1505, 1973.
96. BRANCH RA, et al: The reduction of lidocaine clearance by dl-propranolol: an example of hemodynamic drug interaction. J Pharmacol Exp Ther 184:515, 1973.
97. MELANDER A, et al: Enhancement of the bioavailability of propranolol and metoprolol by food. Clin Pharmacol Ther 22:108, 1977.
98. SHAND DG, et al: Plasma propranolol levels in adults: with observations in four children. Clin Pharmacol Ther 11:112, 1970.
99. OLSEN H, MORLAND J: Ethanol-induced increase in procainamide acetylation in man. Br J Clin Pharmacol 13:203, 1982.
100. REIDENBERG MM, et al: Polymorphic acetylation of procainamide in man. Clin Pharmacol Ther 17:722, 1975.
101. DOBBS JH, et al: Effects of aluminum hydroxide on the absorption of propranolol. Curr Ther Res 21:887, 1977.
102. HURWITZ A, et al: Effects of antacids on gastric emptying. Gastroenterology 71:268, 1976.
103. KOSINSKI EJ, MALINDZAK GS: Glucagon and isoproterenol in reversing propranolol toxicity. Arch Intern Med 132:840, 1973.
104. HAWORTH E, BURROUGHS AK: Disopyramide and warfarin interaction. Br Med J 4:866, 1977.
105. TILSTONE WJ, et al: Effects of furosemide on glomerular filtration rate and clearance of practolol, digoxin, cephaloridine, and gentamicin. Clin Pharmacol Ther 22:389, 1977.
106. ALVAN G, et al: Effect of pentobarbital on the disposition of alprenolol. Clin Pharmacol Ther 22:316, 1977.
107. McLAREN EH: Severe hypertension produced by interaction of phenylpropanolamine with methyldopa and oxprenolol. Br Med J 3:283, 1976.

References (CONT.)

108. EMBIL K, et al: Effect of orange juice consumption on urinary pH. Am J Hosp Pharm 33:1294, 1976.
109. DEISSEROTH A, et al: Quinidine-induced liver disease. Ann Intern Med 77:595, 1972.
110. WINKLER JW Jr: Quinidine hepatotoxicity? (Letter). Ann Intern Med 78:460, 1973.
111. DUJOVNE CA, SHOEMAN DW: Surfactant laxatives and hepatotoxicity (Letter). Ann Intern Med 79:137, 1973.
112. CAIRNS SA, MARSHALL AJ: Clonidine withdrawal (Letter). Lancet 1:368, 1976.
113. DOLLERY CT: Physiological and pharmacological interactions of antihypertensive drugs. Proc R Soc Med 58:983, 1965.
114. SHAFER N: Hypotension due to nitroglycerin combined with alcohol (Letter). N Engl J Med 273:1169, 1965.
115. ALLISON RD, et al: Effects of alcohol and nitroglycerin on vascular responses in man. Angiology 22:211, 1971.
116. DURAO V, et al: Modification of antihypertensive effect of β-adrenoreceptor-blocking agents by inhibition of endogenous prostaglandin synthesis. Lancet 2:1005, 1977.
117. LEE G, et al: Effects of long-term oral administration of isosorbide dinitrate on the antianginal response to nitroglycerin. Am J Cardiol 41:82, 1978.
118. BAILEY RR, NEALE TJ: Rapid clonidine withdrawal with blood pressure overshoot exaggerated by beta-blockade. Br Med J 2:942, 1976.
119. EJVINSSON G: Effect of quinidine on plasma concentrations of digoxin. Br Med J 1:279, 1978.
120. LEAHEY EB, et al: Interaction between quinidine and digoxin. JAMA 240:533, 1978.
121. TARTINI R, et al: Dangerous interaction between amoidarone and quinidine. Lancet 1:1327, 1982.
122. CUMMING AD, ROBERTSON C: Interaction between disopyramide and practolol. Br Med J 2:1204, 1979.
123. CATHCART-RAKE W, et al: The pharmacodynamics of concurrent disopyramide and propanolol. Clin Pharmacol Ther 25:217, 1979.
124. KARIM A, et al: Clinical pharmacokinetics of disopyramide. J Pharmacokinet Biopharm 10:465, 1982.
125. SYLVEN C, ANDERSON P: Evidence that disopyramide does not interact with warfarin. Br Med J 286:1181, 1983.
126. RYLL C, DAVIS LJ: Warfarin-disopyramide interactions. Drug Intell Clin Pharm 13:260, 1979
127. NAPPI JM, et al: Severe hypoglycemia association with disopyramide. West J Med 138:95, 1983.
128. GOLDBERG IJ, et al: Disopyramide (Norpace)-induced hypoglycemia. Am J Med 69:463, 1980.
129. LEAHEY EB, et al: The effect of quinidine and other antiarrhythmic drugs on serum digoxin. A prospective study. Ann Intern Med 92:605, 1980.
130. DOERING W: Quinidine-digoxin interaction. Pharmacokinetics, underlying mechanism and clinical implications. N Engl J Med 301:400, 1979.
131. WELLENS HJJ, et al: Effect of oral disopyramide on serum digoxin levels. A prospective study. Am Heart J 100:934, 1980.
132. ELLRODT G, SINGH BN: Adverse effects of disopyramide (Norpace):

References (CONT.)

toxic interactions with other antiarrhythmic agents. Heart Lung 9:469, 1980.

133. AITIO ML, VUORENMAA T: Enhanced metabolism and diminished efficacy of disopyramide by enzyme induction? Br J Clin Pharmacol 9:149, 1980.

134. AITIO ML, et al: The effect of enzyme induction on the metabolism of disopyramide in man. Br J Clin Pharmacol 11:279, 1981.

135. KESSLER JM, et al: Disopyramide and phenytoin interaction. Clin Pharm 1:263, 1982.

136. MADDUX BD, WHITING RB: Toxic synergism of disopyramide and hyperkalemia. Chest 78:654, 1980.

137. BAKER B, et al: Concurrent use of quinidine and disopyramide: evaluation of serum concentrations and electrocardiographic effects. Am Heart J 105:12, 1983.

138. MORADY F, et al: Drugs five years later. Disopyramide. Ann Intern Med 96:337, 1982.

139. CUNNINGHAM JL, et al: The effect of urine pH and plasma protein binding on the renal clearance of disopyramide. Clin Pharmacokinet 2:373, 1977.

140. CATHCART-RAKE WF, et al: The effect of concurrent oral administration of propranolol and disopyramide on cardiac function in healthy men. Circulation 61:938, 1980.

141. KEIDAR S, et al: Sinoatrial arrest due to lidocaine injection in sick sinus syndrome during amiodarone administration. Am Heart J 104:1384, 1982.

142. KNAPP AB, et al: The cimetidine-lidocaine interaction. Ann Intern Med 98:174, 1983.

143. PERUCCA E, RICHENS A: Reduction of oral bioavailability of lignocaine by induction of first pass metabolism in epileptic patients. Br J Clin Pharmacol 8:21, 1979.

144. PERUCCA E, et al: Effect of low-dose phenobarbitone on five indirect indices of hepatic microsomal enzyme induction and plasma lipoproteins in normal subjects. Br J Clin Pharmacol 12:592, 1981.

145. LELORIER J: Lidocaine and pentobarbital: a potentially lethal drug-drug interaction. Toxicol Appl Pharmacol 44:657, 1978.

146. OCHS HR, et al: Reduction in lidocaine clearance during continuous infusion and by coadministration of propranolol. N Engl M Med 303:373, 1980.

147. GRAHAM CF, et al: Lidocaine-propranolol interactions. N Engl J Med 304:1301, 1981.

148. CONRAD KA, et al: Lidocaine elimination: effects of metoprolol and of propranolol. Clin Pharmacol Ther 33:133, 1983.

149. DEACON CS, et al: Inhibition of oxidative drug metabolism by β-adrenoreceptor antagonists is related to their lipid solubility. Br J Clin Pharmacol 12:429, 1981.

150. BOUDOULAS H, et al: Negative inotropic effect of lidocaine in patients with coronary arterial disease and normal subjects. Chest 71:170, 1977.

151. GREENBLATT DJ, et al: Impairment of antipyrine clearance in humans by propranolol. Circulation 57:1161, 1978.

152. SONNEVILLE PF, et al: Effect of lidocaine on the absorption, disposi-

References (CONT.)

tion and tolerance of intramuscularly administered cefoxitin. Eur J Clin Pharmacol 12:273, 1977.

153. FEELY J, et al: Increased toxicity and reduced clearence of lidocaine by cimetidine. Ann Intern Med 96:592, 1982.

154. KNAPP AB, et al: The cimetidine-lidocaine interaction. Ann Intern Med 98:174, 1983.

155. FEELY J, et al: Reduction of liver blood flow and propranolol metabolism by cimetidine. N Engl J Med 304:692, 1981.

156. FEELY J, GUY E: Lack of effect of ranitidine on the disposition of lignocaine. Br J Clin Pharmacol 15:378, 1983.

157. JACKSON JE, et al: The effects of H_2 blockers on lidocaine disposition. Clin Pharmacol Ther 33:255, 1983.

158. DOERING W: Quinidine-digoxin interaction. Pharmacokinetics, underlying mechanism and clinical implications. N Engl J Med. 301:400, 1979.

159. BRUCKNER J, et al: Neuromuscular drug interactions of clinical importance. Anesth Analg 59:678, 1980.

160. HUET P-M, LELORIER J: Effects of smoking and chronic hepatitis B on lidocaine and indocyanine green kinetics. Clin Pharmacol Ther 28:208, 1980.

161. REMON JP, et al: Interaction of antacids with antiarrhythmics. V. Effect of aluminum hydroxide and magnesium oxide on the bioavailability of quinidine, procainamide and propranolol in dogs. Arzneimittelforsch 33:117, 1983.

162. SOMOGYI A, HEINZOW B: Cimetidine reduces procainamide elimination (Letter). N Engl J Med 307:1080, 1982.

163. DRAYER DE, et al: Cumulation of N-acetylprocainamide, an active metabolite of procainamide, in patients with impaired renal function. Clin Pharmacol Ther 22:63, 1977.

164. REIDENBERG MM, et al: Aging and renal clearance of procainamide and acetylprocainamide. Clin Pharmacol Ther 28:732, 1980.

165. ROMANKIEWICZ JA, et al: The noninterference of aluminum hydroxide gel with quinidine sulfate absorption: an approach to control quinidine-induced diarrhea. Am Heart J 96:518, 1978.

166. CHAPRON DJ, et al: Apparent quinidine-induced digoxin toxicity after withdrawal of pentobarbital. A case of sequential drug interactions. Arch Intern Med 139:363, 1979.

167. SUMMERS WK, et al: Does physostigmine reverse quinidine delirium? West J Med 135:411, 1981.

168. POLISH LB, et al: Digitoxin-quinidine interaction:potentiation during administration of cimetidine. South Med J 74:633, 1981.

169. KOLB KW, et al: The effect of cimetidine on urinary pH and quinidine clearance (Abstract). American Society of Hospital Pharmacists Midyear Clinical Meeting Abstracts, P-64, December, 1982.

170. GREEN J, et al: Nifedipine-quinidine interaction (Abstract). American Society of Hospital Pharmacists, Midyear Clinical Meeting Abstracts, P-45, December, 1982.

171. KROBOTH FJ, et al: Phenytoin-theophylline-quinidine interaction (Letter). N Engl J Med 308:725, 1983.

172. JAILLON, P, DATES RE: Phenytoin-induced changes in quinidine and 3-hydroxyquinidine pharmacokinetics in conscious dogs. J Pharmacol Exp Ther 213:33, 1980.

References (CONT.)

173. TWUM-BARIMA Y, CARRUTHERS SG: Quinidine-rifampin interaction. N Engl J Med 304:1466, 1981.
174. AHMAD D, et al: Rifampicin-quinidine interaction. Br J Dis Chest 73:409, 1979.
175. FENSTER PE, et al: Digoxin-quinidine interaction in patients with chronic renal failure. Circulation 66:1277, 1982.
176. HOOYMANS PM, MERKUS FWHM: The mechanism of the interaction between digoxin and quinidine. Pharmaceutisch Weekblad 1:212, 1979.
177. MUNGALL DR, et al: Effects of quinidine on serum digoxin concentration. Ann Intern Med 93:689, 1980.
178. HAGER WD, et al: Digoxin-quinidine interaction. N Engl J Med 301:400, 1979.
179. DOERING W: Quinidine-digoxin interaction. N Engl J Med 301:400, 1979.
180. LEAHEY EB, et al: The effect of quinidine and other oral antiiarrythmic drugs on serum digoxin. Ann Intern Med 92:605, 1980.
181. PEDERSEN KE, et al: The effect of quinidine on digoxin kinetics in cardiac patients. Acta Med Scand 207:291, 1980.
182. CHEN T-S, FRIEDMAN HS: Alteration of digoxin pharmacokinetics by a single dose of quinidine. JAMA 244:669, 1980.
183. LEAHEY EB, et al: Enhanced cardiac effect of digoxin during quinidine treatment. Arch Intern Med 139:519, 1979.
184. DOERING W, et al: Quinidine-digoxin interaction: evidence for involvement of an extrarenal mechanism. Eur J Clin Pharmacol 21:281, 1982.
185. BUSSEY HI: The influence of quinidine and other agents on digitalis glycosides. Am Heart J 104:289, 1982.
186. LEAHEY EB, et al: Quinidine-digoxin interaction: time course and pharmacokinetics. Am J Cardiol 48:1141, 1981.
187. OCHS HR, et al: Impairment of digoxin clearance by coadministration of quinidine. J Clin Pharmacol 21:396, 1981.
188. FRIEDMAN HS, CHEN T-S: Use of control steady-state serum digoxin levels for predicting serum digoxin concentration after quinidine administration. Am Heart J 104:72, 1982.
189. BELZ GG, et al: Quinidine-digoxin interaction: cardiac efficacy of elevated serum digoxin concentration. Clin Pharmacol Ther 31:548, 1982.
190. MANYARI DE, et al: Quinidine therapy and digitalis toxicity. J Am Geriatr Soc 29:31, 1981.
191. SCHENCK-GUSTAFSSON K, et al: Effect of quindine on digoxin concentration in skeletal muscle and serum in patients with atrial fibrillation. N Engl J Med 305:209, 1981.
192. PIERONI RE, MARSHALL J: Fatal digoxin-quinidine interaction in an elderly woman. J Am Geriatr Soc 29:422, 1981.
193. GARTY M, et al: Digitoxin elimination reduced during quinidine therapy. Ann Intern Med 94:35, 1981.
194. FENSTER PE, et al: Digoxin-quinidine interaction: pharmacokinetic evaluation. Ann Intern Med 93:698, 1980.
195. OCHS HR, et al: Noninteraction of digitoxin and quinidine. N Engl J Med 303:672, 1980.

References (CONT.)

196. FENSTER PE, et al: Combined digitoxin-quinidine administration pharmacokinetic evaluation. Clin Res 28:235, A, 1980.
197. THATCHER SK, LEMBERG L: Digitalist-quinidine interaction. Heart Lung 9:352, 1980.
198. SMALL RE, MARSHALL JH: Quinidine-digoxin interaction. Drug Intell Clin Pharm 13:286, 1979.
199. HOLT DW, et al: Clinically significant interaction between digoxin and quinidine. Br Med J 2:1401, 1979.
200. HAGER WD, et al: Digoxin bioavailability during quinidine administration. Clin Pharmacol Ther 30:594, 1981.
201. PEDERSEN KE, et al: Effect of quinidine on digoxin bioavailability. Eur J Clin Pharmacol 24:41, 1983.
202. STEINESS E, et al: Reduction of digoxin-induced inotropism during quinidine administration. Clin Pharmacol Ther 27:791, 1980.
203. SCHENCK-GUSTAFSSON K, DAHLQVIST R: Pharmacokinetics digoxin in patients subjected to the quinidine-digoxin interaction. Br J Clin Pharmacol 11:181, 1981.
204. WILLIAMS JF, MATHEW B: Effect of quinidine on positive inotropic action of digoxin. Am J Cardiol 47:1052, 1981.
205. LASH RE, et al: Mechanism of additive effects of digoxin and quinidine on contractility in isolated cardiac muscle. Am J Cardiol 50:483, 1982.
206. GEIGER JD, et al: Digoxin-quinidine interaction in unanesthetized guinea pigs. Pharmacology 25:177, 1982.
207. GESSMAN L, et al: An electrophysiologic study of the digoxin-quinidine interaction. J Clin Pharmacol 23:16, 1983.
208. RODENSKY PL, et al: The effect of quinidine on tolerance to digoxin. Am J Cardiol 5:498, 1960.
209. DOHERTY JE, et al: Digoxin-quinidine interaction changes in canine tissue concentration from steady state with quinidine. Am J Cardiol 45:1196, 1980.
210. BALL WJ, et al: Effect of quinidine on the digoxin receptor in vitro. J Clin Invest 68:1065, 1981.
211. HOROWITZ JD, et al: Lack of interaction between digoxin and quinidine in cultured heart cells. J Pharmacol Exp Ther 220:488, 1982.
212. KAPLINSKY C, et al: Digoxin-quinidine: in vitro studies in rat tissue. J Lab Clin Med 96:592, 1980.
213. WEIDLER DJ, et al: The effect of long-term propranolol administration on the pharmacokinetics of procainamide in humans (Abstract). Clin Pharmacol Ther 29:289, 1981.
214. LEGROS, J: Animal studies—a theoretical basis for treatment. J Int Med Res 4(Suppl. 4):46, 1976.
215. CONRAD KA, PROSNITZ EH: Cardiovascular effects of theophylline before and during beta blockade with metroprolol (Abstract). Clin Pharmacol Ther 27:249, 1980.
216. CONRAD KA, NYMAN DW: Effects of metroprolol and propranolol on theophylline elimination. Clin Pharmacol Ther 28:463, 1980.
217. CONRAD KA, PROSNITZ EH: Cardiovascular effects of theophylline. Partial attenuation by beta-blockade. Eur J Clin Pharmacol 21:109, 1981.
218. URBANO AM: Phenytoin-quinidine interaction in a patient with recurrent ventricular tachyarrhythmias (Letter). N Engl J Med 308:225,1982.

References (CONT.)

219. Bax NDS, et al: Inhibition of antipyrine metabolism by beta-adrenoceptor antagonists. Br J Clin Pharmacol 12:779, 1981.
220. Daneshmend TK, Roberts CJC: The short term effects of propranolol, atenolol and labetalol on antipyrine kinetics in normal subjects. Br J Clin Pharmacol 13:817, 1982.
221. Greenblatt DJ, et al: Impairment of antipyrine clearance in humans by propranolol. Circulation 57:1161, 1978.
222. Schafer-Korting Monika, et al: Atenolol interaction with aspirin, allopurinol, and ampicillin. Clin Pharmacol Ther 33:283, 1983.
223. Ponten J, et al: Beta-receptor blockade and spinal anaesthesia. Withdrawal versus continuation of long-term therapy. Acta Anaesthesiol Scand 76:62, 1982.
224. Ponten J, et al: Bupivacaine for intercostal nerve blockade in patients on long-term beta-receptor blocking therapy. Acta Anaesthesiol Scand 76:70, 1982.
225. Regardh CG, et al: The effect of antacid, metoclopramide, and propantheline on the bioavailability of metoprolol and atenolol. Biopharm Drug Dispos 2:79, 1981.
226. Kirch W, et al: Interaction of atenolol with furosemide and calcium and aluminum salts. Clin Pharmacol Ther 30:429, 1981.
227. McElnay JC: Buccal partitioning of propranolol while in the presence and absence of aluminum hydroxide gel. Drug Intell Clin Pharmacol 15:481, 1981.
228. Hirshman, CA Downes H: A possible undesirable interaction of propranolol and atropine. Anesthesiology 53:521, 1980.
229. Hansten PD: Beta-blocking agents and antidiabetic drugs. Drug Intell Clin Pharmacol 14:46, 1980.
230. Popp DA, et al: Role of epinephrine mediated beta-adrenergic mechanisms in hypoglycemic glucose counterregulation and post-hypoglycemic hyperglycemia in insulin-dependent diabetes mellitus. J Clin Invest 69:315, 1982.
231. Santiago, JV, et al: Epinephrine, norepinephrine, glucagon and growth hormone release in association with physiological decrements in the plasma glucose concentration in normal and diabetic man. J Clin Endocrinol Metab 51:877, 1980.
232. Grajower MM, et al: Hypoglycemia in chronic hemodialysis patients: association with propranolol use. Nephron 26:126, 1980.
233. Kallen RJ, et al: A complication of treatment of hypertension with propranolol. Clin Pediatr 19:567, 1980.
234. Wray R, Sutcliffe SBJ: Propranolol-induced hypoglycaemia and myocardial infarction (Letter). Br Med J 2:592, 1972.
235. Holm G, et al: Severe hypoglycaemia during physical exercise and treatment with beta-blockers. Br Med J 282:1360, 1981.
236. Pelsor DA, et al: Propranolol-induced hypoglycemia during growth hormone testing. J Pediatr 99:157, 1981.
237. Hesse B, Pedersen JT: Hypoglycaemia after propranolol in children. Acta Med Scand 193:551, 1973.
238. Newman RJ: Comparison of propranolol, metoprolol, and acebutolol on insulin-induced hypoglycaemia. Br Med J 2:447, 1976.
239. Davidson N, et al: Observation in man of hypoglycaemia during selective and non-selective beta-blockade. Scott Med J 22:69, 1976.
240. Deacon SP, et al: Acebutolol, atenolol, and propranolol and meta-

References (CONT.)

bolic responses to acute hypoglycaemia in diabetics. Br Med J 2:1255, 1977.
241. DEACON SP, BARNETT D: Comparison of atenolol and propranolol during insulin-induced hypoglycaemia. Br Med J 2:272, 1976.
242. SHARMA SD, et al: Comparison of penbutolol and propranolol during insulin-induced hypoglycaemia. Curr Ther Res 26:252, 1979.
243. SAUNDERS J, et al: A comparison between propranolol, practolol and betaxolol (SL75212) on the circulatory and metabolic responses to insulin-induced hypoglycaemia. Eur J Clin Pharmacol 21:177, 1981.
244. RYAN JR, et al: Response of diabetics treated with atenolol or poropranolol to insulin-induced hypoglyceamia (Abstract). Clin Pharmacol Ther 31:266, 1982.
245. OSTMAN J, et al: Effect of metoprolol and alprenolol on the metabolic, hormonal, and haemodynamic response to insulin-induced hypoglycaemia in hypertensive, insulin-dependent diabetics. Acta Med Scand 211:381, 1982.
246. SHEPHERD AMM, et al: Hypoglycemia-induced hypertension in a diabetic patient on metoprolol. Ann Intern Med 94:357, 1981.
247. MEYERS MG, HOPE-GILL HF: Effect of d- and dl-propranolol on glucose-stimulated insulin release. Clin Pharmacol Ther 25:303, 1979.
248. SCANDELLARI C, et al: The effect of propranolol on hypoglycaemia. Diabetologia 15:297, 1978.
249. BLUM I, et al: Prevention of hypoglycemic attacks by propranolol in a patient suffering from insulinoma. Diabetes 24:535, 1975.
250. BLUM I, et al: Suppression of hypoglycemia by dl-propranolol in malignant insulinoma. N Engl J Med 299:487, 1978.
251. MOHLER H, et al: Glucose intolerance during chronic beta-adrenergic blockade in man. Clin Pharmacol Ther 25:237, 1979.
252. NARDONE DA, BOUMA DJ: Hyperglycemia and diabetic coma: possible relationship to diuretic-propranolol therapy. South Med J 72:1607, 1979.
253. GROOP L, et al: Influence of beta-blocking drugs on glucose metabolism in patients with non-insulin dependent diabetes mellitus. Acta Med Scand 211:7, 1982.
254. REEVES RL, et al: The effect of metoprolol and propranolol on pancreatic insulin release. Clin Pharmacol Ther 31:262, 1982.
255. WAAL-MANNING HJ: Metabolic effects of beta-adrenoreceptor blockers. Drugs 11:121, 1976.
256. GROOP L, et al: Influence of beta-blocking drugs on glucose metabolism in hypertensive, non-diabetic patients. Acta Med Scand 213:9, 1983.
257. WOOD AJJ: How the beta-blockers differ: a pharmacologic comparison. Drug Ther 13:59, 1983.
258. WAAL-MANNING HJ: Can beta-blockers be used in diabetic patients? Drugs 17:157, 1979.
259. SMITH U, LAGER I: Beta blockage in diabetes. N Engl J Med 299:1467, 1978.
260. EKBERG G, HANSSON B-G: Glucose tolerance and insulin release in hypertensive patients treated with the cardioselective beta-receptor blocking agent metoprolol. Acta Med Scand 202:393, 1977.
261. ANGELO-NELSEN K, et al: Timolol topically and diabetes mellitus. JAMA 244:2263, 1980.

References (CONT.)

262. WAAL-MANNING HJ: Atenolol and three nonselective beta-blockers in hypertension. Clin Pharmacol Ther 25:8, 1979.
263. COLLSTE P, et al: Influence of pentobarbital on effect and plasma levels and alprenolol and 4-hydroxy-alprenolol. Clin Pharmacol Ther 25:423, 1979.
264. HAGLUND K, et al: Influence of pentobarbital on metoprolol plasma levels. Clin Pharmacol Ther 26:326, 1979.
265. SOTANIEMI EA, et al: Plasma clearance of propranolol and sotalol and hepatic drug-metabolizing enzyme activity. Clin Pharmacol Ther 26:153, 1979.
266. SCHWARTZ DE, et al: Bioavailability of propranolol following administration of cholestyramine. Clin Pharmacol Ther 31:268, 1982.
267. TIULA E, NEUVONEN PJ: Antiepileptic drugs and alpha$_1$-acid glycoprotein. New Engl J Med 307:1148, 1982.
268. PATWARDHAN RV, et al: Effects of caffeine on plasma free fatty acids, urinary catecholamines, and drug binding. Clin Pharmacol Ther 28:398, 1980.
269. FEELY J, et al: Reduction of liver blood flow and propranolol metabolism by cimetidine. New Engl J Med 304:692, 1981.
270. KIRCH W, et al: Interaction of metoprolol, propranolol and atenolol with concurrent administration of cimetidine. Klin Wochenschr 60:1401, 1982.
271. WARBURTON S, et al: Does cimetidine alter the cardiac response to exercise and propranolol? Safr Med J 55:1125, 1979.
272. HEAGERTY AM, et al: Influence of cimetidine on pharmacokinetics of propranolol. Br Med J 282:1917, 1981.
273. REIMANN IW, et al: Cimetidine increases steady plasma levels of propranolol. Br J Clin Pharmacol 12:785, 1981.
274. DONOVAN MA, et al: Cimetidine and bioavailability of propranolol. Lancet 1:164, 1981.
275. HOUTZAGERS JJR, et al: The effect of pretreatment with cimetidine on the bioavailability and disposition of atenolol and metoprolol. Br J Clin Pharmacol 14:67, 1982.
276. DANESHMEND TK, ROBERTS CJC: Cimetidine and bioavailability of labetalol. Lancet 1:565, 1981.
277. YUDKIN JS: Withdrawal of clonidine. Lancet 1:546, 1977.
278. STRAUSS FG, et al: Withdrawal of antihypertensive therapy. JAMA 238:1734, 1977.
279. BRUCE DL, et al: Preoperative clonidine withdrawal syndrome. Anesthesiology 51:90, 1979.
280. VERNON C, SAKULA A: Fatal rebound hypertension after abrupt withdrawal of clonidine and propranolol. Br J Clin Pract 33:112, 1979.
281. WARREN SE, et al: Clonidine and propranolol paradoxical hypertension. Arch Intern Med 139:253, 1979.
282. GARVEY HL, WOODHOUSE BL: Reversal of clonidine-induced hypotension by beta-adrenoceptor blocking drugs. Eur J Pharmacol 65:55, 1980.
283. LILJA M, et al: Interaction of clonidine and beta-blockers. Acta Med Scand 207:173, 1980.
284. ROSENTHAL T, et al: use of Labetalol in hypertensive patients during discontinuation of clonidine therapy. Eur J Clin Pharmacol 20:237, 1981.

References (CONT.)

285. Saarimaa H: Combination of clonidine and sotalol in hypertension. Br Med J 1:810, 1976.
286. Kendall MJ, et al: Metoprolol pharmacokinetics and the oral contraceptive pill. Br J Clin Pharmacol 14:120, 1982.
287. Hung J-S, et al: Digoxin, propranolol, and atrioventricular reentrant tachycardia in the Wolff-Parkinson-White syndrome. Ann Intern Med 97:175, 1982.
288. Lorenzi M, et al: Dopamine during alpha- or beta-adrenergic blockade in man. J Clin Invest 63:310, 1979.
289. Gay GR, et al: Modification of cardiopressor and respirogenic effects of doxapram by propranolol. Clin Toxicol 13:487, 1978.
290. Newman BR, Schultz LK: Epinephrine-resistant anaphylaxis in a patient taking propranolol hydrochloride. Ann Allergy 47:35, 1981.
291. Jacobs RL, et al: Potentiated anaphylaxis in patients with drug-induced beta-adrenergic blockade. J Allergy Clin Immunol 68:125, 1981.
292. Hannaway PJ, Hopper GDK: Severe anaphylaxis and drug-induced beta-blockade. New Engl J Med 302:1536, 1983.
293. Houben H, et al: Effect of low-dose epinephrine infusion on hemodynamics after selective and nonselective beta-blockade in hypertension. Clin Pharmacol Ther 31:685, 1982.
294. Houben H, et al: Influence of selective and non-selective beta-adrenoreceptor blockade on the haemodynamic effect of adrenaline during combined antihypertensive drug therapy. Clin Science 57:397s, 1979.
295. Van Herwaarden CLA, et al: Haemodynamic effects of adrenaline during treatment of hypertensive patients with propranolol and metoprolol. Eur J Clin Pharmacol 12:397, 1977.
296. Yasue H, et al: Prinzmetal's variant form of angina as a manifestation of alpha-adrenergic receptor-mediated coronary artery spasm: documentation by coronary arteriography. Am Heart J 91:148, 1976.
297. Hansbrough JF, Near A: Propranolol-epinephrine antagonism with hypertension and stroke. Ann Intern Med 92:717, 1980.
298. Lampman RM, et al: Cardiac arrhythmias during epinephrine-propranolol infusions for measurement of in vivo insulin resistance. Diabetes 30:618, 1981.
299. Richards DA, et al: Circulatory effects of noradrenaline and adrenaline before and after labetalol. Br J Clin Pharmacol 7:371, 1979.
300. Sotaniemi EA, et al: Propranolol and sotalol metabolism after a drinking party. Clin Pharmacol Ther 29:705, 1981.
301. Grabowski BS, et al: Effects of acute alcohol administration on propranolol absorption. Int J Clin Pharmacol Ther Toxicol 18:317, 1980.
302. Dorian P, et al: Propranolol-ethanol pharmacokinetic interaction. Clin Pharmacol Ther 31:219, 1982.
303. Wagner JG, et al: New method for detecting and quatitating pharmacokinetic drug-drug interactions applied to ethanol-propranolol. Res Commun Chem Pathol Pharmacol 13:9, 1976.
304. Chiariello M, et al: Effect of furosemide on plasma concentration and beta-blockade by propranolol. Clin Pharmacol Ther 26:433, 1979.
305. Wood AJJ, et al: Elevated plasma free drug concentrations of propranolol and diazepam during cardiac catheterization. Circulation 62:1119, 1980.

References (CONT.)

306. NARANJO CA, et al: Nonfatty acid-modulated variations in drug binding due to heparin. Clin Pharmacol Ther 31:746, 1982.
307. BROWN JE, et al: The artifactual nature of heparin-induced drug protein-binding alterations. Clin Pharmacol Ther 30:636, 1981.
308. DELEVE LD, PIAFSKY KM: Lack of heparin effect on propranolol-induced beta-adrenoceptor blockade. Clin Pharmacol Ther 31:216, 1982.
309. JACK DB, et al: The effect of hydralazine on the pharmacokinetics of three different beta adrenoceptor antagonists: metoprolol, nadolol, and acebutolol. Biopharm Drug Dispos 3:47, 1982.
310. McLEAN AJ, et al: Interaction between oral propranolol and hydralazine. Clin Pharmacol Ther 27:726, 1980.
311. HORN J: Case reports. Bulletin of the Mason Clinic. 35:160, 1981–1982.
312. SCHAFER-KORTING M, et al: Pharmacokinetics of bendroflumethiazide alone and in combination with propranolol and hydralazine. Eur J Clin Pharmacol 21:315, 1982.
313. WATKINS, J, et al: Attenuation of hypotensive effect of propranolol and thiazide diuretics by indomethacin. Br Med J 281:702, 1980.
314. SALVETTI A, et al: Interaction between oxprenolol and indomethacin on blood pressure in essential hypertensive patients. Eur J Clin Pharmacol 22:197, 1982.
315. FRIEDMAN PL, et al: Coronary vasoconstrictor effect of indomethacin in patients with coronary-artery disease. New Engl J Med 305:1171, 1981.
316. PERRUCA E, et al: Effect of atenolol, metoprolol, and propranolol on isoproterenol-induced tremor and tachycardia in normal subjects. Clin Pharmacol Ther 29:425, 1981.
317. ZEHNIE CG: Paradoxical hypertension experienced during methyldopa therapy. Am J Hosp Pharm 38:1774, 1981.
318. CHARLES BG, et al: Effect of metoclopramide on the bioavailability of long-acting propranolol. Br J Clin Pharmacol 11:517, 1981.
319. DAVIS WM, HATOUM NS: Lethal synergism between morphine or other narcotic analgesics and propranolol. Toxicology 14:141, 1979.
320. WINTER JC: Propranolol and morphine: A lethal interaction. Arch Int Pharmacodyn Ther 212:195, 1974.
321. DAVIS WM, HATOUM NS: Possible toxic interaction of propranolol and narcotic analgesics. Drug Intell Clin Pharm 15:290, 1981.
322. KIEVAL J, et al: The effects of intravenous verapamil on hemodynamic status of patients with coronary artery disease receiving propranolol. Circulation 65:653, 1982.
323. PACKER M, et al: Hemodynamic consequences of combined beta-adrenergic and slow calcium channel blockade in man. Circulation 65:660, 1982.
324. PACKER M, et al: Hemodynamic and clinical effects of combined verapamil and propranolol therapy in angina pectoris. Am J Cardiol 50:903, 1982.
325. WINNIFORD MD, et al: Randomized, double-blind comparison of propranolol alone and a propranolol-verapamil combination in patients with severe angina of effort. J Am Coll Cardiol 1:492, 1983.
326. WINNIFORD MD, et al: Hemodynamic and electrophysiologic effects of verapamil and nifedipine in patients on propranolol. Am J Cardiol 50:704, 1982.

References (CONT.)

327. WAYNE VS, et al: Adverse interaction between beta-adrenergic blocking drugs and verapamil—report of three cases. Aust NZ J Med 12:285, 1982.
328. SUBRAMANIAN B, et al: Combined therapy with verapamil and propranolol in chronic stable angina. Am J Cardiol 49:125, 1982.
329. KRIKLER DM, et al: Calcium-channel blockers and beta-blockers: advantages and disadvantages of combination therapy in chronic stable angina pectoris. Am Heart J 104:702, 1982.
330. YOUNG KD, MacDONALD G: Treatment of angina pectoris in general practice with a combination of nifedipine and beta-blocker. Br J Clin Pract 36:103, 1982.
331. DALY K, et al: Beneficial effect of adding nifedipine to beta-adrenergic blocking therapy in angina pectoris. Eur Heart J 3:42, 1982.
332. CHRISTENSEN CK, et al: Renal effects of acute calcium blockade with nifedipine in hypertensive patients receiving beta-adrenoceptor-blocking drugs. Clin Pharmacol Ther 32:572, 1982.
333. DARGIE HJ, et al: Nifedipine and propranolol: a beneficial drug interaction. Am J Med 71:676, 1981.
334. PFISTERER M, et al: Combined acebutolol/nifedipine therapy in patients with chronic coronary artery disease: additional improvement of ischemia-induced left ventricular dysfunction. Am J Cardiol 49:1259, 1982.
335. EGGERTSEN R, HANSSON L: Effects of treatment with nifedipine and metoprolol in essential hypertension. Eur J Clin Pharmacol 21:389, 1982.
336. DEAN S, KENDALL MJ: Adverse interaction between nifedipine and beta-blockade. Br Med J 282:1322, 1981.
337. DEPONTI C, et al: Effects of nifedipine, acebutolol, and their association on exercise tolerance in patients with effort angina. Cardiology 68:195, 1981.
338. HUSTED SE, et al: Long-term therapy of arterial hypertension with nifedipine given alone or in combination with a beta-adrenoceptor blocking agent. Eur J Clin Pharmacol 22:101, 1982.
339. JOSHI PI, et al: Nifedipine and left ventricular function in beta-blocked patients. Br Heart J 45:457, 1981.
340. ROBSON RH, VISHWANATH MC: Nifedipine and beta-blockade as a cause of cardiac failure. Br Med J 284:104, 1982.
341. STAFFURTH JS, EMERY P: Adverse interaction between nifedipine and beta-blockade. Br Med J 282:225, 1981.
342. ANASTASSIADES C: Nifedipine and beta-blockade as a cause of cardiac failure. Br Med J 284:506, 1982.
343. OPIE LH, WHITE DA: Adverse interaction between nifedipine and beta-blockade. Br Med J 281:1462, 1980.
344. ANASTASSIADES CJ: Nifedipine and beta-blocker drugs. Br Med J 281:1251, 1980.
345. CASS E, et al: Hazards of phenylephrine topical medication in persons taking propranolol. Can Med Assoc J 120:1261, 1979.
346. BROWN MM, et al: Lack of side effects from topically administered 10% phenylephrine eyedrops. Arch Ophthalmol 98:487, 1980.
347. ALDER AG, et al: Systemic effects of eye drops. Arch Intern Med 142:2293, 1982.
348. MYERS MG, IAZZETTA JJ: Intranasally administered phenylephrine and blood pressure. Can Med Assoc J 127:365, 1982.

References (CONT.)

349. Vestal RE, et al: Inhibition of propranolol metabolism by chlorpromazine. Clin Pharmacol Ther 25:19, 1979.
350. Peet M, et al: Pharmacokinetic interaction between propranolol and chlorpromazine in schizophrenic patients. Lancet 2:978, 1980.
351. Miller FA: Adverse effects of combined propranolol and chlorpromazine therapy. Am J Psychiatry 139:1198, 1982.
352. Graham RM, et al: Prazosin: the first-dose phenomenon. Br Med J 4:1293, 1976.
353. Elliott HL, et al: Immediate cardiovascular responses to oral prazosin—effects of concurrent beta-blockers. Clin Pharmacol Ther 29:303, 1981.
354. Seideman P, et al: Prazosin first dose phenomenon during combined treatment with a beta-adrenoceptor in hypertensive patients. Br J Clin Pharmacol 13:865, 1982.
355. Rubin P, et al: Studies on the clinical pharmacology of prazosin. II: The influence of indomethacin and of propranolol on the action and disposition of prazosin. Br J Clin Pharmacol 10:33, 1980.
356. Lundborg P, et al: The effect of propoxyphene pretreatment on the disposition of metoprolol and propranolol. Clin Pharmacol Ther 29:263, 1981.
357. Hillestad L, Storstein O: Conversion of chronic atrial fibrillation to sinus rhythm with combined propranolol and quinidine treatment. Am Heart J 77:137, 1969.
358. Kates RE, Blanford MF: Disposition kinetics of oral quinidine when administered concurrently with propranolol. J Clin Pharmacol 19:378, 1979.
359. Fors WJ, et al: Evaluation of propranolol and quinidine in the treatment of quinidine-resistant arrhythmias. Am J Cardiol 27:190, 1971.
360. Kessler KM, et al: Quinidine pharmacokinetics in patients with cirrhosis or receiving propranolol. Am Heart J 96:627, 1978.
361. Fenster P, et al: Kinetic evaluation of the propranolol-quinidine combination. Clin Pharmacol Ther 27:450, 1980.
362. Reimann IW, et al: Effects cimetidine and rantidine on steady-state propranolol kinetics and dynamics. Clin Pharmacol Ther 32:749, 1982.
363. Heagerty AM, et al: Failure of ranitidine to interact with propranolol. Br Med J 284:1304, 1982.
364. Heagerty AM, et al: The influence of histamine (H_2) antagonists on propranolol pharmacokinetics. Int J Clin Pharmacol Res 2:203, 1982.
365. Patel L, Weerasuriya K: Effect of cimetidine and ranitidine on propranolol clearance. Br J Clin Pharmacol 15:152P, 1983.
366. Kirch W, et al: 14th Congress of the European Society of Toxicology. Rome, 28–30 March 1983.
367. Spahn H, et al: Influence of ranitidine on plasma metoprolol and atenolol concentrations. Br Med J 286:1546, 1983.
368. Moysey JO, et al: Amiodarone increases plasma digoxin concentrations. Br Med J 282:272, 1981.
369. Achilli A, Serra N: Amiodarone increases plasma digoxin concentrations. Br Med J 282:1630, 1981.
370. McGovern B, et al: Sinus arrest during treatment with amiodarone. Br Med J 284:160, 1982.

References (CONT.)

371. McGovern B, et al: Sinus arrest during treatment with amiodarone. Br Med J 284:1120, 1982.
372. Southworth W, et al: Possible amiodarone-aprindine interaction. Am Heart J 104:323, 1982.
373. Rees A, et al: Dangers of amiodarone and anticoagulant treatment. Br Med J 282:1756, 1981.
374. Serlin MJ, et al: Danger of amiodarone and anticoagulant treatment. Br Med J 283:58, 1981.
375. Harris L: Dangers of amiodarone and anticoagulant treatment. Br Med J 282:1973, 1981.
376. Martinowitz U, et al: Interaction between warfarin sodium and amiodarone. N Engl J Med 304:671, 1981.
377. Hamer A, et al: The potentiation of warfarin anticoagulation by amiodarone. Circulation 65:1025, 1982.
378. Bennett PN, et al: Effects of rifampin on metoprolol and antipyine kinetics. Br J Clin Pharmacol 13:387, 1982.
379. Bobik A, et al: Low oral bioavailability of dihydroergotamine and first-pass extraction in patients with orthostatic hypotension. Clin Pharmacol Ther 30:673, 1981.
380. Powell JR, et al: Lack of cimetidine-lidocaine interaction in patients with suspected myocardial infarction. Drug Intell Clin Pharm 17:445, 1983.
381. Foster CA, Aston SJ: Propranolol-epinephrine interaction: a potential disaster. Plast Reconstr Surg 72:74, 1983.
382. Smits P, et al: Hemodynamic and humoral effects of coffee after β_1-selective and nonselective β-blockade. Clin Pharmacol Ther 34:153, 1983.
383. Green JA, et al: Nifedipine-quinidine interaction. Clin Pharm 2:461, 1983.
384. Risler T, et al: On the interaction between digoxin and disopyramide. Clin Pharmacol Ther 34:176, 1983.
385. DuSouich P, et al: Enhancement of nadolol elimination by activated charcoal and antibiotics. Clin Pharmacol Ther 33:585, 1983.
386. Ochs HR, et al: Do beta-blockers alter the kinetics of procainamide? Clin Pharmacol Ther 33:209, 1983.
387. Hardy BG, et al: Effect of cimetidine on the pharmacokinetics and pharmacodynamics of quinidine. Am J Cardiol 52:172, 1983.
388. Bussey HI, et al: Influence of rifampin (R) on quinidine (Q) and digoxin (D). Drug Intell Clin Pharm 17:436, 1983.
389. Strathman I, et al: Hypoglycemia in patients receiving disopyramide phosphate. Drug Intell Clin Pharm 17:635, 1983.

CHAPTER 2

Oral Anticoagulant Drug Interactions

ORAL ANTICOAGULANT INTERACTIONS

DRUGS	DISCUSSION

Acetaminophen (Datril) (Tylenol) (Nebs)[5,85,86,232]

MECHANISM: Not established.

CLINICAL SIGNIFICANCE: In one study, acetaminophen (2.6 g/day for 2 weeks) was given to patients on various oral anticoagulants and resulted in a mean increase of 3.7 seconds in the prothrombin time when compared to effects from a placebo.[85] A subsequent study found acetaminophen (3 g/day for 2 weeks) to have no effect on the prothrombin time response to warfarin.[5] Others[86] found two doses of 650 mg of acetaminophen to have no effect on the prothrombin time response to oral anticoagulants. In another study, 10 of 20 patients on chronic oral anticoagulants were given acetaminophen (2.0 g/day for 3 weeks), and the other 10 were given placebo.[232] There was a moderate increase in the hypoprothrombinemic response in the patients given acetaminophen. However, none of the patients was receiving warfarin, and it is not clear that the results can be applied to warfarin. In summary, there is evidence that repeated doses of acetaminophen may produce a mild to moderate increase in the hypoprothrombinemic response to oral anticoagulants in some patients. However, acetaminophen lacks the adverse effects of aspirin on the gastric mucosa and platelets, and is thus safer than aspirin in anticoagulated patients.

MANAGEMENT: Watch for evidence of enhanced hypoprothrombinemic response to oral anticoagulants if acetaminophen is used concurrently. Lower anticoagulant dosage as needed.

Alcohol, Ethyl (Ethanol)[5,15,160,210,259,260]

MECHANISM:
1. No mechanism has been established for the purported enhancement of oral anticoagulant effect by ethanol.
2. The increase in warfarin metabolism in heavy drinkers is probably due to ethanol-induced stimulation of hepatic microsomal enzymes.[15]

CLINICAL SIGNIFICANCE: Ethanol-induced increases in the hypoprothrombinemic response to oral anticoagulants have apparently been

DRUGS	DISCUSSION

noted clinically for many years, but few cases have been reported. It is clear, however, that many patients on oral anticoagulants are not affected by moderate ethanol intake. In ten patients on chronic warfarin therapy, only one developed enhanced hypoprothrombinemia following 8 oz of vodka daily for 2 weeks.[5] In another study, 80 g of ethanol did not affect the hypoprothrombinemic response in healthy subjects maintained on Marcoumar.[160] Further, daily ingestion of 592 ml of table wine or 296 ml of fortified wine (20% ethanol) did not affect the hypoprothrombinemic response to warfarin in healthy subjects.[259,260] Additional study in patients with "coronary disease" indicated a slight increase in hypoprothrombinemic response to Marcoumar in some patients following administration of moderate amounts of ethanol. Enhanced metabolism of warfarin may occur in alcoholics,[15] but this would be expected to occur while the patient is not intoxicated. In summary, occasional patients on oral anticoagulants may manifest enhanced hypoprothrombinemia with ingestion of large amounts of ethanol. Small to moderate ethanol intake does not seem likely to cause such increases.

MANAGEMENT: It would be prudent for patients on oral anticoagulants to avoid ingestion of large amounts of ethanol, but 2 to 3 drinks per day are unlikely to affect warfarin response.

Allopurinol (Zyloprim)[11,161–163,183,225,258]

MECHANISM: It is proposed that allopurinol inhibits the hepatic metabolism of oral anticoagulants.

CLINICAL SIGNIFICANCE: Allopurinol administration (2.5 mg/kg twice a day for 14 days) to six healthy medical students resulted in a prolongation in the half-life of a single dose of dicumarol in each case.[11] However, in a subsequent study in healthy subjects only one of three developed a prolonged dicumarol half-life during allopurinol, and warfarin disposition was not affected.[161] Another study demonstrated a decrease in warfarin elimination in only one of six subjects given allopurinol.[183] Two patients on chronic phenprocoumon therapy developed excessive hypoprothrombinemia and bleeding following initiation of allopurinol therapy.[225] These findings, along with isolated case reports of enhanced response to warfarin[162,163,258] and cases I have observed, indicate that occasional patients on oral anticoagulants and allopurinol will develop enhanced anticoagulant effect.

MANAGEMENT: One should be alert for alteration in hypoprothrombinemic response to oral anticoagulants if allopurinol is initiated or discontinued. Adjust oral anticoagulant dosage as needed.

Aminoglycosides[2,3,5,6,92,173,177,198,213,261,262]

MECHANISM: It is proposed that aminoglycosides may reduce vitamin K production by gut bacteria, thus enhancing the hypoprothrom-

DRUGS	DISCUSSION

binemic response to oral anticoagulants. Impaired vitamin K *absorption* due to oral neomycin has also been proposed. Streptomycin has been implicated in the production of a factor V inhibitor in several patients,[2,177] which would theoretically add to the anticoagulant effect of oral anticoagulants. Also, animal studies indicate that oral neomycin may inhibit the enterohepatic circulation of warfarin, thus reducing plasma warfarin levels.[261]

CLINICAL SIGNIFICANCE: In patients with sufficient dietary vitamin K, the reduction of bacterial vitamin K by aminoglycosides is probably of minor significance. However, combined dietary vitamin K deficiency and aminoglycoside therapy (especially oral) may be more likely to produce or enhance hypoprothrombinemia.[262] In one study,[5] six of ten patients on warfarin therapy exhibited increased prothrombin times (mean, 5.6 sec) with oral neomycin (2 g/day for 2 weeks). In another study oral neomycin (1, 1.5, or 2 g/day for 18 weeks) failed to alter anticoagulant requirements in seven patients[198] but few details were given. The association of streptomycin therapy with a factor V inhibitor has now been reported several times, but the nature of the association and the incidence are not clear. In summary, aminoglycosides appear to enhance the hypoprothrombinemic response to oral anticoagulants only in certain predisposed patients. Possible predisposing factors include oral administration and/or large doses of the aminoglycoside, a deficiency of dietary vitamin K, and impaired hepatic function with reduced synthesis of clotting factors.

MANAGEMENT: Since many patients appear unaffected by this interaction, concomitant use need not be avoided. However, more careful monitoring of hypoprothrombinemia appears warranted with oral aminoglycoside administration and/or dietary vitamin K deficiency.

Aminosalicylic Acid (PAS)[10,16,17]

MECHANISM:
1. Aminosalicylic acid reportedly decreases prothrombin formation by the liver.[17]
2. Animal studies indicate that isoniazid and PAS enhance dicumarol blood levels and hypoprothrombinemic effect.

CLINICAL SIGNIFICANCE: There has been one patient in whom the administration of aminosalicylic acid appeared to enhance the hypoprothrombinemic effect of warfarin.[16] It should be noted that the patient was also receiving isoniazid, a drug that appears to increase blood levels of dicumarol in animal studies.[10]

MANAGEMENT: Concomitant use need not be avoided, but some patients may require a reduction in oral anticoagulant dosage.

Anabolic Steroids[57,60,83,116–118,143,203,263]

MECHANISM: Among the mechanisms proposed are decreased clotting factor formation, increased clotting factor degradation, and increased

DRUGS	DISCUSSION

affinity of receptor site for the anticoagulant. Also, the fibrinolytic activity of anabolic steroids may have been involved in the patients who have developed hemorrhages.

CLINICAL SIGNIFICANCE: Well documented. A number of patients receiving both oral anticoagulants and anabolic steroids have developed hemorrhages. There is evidence to indicate that 17-alpha-alkylated anabolic steroids such as methandrostenolone (Dianabol), norethandrolone (Nilevar), methyltestosterone (Metandren), and oxymetholone (Anadrol) are more likely to potentiate oral anticoagulants than anabolic steroids that are not so substituted. One case of enhanced warfarin hypoprothrombinemia following a 2% testosterone propionate ointment has also been reported.[263]

MANAGEMENT: Concomitant use of oral anticoagulants and anabolic steroids should be avoided if possible. With concurrent use, patients should be monitored more carefully for excessive anticoagulant response.

Antacids (Oral)[18,120]

MECHANISM: It has been proposed that concomitant magnesium hydroxide and dicumarol administration can result in the formation of a magnesium chelate of dicumarol that is more readily absorbed than dicumarol itself.

CLINICAL SIGNIFICANCE: In one study, peak plasma levels of dicumarol were earlier and higher when the dicumarol was given with magnesium hydroxide than when it was given with water.[18] Aluminum hydroxide does not appear to affect dicumarol blood levels.[18] Warfarin plasma levels do not appear to be affected by aluminum hydroxide,[18] magnesium hydroxide,[18] or a mixture of the two antacids.[120]

MANAGEMENT: In patients requiring antacids as well as oral anticoagulants, warfarin should probably be used rather than dicumarol.

Antidepressants, Tricyclic[11,153,164,192,264,265]

MECHANISM: Impairment of dicumarol metabolism by tricyclic antidepressants has been proposed[11] but not confirmed.[164] The bioavailability of dicumarol might be increased by tricyclic-antidepressant-induced slowing of intestinal motility.[164] Animal studies indicate that amitriptyline and nortriptyline inhibit the hepatic metabolism of warfarin.[264]

CLINICAL SIGNIFICANCE: Clinically significant alteration in anticoagulant response to warfarin reportedly may occur due to amitriptyline,[153] and others have noted a greater degree of instability in anticoagulant control in patients receiving tricyclic antidepressants.[192] However, a study in normal volunteers indicating that nortriptyline inhibits dicumarol metabolism[11] was not confirmed in subsequent work.[164] Warfarin metabolism also appeared to be

DRUGS	DISCUSSION

unaffected. In another study, mianserin did not affect the anticoagulant response to phenprocoumon in 60 patients.[265] If an interaction between oral anticoagulants and tricyclic antidepressants does occur, it is probably significant in only an occasional patient.

MANAGEMENT: It does not seem necessary to avoid concomitant use, but patients should be watched for altered anticoagulant response.

Antidiabetics[19-24,112,134,153,165,197,204,211]

MECHANISM:
A. Effect of anticoagulant on antidiabetic drugs:
1. Dicumarol appears to inhibit the hepatic metabolism of tolbutamide.[20,24]
2. Dicumarol may result in increased serum chlorpropamide levels due to impaired hepatic metabolism and/or reduced renal clearance of chlorpropamide.[22]
B. Effect of antidiabetic drugs on anticoagulants: Tolbutamide may initially enhance the anticoagulant effect of dicumarol due to displacement of dicumarol from plasma protein binding. Continued therapy with both drugs may result in decreased plasma levels and anticoagulant effect of dicumarol (based on animal studies).[112] This could be due to more rapid metabolism of dicumarol because of the protein-binding displacement and/or tolbutamide-induced enzyme induction.

CLINICAL SIGNIFICANCE:
A. Effect of anticoagulant on antidiabetic drugs: dicumarol has been shown to produce an appreciable increase in the half-life of tolbutamide in both patients[24,211] and healthy subjects.[20] Also, plateau levels of tolbutamide may be increased by dicumarol.[197] This increase is accompanied by the expected enhanced hypoglycemic effect. Several cases of hypoglycemic reactions have been reported with the concomitant use of these two drugs.[23,24] Although it is not as well documented as the dicumarol-tolbutamide interaction, dicumarol also appears to enhance the effect of chlorpropamide. The increase in serum chlorpropamide levels following dicumarol therapy has been demonstrated in three diabetic patients.[22] Finally, an increased chlorpropamide half-life was noted in a single patient following the administration of acenocoumarol.[19] Tolbutamide metabolism does *not* appear to be affected by warfarin, phenindione, or phenprocoumon.[211]
B. Effect of antidiabetic drugs on anticoagulants: In 1958, Chaplin and Cassell described two patients stabilized on dicumarol therapy who manifested hypoprothrombinemia following initiation of tolbutamide therapy.[21] However, subsequent observation of three similar patients revealed no sign of interaction.[21] Three additional cases of possible enhancement of dicumarol by tolbutamide were apparently reported to the Upjohn Company but no details were given.[134] The retrospective study of Poucher and Vecchio showed no enhancement of dicumarol or warfarin effect

DRUGS	DISCUSSION

by tolbutamide,[134] but none would be expected since they used records from patients maintained on tolbutamide who were then given an anticoagulant. Finally, in a study of four normal volunteers, tolbutamide altered dicumarol pharmacokinetics but did not alter the anticoagulant response.[197] Neither the half-life nor the plasma levels of phenprocoumon appear to be affected by tolbutamide, insulin, glibenclamide, or glibornuride as measured in diabetics, nondiabetic aged patients, or healthy young volunteers.[204]

MANAGEMENT: Most of the preceding interactions described involved the use of dicumarol. Thus, the use of warfarin may decrease the chance of interactions with antidiabetic drugs. Patients maintained on either an oral anticoagulant or an antidiabetic should be observed more closely during the initiation or discontinuation of therapy with a drug from the other class.

Antipyrine[8]

MECHANISM: It is proposed that antipyrine stimulates hepatic warfarin metabolism. The concomitant increases seen in serum gamma-glutamyl transpeptidase activity are consistent with antipyrine-induced hepatic microsomal enzyme induction.

CLINICAL SIGNIFICANCE: Decreases in plasma warfarin concentration have been noted in several patients on long-term warfarin therapy who were subsequently given antipyrine.[8] Determination of the magnitude of the effect must await further study.

MANAGEMENT: Watch for altered anticoagulant effect when antipyrine therapy is started or stopped in a patient receiving oral anticoagulants.

Ascorbic Acid (Vitamin C)[25,26,149,150,155,191]

MECHANISM: Not established. It has been proposed that very large doses of ascorbic acid (e.g., 10g/day or more) might impair gastrointestinal absorption of warfarin due to the diarrhea produced.[191]

CLINICAL SIGNIFICANCE: Two case reports appeared which indicated that ascorbic acid impaired the response to warfarin.[149,155] In a subsequent study involving 19 patients, 3, 5, or 10g of ascorbic acid failed to produce a clinically significant effect on the hypoprothrombinemic response to warfarin,[191] although plasma warfarin decreased slightly.

MANAGEMENT: No special precautions appear necessary.

Azapropazone[207,218]

MECHANISM: Not established. In-vitro protein binding studies indicate that azapropazone may displace warfarin from human serum albumin,[218] but it is not known whether such displacement is important clinically.

DRUGS	DISCUSSION

CLINICAL SIGNIFICANCE: A patient stabilized on warfarin developed hematemesis and markedly prolonged prothrombin time after receiving azapropazone (1.2g/day for 4 days).[207] The azapropazone appeared to be responsible for the bleeding episode in this patient, but additional studies are needed to determine the incidence of magnitude of this interaction. The fact that azapropazone resembles phenylbutazone lends support to the possibility that the interaction is real.

MANAGEMENT: Concomitant use of azapropazone and oral anticoagulants would be best avoided until this potential interaction is better described. Patients treated with the combination should be monitored closely for excessive hypoprothrombinemia.

Barbiturates[1,8,12,27−30,43,62,70,75,77,78,82,101−103,111,112,166,192,202,266]

MECHANISM: Barbiturates appear to induce hepatic microsomal enzymes resulting in increased metabolism of coumarin anticoagulants. Barbiturates may also decrease gastrointestinal absorption of dicumarol,[101,102] although the absorption of warfarin is not likely to be significantly affected.

CLINICAL SIGNIFICANCE: Well documented. Phenobarbital, butabarbital, heptabarbital, secobarbital, and amobarbital have been shown to decrease the response to coumarin anticoagulants in man. Most barbiturates probably have this ability. A patient on both barbiturate and coumarin anticoagulant therapy who stops taking the barbiturate runs the risk of hemorrhage if his anticoagulant dosage is not readjusted. The effect may be dose related; one patient showed no effect when on plasma warfarin with 100 mg of secobarbital daily, but manifested a considerable decrease in plasma warfarin when the dosage was increased to 200 mg daily.[8] However, in six healthy subjects 100 mg of secobarbital daily was sufficient to enhance warfarin metabolism.[266] Decreasing anticoagulant response usually develops gradually after starting the barbiturate, with maximal effect by about 2 weeks. The time course following discontinuation of the barbiturate is similar: the results of enzyme induction usually begin to diminish by within a week, with little induction remaining by 2 to 3 weeks. (Note that specific patients may not conform to these "average" durations.)

MANAGEMENT: In a patient receiving an oral anticoagulant no barbiturate therapy should be stopped or started without careful attention to possible readjustment of anticoagulant dosage. Because of the problems of oral anticoagulant dosage control in such patients, it would be wise to avoid barbiturates and other interacting hypnotics completely. Current evidence shows that possible alternative hypnotic drugs would include flurazepam (Dalmane), chlordiazepoxide (Librium), diazepam (Valium), or diphenhydramine (Benadryl). The consistent use of stable doses of barbiturates, as in epileptic patients, does not appear to interfere significantly with anticoagulant control.[192]

ORAL ANTICOAGULANT INTERACTIONS (CONT.)

DRUGS	DISCUSSION

Bumetanide (Bumex)[223,267]

MECHANISM: None.

CLINICAL SIGNIFICANCE: Two studies involving a total of 21 healthy subjects indicated that bumetanide (1.0 to 2.0 mg/day) does not affect the disposition or hypoprothrombinemic response to warfarin.[223,267]

MANAGEMENT: No special precautions appear necessary.

Carbamazepine (Tegretol)[148,268]

MECHANISM: Carbamazepine appears to enhance warfarin metabolism by induction of hepatic microsomal enzymes.

CLINICAL SIGNIFICANCE: In a preliminary study, each of the patients receiving warfarin developed decreased serum warfarin and impaired hypoprothrombinemic response when carbamazepine therapy was given.[148] Also, in two of three patients warfarin half-lives decreased after carbamazepine therapy. A patient on chronic warfarin therapy developed a complete reversal of hypoprothrombinemic response following addition of carbamazepine therapy, 400 mg daily.[268]

MANAGEMENT: Watch for altered anticoagulant effect when carbamazepine therapy is started or stopped in a patient receiving oral anticoagulants.

Chloral Hydrate (Noctec, Somnos)[4,5,63,70,82,124-131,166-168]

MECHANISM: Trichloroacetic acid, a major metabolite of chloral hydrate, appears to displace warfarin from plasma protein binding. This results in a transient increase in the amount of free (active) plasma warfarin and also an increase in its rate of metabolism. It is likely that dicumarol is affected similarly, but almost all available data deal with warfarin.

CLINICAL SIGNIFICANCE: Results from several clinical studies indicate that chloral hydrate temporarily increases the hypoprothrombinemic effect of warfarin in some patients.[124,126-128,167] Reports to the contrary[125,131] have dealt more with longer range effects, thus demonstrating that continued administration of the two drugs tends to result in normalization of the hypoprothrombinemic effect of warfarin. Although most patients appear to be minimally affected by this interaction one cannot assume that chloral hydrate can be administered with impunity to patients receiving oral anticoagulants. Based on experience with many other drug interactions, one would expect an occasional predisposed patient to develop a considerable increase in hypoprothrombinemic response with addition of chloral hydrate therapy.

MANAGEMENT: Statements on the safety of concomitant use of chloral hydrate and oral anticoagulants notwithstanding, it would be preferable to use hypnotic drugs that do not appear to interact such as flur-

DRUGS	DISCUSSION

azepam (Dalmane) or diazepam (Valium). If chloral hydrate is given to a patient receiving an oral anticoagulant, the patient should be monitored for excessive hypoprothrombinemia during the first several days of chloral hydrate therapy. However, long-term coadministration of the two drugs probably does not represent any significantly greater hazard of bleeding than oral anticoagulant therapy alone.

Chloramphenicol (Chloromycetin)[2,3,6,90,109,113,114,213]

MECHANISM:
1. Chloramphenicol has been shown to inhibit the metabolism of dicumarol, probably by inhibiting hepatic microsomal enzymes.[90]
2. It has been proposed that chloramphenicol may decrease vitamin K production by gut bacteria. However, bacterial production of vitamin K appears less important than dietary intake,[109,113,114] and chloramphenicol does not usually have much effect on bowel flora.[6]
3. Chloramphenicol might affect the production of prothrombin by an effect within the hepatic cell.[3]

CLINICAL SIGNIFICANCE: Chloramphenicol produced a two- to fourfold increase in the half-life of dicumarol in four patients.[90] The effect of chloramphenicol on warfarin or other oral anticoagulant metabolism has not been established. The significance of the proposed effect of chloramphenicol on vitamin K production by gut bacteria or on prothrombin production in the liver remains speculative. Vitamin K deficiency associated with antibiotics has been reported, but concomitant dietary deficiency of vitamin K seems to be an important contributing factor in most cases.[213]

MANAGEMENT: Concomitant use of chloramphenicol and dicumarol should probably be avoided. If chloramphenicol must be used, warfarin might be less likely to interact. However, more frequent prothrombin determinations would still be desirable.

Chlordiazepoxide (Librium)[8,70,84,169]

MECHANISM: None.

CLINICAL SIGNIFICANCE: Several studies have appeared which demonstrate a lack of interaction between chlordiazepoxide and oral anticoagulants.[8,70,84,169]

MANAGEMENT: No special precautions appear necessary.

Chlorinated Hydrocarbon Insecticides[200]

MECHANISM: It is proposed that exposure to chlorinated hydrocarbon insecticides may stimulate the metabolism of warfarin.

CLINICAL SIGNIFICANCE: Loss of hypoprothrombinemic response to warfarin was noted in one patient following intense exposure to a

DRUGS	DISCUSSION

combination of toxaphene and gamma benzene hexachloride.[200] Re-exposure inhibited oral anticoagulant response again. Various insecticides seem to affect drug metabolism, and exposure to such agents should be considered a potential factor in patients with altered response to oral anticoagulants.

MANAGEMENT: It may occasionally be necessary for patients on oral anticoagulants to avoid exposure to insecticides.

Chlorthalidone (Hygroton)[135]

MECHANISM: It has been proposed that chlorthalidone diuresis with consequent decrease in plasma water results in concentration of clotting factors, thus decreasing the response to oral anticoagulants.

CLINICAL SIGNIFICANCE: In one study in six subjects, chlorthalidone reduced the hypoprothrombinemic response to a single dose of warfarin (1.5 mg/kg body weight) as compared to the same dose of warfarin given alone.[135] However, no studies have appeared describing an effect of chlorthalidone in patients on chronic oral anticoagulant therapy.

MANAGEMENT: Concomitant use need not be avoided, and chronic use of both drugs would not appear to require any more frequent monitoring of hypoprothrombinemic effect. When starting or stopping chlorthalidone in an anticoagulated patient, one should check to ensure that anticoagulant requirements have not changed.

Cholestyramine (Cuemid) (Questran)[31,91,108,119-122,161,198,212,226]

MECHANISM:
1. Cholestyramine may bind oral anticoagulants in the gut, resulting in impaired absorption. The binding may also interfere with enterohepatic circulation of oral anticoagulants.[212,226]
2. Hypoprothrombinemia with bleeding has occurred rarely in persons treated with cholestyramine but not on oral anticoagulant therapy. This is presumably due to inhibition of vitamin K absorption.

CLINICAL SIGNIFICANCE: Preliminary clinical study indicates that when warfarin and cholestyramine are given concomitantly or 3 hours apart, warfarin absorption is decreased.[120] This appears to represent an actual decrease in *amount* of warfarin absorbed rather than merely a decrease in absorption *rate*. In another study in healthy subjects the clearance of intravenous phenprocoumon was enhanced by the concomitant administration of cholestyramine (12 g/day),[212] indicating that phenprocoumon undergoes enterohepatic circulation that is impaired by cholestyramine. Similar results were found with intravenous warfarin and oral cholestyramine.[226] The possible hypoprothrombinemia (Mechanism #2) that may occur following cholestyramine therapy alone is probably seldom an important clinical problem.

DRUGS	DISCUSSION

MANAGEMENT: Giving warfarin at least 6 hours after the cholestyramine reportedly avoids the impaired warfarin absorption (Mechanism #1).[122] However, any anticoagulant that undergoes enterohepatic circulation would theoretically be inhibited by cholestyramine therapy even if the doses were separated. If possible, concomitant use should probably be avoided. If concurrent use is necessary, the patient should be monitored more frequently for altered anticoagulant response.

Cimetidine (Tagamet)[93,289-294]

MECHANISM: Inhibition of the hepatic metabolism of the oral anticoagulant.

CLINICAL SIGNIFICANCE: Cimetidine regularly produces a clinically important increase in the hypoprothrombinemic response to oral anticoagulants.[93,289-291] In a patient receiving warfarin, the addition of cimetidine results in a gradual increase in hypoprothrombinemia over 1 to 2 weeks, and it takes about 1 week for the prothrombin time to return to pre-cimetidine levels when cimetidine is discontinued. Ranitidine (Zantac) does not appear to affect the hypoprothrombinemic response to warfarin,[292,293] and phenprocoumon (Liquamar) does not appear to be affected by cimetidine.[294]

MANAGEMENT: If possible, avoid concurrent use of cimetidine and oral anticoagulants. If the combination is used, the hypoprothrombinemic response to the oral anticoagulant should be carefully monitored when cimetidine is initiated, discontinued, or changed in dosage.

Clofibrate (Atromid S)[1,5,32-34,60,75,161,170,192,201]

MECHANISM: Not established. Available evidence indicates that clofibrate may enhance the effect of warfarin on vitamin K dependent clotting factor synthesis and/or affect the turnover of vitamin K.

CLINICAL SIGNIFICANCE: It is well documented that some patients manifest an increased anticoagulant effect when clofibrate is also taken;[1,5,32-34,60] loss of anticoagulant control with hemorrhage may occur. At least one death from massive hemorrhage has been attributed to this interaction.[32] Not all patients receiving this combination manifest evidence of interaction,[1,5] and it may be that certain predisposing factors increase the likelihood of interaction (e.g., large clofibrate dose, hyperlipidemia, increasing age[33]). Certainly, the interaction of the drugs should be assumed in a given patient until proved otherwise.

MANAGEMENT: Concomitant therapy with clofibrate and oral anticoagulants should be avoided if possible. If oral anticoagulant therapy is begun in a patient receiving clofibrate, doses of anticoagulant should probably be conservative until the maintenance dose is established. Initiation or discontinuation of clofibrate therapy in a patient stabilized on an oral anticoagulant may necessitate a change in the maintenance anticoagulant dose.

DRUGS	DISCUSSION

Contraceptives, Oral[64,269]

MECHANISM: Oral contraceptives may increase the activity of certain clotting factors in the blood. However, oral contraceptives have also been shown to inhibit drug metabolism, and it is possible that oral anticoagulants are affected.

CLINICAL SIGNIFICANCE: Oral contraceptives have been shown clinically to decrease the anticoagulant response to bishydroxycoumarin.[64] However, a subsequent study found that the response to acenocoumarol (Sintrom) was enhanced in the presence of oral contraceptives.[269] Little information is available concerning the effect of oral contraceptives on the response to warfarin.

MANAGEMENT: Oral contraceptive administration may require an alteration in oral anticoagulant dosage.

Corticosteroids[7,35,65,139,140]

MECHANISM: Corticosteroids have been shown to produce hypercoagulability of the blood.[35] Thus, the possibility exists that the effects of anticoagulants could be antagonized by corticosteroids. Conversely, an adverse effect of corticosteroids on vascular integrity has been proposed[139,140] which could increase the danger of hemorrhage at a given level of anticoagulation.

CLINICAL SIGNIFICANCE: Clinical evidence from some investigators indicates that corticosteroids or corticotropin may increase oral anticoagulant requirements[65] while others reported hemorrhage due to combined corticotropin and ethyl biscoumacetate therapy[140] and increased warfarin sensitivity in a patient receiving prednisone.[7] These studies were limited, and the results are not necessarily conflicting. It may be that corticosteroids both antagonize the hypoprothrombinemic effect of oral anticoagulants and increase the risk of hemorrhage in some patients due to vascular effects. Certainly, many other factors such as diseases and drug doses are likely to be important. The purported ulcerogenic potential of corticosteroids could also be dangerous in an anticoagulated patient, but it may be that corticosteroid-induced ulceration is less common than previously thought. Much more study is needed to resolve the clinical significance of concomitant use of corticosteroids and oral anticoagulants.

MANAGEMENT: The dangers of corticosteroid-induced gastrointestinal ulceration and possible increased hemorrhagic potential (not related to prothrombin time) should be kept in mind in patients receiving oral anticoagulants even though evidence for the latter effect is quite scanty. Also, the initiation or discontinuation of corticosteroid therapy in patients receiving oral anticoagulants should alert the physician to the possibility of the need for adjustment of anticoagulant dosage.

Cyclophosphamide (Cytoxan)[276]

MECHANISM: Not established.

DRUGS	DISCUSSION

CLINICAL SIGNIFICANCE: A patient on warfarin and cyclophosphamide (450 mg/day) developed a marked increase in prothrombin time when cyclophosphamide was discontinued.[276] Although the cyclophosphamide may have been responsible for the reduced warfarin effect in this patient, confirmation is needed.

MANAGEMENT: Until more is known about this potential interaction monitor prothrombin time carefully if cyclophosphamide is initiated or discontinued in the presence of oral anticoagulant therapy.

Danazol[270,271]

MECHANISM: Not established.

CLINICAL SIGNIFICANCE: Danazol therapy has been associated with excessive hypoprothrombinemia and bleeding in two women on chronic warfarin therapy.[270,271] Anabolic steroids are known to increase the hypoprothrombinemic response to oral anticoagulants, and it seems likely that danazol is no exception.

MANAGEMENT: One should be alert for evidence of enhanced hypoprothrombinemic response to oral anticoagulants in the presence of danazol therapy. Oral anticoagulant dosage may need to be reduced.

Dextrothyroxine (Choloxin)[60,69,94,205]

MECHANISM: Not established. It has been proposed that dextrothyroxine increases the affinity of the receptor site for the oral anticoagulant, but animal studies indicate that the mechanism might be an enhanced rate of factor II degradation.[205]

CLINICAL SIGNIFICANCE: Well documented. An increase in the hypoprothrombinemic response to oral anticoagulants is likely to occur.

MANAGEMENT: Concomitant therapy with dextrothyroxine and oral anticoagulants should be avoided if possible. If oral anticoagulant therapy is begun in a patient receiving dextrothyroxine, doses of anticoagulant should probably be conservative until the maintenance dose is established. Initiation or discontinuation of dextrothyroxine therapy in a patient stabilized on an oral anticoagulant is likely to necessitate a change in the maintenance anticoagulant dose.

Diazepam (Valium)[8,67,123,169]

MECHANISM: None.

CLINICAL SIGNIFICANCE: Although an early case report indicated that diazepam might interact with dicumarol,[67] subsequent studied have shown that diazepam probably has no significant effect on the action of warfarin.[8,123,169]

ORAL ANTICOAGULANT INTERACTIONS (CONT.)

DRUGS	DISCUSSION

MANAGEMENT: No special precautions appear to be necessary.

Diazoxide (Hyperstat)[76,110]

MECHANISM: It is proposed that the high blood levels of diazoxide required in treatment of severe hypertension could displace coumarin anticoagulants from plasma protein binding.

CLINICAL SIGNIFICANCE: Clinical examples of this interaction have not appeared in the literature; it is based primarily on theoretical considerations and in-vitro studies.

MANAGEMENT: Watch for altered anticoagulant effect when diazoxide is started or stopped in a patient receiving oral anticoagulants.

Diclofenac[219]

MECHANISM: None.

CLINICAL SIGNIFICANCE: A cross-over study in 32 patients receiving oral anticoagulants indicates that diclofenac does not significantly affect the hypoprothrombinemic response.[219]

MANAGEMENT: No special precautions appear necessary.

Diflunisal (Dolobid)[209,233-239]

MECHANISM: Not established. Displacement from plasma protein binding may be involved.

CLINICAL SIGNIFICANCE: Five healthy subjects received a subtherapeutic dose of warfarin for 6 weeks, with diflunisal (500 mg bid) added during the third and fourth weeks.[233] The hypoprothrombinemic response to warfarin was not affected during diflunisal administration; however, following discontinuation of the diflunisal, there was a substantial reduction in the hypoprothrombinemic response to warfarin which took place over several days and lasted for at least 2 weeks. Because this study used five healthy subjects receiving subtherapeutic warfarin doses, the results cannot automatically be applied to the clinical situation. Further, we cannot yet rule out the possibility that an increase in hypoprothrombinemia may occur in certain predisposed patients when diflunisal is used concurrently with oral anticoagulants. Three out of six patients stabilized on acenocoumarol reportedly developed enhanced hypoprothrombinemia when diflunisal was added (375 mg twice daily),[209] but details of the study were not presented. Other cases of possible diflunisal-induced increases in prothrombin time have apparently occurred. Although diflunisal appears to have less adverse effect than aspirin on platelet function and the gastrointestinal mucosa,[234-238] larger doses of diflunisal can impair platelet function,[236] and the drug has been reported to occasionally cause gastrointestinal hemorrhage.[234,239] In summary, diflunisal is potentially dangerous in patients receiving anticoagulants, but data are insufficient to assess the likelihood of difficulty relative to other anti-inflammatory drugs.

MANAGEMENT: Until this purported interaction is better defined, concomitant use should be avoided if possible. Patients should be monitored carefully for excessive anticoagulant response when diflunisal therapy is initiated, and for reduced anticoagulation when diflunisal is discontinued.

Diphenhydramine (Benadryl)[75,105]

MECHANISM: See Clinical Significance.

CLINICAL SIGNIFICANCE: Although antihistamines reportedly can result in induction of hepatic microsomal enzymes, they have not been shown to affect the response to oral anticoagulants. Indeed, one study in dogs demonstrated diphenhydramine to have no effect on warfarin metabolism.[105] Studies in humans are needed to resolve the clinical significance, but present evidence would indicate that diphenhydramine has little or no effect on anticoagulant response.

MANAGEMENT: No special precautions appear to be necessary.

Disulfiram (Antabuse)[40,95,151,152,272]

MECHANISM: Disulfiram may directly increase the activity of warfarin in the liver.[272]

CLINICAL SIGNIFICANCE: Case reports and study in volunteers indicate that disulfiram increases the hypoprothrombinemic effect and plasma levels of warfarin.[40,95,151,152] Research in healthy subjects indicates that most people receiving the combination manifest these increases in warfarin effect.

MANAGEMENT: Concomitant use of disulfiram and oral anticoagulants should be avoided if possible. Patients should be monitored for altered anticoagulant effect when disulfiram is started or stopped in a patient receiving oral anticoagulants. If oral anticoagulant therapy is begun in a patient receiving disulfiram, doses of anticoagulant should be conservative until the maintenance dose is established.

Erythromycin[273–275]

MECHANISM: Not established. Inhibition of warfarin metabolism by erythromycin may be involved.

CLINICAL SIGNIFICANCE: Three cases have been described of enhanced hypoprothrombinemic response to warfarin following erythromycin administration in doses of 1.0 to 2.0 g/day.[273–275] Although the data are insufficient to establish this interaction with certainty, the temporal relationship, the results of animal studies, and the known properties of erythromycin indicate that it is probably real.

DRUGS	DISCUSSION

MANAGEMENT: One should be alert for enhanced hypoprothrombinemic response in patients on oral anticoagulants who also receive erythromycin.

Ethacrynic Acid (Edecrin)[41,110,153,171]

MECHANISM: Ethacrynic acid has been shown, in vitro, to displace warfarin from human albumin binding sites.

CLINICAL SIGNIFICANCE: The clinical evidence to support this interaction consists primarily of occasional case reports.[153,171] In at least one of the cases hypoalbuminemia was present, which may have predisposed to the enhanced hypoprothrombinemia.[171] Renal insufficiency or large doses of ethacrynic acid might also be expected to increase the likelihood of interaction. The possibility of an increased incidence of gastrointestinal bleeding in patients receiving ethacrynic acid[41] is also worth consideration in the patient receiving oral anticoagulants.

MANAGEMENT: Ethacrynic acid should be given with caution to patients receiving oral anticoagulants, especially in the presence of hypoalbuminemia, large doses of ethacrynic acid, or renal impairment. Reduction in anticoagulant dosage may be required. It is possible that furosemide (Lasix) may be a suitable alternative, although little is known of its effect on oral anticoagulants.

Ethchlorvynol (Placidyl)[61,81]

MECHANISM: Ethchlorvynol appears to increase metabolism of coumarin anticoagulants by induction of hepatic microsomal enzymes.

CLINICAL SIGNIFICANCE: In one patient receiving warfarin, a marked decrease in prothrombin activity following ethchlorvynol administration.[61] In another study of six patients on dicumarol, ethchlorvynol (1.0 g/day for 18 days) inhibited the hypoprothrombinemic response.[81]

MANAGEMENT: Watch for altered anticoagulant effect when ethchlorvynol is started or stopped in a patient receiving oral anticoagulants.

Fenoprofen (Nalfon)[240]

MECHANISM: None established.

CLINICAL SIGNIFICANCE: Although fenoprofen is highly bound to plasma albumin and in high concentrations displaces warfarin from protein binding in vitro,[240] little clinical information is available regarding the effect of fenoprofen on the hypoprothrombinemic response to oral anticoagulants. However, fenoprofen has caused gastrointestinal bleeding and may inhibit platelet function somewhat.

MANAGEMENT: Monitor for altered anticoagulant response if fenoprofen is initiated or discontinued in a patient receiving oral anticoagulants.

ORAL ANTICOAGULANT INTERACTIONS (CONT.)

Flurazepam (Dalmane)[42]

MECHANISM: None.

CLINICAL SIGNIFICANCE: In a study of eight normal subjects, fluraze-pam did not affect plasma warfarin levels.[42] A slight decrease in the hypoprothrombinemic effect of warfarin seen in these subjects was not substantiated by subsequent observations of twelve patients maintained on chronic warfarin therapy. The lack of interaction found in this published study is consistent with my observations of patients receiving this combination.

MANAGEMENT: No special precautions appear to be necessary.

Furosemide (Lasix)[223]

MECHANISM: None described.

CLINICAL SIGNIFICANCE: In a study in 11 normal subjects, furosemide did not affect either warfarin half-life or hypoprothrombinemic response.[223]

MANAGEMENT: No special precautions appear necessary.

Glucagon[106,107]

MECHANISM: Not established, although a number of possible mechanisms have been proposed.[106]

CLINICAL SIGNIFICANCE: In eight patients who received glucagon for 2 or more days in a total dose of more than 50 mg, marked enhancement of the hypoprothrombinemic response to warfarin was noted.[106] Three of these eight patients had bleeding episodes, presumably as a result of the interaction. A similar potentiating effect of acenocoumarin by glucagon has been demonstrated in animals.[107]

MANAGEMENT: Concomitant administration of oral anticoagulants and glucagon should be undertaken cautiously. If the dose of glucagon exceeds 25 mg per day for 2 or more days, it may be wise to lower the dose of warfarin and observe the prothrombin times of the patient closely.[106]

Glutethimide (Doriden)[12,43,75,82,166]

MECHANISM: Glutethimide appears to increase the metabolism of oral anticoagulants by induction of hepatic microsomal enzymes.

CLINICAL SIGNIFICANCE: Glutethimide has been shown to decrease plasma warfarin levels and warfarin half-lives in patients and healthy subjects.[43,82] Accordingly, the hypoprothrombinemic response in patients stabilized on warfarin was inhibited by glutethimide administration.[166] These effects of glutethimide appear to be similar in magnitude to those of barbiturates.

DRUGS	DISCUSSION

MANAGEMENT: Watch carefully for altered anticoagulant effect when glutethimide therapy is started or stopped in a patient receiving oral anticoagulants. Benzodiazepines such as flurazepam (Dalmane) or diazepam (Valium) are preferable to glutethimide as hypnotics in patients on oral anticoagulants. (And in most other patients for that matter).

Griseofulvin[5,61]

MECHANISM: Not established. It has been proposed that griseofulvin induces hepatic microsomal enzymes resulting in enhanced metabolism of oral anticoagulants.

CLINICAL SIGNIFICANCE: Three patients have been described in whom griseofulvin appeared to inhibit the effect of warfarin, but no effect was seen in a healthy volunteer given the combination.[61] Udall[5] found that only four of ten patients on chronic warfarin therapy had decreased prothrombin times (mean, 4.2 seconds) when placed on griseofulvin (1.0 g/day for 2 weeks). Thus, it appears likely that the interactions is real but occurs only in some patients.

MANAGEMENT: In a patient receiving oral anticoagulants, watch for altered anticoagulant effect when griseofulvin therapy is started or stopped.

Haloperidol (Haldol)[73]

MECHANISM: Not established.

CLINICAL SIGNIFICANCE: A single case has been reported in which haloperidol appeared to antagonize the anticoagulant effect of phenindione.[73] Confirmation of this finding is needed to assess the clinical significance of this interaction.

MANAGEMENT: No special precautions appear to be necessary.

Heparin[68]

MECHANISM: Heparin administration may further prolong the prothrombin time in patients receiving oral anticoagulants.

CLINICAL SIGNIFICANCE: Bolus intravenous administration of heparin prolongs the prothrombin time considerably, while subcutaneous administration of the same dose (e.g., 10,000 units) results in only a modest prolongation (e.g., 1 or 2 seconds).

MANAGEMENT: To avoid confusing laboratory values resulting in improper selection of oral anticoagulant dosage, blood for prothrombin times should not be drawn within about 5 or 6 hours of intravenous heparin administration.

Ibuprofen (Motrin)[156,172,187,193]

MECHANISM: See Clinical Significance.

ORAL ANTICOAGULANT INTERACTIONS (CONT.)

DRUGS	DISCUSSION

Clinical Significance: In 24 patients stabilized on long-term phenprocoumon (Liquamar), the administration of ibuprofen under double-blind conditions did not affect the anticoagulant response to phenprocoumon as measured by the Thrombotest.[156] A similar lack of interaction between ibuprofen and phenoprocoumon has been shown by other workers.[172] It has also been shown that ibuprofen does not affect the hypoprothrombinemic response to warfarin.[187] A case of a drug interaction between warfarin and ibuprofen has apparently been reported, but no details were given other than that the result was a "coagulation defect."[193] Thus, a majority of evidence indicates that the hypoprothrombinemic response to oral anticoagulants is not affected by ibuprofen. However, as with any nonsteroidal anti-inflammatory agent, one must consider the possible detrimental effects of ibuprofen on the gastrointestinal mucosa and on platelet function.

Management: No special precautions appear to be necessary at this time.

Indomethacin (Indocin)[74,80,153,154,158,162,193,241]

Mechanism: Indomethacin is ulcerogenic and may inhibit platelet function.[154] Both of these effects may be dangerous in patients receiving anticoagulants. The possibility that indomethacin may displace coumarin anticoagulants from plasma protein binding[74] has not been proved.

Clinical Significance: At least two studies have indicated that indomethacin has little effect on hypoprothrombinemic response to oral anticoagulants.[80,158] Indomethacin (25 mg tid for 3 weeks) was given to 16 patients stabilized on phenprocoumon (Liquamar).[80] There was no mean change in the hypoprothrombinemic response to phenprocoumon during indomethacin administration. In another study, indomethacin (100 mg/day for 5 days) failed to affect the hypoprothrombinemic response to warfarin given chronically to 16 healthy subjects, and indomethacin (100 mg/day for 11 days) failed to affect either the hypoprothrombinemic response or plasma half-life of single doses of warfarin in 19 healthy subjects.[158] It is clear from these studies that indomethacin is not likely to affect the hypoprothrombinemic response to oral anticoagulants, at least at indomethacin doses up to 100 mg/day. Isolated cases of possible indomethacin-induced increases in warfarin hypoprothrombinemia have been reported,[153,162,193,241] so one should consider the possibility that such a reaction may occur, albeit rarely. Further, indomethacin can cause gastrointestinal bleeding and can inhibit platelet function somewhat. In summary, indomethacin appears to have minimal effects on the anticoagulant response to oral anticoagulants in the majority of patients, but the combination should be used with caution due to the gastrointestinal and platelet effects of indomethacin.

Management: Based on the studies cited above, it would not seem necessary to perform more frequent prothrombin times in patients

DRUGS	DISCUSSION

receiving indomethacin and oral anticoagulants. However, careful attention to clinical detection of bleeding, especially of the gastrointestinal tract, would seem warranted.

Influenza Vaccination[231,310,311]

MECHANISM: It is proposed that influenza vaccination may inhibit the hepatic metabolism of warfarin.

CLINICAL SIGNIFICANCE: Brief mention has been made of a patient well controlled on warfarin for several years who developed a serious bleeding episode following the administration of an influenza vaccination.[231] In another study, influenza vaccine tended to increase the hypoprothrombinemic response in eight patients on chronic warfarin,[310] but a subsequent study in 21 patients found no effect.[311] The reason for the disparate results is not clear; more study is needed.

MANAGEMENT: Until more information is available, one should watch for evidence of an enhanced effect of oral anticoagulants following influenza vaccination.

Isoniazid (INH)[10,146,221,295]

MECHANISM: Animal studies indicate that isoniazid may inhibit dicumarol metabolism, but other possible mechanisms have not been excluded.

CLINICAL SIGNIFICANCE: A patient stabilized on warfarin (Coumadin) developed excessive hypoprothrombinemia and bleeding about 10 days after his isoniazid (INH) dose was increased from 300 mg/day to 600 mg/day.[221] Data from animal studies are conflicting. Isoniazid 15 mg/kg body weight) increased the plasma levels and hypoprothrombinemic response to dicumarol in dogs,[10] but the same dose of INH failed to alter plasma warfarin or hypoprothrombinemia in rabbits.[146] Considering these reports and the known properties of INH, it would be prudent to assume that at least occasional patients receiving oral anticoagulants will develop exaggerated anticoagulant responses when INH is added to their drug regimen. Slow INH acetylators taking large doses of INH are probably predisposed to this interaction. Furthermore, INH therapy alone has resulted in severe bleeding in several patients due to production of an inhibitor of fibrin stabilization.[295] This latter reaction is probably quite rare, but should be considered in patients on INH who develop bleeding.

MANAGEMENT: Patients stabilized on oral anticoagulants should probably be monitored somewhat more closely during initiation of isoniazid therapy. Based on current information, initiation of oral anticoagulant therapy in a patient already on chronic isoniazid should not pose difficulty since the patient would be titrated to the proper dose of anticoagulant.

ORAL ANTICOAGULANT INTERACTIONS (CONT.)

Laxatives[87-89]

MECHANISM: It has been proposed that laxative-induced increased speed of the contents through the intestinal tract may result in decreased absorption of vitamin K and/or oral anticoagulants.

CLINICAL SIGNIFICANCE: Little evidence exists to support decreased absorption of either vitamin K or oral anticoagulants in patients receiving laxatives. No evidence of hypoprothrombinemia was noted in several patients not on oral anticoagulants who abused laxatives.[87-89] If this purported interaction were to occur, it would probably be more likely with dicumarol than warfarin since the former is more erratically and more poorly absorbed (see also Mineral Oil, p. 89).

MANAGEMENT: Although there is little evidence of interaction, it would be prudent to watch for altered anticoagulant effect in patients ingesting large quantities of laxatives.

Meclofenamate (Meclomen)[242,243]

MECHANISM: Not established.

CLINICAL SIGNIFICANCE: The hypoprothrombinemic response to warfarin is reportedly increased by meclofenamate,[242,243] but details of the studies are not given.

MANAGEMENT: Monitor patient carefully for enhanced hypoprothrombinemic response. Consider use of a nonsteroidal anti-inflammatory agent, such as ibuprofen, naproxen, or tolmetin, which has a minimal effect on the anticoagulant response.

Mefenamic Acid (Pontstel)[79,110,127,132]

MECHANISM: Mefenamic acid probably displaces warfarin from albumin binding sites, thus increasing hypoprothrombinemic activity.

CLINICAL SIGNIFICANCE: The earlier suggestion that mefenamic acid may have enhanced the response to oral anticoagulants clinically[79] has been substantiated by a preliminary clinical study in 12 healthy volunteers.[132] In the latter study a small but significant decrease in prothrombin concentration occurred when the warfarin-treated volunteers were given mefenamic acid (500 mg qid). Although more evidence is needed, mefenamic acid appears likely to be proved capable of enhancing the effect of coumarin anticoagulants. The possibility of mefenamic-acid induced gastrointestinal hemorrhage should also be kept in mind in the patient receiving oral anticoagulants.

MANAGEMENT: Mefenamic acid should probably be avoided in patients receiving oral anticoagulants. Consider use of a nonsteroidal anti-inflammatory agent such as ibuprofen, naproxen, or tolmetin which has minimal effect on the anticoagulant response.

Meprobamate (Equanil) (Miltown)[75,141,142,169]

MECHANISM: See Clinical Significance.

ORAL ANTICOAGULANT INTERACTIONS (CONT.)

DRUGS	DISCUSSION

CLINICAL SIGNIFICANCE: Although meprobamate has been said to decrease the action of oral anticoagulants, studies in humans have not shown any clinically significant effect,[141,142,169] even at the maximum recommended dose.[142]

MANAGEMENT: No special precautions appear to be necessary.

Mercaptopurine (Purinethol)[220,224]

MECHANISM: Not established. Animal studies indicate that mercaptopurine increases prothrombin synthesis or activation.[224]

CLINICAL SIGNIFICANCE: A patient well controlled on chronic warfarin therapy developed a reduced hypoprothrombinemic response during mercaptopurine therapy.[220] When the mercaptopurine was stopped, the response to warfarin returned to normal, and a subsequent administration of mercaptopurine produced changes similar to the first episode. Although it appears quite likely that mercaptopurine reduced the hypoprothrombinemic response to warfarin in this patient, it is not known how frequently this would appear in other patients receiving the combination. Since azathioprine (Imuran) is metabolized to mercaptopurine, azathioprine may also inhibit the hypoprothrombinemic response to oral anticoagulants.

MANAGEMENT: It does not seem necessary to avoid concomitant use since adjustment of warfarin dose may allow proper control of anticoagulation. However, patients receiving oral anticoagulants should be monitored more closely when mercaptopurine is started or stopped.

Methaqualone (Parest, Quaalude, Sopor)[8,12,166]

MECHANISM: Methaqualone appears to have a minor stimulatory effect on the metabolism of warfarin.

CLINICAL SIGNIFICANCE: In ten patients on chronic warfarin therapy, methaqualone (0.3 g/day for 4 weeks) was associated with a slight decrease in the hypoprothrombinemic response.[166] However, the change was not clinically significant. Whitfield[8] found no effect of methaqualone on plasma warfarin levels in one patient, but an increase in plasma gamma-glutamyl transpeptidase activity (which can be a sign of enzyme induction) was seen. In rats, methaqualone did appear to enhance dicumarol metabolism, but the effect was less than when phenobarbital or glutethimide was given with the dicumarol.[12] In summary, methaqualone appears to slightly decrease the hypoprothrombinemic response to oral anticoagulants in many patients, but the magnitude of the change is generally insufficient to interfere with anticoagulant therapy.

MANAGEMENT: Based on current evidence the concomitant use of methaqualone and oral anticoagulants should seldom cause adverse effects. Benzodiazepines such as flurazepam (Dalmane) or diazepam (Valium) would be more appropriate sedative-hypnotics to use whether or not the patient was receiving oral anticoagulants.

ORAL ANTICOAGULANT INTERACTIONS (CONT.)

DRUGS	DISCUSSION

Metronidazole (Flagyl)[195,199,296]

MECHANISM: It is proposed that metronidazole inhibits the metabolism of the S(−) form of warfarin, but has no effect on the R(+) form.[195] Since commercially available warfarin consists of both S(−) and R(+), metronidazole enhances the hypoprothrombinemic effect.

CLINICAL SIGNIFICANCE: In eight subjects, a single dose of the commercially available racemic warfarin (1.5 mg/kg body weight) was given with and without pretreatment with metronidazole (750 mg/day for 7 days).[195] Metronidazole increased the hypoprothrombinemic response and plasma warfarin levels. S(−) warfarin (0.75 mg/kg body weight) was similarly enhanced by metronidazole, but R(+) warfarin was not affected. Also, two patients on chronic warfarin therapy developed prolonged prothrombin times and bleeding episodes after receiving metronidazole.[199,296] It appears that metronidazole is a potential hazard when given concomitantly with oral anticoagulants.

MANAGEMENT: Concomitant use of metronidazole and oral anticoagulants should be avoided if possible. Patients should be monitored for altered anticoagulant effect when metronidazole is started or stopped in a patient receiving oral anticoagulants. If oral anticoagulant therapy is begun in a patient receiving metronidazole, anticoagulant doses should be conservative until the maintenance dose is established.

Methylphenidate (Ritalin)[96,133]

MECHANISM: It has been proposed that methylphenidate inhibits the metabolism of ethyl biscoumacetate.[96]

CLINICAL SIGNIFICANCE: The results of a preliminary study in four volunteers showing a prolongation of the half-life of ethyl biscoumacetate due to methylphenidate[96] could not be confirmed by a subsequent doubled-blind study in 12 healthy volunteers.[133] Thus, available evidence is not sufficient to support the existence of a clinically significant interaction between these drugs.

MANAGEMENT: No special precautions appear necessary.

Miconazole (Monistat)[228-230]

MECHANISM: Not established.

CLINICAL SIGNIFICANCE: Several patients have developed an enhanced hypoprothrombinemic response to warfarin following miconazole therapy.[228-230] Although clinical information is limited, at least two of the patients exhibited a positive rechallenge.

MANAGEMENT: One should be alert for an altered hypoprothrombinemic response to oral anticoagulants if miconazole therapy is initiated or discontinued. Adjust oral anticoagulant dose as necessary.

ORAL ANTICOAGULANT INTERACTIONS (CONT.)

Mineral Oil[72,97,109]

MECHANISM: Mineral oil is said to reduce absorption of fat-soluble nutrients such as vitamin K. Such a decrease could enhance the hypoprothrombinemia produced by oral anticoagulants. However, the possibility exists that mineral oil could also impair oral anticoagulant absorption (see also Laxatives, p. 86).

CLINICAL SIGNIFICANCE: Not established. Very little clinical information is available on either of the two possible mechanisms mentioned.

MANAGEMENT: Although the importance of this purported interaction is not clear, it might be prudent to discourage patients receiving oral anticoagulants from the ingestion of large amounts of mineral oil.

Nalidixic Acid (Neg Gram)[110,159,297]

MECHANISM: Nalidixic acid has been shown, in vitro, to displace warfarin from human albumin binding sites.

CLINICAL SIGNIFICANCE: A patient stabilized on warfarin developed excessive hypoprothrombinemia, purpura, and bruising a few days after nalidixic acid was started.[159] Another patient on nicoumalone developed increased hypoprothrombinemia after treatment with nalidixic acid (1 g daily).[297] Although these reactions might have been due to drug interactions, there is little information to indicate how frequently it would occur in patients receiving the two drugs concurrently.

MANAGEMENT: The evidence does not seem sufficient to recommend avoiding concomitant use, but one should watch for altered anticoagulant effect when nalidixic acid therapy is started or stopped in patients receiving oral anticoagulants.

Naproxen (Anaprox, Naprosyn)[244,245]

MECHANISM: None.

CLINICAL SIGNIFICANCE: Ten healthy subjects on oral warfarin for 25 days were given naproxen (375 mg BID) from day 11 to day 20.[244] Naproxen administration was not associated with changes in the disposition or the hypoprothrombinemic response to warfarin. In another study, naproxen (375 mg BID for 17 days) did not affect the pharmacokinetics or anticoagulant effect of a single 50-mg dose of warfarin.[245] Thus, available evidence indicates that naproxen has minimal effects on oral anticoagulants in healthy subjects. However, one must still consider the possibility that an occasional patient might manifest an enhanced anticoagulant response, and that naproxen may cause gastrointestinal bleeding and impair platelet function.

MANAGEMENT: Naproxen is probably one of the safer nonsteroidal anti-inflammatory drugs (NSAID) to use in a patient on oral anticoag-

DRUGS	DISCUSSION

ulants, but one should monitor carefully for evidence of bleeding when any NSAID is given to a patient on oral anticoagulants.

Narcotic Analgesics[66]

MECHANISM: Not established.

CLINICAL SIGNIFICANCE: Narcotic analgesics reportedly may enhance the response to oral anticoagulants. However, the clinical significance has not been established, and there is little evidence that short-term narcotic administration has an appreciable effect on the response to oral anticoagulants.

MANAGEMENT: No special precautions appear necessary.

Nitrazepam (Mogadon)[8,147]

MECHANISM: See Clinical Significance.

CLINICAL SIGNIFICANCE: A double-blind study in 22 volunteers has shown nitrazepam to have no significant effect on long-term anticoagulant therapy with phenprocoumon.[147] One patient on long-term warfarin therapy did not manifest changes in plasma warfarin levels when nitrazepam was given.[8] Finally, the lack of effect of other benzodiazepines on oral anticoagulant therapy further supports the likelihood that nitrazepam does not interact with oral anticoagulants.

MANAGEMENT: No special precautions appear to be necessary.

Oxyphenbutazone (Tandearil)

See phenylbutazone below; the same discussion applies.

Phenformin[139]*

MECHANISM: It has been proposed that the phenformin-induced increase in fibrinolytic activity can produce a tendency to hemorrhage in patients receiving oral anticoagulants, even in the absence of excessively prolonged prothrombin times.

CLINICAL SIGNIFICANCE: Not established. A single case has been reported in which a patient on warfarin therapy developed severe hematuria 3 months after initiation of phenformin therapy.[139] Coagulation tests were within the therapeutic range, but there was evidence of increased fibrinolytic activity. More information is needed.

MANAGEMENT: Although evidence is scanty, it would be prudent to watch patients on combined phenformin and oral anticoagulant therapy more closely for signs of hemorrhage. Theoretically, prothrombin times may not be excessively prolonged in patients who develop hemorrhage as a result of this interaction.

*Removed from general use in the United States.

DRUGS	DISCUSSION

Phenothiazines[66]

MECHANISM: Not established.

CLINICAL SIGNIFICANCE: Although chlorpromazine may enhance the hypoprothrombinemic effect of acenocoumarol (Sintrom) in animals,[66] studies in humans are lacking.

MANAGEMENT: No special precautions appear to be necessary.

Phenylbutazone (Butazolidin)[5,7,13,44-46,71,74,112,115,154,174,186,190,246-248]

MECHANISM: Phenylbutazone appears to inhibit the metabolism of the more potent S(−) isomer of warfarin and may also displace warfarin from plasma protein binding. Phenylbutazone may also produce gastrointestinal ulceration and impair platelet function.

CLINICAL SIGNIFICANCE: This is probably the most critical interaction of coumarin anticoagulants. The enhanced anticoagulant response is marked and occurs in nearly all patients treated with both drugs. In patient stabilized on oral anticoagulants, enhanced hypoprothrombinemia may occur as early as 1 to 2 days following the start of phenylbutazone therapy. In one study[5] all of ten patients on warfarin therapy exhibited increased prothrombin times (mean, 14.4 seconds) with phenylbutazone administration (300 mg/day for 2 weeks). A number of bleeding episodes have occurred in patients receiving both oral anticoagulants and phenylbutazone. Also, the possible phenylbutazone-induced peptic ulcer and impaired platelet function are added hazards to the patient receiving anticoagulants.

MANAGEMENT: Every effort should be made to avoid phenylbutazone or oxyphenbutazone treatment in patients receiving oral anticoagulants. It is not likely that a condition exists in which the benefit of phenylbutazone therapy outweighs the serious risk of concomitant therapy with oral anticoagulants. Consider the use of a nonsteroidal anti-inflammatory agent that has a minimal effect on the anticoagulant response such as ibuprofen, naproxen, or tolmetin.

Phenyramidol[59,98]

MECHANISM: Phenyramidol appears to inhibit the metabolism of oral anticoagulants.

CLINICAL SIGNIFICANCE: Well documented. In one study,[59] phenyramidol (800 to 1600 mg/day) given to nine patients on various oral anticoagulants caused increased prothrombin times in all patients, usually within 3 to 7 days. However, phenyramidol is no longer commerically available in the United States.

MANAGEMENT: The dose of anticoagulant is likely to need reduction to avoid excessive prolongation of the prothrombin time if phenyramidol is also given.

ORAL ANTICOAGULANT INTERACTIONS (CONT.)

DRUGS	DISCUSSION

Phenytoin (*Dilantin*)[9,36–39,211,298,299]

MECHANISM: The interrelationships of these two drugs are exceedingly complex, with several different mechanisms apparently involved.
1. Dicumarol and probably phenprocoumon inhibit the parahydroxylation of phenytoin in the liver.
2. Phenytoin may stimulate the metabolism of dicumarol due to enzyme induction.
3. Phenytoin may have the ability to displace dicumarol from plasma protein binding.
4. Phenytoin alone may prolong the prothrombin time in some patients.[36,37] The overall effect of these (and perhaps other) mechanisms on half-lives, blood levels, and therapeutic effect of the two drugs will require much more study.

CLINICAL SIGNIFICANCE: On the basis of current knowledge, the following clinical effects may be expected:
1. If dicumarol or phenprocoumon is given to a patient maintained on phenytoin:
   a. Serum levels of phenytoin are likely to increase, perhaps to a point where signs of phenytoin intoxication occur.
   b. Higher than normal doses of anticoagulant might be required, but this has not yet been documented clinically.
2. If phenytoin is given to a patient maintained on oral anticoagulants:
   a. A transient initial increase in anticoagulant effect due to displacement of the oral anticoagulant might take place. Isolated cases of this have been reported.[298,299]
   b. A decrease in anticoagulant effect might take place, possibly due to enzyme induction, within a week or two of initiation of phenytoin therapy.

MANAGEMENT: Due to the complex nature of the interaction between phenytoin and dicumarol, it would be best to avoid concomitant use of these drugs. Warfarin may be less likely to interact and is probably preferable in the patient receiving phenytoin (and other patients, for that matter). If phenytoin is given with oral anticoagulants the effects of both agent should be monitored closely and dosage adjustments made as necessary.

Piroxicam (Feldene)[249,250]

MECHANISM: Not established.

CLINICAL SIGNIFICANCE: A slight increase in the hypoprothrombinemic response was reportedly noted in four of ten subjects given piroxicam (20 mg/day) in addition to acenocoumarol.[249] More study is needed to determine the clinical significance of any interaction between piroxicam and warfarin. The ability of piroxicam to produce gastrointestinal bleeding and inhibition of platelet function must also be considered when anticoagulants are used.[249,250]

DRUGS	DISCUSSION

MANAGEMENT: Watch for increased anticoagulant response if piroxicam is given to patients on oral anticoagulants. Until more is known about this potential interaction, consider the use of a nonsteroidal anti-inflammatory agent with minimal effects on the hypoprothrombinemic response to oral anticoagulants such as ibuprofen, naproxen, or tolmetin.

Propoxyphene (Darvon)[182,300]

MECHANISM: It has been proposed that propoxyphene inhibits the metabolism of warfarin.

CLINICAL SIGNIFICANCE: Two patients stabilized on warfarin developed bleeding episodes following administration of a preparation containing propoxyphene and acetaminophen.[182] A similar case was subsequently reported.[300] Since the product involved in these three cases also contained acethaminophen, it is not possible to determine which drug was primary responsible (if, in fact, a drug interaction was involved).

MANAGEMENT: The evidence does not seem sufficient to recommend avoiding concomitant use, but patients should be monitored more closely if propoxyphene is started or stopped in a patient receiving oral anticoagulants.

Psyllium (Metamucil)[120]

MECHANISM: See Clinical Significance.

CLINICAL SIGNIFICANCE: In six normal subjects, psyllium (As Metamucil) failed to affect the absorption of concomitantly administered warfarin.[120]

MANAGEMENT: It appears that psyllium may be given to patients receiving warfarin therapy without fear of altered warfarin absorption.

Reserpine[66,175]

MECHANISM: Not established.

CLINICAL SIGNIFICANCE: Although it has been suggested that long-term reserpine therapy may enhance the effect of oral anticoagulants, convincing evidence in humans is lacking. Short-term therapy in rats has been shown to *inhibit* the hypoprothrombinemic response to ethylbiscoumacetate.[175]

MANAGEMENT: No special precautions appear necessary.

Rifampin (Rifadin) (Rimactane)[145,157,176,188,189,196,301]

MECHANISM: Rifampin appears to stimulate the metabolism of warfarin by induction of hepatic microsomal enzymes.

ORAL ANTICOAGULANT INTERACTIONS (CONT.)

CLINICAL SIGNIFICANCE: In a study of ten normal subjects, O'Reilly[157] found a considerable increase in elimination of a single dose of warfarin when rifampin was also given. The hypoprothrombinemic response to warfarin was also inhibited by rifampin. Subsequent study in eight subjects given chronic warfarin showed a similar decrease in the hypoprothrombinemic effect of warfarin.[188] In addition, a number of cases have been reported describing rifampin-induced inhibition of the anticoagulant effect of warfarin,[176,196] phenprocoumon,[189] and acenocoumarol. In two cases [176,196] the dose of warfarin had to be reduced by 50% or more when rifampin was discontinued. In another brief report, initiation of rifampin therapy necessitated a two- to threefold increase in warfarin dosage.[301] Based on studies to date, rifampin-induced inhibition of warfarin hypoprothrombinemia is maximal at 5 to 10 days after starting rifampin. In summary, it appears that rifampin can be expected to produce a clinically significant reduction in the hypoprothrombinemic effect of oral anticoagulants in a majority of patients.

MANAGEMENT: Rifampin therapy should not be started or stopped in a patient receiving an oral anticoagulant without attention to possible readjustment of anticoagulant dosage.

Salicylates[1,5,47,48,99,100,132,135-138,251-253]

MECHANISM: Large doses of salicylates tend to reduce plasma prothrombin levels. It is also possible that salicylates may displace coumarin anticoagulants from plasma protein binding. Other factors to consider are the gastrointestinal bleeding that salicylates may produce and the ability of aspirin to impair primary hemostasis (effects on platelets, etc.).

CLINICAL SIGNIFICANCE: Conflicting reports have appeared with regard to the effect of salicylates on the response to oral anticoagulants. It appears that some subjects receiving warfarin manifest additive hypoprothrombinemic effects with doses of about 2 g per day of aspirin. With doses of 3 to 4 g per day of aspirin, it is more likely that the hypoprothrombinemic effects of oral anticoagulants would be enhanced in a majority of patients. However, probably more important than these additive effects is the ability of aspirin to impair primary hemostasis and its ability to produce gastrointestinal bleeding. These latter two effects may occur with doses of aspirin below 2 g per day. A study in 534 patients with prosthetic heart valves showed that excessive bleeding was about three times more common with warfarin plus aspirin (500 mg/day) than with either warfarin plus dipyridamole (400 mg/day) or warfarin alone.[251] The authors suggest that combined use of warfarin and aspirin is contraindicated. In another study, 2 of 11 patients on warfarin and dipyridamole developed enhanced hypoprothrombinemia during the first few days of aspirin therapy (1.0 g/day)[252] Others have also noted bleeding episodes that may have been due to concurrent therapy with aspirin and oral anticoagulants.[1,253]

ORAL ANTICOAGULANT INTERACTIONS (CONT.)

DRUGS	DISCUSSION

MANAGEMENT: When all of the evidence is taken together it is clear that patients receiving warfarin should avoid aspirin-containing products if possible. If a salicylate is necessary, nonaspirin salicylates such as choline salicylate (Arthropan), salsalate (Disalcid), sodium salicylate, and magnesium salicylate would theoretically be preferable since they have little effect on platelet function and are probably less likely than aspirin to cause gastrointestinal bleeding. If a mild analgesic is needed, acetaminophen is preferable to a salicylate.

Simethicone (Mylicon)[144]

MECHANISM: It has been proposed that this agent impairs absorption of oral anticoagulants.

CLINICAL SIGNIFICANCE: Not established. Several patients who had eaten potato chips cooked in an oil-containing methyl polysiloxane (simethicone) appeared to manifest antagonism of hypoprothrombinemic effect of warfarin or phenindione, but a causal relationship was not established.

MANAGEMENT: No special precautions appear necessary.

Spironolactone (Aldactone)[277]

MECHANISM: Spironolactone diuresis probably results in concentration of clotting factors in the blood.

CLINICAL SIGNIFICANCE: In nine normal subjects, spironolactone (200 mg/day) reduced the hypoprothrombinemic response to a single 1.5 mg/kg body weight dose of warfarin.[277] The plasma warfarin concentration was not changed but the hematocrit was increased, indicating that the interaction was caused by diuresis and the resultant concentration of clotting factors. Because this report involved healthy subjects, it is not known whether the interaction would have been observed in volume overloaded patients who needed a diuretic. Furthermore, therapy with spironolactone was short-term and it is not known whether this drug interaction would be clinically significant if spironolactone therapy had been initiated well before the anticoagulant or continued chronically. Situations which would reduce the likelihood of a clinically important effect include (1) chronic therapy with spironolactone prior to the initiation of the anticoagulant; (2) spironolactone initiated as a replacement for another diuretic (clotting factors would already be concentrated); and (3) close monitoring of a patient's response to the anticoagulant in a hospital setting (any effect of spironolactone would be compensated for by a change in dose of the anticoagulant).

MANAGEMENT: Monitor prothrombin time if spironolactone is initiated or discontinued, and adjust oral anticoagulant dosage as needed.

ORAL ANTICOAGULANT INTERACTIONS (CONT.)

Sucralfate (Carafate)[227]

MECHANISM: Not established. Sucralfate may inhibit the absorption of warfarin and possibly other oral anticoagulants.

CLINICAL SIGNIFICANCE: When a 59-year-old man on chronic warfarin therapy (prothrombin times, 26 to 29 seconds) developed upper gastrointestinal bleeding, the warfarin was stopped and sucralfate started.[227] When the warfarin was restarted and given at the same time as the sucralfate, the prothrombin time was subtherapeutic (12.5 to 14.5 seconds). Discontinuation of the sucralfate was accompanied by a return of the previous hypothrombinemic response to warfarin. It seems likely that the sucralfate reduced the effect of warfarin in this patient. However, few conclusions can be drawn from a single case report.

MANAGEMENT: Until this interaction is better studied, one should separate the doses of sucralfate and oral anticoagulants as much as possible. Since warfarin undergoes enterohepatic circulation, some reduction in warfarin effect could still occur.

Sulfinpyrazone (Anturane)[278-288]

MECHANISM: The primary mechanism is inhibition of hepatic warfarin metabolism, although sulfinpyrazone-induced platelet inhibition and protein-binding competition with warfarin may also be involved.

CLINICAL SIGNIFICANCE: Numerous cases have been reported of substantial increases in the hypoprothrombinemic response to warfarin following sulfinpyrazone.[278-284] Bleeding occurred in several patients. Controlled studies have confirmed that warfarin and acenocoumarol response is enhanced by sulfinpyrazone,[285-287] but phenprocoumon (Liquamar) does not appear to be affected.[288]

MANAGEMENT: Be alert for the need to change warfarin dose if sulfinpyrazone therapy is started or stopped. In patients receiving sulfinpyrazone in whom warfarin therapy is initiated, increased sensitivity to warfarin's hypoprothrombinemic effect may be observed. Phenprocoumon apparently does not interact with sulfinpyrazone and may be preferable to warfarin in this situation.

Sulfonamides[14,49,92,173,178,179,185,194,222,302-306]

MECHANISM: Sulfonamides appear to impair the hepatic metabolism of oral anticoagulants. Competition for plasma protein binding may play an additional role. Although sulfonamides reportedly decrease vitamin K production by gut bacteria, evidence for such an effect is lacking.

CLINICAL SIGNIFICANCE: Several reports have appeared describing enhanced hypoprothrombinemic response to warfarin when sulfamethoxazole (in combination with trimethoprim) was added to the patient's therapy.[185,222,302-304] Two pharmacokinetic studies in

DRUGS	DISCUSSION

healthy subjects confirmed that trimethoprim-sulfamethoxazole enhances the hypoprothrombinemic response to warfarin in most people.[305,306] Although the sulfamethoxazole seems more likely to have been responsible than the trimethoprim, a trimethoprim effect cannot be ruled out. Preliminary clinical evidence also indicates that sulfamethizole inhibits warfarin metabolism[194] and that sulfaphenazole enhances the hypoprothrombinemic response to phenindione.[179] The latter effect on phenindione appeared to be more pronounced in patients with hypoalbuminemia. In summary, some sulfonamides appear to enhance the hypoprothrombinemic response to oral anticoagulants in predisposed patients.

MANAGEMENT: It does not seem necessary to avoid the use of sulfonamides in patients receiving oral anticoagulants. However, the hypoprothrombinemic response of patients receiving concomitant therapy should be monitored closely, especially during initiation or discontinuation of the sulfonamide.

Sulindac (Clinoril)[254-256]

MECHANISM: Not established.

CLINICAL SIGNIFICANCE: The hypoprothrombinemic response to chronic warfarin was not significantly different in ten subjects on sulindac (400 mg/day for 10 days) when compared to the response in nine control subjects on placebo.[254] However, several cases have been reported describing enhanced hypoprothrombinemia and bleeding when sulindac was added to warfarin therapy.[254-256] Thus, it appears that occasional patients develop the interaction, but the factors that predispose to this interaction have not been established. As with other nonsteroidal anti-inflammatory agents, the potential adverse effects of sulindac on the gastrointestinal mucosa and platelet function should be considered.

MANAGEMENT: Monitor patients for enhanced hypoprothrombinemia and for clinical evidence of bleeding. Consider the use of a nonsteroidal anti-inflammatory drug that may be less likely to affect the hypoprothrombinemic response such as ibuprofen, naproxen, or tolmetin.

Tetracyclines[3,6,58,92,104,173,307,308]

MECHANISM:
1. Intravenous tetracycline therapy may result in a reduction of plasma prothrombin activity, possibly by impairing prothrombin utilization.[58]
2. Tetracyclines purportedly may decrease vitamin K production by gut bacteria, but this is of questionable significance (see Clinical Significance).
3. Animal studies indicate that a combination of tetracycline, neomycin, and bacitracin may inhibit the enterohepatic circulation of warfarin.[308]

DRUGS	DISCUSSION

CLINICAL SIGNIFICANCE: The proposed anticoagulant activity of intravenous tetracycline could theoretically add to the anticoagulant activity of oral anticoagulants. However, more work needs to be done to substantiate the earlier findings[58] on this effect of tetracyclines. A case of possible doxycycline-induced increase in warfarin hypoprothrombinemia has been reported.[307] The effect of tetracyclines on vitamin K production by gut bacteria has not been shown to be a significant problem. It is possible (but not proven) that this effect might be found to be significant in patients on anticoagulant therapy with deficient vitamin K intake.

MANAGEMENT: Although limited clinical evidence for an interaction exists, one should probably watch for enhanced anticoagulant effect when tetracyclines are used in a patient receiving oral anticoagulants.

Thiazide Diuretics[70,114,135]

MECHANISM: It has been proposed that thiazides may antagonize the effect of oral anticoagulants by
1. concentrating circulating clotting factors due to a decrease in plasma water.
2. reducing hepatic congestion in some patients, which may improve hepatic function and increase clotting factor synthesis.

CLINICAL SIGNIFICANCE: One study in eight subjects indicated that treatment with chlorothiazide (1 g/day for 21 days) did not alter the hypoprothrombinemia or plasma warfarin concentration following single doses of warfarin.[70] However, a study of thiazide administration to patients on chronic oral anticoagulant therapy seems more appropriate to detect effects based on preceding Mechanism #1. Effects based on Mechanism#2 apparently have been documented clinically.[135] In summary, thiazides probably have relatively minor effects on the hypoprothrombinemic response to oral anticoagulants in most patients.

MANAGEMENT: Patients on chronic oral anticoagulant therapy might be watched for increase in anticoagulant requirements during initiation of diuretic therapy. Such an effect in probably more likely in cardiac patients with hepatic congestion (see also Chlorthalidone, p. 75).

Thyroid Preparations[50–55,180,181,184,208]

MECHANISM: Thyroid hormones appear to increase catabolism of vitamin-K-dependent clotting factors. If oral anticoagulants are also being given, compensatory increases in clotting factor synthesis are impaired. A detailed description of the proposed mechanisms involved has appeared.[50]

CLINICAL SIGNIFICANCE: Patients with hypothyroidism are usually "warfarin resistant," and require larger doses of warfarin to achieve therapeutic levels of anticoagulation. Subsequent thyroid replace-

DRUGS	DISCUSSION

ment therapy in such a patient increases clotting factor catabolism without affecting clotting factor synthesis (suppressed by warfarin), and results in excessive anticoagulation and possibly a hemorrhagic episode. On the other hand, a patient rendered euthyroid by maintenance thyroid replacement therapy will respond like any other euthyroid patient to the initiation of oral anticoagulant therapy. Thus, changes in the thyrometabolic status of the patient cause changes in anticoagulant requirements. This should be kept in mind when evaluating this interaction in specific patients.

MANAGEMENT: Patients stabilized on oral anticoagulants who are found to require thyroid replacement therapy should be watched very closely when the thyroid is started. If the patient is truly hypothyroid, it is likely that a reduction in anticoagulant dosage will be required. No special precautions appear to be necessary when oral anticoagulant therapy is begun in a patient already stabilized on maintenance thyroid replacement therapy.

Tolmetin (Tolectin)[257]

MECHANISM: Not established.

CLINICAL SIGNIFICANCE: In doses of 800 to 1200 mg/day, tolmetin does not appear to affect the hypoprothrombinemic response to oral anticoagulants.[257] However, the potential adverse effects of tolmetin on the gastrointestinal tract and platelet function should be considered.

MANAGEMENT: Based on the evidence available, tolmetin appears to be one of the safer nonsteroidal anti-inflammatory drugs (NSAID) to use in a patient on oral anticoagulants. However, one should monitor carefully for evidence of bleeding when any NSAID is given to an anticoagulated patient.

Triclofos (Triclos)[4,56]

MECHANISM: It is proposed that a metabolite of triclofos (trichloroacetic acid) displaces warfarin from plasma protein binding.

CLINICAL SIGNIFICANCE: In a study involving seven healthy subjects stabilized on warfarin, triclofos considerably increased the hypoprothrombinemic response initially, with a gradual diminution of this effect after the first week.[56] Thus, the authors propose that patients receiving chronic oral anticoagulant therapy who are started on triclofos are only at risk of hemorrhage during the first 2 weeks of combined therapy.

MANAGEMENT: In patients on chronic oral anticoagulant therapy who require sedative-hypnotics, it would be preferable to use drugs that do not interact such as flurazepam (Dalmane) or diazepam (Valium). If triclofos is used, the patient should be monitored closely during the first 2 weeks of triclofos therapy.

ORAL ANTICOAGULANT INTERACTIONS (CONT.)

DRUGS	DISCUSSION

Vitamin E[170,206,309]

MECHANISM: Not established. It has been proposed that vitamin E may interfere with the effect of vitamin K in the production of clotting factors.[170]

CLINICAL SIGNIFICANCE: Vitamin E (800 IU/day) appeared to enhance the hypoprothrombinemic response to warfarin in one patient.[170] In a subsequent case, vitamin E (up to 1200 units/day) was associated with an excessive hypoprothrombinemic response to warfarin and bleeding.[309] There was a positive challenge and dechallenge under controlled conditions. Another study in three healthy subjects showed a mild increase in the hypoprothrombinemic response to dicumarol (150 mg) when the patients were given vitamin E (42 IU/day for 30 days).[206] Study in rats also indicated that vitamin E administration can enhance the anticoagulant response to warfarin.[206] Thus, it appears that vitamin E may enhance the hypoprothrombinemic response to oral anticoagulants in some patients.

MANAGEMENT: Patients receiving oral anticoagulants should avoid vitamin E therapy. If an anticoagulated patient has a legitimate need for vitamin E (highly unlikely), the hypoprothrombinemic response should be monitored carefully.

Vitamin K (in Foods)[214-217]

MECHANISM:
1. It is proposed that excessive dietary intake of vitamin K could offset oral anticoagulant-induced depression of clotting factor synthesis.
2. The delay in the absorption of warfarin caused by food could be due to a decrease in the rate of stomach emptying or a reduction of the dissolution rate of the drug.

CLINICAL SIGNIFICANCE: Inhibition of the hypoprothrombinemic response to oral anticoagulants may occur with excessive intake of foods with high vitamin K content. Foods which reportedly have a high vitamin K content include asparagus, broccoli, cabbage, lettuce, turnip green, beef liver, green tea, spinach, watercress, tomato, and coffee.[214] A study involving six healthy male volunteers demonstrated that food (high protein meal, high carbohydrate meal or high fat meal) significantly decreased the absorption rate of warfarin sodium but did not affect the total amount of warfarin absorbed.[216]

MANAGEMENT: Patients should be cautioned about sudden increases in intake of leafy vegetables or other foods high in vitamin K content. Warfarin requirements should not be altered if patients are consistent in their intake of these foods. Since meals do not appear to affect total absorption of warfarin, timing of administration with regard to meals does not seem necessary.

References

1. STARR KJ, PETRIE JC: Drug interactions in patients on long term oral anticoagulant and antihypertensive adrenergic neuron-blocking drugs. Br Med J 4:133, 1972.
2. FEINSTEIN DI, et al: Factor V inhibitor: report of a case, with comments on a possible effect of streptomycin. Ann Intern Med 78:385, 1973.
3. KIPPEL AP, PITSINGER B: Hypoprothrombinemia secondary to antibiotic therapy and manifested by massive gastrointestinal hemorrhage. Report of three cases. Arch Surg 96:266, 1968.
4. BELILES RP, FOSTER GV, Jr: Interaction of bishydroxycoumarin with chloral hydrate and trichloroethyl phosphate. Toxicol Appl Pharmacol 27:225, 1974.
5. UDALL, JA: Drug interference with warfarin therapy. Clin Med 77:20, 1970.
6. FINEGOLD SM: Interaction of antimicrobial therapy and intestinal flora. Am J Clin Nutr 23:1466, 1970.
7. BROZOVIC M, CURD LJ: Prothrombin during warfarin treatment. Br J Haematol 24:579, 1973.
8. WHITFIELD JB, et al: Changes in plasma α-glutamyl transpeptidase activity associated with alterations in drug metabolism in man. Br Med J 1:316, 1973.
9. HANSEN JM, et al: Dicumarol-induced diphenylhydantoin intoxication. Lancet 2:265, 1966.
10. EADE NR, et al: Potentiation of bishydroxycoumarin in dogs by isoniazid and p-aminosalicylic acid. Am Rev Respir Dis 103:792, 1971.
11. VESELL ES, et al: Impairment of drug metabolism in man by allopurinol and nortriptyline. N Engl J Med 283:1484, 1970.
12. ZAROSLINSKI J, et al: Effect of subacute administration of methaqualone, phenobarbital and glutethimide on plasma levels of bishydroxycoumarin. Arch Int Pharmacodyn Ther 195:185, 1972.
13. PACKHAM MA, et al: Alteration of the response of platelets to surface stimuli by pyrazole compounds. J Exp Med 126:171, 1967.
14. SOLOMON HM, SCHROGIE JJ: The effect of various drugs on the binding of warfarin-^{14}C to human albumin. Biochem Pharmacol 16:1219, 1967.
15. KATER RHM, et al: Increased rate of clearance of drugs from the circulation of alcoholics. Am J Med Sci 258:35, 1969.
16. SELF TH: Interaction of warfarin and aminosalicylic acid (Letter). JAMA 223:1285, 1973.
17. WEINSTEIN L: Drugs used in the chemotherapy of leprosy and tuberculosis. In Goodman LS, Gilman A (Eds): The Pharmacological Basis of Therapeutics. 4th Ed. New York, Macmillan, 1970, pp. 1320–1324.
18. AMBRE JJ, FISCHER LJ: Effect of coadministration aluminum and magnesium hydroxides on absorption of anticoagulants in man. Clin Pharmacol Ther 14:231, 1973.
19. PETITPIERRE B, et al: Behaviour of chlorpropamide in renal insufficiency and under the effect of associated drug therapy. Int J Clin Pharmacol Ther Toxicol 6:120, 1972.
20. SOLOMON HM, SCHROGIE JJ: Effect of phenyramidol and bishydroxycoumarin on the metabolism of tolbutamide in human subjects. Metabolism 16:1029, 1967.

References (CONT.)

21. CHAPLIN H, Jr, CASSELL M: Studies on the possible relationship of tolbutamide to dicumarol in anticoagulant therapy. Am J Med Sci 235:706, 1958.
22. KRISTENSEN M, HANSEN JM: Accumulation of chlorpropamide caused by dicumarol. Acta Med Scand 183:83, 1968.
23. SPURNEY OM, et al: Protracted tolbutamide-induced hypoglycemia. Arch Intern Med 115:53, 1965.
24. KRISTENSEN M, HANSEN JM: Potentiation of the tolbutamide effect of dicumarol. Diabetes 16:211, 1967.
25. DECKERT FW: Ascorbic acid and warfarin (Letter). JAMA 223:440, 1973.
26. WEINTRAUB M, GRINER PF: Warfarin and ascorbic acid: lack of evidence for a drug interaction. Toxicol Appl Pharmacol 28:53, 1974.
27. ANON: Therapeutic conferences. Drug Interaction. Brit Med J 1:389, 1971.
28. BRECKENRIDGE A, et al: Dose-dependent enzyme induction. Clin Pharmacol Ther 14:514, 1973.
29. CUCINELL SA, et al: Drug interactions in man. I. Lowering effect of phenobarbital on plasma levels of bishydroxycoumarin (Dicumarol) and diphenylhydantoin (Dilantin). Clin Pharmacol Ther 6:420, 1965.
30. O'REILLY RA, AGGELAR PM: Effect of barbiturates on oral anticoagulants (Abstract). Clin Res 17:153, 1969.
31. BENJAMIN D, et al: Cholestyramine binding of warfarin in man and *in vitro* (Abstract). Clin Res 18:336, 1970.
32. SOLOMON RB, ROSNER F: Massive hemorrhage and death during treatment with clofibrate and warfarin. NY State J Med 73:2002, 1973.
33. EASTHAM RD: Warfarin dosage influenced by clofibrate plus age (Letter). Lancet 1:1450, 1973.
34. OLIVER MF, et al: Effect of atromid and ethyl chlorophenoxy-isobutyrate on anticoagulant requirements. Lancet 1:143, 1963.
35. WADMAN B, WERNER I: Thromboembolic complications during corticosteroid treatment of temporal arteritis (Letter). Lancet 1:907, 1972.
36. ANDREASEN PB, et al: Abnormalities in liver function tests during long-term diphenylhydantoin therapy in epileptic outpatients. Acta Med Scand 194:261, 1973.
37. SOLOMON GE, et al: Coagulation defects caused by diphenylhydantoin. Neurology 22:1165, 1972.
38. HANSEN JM, et al: Effect on diphenylhydantoin on the metabolism of dicumarol in man. Acta Med Scand 189:15, 1971.
39. ROTHERMICH NO: Diphenylhydantoin intoxication (Letter). Lancet 2:640, 1966.
40. O'REILLY RA: Interaction of sodium warfarin and disulfiram (Antabuse®) in man. Ann Intern Med 78:73, 1973.
41. SLONE D, et al: Intravenously given ethacrynic acid and gastrointestinal bleeding. A finding resulting from comprehensive drug surveillance. JAMA 209:1668, 1969.
42. ROBINSON DS, AMIDON EL: Interaction of benzodiazepines with warfarin in man. Presented at the Annual Symposium on Benzodiazepines in Milan, Italy. November 2–4, 1971.
43. CORN M: Effect of phenobarbital and glutethimide on biological half-life of warfarin. Thromb Diath Haemorrh 16:606, 1966.

References (CONT.)

44. Wosilait WD, Eisenbrandt LL: The effect of oxyphenbutazone on the excretion of ^{14}C-warfarin in the bile of rat. Res Commun Chem Pathol Pharmacol 4:413, 1972.
45. Weiner M, et al: Drug interactions: the effect of combined administration on the half-life of coumarin and pyrazolone drugs in man (Abstract). Fed Proc 24:153, 1965.
46. O'Reilly RA: The binding of sodium warfarin to plasma albumin and its displacement by phenylbutazone. Ann NY Acad Sci 226:293, 1973.
47. Chignell CF, Starkweather DK: Optical studies of drug-protein complexes. V. The interaction of phenylbutazone, flufenamic acid, and dicumarol with acetylsalicylic acid-treated human serum albumin. Mol Pharmacol 7:229, 1971.
48. Coldwell BB, Thomas BH: Effect of aspirin on the fate of bishydroxycoumarin in the rat (Letter). J Pharm Pharmacol 23:226, 1971.
49. Anton AH: Increasing activity of sulfonamides with displacing agents: a review. Ann NY Acad Sci 226:273, 1973.
50. Hansten PD: Oral anticoagulant therapy in the patient with altered thyroid function. Northwest Med J 1:39 (April), 1974.
51. Loeliger EA, et al: The biological disappearance rate of prothrombin, factors VII, IX and X from plasma in hypothyroidism, hyperthyroidism and during fever. Thromb Diath Haemorrh 10:267, 1964.
52. Walters MB: The relationship between thyroid function and anticoagulant therapy. Am J Cardiol 11:112, 1963.
53. Vagenakis AG, et al: Enhancement of warfarin-induced hypoprothrombinemia by thyrotoxicosis. Johns Hopkins Med J 131:69, 1972.
54. McIntosh TJ, et al: Increased sensitivity to warfarin in thyrotoxicosis (Abstract). J Clin Invest 49:63a, 1970.
55. Rice AJ, et al: Decreased sensitivity to warfarin in patients with myxedema. Am J Med Sci 262:211, 1971.
56. Sellers EM, et al: Enhancement of warfarin-induced hypoprothrombinemia by triclofos. Clin Pharmacol Ther 13:911, 1972.
57. Murakami M, et al: Effects of anabolic steroids on anticoagulant requirements. Jpn Circ J 29:243, 1965.
58. Searcy RL, et al: Blood clotting anomalies associated with intensive tetracycline therapy. Clin Res 12:230, 1964.
59. Carter SA: Potentiation of the effect of orally administered anticoagulants by phenyramidol hydrochloride. N Engl J Med 273:423, 1965.
60. Schrogie JJ, Solomon HM: The anticoagulant response to bishydroxycoumarin. II The effect of D-thyroxine, clofibrate, and norethandrolone. Clin Pharmacol Ther 8:70, 1967.
61. Cullen SI, Catalano PM: Griseofulvin-warfarin antagonism. JAMA 199:582, 1967.
62. Robinson DS, MacDonald MG: The effect of phenobarbital administration on the control of coagulation achieved during warfarin therapy in man. J Pharmacol Exp Ther 153:250, 1966.
63. Cucinell SA, et al: The effect of chloral hydrate on bishydroxycoumarin metabolism. JAMA 197:366, 1966.
64. Schrogie JJ, et al: Effect of oral contraceptives on vitamin K-dependent clotting activity. Clin Pharmacol Ther 8:670, 1967.
65. Chatterjea JB, Salomon L: Antagonistic effect of ACTH and corti-

References (CONT.)

sone on the anticoagulant activity of ethyl biscoumacetate. Br Med J 2:790, 1954.

66. WEINER M: Effect of centrally active drugs on the action of coumarin anticoagulants. Nature 212:1599, 1966.

67. TAYLOR PJ: Hemorrhage while on anticoagulant therapy precipitated by drug interaction. Arizona Med 24:697, 1967.

68. MOSER KM, HAJJAR GC: Effect of heparin on the one-stage prothrombin time. Source of artifactual "resistance" to prothrombinopenic therapy. Ann Intern Med 66:1207, 1967.

69. SOLOMON HM, SCHROGIE JJ: Change in receptor site affinity: a proposed explanation for the potentiating effect of D-thyroxine on the anticoagulant response to warfarin. Clin Pharmacol Ther 8:797, 1967.

70. ROBINSON DS, SYLWESTER D: Interaction of commonly prescribed drugs and warfarin. Ann Intern Med 72:853, 1970.

71. AGGELER PM, et al: Potentiation of anticoagulant effect on warfarin by phenylbutazone. N Engl J Med 276:496, 1967.

72. BECKER GL: The case against mineral oil. Am J Dig Dis 19:344, 1952.

73. OAKLEY DP, LAUTCH H: Haloperidol and anticoagulant treatment (Letter). Lancet 2:1231, 1963.

74. HOFFBRAND BI, KININMONTH DA: Potentiation of anticoagulants (Letter). Br Med J 2:838, 1967.

75. HUNNINGHAKE DB, AZARNOFF DL: Drug interactions with warfarin. Arch Intern Med 121:349, 1968.

76. SELLERS EM, KOCH-WESER J: Protein binding and vascular activity of diazoxide. N Engl J Med 281:1141, 1969.

77. ANTLITZ AM, et al: Effect of butabarbital on orally administered anticoagulants. Curr Ther Res 10:70, 1968.

78. MacDONALD MG, ROBINSON DS: Clinical observations of possible barbiturate interference with anticoagulation. JAMA 204:97, 1968.

79. ANON: Today's Drugs. Mefenamic acid. Br Med J 2:1506, 1966.

80. FROST H, HESS H: Concomitant administration of indomethacin and anticoagulants, International Symposium on Inflammation, Freiburg Im Breisgau, Germany, May 4–6, 1966.

81. JOHANSSON S: Apparent resistance to oral anticoagulant therapy and influence of hypnotics on some coagulation factors. Acta Med Scand 184:297, 1968.

82. MacDONALD MG, et al: The effects of phenobarbital, chloral betaine, and glutethimide administration on warfarin plasma levels and hypoprothrombinemic responses in man. Clin Pharmacol Ther 10:80, 1969.

83. DRESDALE FC, HAYES JC: Potential dangers in the combined use of methandrostenolone and sodium warfarin. J Med Soc NJ 64:609, 1967.

84. LACKNER H, HUNT VE: The effect of Librium on hemostasis. Am J Med Sci 256:368, 1968.

85. ANTLITZ AM, et al: Potentiation of oral anticoagulant therapy by acetaminophen. Curr Ther Res 10:501, 1968.

86. ANTLITZ AM, AWALT, LF: A double blind study of acetaminophen used in conjunction with oral anticoagulant therapy. Curr Ther Res 11:360, 1969.

87. FLEISCHER N, et al: Chronic laxative-induced hyperaldosteronism

References (CONT.)

and hypokalemia simulating Bartter's syndrome. Ann Intern Med 70:791, 1969.

88. GOLDFINGER P: Hypokalemia, metabolic acidosis, and hypocalcemic tetany in a patient taking laxatives. J Mt Sinai Hosp 36:113, 1969.

89. HEIZER WD, et al: Protein-losing gastroenteropathy and malabsorption associated with factitious diarrhea. Ann Intern Med 68:839, 1968.

90. CHRISTENSEN LK, SKOVSTED L: Inhibition of drug metabolism by chloramphenicol. Lancet 2:1397, 1969.

91. GROSS I, BROTMAN M: Hypoprothrombinemia and hemorrhage associated with cholestyramine therapy. Ann Intern Med 72:95, 1970.

92. MARTIN WJ: Hemorrhagic diathesis induced by antimicrobials (Questions and Answers). JAMA 205:192, 1968.

93. FLIND AC: Cimetidine and oral anticoagulants (Letter). Br Med J 2:1367, 1978.

94. OWENS JC, et al: Effect of sodium dextrothyroxine in patients receiving anticoagulants. N Engl J Med 266:76, 1962.

95. ROTHSTEIN E: Warfarin effect enhanced by disulfiram (Letter). JAMA 206:1574, 1968.

96. GARRETTSON LK, et al: Methylphenidate interaction with both anticonvulsants and ethyl biscoumacetate. JAMA 207:2053, 1969.

97. MOROWITZ DA: Complications of long-term mineral oil intake. (Questions and Answers). JAMA 204:937, 1968.

98. SOLOMON HM, SCHROGIE JJ: The effect of phenyramidol on the metabolism of bishydroxycoumarin. J Pharmacol Exp Ther 154:660, 1966.

99. Editorial: Aspirin and gastrointestinal bleeding. JAMA 207:2430, 1969.

100. BARROW MV, et al: Salicylate hypoprothrombinemia in rheumatoid arthritis with liver disease. Arch Intern Med 120:620, 1967.

101. AGGELER PM, O'REILLY RA: Effect of heptabarbital on the response to bishydroxycoumarin in man. J Lab Clin Med 74:229, 1969.

102. LEWIS RJ: Effect of barbiturates on anticoagulant therapy (Letter). N Engl J Med 274:110, 1966.

103. GOSS JE, DICKHAUS DW: Increased bishydroxycoumarin requirements in patients receiving phenobarbital. N Engl J Med 273:1094, 1965.

104. SEARCY RL, et al: Evaluation of the blood-clotting mechanism in tetracycline-treated patients. Antimicrob Agents Chemother—1964. pp. 179–183, 1965.

105. CONNEY AH: Pharmacological implications of microsomal enzyme induction. Pharmacol Rev 19:317, 1967.

106. KOCH-WESER J: Potentiation of glucagon of the hypoprothrombinemic action of warfarin. Ann Intern Med 72:331, 1970.

107. WEINER M, MOSES D: The effect of glucagon and insulin on the prothrombin response to coumarin anticoagulants. Proc Soc Exp Biol Med 127:761, 1968.

108. CASDORPH HR: Safe uses of cholestyramine (Letter). Ann Intern Med 72:759, 1970.

109. O'REILLY RA, AGGELER PM: Determinants of the response to oral anticoagulant drugs in man. Pharmacol Rev 22:35, 1970.

110. SELLERS EM, KOCH-WESER J: Displacement of warfarin from human albumin by diazoxide and ethacrynic, mefenamic and nalidixic acids. Clin Pharmacol Ther 11:524, 1970.

References (CONT.)

111. Levy G, et al: Pharmacokinetic analysis of the effect of barbiturate on the anticoagulant action of warfarin in man. Clin Pharmacol Ther 11:372, 1970.
112. Welch RM, et al: An experimental model in dogs for studying interactions of drugs with bishydroxycoumarin. Clin Pharmacol Ther 10:817, 1969.
113. Koch-Weser J, Sellers EM: Drug interactions with coumarin anticoagulants (First of two parts). N Engl J Med 285:487, 1971.
114. Koch-Weser J, Sellers EM: Drug interactions with coumarin anticoagulants (Second of two parts). N Engl J Med 285:547, 1971.
115. Kleinman PD, Griner PF: Studies of the epidemiology of anticoagulant-drug interactions. Arch Intern Med 126:522, 1970.
116. Robinson BHB, et al: Decreased anticoagulant tolerance with oxymetholone (Letter). Lancet 1:1356, 1971.
117. Longridge RGM, et al: Decreased anticoagulant tolerance with oxymetholone (Letter). Lancet 2:90, 1971.
118. Edwards MS, Curtis JR: Decreased anticoagulant tolerance with oxymetholone (Letter). Lancet 2:221, 1971.
119. Casdorph HR: The efficacy and safety of cholestyramine therapy in hyperlipidemic patients (Abstract). Ann Intern Med 74:818, 1971.
120. Robinson DS, et al: Interaction of warfarin and nonsystemic gastrointestinal drugs. Clin Pharmacol Ther 12:491, 1971.
121. Lutz EE, Margolis AJ: Obstetric hepatosis: treatment with cholestyramine and interim response to steroids. Obstet Gynecol 33:64, 1969.
122. Anon: Scheduling avoids interaction problem (Medical News). JAMA 215:876, 1971.
123. Solomon HM, et al: Mechanisms of drug interactions. JAMA 216:1997, 1971.
124. Sellers EM, Koch-Weser J: Potentiation of warfarin-induced hypoprothrombinemia by chloral hydrate. N Engl J Med 283:827, 1970.
125. Griner PF, et al: Chloral hydrate and warfarin interaction: clinical significance? Ann Intern Med 74:540, 1971.
126. Weiner M: Species differences in the effect of chloral hydrate on coumarin anticoagulants. Ann NY Acad Sci 179:226, 1971.
127. Sellers EM, Koch-Weser J: Kinetics and clinical importance of displacement of warfarin from albumin by acidic drugs. Ann NY Acad Sci 179:213, 1971.
128. Boston Collaborative Drug Surveillance Program: Interaction between chloral hydrate and warfarin. N Engl J Med 286:53, 1972.
129. Rickles FR, Griner PF: Chloral hydrate and warfarin (Letter). N Engl J Med 286:611, 1972.
130. Anon: Chloral hydrate and oral anticoagulants. Lancet 1:524, 1972.
131. Udall JA: Chloral hydrate and warfarin therapy (Letter). Ann Intern Med 75:141, 1971.
132. Holmes EL: Pharmacology of the fenamates. IV. Toleration by normal human subjects. Ann Phys Med (Supplement) 9:36, 1967.
133. Hague DE, et al: The effect of methylphenidate and prolintane on the metabolism of ethyl biscoumacetate. Clin Pharmacol Ther 12:259, 1971.
134. Poucher RL, Vecchio TJ: Absence of tolbutamide effect on anticoagulant therapy. JAMA 197:1069, 1966.

References (CONT.)

135. O'REILLY RA, et al: Impact of aspirin and chlorthalidone on the pharmacodynamics of oral anticoagulant drugs in man. Ann NY Acad Sci 179:173, 1971.
136. FAUSA O: Salicylate-induced hypoprothrombinemia. A report of four cases. Acta Med Scand 188:403, 1970.
137. ANON: Aspirin and bleeding (Editorial). JAMA, 218:89, 1971.
138. O'BRIEN JR, et al: A comparison of an effect of different anti-inflammatory drugs on human platelets. J Clin Pathol 23:522, 1970.
139. HAMBLIN TJ: Interaction between warfarin and phenformin (Letter). Lancet 2:1323, 1971.
140. VAN CAUWENBERGE H, JAQUES LB: Haemorrhagic effect of ACTH with anticoagulants. Can Med Assoc J 79:536, 1958.
141. UDALL JA: Warfarin therapy not influenced by meprobamate. A controlled study in nine men. Curr Ther Res 12:724, 1970.
142. GOULD L, et al: Prothrombin levels maintained with meprobamate and warfarin. A controlled study. JAMA 220:1460, 1972.
143. DE OYA JC, et al: Decreased anticoagulant tolerance with oxymetholone in paroxysmal nocturnal haemoglobinuria (Letter). Lancet 2:259, 1971.
144. TALBOT JM, HEADE BW: Effect of silicones on the absorption of anticoagulant drugs (Letter). Lancet 1:1292, 1971.
145. MICHOT F, et al: Rimactan (Fifampizin) und Antikoagulatientherapie. Schweiz Med Wochenschr 100:583, 1970. (From De Haen, Drugs in Use, U7945/33).
146. KIBLAWI SS, et al: Influence of isoniazid on the anticoagulant effect of warfarin. Clin Ther 2:235, 1979.
147. BIEGER R, et al: Influence of nitrazepam on oral anticoagulation with phenprocoumon. Clin Pharmacol Ther 13:361, 1972.
148. HANSEN JM, et al: Carbamazepine-induced acceleration of diphenylhydantoin and warfarin metabolism in man. Clin Pharmacol Ther 12:539, 1971.
149. ROSENTHAL G: Interaction of ascorbic acid and warfarin (Letter). JAMA 215:1671, 1971.
150. HUME R, et al: Interaction of ascorbic acid and warfarin (Letter). JAMA 219:1479, 1972.
151. ROTHSTEIN E: Warfarin effect enhanced by disulfiram (Antabuse) (Letter). JAMA 22:1052, 1972.
152. O'REILLY RA: Potentiation of anticoagulant effect by disulfiram. Clin Res 19:180, 1971.
153. KOCH-WESER J: Hemorrhagic reactions and drug interactions in 500 warfarin-treated patients (Abstract). Clin Pharmacol Ther 14:139, 1973.
154. ZUCKER MB, PETERSON J: Effect of acetylsalicylic acid, other nonsteroidal antiinflammatory agents, and dipyridamole on human blood platelets. J Lab Clin Med 76:66, 1970.
155. SMITH EC, et al: Interaction of ascorbic acid and warfarin (Letter). JAMA 221:1166, 1972.
156. BOEKHOUT-MUSSERT MJ, LOELIGER EA: Influence of ibuprofen on oral anticoagulation with phenprocoumon. J Int Med Res 2:279, 1974.
157. O'REILLY RA: Interaction of sodium warfarin and rifampin. Studies in man. Ann Intern Med 81:337, 1974.
158. VESELL ES, et al: Failure of indomethacin and warfarin to interact in normal human volunteers. J Clin Pharmacol 15:486, 1975.

References (CONT.)

159. HOFFBRAND BI: Interaction of nalidixic acid and warfarin (Letter). Br Med J 2:666, 1974.

160. WARIS E: Effect of ethyl alcohol on some coagulation factors in man during anticoagulant therapy. Ann Med Exp Biol Fenn 41:45, 1963.

161. POND SM, et al: The effects of allopurinol and clofibrate on the elimination of coumarin anticoagulants in man. Aust NZ J Med 5:324, 1975.

162. SELF TH, et al: Drug-enhancement of warfarin activity (Letter). Lancet 2:557, 1975.

163. WEART CW: Coumarin and allopurinol—a drug interaction case report (Abstract). Contributed paper, 32nd annual meeting ASHP, 1975.

164. POND SM, et al: Effects of tricyclic antidepressants on drug metabolism. Clin Pharmacol Ther 18:191, 1975.

165. JUDIS J: Displacement of sulfonylureas from human serum proteins by coumarin derivatives and cortical steroids. J Pharm Sci 62:232, 1973.

166. UDALL JA: Clinical implications of warfarin interactions with five sedatives. Am J Cardiol 35:67, 1975.

167. UDALL JA: Warfarin-chloral hydrate interaction: pharmacological activity and clinical significance. Ann Intern Med 81:341, 1974.

168. GALINSKY RE, et al: "post hoc" and hypoprothrombinemia. Ann Intern Med 83:286, 1975.

169. DeCAROLIS PP, et al: Effect of tranquilizers on prothrombin time response to coumarin. J Clin Pharmacol 15:557, 1975.

170. CORRIGAN JJ, MARCUS PI: Coagulopathy associated with vitamin E ingestion. JAMA 230:1300, 1974.

171. PETRICK RJ, et al: Interaction between warfarin and ethacrynic acid. JAMA 231:843, 1975.

172. THILO D, et al: A study of the effects of the anti-rheumatic drug ibuprofen (brufen) on patients being treated with the oral anti-coagulant phenprocoumon (marcoumar). J Int Med Res 2:276, 1974.

173. MESSINGER WJ, et al: The effect of a bowel sterilizing antibiotic on blood coagulation mechanisms. Angiology 16:29, 1965.

174. LEWIS RJ, et al: Warfarin. Stereochemical aspects of its metabolism and the interaction with phenylbutazone. J Clin Invest 53:1607, 1974.

175. HRDINA P, et al: Effect of reserpine and some adrenolytics on the anticoagulant activity of pelentan (ethylbiscoumacetate). Thromb Diath Haemorrh 18:759, 1967.

176. SELF TH, et al: Interaction of rifampin and warfarin. Chest 67:490, 1975.

177. STENBJERG S, et al: A circulating factor V inhibitor: possible side effect of treatment with streptomycin. Scand J Haematol 14:280, 1975.

178. SELF TH, et al: Interaction of sulfisoxazole and warfarin. Circulation 52:528, 1975.

179. VARMA DL, et al: Prothrombin response to phenindione during hypoalbuminaemia (Letter). Br J Clin Pharmacol 2:467, 1975.

180. SELF T, et al: Warfarin-induced hypoprothrombinemia: potentiation by hyperthyroidism. JAMA 231:1165, 1975.

References (CONT.)

181. Edson JR, et al: Low platelet adhesiveness and other hemostatic abnormalities in hypothyroidism. Ann Intern Med 82:342, 1975.
182. Orme M, et al: Warfarin and distalgesic interaction. Br Med J 1:200, 1976.
183. Rawlins MD, Smith SE: Influence of allopurinal on drug metabolism in man. Br J Pharmacol 48:693, 1973.
184. Self TH, et al: Effect of hyperthyroidism on hypoprothrombinemic response to warfarin. Am J Hosp Pharm 33:387, 1976.
185. Hassall C, et al: Potentiation of warfarin by co-trimoxazole (Letter). Lancet 2:1155, 1975.
186. Bull J, MacKinnon J: Phenylbutazone and anticoagulant control. Practitioner 215:767, 1975.
187. Penner JA, Abbrecht PH. Lack of interaction between ibuprofen and warfarin. Curr Ther Res 18:862, 1975.
188. O'Reilly RA: Interaction of chronic daily warfarin therapy and rifampin. Ann Intern Med 83:506, 1975.
189. Boekhout-Mussert RJ, et al: Inhibition by rifampicin of the anticoagulant effect of phenprocoumon. JAMA 229:1903, 1974.
190. Chierichetti S, et al: Comparison of feprazone and phenylbutazone interaction with warfarin in man. Curr Ther Res 18:568, 1975.
191. Feetam CL, et al: Lack of a clinically important interaction between warfarin and ascorbic acid. Toxicol Appl Pharmacol 31:544, 1975.
192. Williams JRB, et al: Effect of concomitantly administered drugs on the control of long term anticoagulant therapy. Q J Med 45(No. 177):63, 1976.
193. McQueen EG: New Zealand Committee on adverse drug reactions: tenth annual report, 1975. NZ Med J 82:308, 1975.
194. Lumholtz B, et al: Sulfamethizole-induced inhibition of diphenylhydantoin, tolbutamide, and warfarin metabolism. Clin Pharmacol Ther 17:731, 1975.
195. O'Reilly RA: The stereoselective interaction of warfarin and metronidazole in man. N Engl J Med 295:354, 1976.
196. Ramankiewicz JA, Ehrman M: Rifampin and warfarin: a drug interaction. Ann Intern Med 82:224, 1975.
197. Jahnschen E, et al: Pharmacokinetic analysis of the interaction between dicumarol and tolbutamide in man. Eur J Clin Pharmacol 10:349, 1976.
198. Schade RWB, et al: A comparative study of the effects of cholestyramine and neomycin in the treatment of type II hyperlipoproteinaemia. Acta Med Scand 199:175–180, 1976.
199. Kazmier FJ: A significant interaction between metronidazole and warfarin. Mayo Clin Proc 51:782, 1976.
200. Jeffery WH, et al: Loss of warfarin effect after occupational insecticide exposure. JAMA 236:2881, 1976.
201. Bjornsson TD, et al: Interaction of clofibrate with warfarin: studies using radiolabeled vitamin K (Abstract). Clin Pharmacol Ther 21:99, 1977.
202. Orme M, Breckenridge A: Enantiomers of warfarin and phenobarbital (Letter). N Engl J Med 295:1482, 1976.
203. Husted S, et al: Increased sensitivity to phenprocoumon during methyltestosterone therapy. Eur J Clin Pharmacol 10:209, 1976.

References (CONT.)

204. HEINE P, et al: The influence of hypoglycaemic sulphonylureas on elimination and efficacy of phenprocoumon following a single oral dose in diabetic patients. Eur J Clin Pharmacol 10:31, 1976.
205. WEINTRAUB M, et al: The effects of dextrothyroxine on the kinetics of prothrombin activity: proposed mechanism of the potentiation of warfarin by D-thyroxine. J Lab Clin Med 81:273, 1973.
206. SCHROGIE, JJ, et al: Coagulopathy and fat-soluble vitamins (Letter). JAMA 232:19, 1975.
207. POWELL-JACKSON PR: Interaction between azapropazone and warfarin. Br Med J 1:1193, 1977.
208. VAN DOSTEROM AT, et al: The influence of the thyroid function on the metabolic rate of prothrombin, factor VII, and factor X in the rat. Thromb Haemost 3:607, 1976.
209. TEMPERO KF, et al: Diflunisal: a review of pharmacokinetic and pharmacodynamic properties, drug interactions, and special tolerability studies in humans. Br J Clin Pharmacol 4:31S, 1977.
210. BRECKENRIDGE A: Pathophysiological factors influencing drug kinetics. Acta Pharmacol Toxicol 29(Supplement 3):225, 1971.
211. SKOVSTED L, et al: The effect of different oral anticoagulants on diphenylhydantoin (DPH) and tolbutamide metabolism. Acta Med Scand 199:513, 1976.
212. MEINERTZ T, et al: Interruption of the enterohepatic circulation of phenprocoumon by cholestyramine. Clin Pharmacol Ther 21:731, 1977.
213. ANSELL JE, et al: The spectrum of vitamin K deficiency. JAMA 238:40, 1977.
214. FLETCHER DC: Do clotting factors in vitamin K-rich vegetables hinder anticoagulant therapy? (Questions and Answers) JAMA 237:1871, 1977.
215. QUICK A: Leafy vegetables in diet alter prothrombin time in patients taking anticoagulant drugs. JAMA 187:27, 1964.
216. MUSA MN, LYONS LL: Absorption and distribution of warfarin: effects of food and liquids. Curr Ther Res 20:630, 1976.
217. TALBOT JM, MEAD BW: Effect of silicones on the absorption of anticoagulant drugs. Lancet 1:1292, 1971.
218. McELNAY JC, D'ARCY PF: Interaction between azapropazone and warfarin (Letter). Br Med J 2:773, 1977.
219. MICHOT F, et al: A double-blind clinical trial to determine if an interaction exists between diclofenac sodium and the oral anticoagulant acenocoumarol (nicoamalone). J Int Med Res 3:153, 1975.
220. SPIERS ASD, MISBASHAN RS: Increased warfarin requirement during mercaptopurine therapy: a new drug interaction (Letter). Lancet 2:221, 1974.
221. ROSENTHAL, AR, et al: Interaction of isoniazid and warfarin. JAMA 238:2177, 1977.
222. TILSTONE WJ, et al: Interaction between warfarin and sulphamethoxazole. Postgrad Med J 53:388, 1977.
223. NILSSON CM, et al: The effect of furosemide and bumetanide on warfarin metabolism and anticoagulant response. J Clin Pharmacol 18:91, 1978.

References (CONT.)

224. Martini A, Jahnchen, E: Studies in rats on the mechanisms by which 6-mercaptopurine inhibits the anticoagulant effect of warfarin. J Pharmacol Exp Ther 201:547, 1977.
225. Jahnchen E, et al: Interaction of allopurinol with phenprocoumon in man. Klin Wschr 55:759, 1977.
226. Jahnchen E, et al: Enhanced elimination of warfarin during treatment with cholestyramine. Br J Clin Pharmacol 5:437, 1978.
227. Mungall D, et al: Effects of quinidine on serum digoxin concentration. Ann Intern Med 93:689, 1980.
228. Watson PG, et al: Drug interaction with coumarin derivative anticoagulants. Br Med J 285:1045, 1982.
229. Goenen M, et al: A case of candida albicans endocarditis 3 years after an aortic valve replacement. Successful combined medical and surgical therapy. J Cardiovasc Surg 18:391, 1977.
230. Deresinski SC, et al: Miconazole treatment of human coccidioidomycosis: status report. In Ajello L (Ed) Coccidioidomycosis: Current Clinical and Diagnostic Status. Proceedings of the Third International Coccidioidomycosis Symposium, Tucson, Arizona, November 1976. Miami, Symposia Specialists, 1977:267–92.
231. Sumner HW, et al: Drug induced liver disease. Geriatrics 36:83, 1981.
232. Boeijinga JJ, et al: Interaction between paracetamol and coumarin anticoagulants. Lancet 1:506, 1982.
233. Serlin MJ, et al: Interaction between difusinal and warfarin. Clin Pharmacol Ther 28:493, 1980.
234. Davies RO: Review of the animal and clinical pharmacology of diflunisal. Pharmacotherapy 3(Supp 1):9S, 1983.
235. Rider JA: Comparison of fecal blood loss after use of aspirin and diflunisal. Pharmacotherapy 3(Supp 1):61S, 1983.
236. Green D, et al: Effects of diflunisal on platelet function and fetal blood loss. Clin Pharmacol Ther 30:378, 1981.
237. Petrillo M: Diflunisal, aspirin, and gastric mucosa. Lancet 2:638, 1979.
238. Ghosh ML, et al: Platelet aggregation in patients treated with diflunisal. Curr Med Res Opin 6:510, 1980.
239. Admani AK, et al: Gastrointestinal haemorrhage associated with diflunisal. Lancet 1:1247, 1979.
240. Rubin A, et al: Physiological disposition of fenoprofen in man. J Pharmacol Exp Ther 183:449, 1972.
241. Self TH, et al: Possible interaction of indomethacin and warfarin. Drug Intell Clin Pharm 12:580, 1978.
242. AMA Drug Evaluations: 5th Ed. American Medical Association, 1983, p. 123. Chicago, Illinois.
243. Meclomen: Product Information, 1983.
244. Jain A, et al: Effect of haproxen on the steady-state serum concentration and anticoagulants of warfarin. Clin Pharmacol Ther 25:61, 1979.
245. Slattery JT, et al: Effect of naproxen on the kinetics of elimination and anticoagulant activity of single dose warfarin. Clin Pharmacol Ther 25:51, 1979.

References (CONT.)

246. O'REILLY RA: Phenylbutazone and sulfinpyrazone interaction with oral anticoagulant phenprocoumon. Arch Int Med 142:1634, 1982.
247. O'REILLY RA, et al: Comparative interaction of sulfinpyrazone and phenylbutazone with racemic warfarin: alteration in vivo of free fraction of plasma warfarin. J Pharmacol Exp Ther 219:691, 1981.
248. O'REILLY RA, et al: Stereoselective interaction of phenylbutazone with [$^{12}C/^{13}C$] warfarin pseudoracemates in man. J Clin Invest 6S:746, 1980.
249. DAHL SL: Pharmacology, clinical efficacy, and adverse effects of piroxicam, a new nonsteroidal antiinflammatory agent. Pharmacotherapy 2:80, 1982.
250. EMERGY P: Gastrointestinal blood loss and piroxicam. Lancet 1:1302, 1982.
251. CHESEBRO JH, et al: Trial of combined warfarin plus dipyridamole or ASA therapy in prosthetic heart valve replacement: Danger of ASA compared with Dipyridamole. Am J Cardiol 51:1537, 1983.
252. DONALDSON DR, et al: Assessment of the interaction of warfarin with aspirin and dipyridamole. Thromb Haemostas 47:77, 1982.
253. TRUNET P, et al: The role of iatrogenic disease in admissions to intensive care. JAMA 244:2617, 1980.
254. LOFTIN JP: Interaction between sulindac and warfarin: Different results in normal subjects and in an unusual patient with a potassium-losing renal tubular defect. J Clin Pharmacol 19:733, 1979.
255. ROSS JRY, et al: Sublindac, prothrombin time, and anticoagulants. Lancet 2:1075, 1979.
256. CARTER SA: Potential effect of sulindac on response of prothrombin-time to oral anticoagulants. Lancet 2:698, 1979.
257. PULLAR T: Interaction between oral anti-coagulant drugs and non-steroidal anti-inflammatory agents: A review. Scot Med J 28:42, 1983.
258. McINNES GT, et al: Acute adverse reactions attributed to allopurinol in hospitalized patients. Ann Rheum Dis 40:245, 1981.
259. O'REILLY RA: Lack of effect of mealtime wine on the hypoprothrombinemia of oral anticoagulants. Am J Med Sci 277:189, 1979.
260. O'REILLY RA: Lack of effect of fortified wine ingested during fasting and anticoagulant therapy. Arch Intern Med 141:458, 1981.
261. REMMEL RP, ELMER GW: The effect of broad-spectrum antibiotics on warfarin excretion and metabolism in the rat. Res Commun Chem Pathol Pharmacol 34:503, 1981.
262. RODRIGUEZ-ERDMANN F, et al: Interaction of antibiotics with vitamin K. JAMA 246:937, 1981.
263. WEIBERT RT, McQUADE SE: Potentiation of warfarin anticoagulation by topical testosterone ointment. Midyear Clinical Meeting Abstracts, American Society of Clinical Pharmacists, Los Angeles, December 1982, p. 134.
264. LOOMIS CW, RACZ WJ: Drug interactions of amitriptyline and nortriptyline with warfarin in the rat. Res Commun Chem Pathol Pharmacol 30:41, 1980.
265. KOPERA H, et al: Phenprocoumon requirement, whole blood coagulation time, bleeding time and plasma gamma- GT in patients receiving mianserin. Eur J Clin Pharmacol 13:351, 1978.

266. O'REILLY RA, et al: Interaction of secobarbital with warfarin pseudoracemates. Clin Pharmacol Ther 28:187, 1980.
267. NIPPER H, et al: The effect of bumetanide on the serum disappearance of warfarin sodium. J Clin Pharmacol 21:654, 1981.
268. KENDALL AG, BOIVIN M: Warfarin-carbamazepine interaction. Ann Intern Med 94:280, 1981.
269. DE TERESA E, et al: Interaction between anticoagulants and contraceptives: An unexpected finding. Br Med J 2:1260, 1979.
270. GOULBOURNE IA, MACLEOD DAD: An interaction between danazol and warfarin. Case report. Br J Obstet Gynaecol 88:950, 1981.
271. SMALL M, et al: Danazol and oral anticoagulants. Scott Med J 27:331, 1982.
272. O'REILLY RA: Dynamic interaction between disulfiram and separated enantiomorphs of racemic warfarin. Clin Pharmacol Ther 29:332, 1981.
273. SCHWARTZ J, et al: Interaction between warfarin and erythromycin. South Med J 1983; 76:91.
274. FRIEDMAN HS, BONVENTRE MV: Erythromycin-induced digoxin toxicity. Chest 82:202, 1982.
275. BARTLE WR: Possible warfarin-erythromycin interaction. Arch Intern Med 140:985, 1980.
276. TASHIMA CK: Cyclophosphamide effect on coumarin anticoagulation. South Med J 72:633, 1979.
277. O'REILLY RA: Spironolactone and warfarin interaction. Clin Pharmacol Ther 27:198, 1980.
278. WEISS M: Potentiation of coumarin effect by sulfinpyrazone. Lancet 1:609, 1979.
279. JAMIL A, et al: Interaction between sulphinpyrazone and warfarin. Chest 79:373, 1981.
280. BAILEY RR, REDDY J: Potentiation of warfarin action by sulphinpyrazone. Lancet 1:254, 1980.
281. DAVIS JW, JOHNS LE: Possible interaction of sulfinpyrazone with coumarins. N Engl J Med 299:955, 1978.
282. GALLUS A, BIRKETT D: Sulphinpyrazone and warfarin: a probable drug interaction. Lancet 1:535, 1980.
283. THOMPSON PL, SERJEANT C: Potentially serious interaction of warfarin with sulfinpyrazone. Med J Aust 1:41, 1981.
284. NENCI GG, et al: Biphasic sulphinpyrazone-warfarin interaction. Br Med J 282:1361, 1981.
285. O'REILLY RA: Stereoselective interaction of sulfinpyrazone with racemic warfarin and its separated enantiomorphs in man. Circulation 65:202, 1982.
286. GIROLAMI A, et al: Potentiation of anticoagulant response to warfarin by sulphinpyrazone: a double-blind study in patients with prosthetic heart values. Clin Lab Haematol 4:23, 1982.
287. MICHOT F, et al: Uber die beeinflussung der gerinnungshemmenden wirkung von acenocoumarol durch sulfinpurazon. Schweiz Med Wochenschr 111:255, 1981.
288. O'REILLY RA: Phenylbutazone and sulfinpurazone interaction with oral anticoagulant phenprocoumon. Arch Intern Med 142:1634, 1982.

References (CONT.)

289. SERLIN MJ, et al: Cimetidine: Interactions with oral anticoagulants in man. Lancet 2:317, 1979.
290. PUURUNEN J, et al: Effect of cimetidine on microsomal drug metabolism in man. Eur J Clin Pharmacol 18:185, 1980.
291. KERLEY B, ALI M: Cimetidine potentiation of warfarin action. Can Med Assoc J 126:116, 1982.
292. SERLIN MJ, et al: Lack of effect of ranitidine on warfarin action. Br J Clin Pharmacol 12:791, 1981.
293. O'REILLY RA: Comparative interaction of cimetidine and ranitidine with racemic warfarin in man. Fed Proc 42:1175, 1983.
294. HARENBERG J, et al: Lack of effect of cimetidine on action of phenprocoumon. Eur J Clin Pharmacol 23:365, 1982.
295. OTIS PT, et al: An acquired inhibitor of fibrin stabilization associated with isoniazid therapy: clinical and biochemical observations. Blood 44:771, 1974.
296. DEAN RP, TALBERT RL: Bleeding associated with concurrent warfarin and metronidazole therapy. Drug Intell Clin Pharm 14:864, 1980.
297. POTASMAN I, BASSAN H: Nicoumalone and nalidixic acid interaction. Ann Intern Med 92:572, 1980.
298. NAPPI JM: Warfarin and phenytoin interaction. Ann Intern Med 90:852, 1979.
299. TAYLOR JW, et al: Oral anticoagulant-phenytoin interactions. Drug Intell Clin Pharm 14:669, 1980.
300. JONES RV: Warfarin and distalgesic interaction. Br Med J 1:460, 1976.
301. Fox P: Warfarin-rifampicin interaction. Med J Aust 1:60, 1982.
302. KAUFMAN JM, FAUVER HE: Potentiation of warfarin by trimethoprim-sulfamethoxazole. Urology 16:601, 1980.
303. ERRICK JK, KEYES PW: Co-trimoxazole and warfarin: case report of an interaction. Am J Hosp Pharm 35:1399, 1978.
304. GREENLAW CW: Drug interaction between co-trimoxazole and warfarin. Am J Hosp Pharm 36:1155, 1979.
305. O'REILLY RA, MOTLEY CH: Racemic warfarin and trimethoprim-sulfamethoxazole interaction in humans. Ann Intern Med 91:34, 1979.
306. O'REILLY RA: Stereoselective interaction of trimethoprim-sulfamethoxazole with the separated enantiomorphs of racemic warfarin in man. N Engl J Med 302:33, 1980.
307. WESTFALL LK, et al: Potentiation of warfarin by tetracycline. Am J Hosp Pharm 37:1620, 1980.
308. REMMEL RP, ELMER GW: The effect of broad-spectrum antibiotics on warfarin excretion and metabolism in the rat. Res Comm Chem Pathol Pharmacol 34:503, 1981.
309. ANON: Vitamin K, vitamin E and the coumarin drugs. Nutr Rev 40:180, 1982.
310. KRAMER P, et al: Effect of influenza vaccine on warfarin anticoagulation. Clin Pharmacol Ther 35:416, 1984.
311. LIPSKY BA, et al: Influenza vaccination and warfarin anticoagulation. Ann Intern Med 100:835, 1984.

CHAPTER 3

Anticonvulsant (General) Interactions

ANTICONVULSANT (GENERAL) INTERACTIONS

DRUGS	DISCUSSION

Antidepressants, Tricyclic[64,84–86,178]

MECHANISM: Tricyclic antidepressants may produce seizures in susceptible patients, especially if large doses are used. High doses may produce seizures even in nonepileptic patients. The effects of tricyclic antidepressants on phenytoin disposition have been conflicting,[86,178] but it appears that increased serum phenytoin levels may occasionally occur[178] (see Phenytoin plus Antidepressants, Tricyclic).

CLINICAL SIGNIFICANCE: Administration of tricyclic antidepressants to predisposed patients has been associated with seizures, in some cases necessitating an increase in anticonvulsant dosage. Factors which reportedly predispose patients to tricyclic antidepressant-induced epileptic seizures include family history of epilepsy, brain damage, cerebral arteriosclerosis, alcoholism, barbiturate withdrawal, and previous electroconvulsive therapy.[64] However, in some seizure-prone individuals tricyclic antidepressants appear to *reduce* seizure activity. It has been proposed that this beneficial response may be due to reduction of depression-induced cerebral excitability.[84] In summary, tricyclic antidepressants have been associated with increased seizure activity in several reports, and occasionally have been associated with reduced seizure activity.

MANAGEMENT: It does not appear necessary to avoid the use of tricyclic antidepressants in epileptic patients controlled on anticonvulsants. However, such patients should be watched more closely for decreased epileptic control when tricyclic antidepressant therapy is initiated.

Contraceptives, Oral[1,50,55,62,63,89,103,107,111,179]

MECHANISM:
A. Effect of oral contraceptives on anticonvulsants: It has been proposed that oral-contraceptive-induced fluid retention could precipitate seizures.[63] It has also been proposed that contraceptive steroids may affect plasma protein binding of anticonvulsants,[62] but Hooper and associates[1] could not find any effect of oral contraceptives on the plasma protein binding of diphenylhydantoin. Finally, it has been proposed that estrogens may inhibit phenytoin metabolism.[50]

ANTICONVULSANT (GENERAL) INTERACTIONS (CONT.)

B. Effect of anticonvulsants on oral contraceptives: Anticonvulsant-induced enzyme induction may enhance the metabolism of oral contraceptives.

CLINICAL SIGNIFICANCE:
A. Effect of oral contraceptives on anticonvulsants: One case of possible oral contraceptive-induced epilepsy has been reported in a patient receiving phenytoin and phenobarbital.[63] However, in another study of 20 epileptics (most of whom were receiving phenytoin), oral contraceptives did not appear to affect seizure frequency compared to placebo.[62] Kutt[50] reports that he found rare clinical cases of estrogen-induced inhibition of phenytoin metabolism, but the incidence and magnitude of this effect cannot be determined with the data presented.

B. Effect of anticonvulsants on oral contraceptives: A few reports have appeared describing unplanned pregnancies in epileptics on anticonvulsants who were taking oral contraceptives correctly.[89,103,107] In a subsequent retrospective study, three of 41 women developed unwanted pregnancy while on oral contraceptives and anticonvulsants, while none of the epileptics on oral contraceptives alone became pregnant.[179] Although these pregnancies could have been merely coincidence, a more likely explanation is that the anticonvulsants were responsible for the diminished contraceptive effect.

MANAGEMENT: Although evidence for an interaction is scanty, one might be alert for increased seizure activity or phenytoin toxicity in patients receiving oral contraceptives and phenytoin concomitantly. If it is important to avoid pregnancy in epileptics receiving enzyme-inducing anticonvulsants such as phenobarbital, phenytoin, or primidone, it would be prudent to use other means of contraception instead of or in addition to oral contraceptives. Patients who are taking oral contraceptives and enzyme-inducing anticonvulsants should be aware that spotting or breakthrough bleeding is an indication that the interaction is occurring.

CARBAMAZEPINE INTERACTIONS

Barbiturates[16,112]

MECHANISM: It has been proposed that phenobarbital may stimulate the metabolism of carbamazepine by hepatic microsomal enzymes.[16]

CLINICAL SIGNIFICANCE: In a study of 123 patients receiving carbamazepine, those patients who were also receiving phenobarbital tended to have lower plasma levels of carbamazepine (mean, 5.5 mg/L) than those who received carbamazepine alone (mean, 6.7 mg/L).[16] Similar differences in plasma levels of carbamazepine were found in a group of 43 children.[112] Those on carbamazepine alone had higher carbamazepine plasma levels than those receiving carbamazepine

DRUGS	DISCUSSION

plus other anticonvulsants (usually phenobarbital and/or phenytoin). The clinical significance of this effect is not clear at this time but would not appear to be great, since the anticonvulsant effect of the barbiturate may more than offset any decrease in plasma carbamazepine levels.

MANAGEMENT: No special precautions appear necessary.

Clonazepam[120]

MECHANISM: None.

CLINICAL SIGNIFICANCE: Study in epileptic patients receiving carbamazepine indicates that clonazepam does not affect carbamazepine serum levels.[120]

MANAGEMENT: No precautions appear necessary.

Erythromycin[146,147]

MECHANISM: Erythromycin probably inhibits the hepatic metabolism of carbamazepine.

CLINICAL SIGNIFICANCE: In eight healthy nonsmokers erythromycin 250 mg orally every 6 hours for 5 days before and 3 days after a single 400 mg dose of carbamazepine reduced the clearance of carbamazepine by 5% to 41%.[146] This is consistent with previous observations of possible carbamazepine toxicity in patients given erythromycin.[147]

MANAGEMENT: Patients receiving carbamazepine and erythromycin should be monitored for evidence of carbamazepine toxicitity (e.g., dizziness, drowsiness, nausea), and carbamazepine dosage reduced as necessary.

Isoniazid (INH)[154–156]

MECHANISM: Isoniazid probably inhibits carbamazepine metabolism. It has also been proposed that carbamazepine stimulates the production of hepatotoxic isoniazid metabolites.

CLINICAL SIGNIFICANCE: A patient receiving carbamazepine (1.0 g/ day) developed serum levels of 5 to 6 mg/ml. After 5 days of therapy with isoniazid (300 mg/day), symptoms of carbamazepine toxicity such as ataxia, headaches, drowsiness, vomiting, and a serum carbamazepine level of 15 mcg/ml were noted.[154] When isoniazid was discontinued, these symptoms subsided within 2 days; after 1 week the serum carbamazepine level had decreased to 6.1 mcg/ml. In another study, ten of 13 patients on carbamazepine developed symptoms of carbamazepine toxicity (disorientation, ataxia, lethargy, drowsiness) following initiation of isoniazid prophylaxis.[155] The toxicity subsided when the carbamazepine dose was reduced. Although serum carbamazepine levels were measured in only three of the patients with toxicity, elevated levels were found in each. In another report, isoniazid

DRUGS	DISCUSSION

300 mg bid was initiated in a patient who was receiving carbamazepine 400 mg qid. Within 24 hours of initiating the isoniazid, the patient developed headache, drowsiness, and nausea; by the second day he was in a stupor. Serum carbamazepine levels were 5 to 8 mg/ml prior to the initiation of isoniazid therapy and 18 to 22 mg/ml by the second and third day of the isoniazid therapy. Following the discontinuation of isoniazid, the patient was able to take the same dose of carbamazepine without toxicity. Subsequent study in this patient indicated that 300 mg/day of isoniazid reduced carbamazepine clearance by 45% and increased the serum concentration of carbamazepine. A daily dose of 150 mg had little effect. Liver enzymes, which were increased when this patient was receiving carbamazepine and 300 mg/day of isoniazid, were attributed to carbamazepine induction of hepatic microsomal enzymes, thus increasing the production of hepatotoxic isoniazid metabolites. In summary, there is substantial evidence that isoniazid increases serum carbamazepine levels and toxicity in most patients. The interaction is more likely to occur with isoniazid doses of 200 mg/day or more, and carbamazepine toxicity may occur within the first day or two of isoniazid therapy. Data are too limited to assess the likelihood of increased isoniazid hepatotoxicity in the presence of carbamazepine.

MANAGEMENT: Isoniazid is likely to reduce the dosage requirements for carbamazepine in a majority of patients. Watch for symptoms of carbamazepine toxicity (e.g., dizziness, drowziness, nausea, vomiting, ataxia, headache, nystagmus, blurred vision), and monitor serum carbamazepine concentrations if possible.

Lithium Carbonate[151-153]

MECHANISM: Not established.

CLINICAL SIGNIFICANCE: Five of ten patients on chronic lithium therapy developed symptoms such as ataxia, dizziness, confusion, and restlessness within a few days of starting carbamazepine in a dose of 300 to 600 mg/day.[151] Similar symptoms occurred in another patient on the combination of lithium and carbamazepine but not with either drug alone.[152] However, the combination has also been reported to produce favorable effects: in three patients acute manic symptoms improved on the combination but not on either drug alone.[153] It is possible that carbamazepine increases the effect of lithium, producing toxicity in some patients and improved response in others.

MANAGEMENT: One should be alert for evidence of lithium toxicity if carbamazepine is given concurrently. It is not yet established whether plasma lithium levels are useful in monitoring this interaction since the carbamazepine might increase the effect of lithium without increasing plasma lithium concentration.

Phenytoin (Dilantin)[16,79,88,112,121,144]

MECHANISM: Carbamazepine appears to enhance phenytoin metabolism by induction of hepatic microsomal enzymes.

CARBAMAZEPINE INTERACTIONS (CONT.)

CLINICAL SIGNIFICANCE: In a preliminary study, carbamazepine appeared to decrease serum phenytoin levels in three of seven patients.[79] In another part of this study, all of five patients manifested decreases in phenytoin half-life as measured by an intravenous dose of phenytoin before and during carbamazepine therapy (600 mg daily). Others have apparently also found lowered phenytoin serum levels in the presence of carbamazepine.[144] In other studies, carbamazepine serum levels have been lower when phenytoin or other anticonvulsants have been given concomitantly as compared to carbamazepine given alone.[16,88,112] Thus, in a patient receiving both drugs, the potential exists for decreased plasma levels of both phenytoin[79] and carbamazepine.[16] The clinical consequences of these effects remain to be determined, but probably will not prove to be great.

MANAGEMENT: No special precautions appear necessary, but this information should be kept in mind when evaluating phenytoin or carbamazepine serum levels in patients on both drugs.

Propoxyphene (Darvon)[127,180,181]

MECHANISM: It is proposed that propoxyphene inhibits the oxidative metabolism of carbamazepine.

CLINICAL SIGNIFICANCE: Following clinical observations suggestive of interaction, seven patients on carbamazepine were given propoxyphene (65 mg three times daily).[127] Plasma carbamazepine levels measured after propoxyphene were considerably higher than before, and signs of carbamazepine toxicity appeared in some of the patients. In another study of six patients on chronic carbamazepine therapy (600 to 800 mg/day), addition of propoxyphene (65 mg three times a day) increased serum carbamazepine levels in all patients (mean increase, 66%).[180] Another report describes a patient who developed 200% to 300% increases in serum carbamazepine levels following propoxyphene.[181] In summary, the evidence is substantial that propoxyphene can elevate serum carbamazepine, and the effect seems to occur in most patients receiving the combination.

MANAGEMENT: Although concomitant use of carbamazepine and propoxyphene is not contraindicated, it would seem prudent to use analgesics other than propoxyphene in carbamazepine-treated patients when possible. If the combination is used, special attention should be directed toward detection of excessive carbamazepine levels.

Troleandomycin (TAO)[125,182]

MECHANISM: It is proposed that troleandomycin (TAO) inhibits the metabolism of carbamazepine.

CLINICAL SIGNIFICANCE: Eight patients maintained on carbamazepine developed apparent signs of carbamazepine intoxication within 24 hours of starting TAO therapy.[125] Plasma carbamazepine levels measured in two of the patients were consistent with the suggestion that

CARBAMAZEPINE INTERACTIONS (CONT.)

DRUGS	DISCUSSION

the adverse reactions represented carbamazepine toxicity. In another study of epileptic patients receiving carbamazepine, troleandomycin (8 to 33 mg/kg body weight/day) was associated with increased plasma carbamazepine levels and evidence of carbamazepine toxicity.[182]

MANAGEMENT: Although concomitant use of carbamazepine and TAO is not contraindicated, it would seem prudent to use antibiotics other than TAO in carbamazepine-treated patients when possible. Since erythromycin is closely related to TAO, one should be alert for increased carbamazepine serum levels if either of these antibiotics is used. Evidence of carbamazepine toxicity includes drowsiness, nausea, vomiting, and dizziness.

CLONAZEPAM INTERACTIONS

DRUGS	DISCUSSION

Barbiturates[120]

MECHANISM: None.

CLINICAL SIGNIFICANCE: Study in epileptic patients receiving barbiturates indicates that clonazepam does not affect barbiturate serum levels.[120]

MANAGEMENT: No precautions appear necessary.

Phenytoin (Dilantin)[120,121]

MECHANISM: None proposed.

CLINICAL SIGNIFICANCE: Study in epileptic patients receiving phenytoin indicated that clonazepam did not affect phenytoin serum levels.[120] In another study, short-term therapy with clonazepam and valproate reportedly was associated with increased phenytoin levels,[121] but it does not seem likely that clonazepam was responsible.

MANAGEMENT: No special precautions appear necessary.

Primidone (Mysoline)[121]

MECHANISM: None proposed.

CLINICAL SIGNIFICANCE: Clonazepam has reportedly been associated with increased serum levels of primidone in epileptic patients,[121] but no details were given.

MANAGEMENT: No special precautions appear necessary.

PHENYTOIN INTERACTIONS

Acetaminophen (Tylenol)[157,158]

MECHANISM: Phenytoin appears to enhance the metabolism of acetaminophen.

CLINICAL SIGNIFICANCE: Patients on combination anticonvulsant therapy (including phenytoin) tend to have reduced acetaminophen bioavailability and half-life.[157] Although little clinical evidence is available, one might expect that phenytoin would tend to increase the hepatotoxicity of acetaminophen overdoses by increasing the production of toxic acetaminophen metabolites. Acetaminophen (1.5 g/day) did not significantly affect serum phenytoin levels in nine epileptic patients on chronic phenytoin therapy.[158]

MANAGEMENT: Until more is known about this interaction, large doses of acetaminophen should be administered with caution to patients on phenytoin.

Acetazolamide (Diamox)[97,128,129]

MECHANISM: Several mechanisms for enhanced anticonvulsant osteomalacia due to acetazolamide have been proposed.[97,129] Among these are acetazolamide-induced increases in urinary excretion of calcium and phosphate, and the tendency of acetazolamide to cause systemic acidosis.

CLINICAL SIGNIFICANCE: Several patients have been described in whom acetazolamide administration appeared to accelerate anticonvulsant osteomalacia.[97,129] In two patients with severe osteomalacia, discontinuation of acetazolamide was associated with a considerable decrease in the rate of urinary calcium excretion.[129] Although more evidence is certainly needed, the clinical and biochemical evidence available to date suggest that acetazolamide can worsen anticonvulsant-induced osteomalacia.

MANAGEMENT: In patients receiving acetazolamide (or other carbonic anhydrase inhibitors) in addition to anticonvulsants such as phenytoin, phenobarbital, primidone, special attention should be given to early detection of osteomalacia. If osteomalacia does occur under these conditions, discontinuation of the acetazolamide and replacement of any phosphate or vitamin D deficiencies may be beneficial.[97,129]

Allopurinol (Zyloprim)[165]

MECHANISM: Allopurinol may inhibit the hepatic metabolism of phenytoin.

CLINICAL SIGNIFICANCE: Allopurinol appeared to inhibit the metabolism of phenytoin in one patient,[165] but the incidence and magnitude of this purported interaction remains to be established. Allopurinol is known to inhibit the hepatic metabolism of other drugs, so it would not be surprising to find that phenytoin is also affected.

DRUGS	DISCUSSION

MANAGEMENT: Until more information is available, one should be alert for evidence of enhanced phenytoin effect (e.g., nystagmus, ataxia, mental impairment) if allopurinol is given concurrently.

Aminosalicylic Acid (PAS)[42,43,68]

MECHANISM: It has been proposed that PAS may inhibit phenytoin metabolism, but it is possible that it only increases the blood levels of concomitantly administered isoniazid, which in turn impairs phenytoin metabolism.

CLINICAL SIGNIFICANCE: More study of patients receiving PAS and phenytoin in the absence of isoniazid is needed to assess clinical significance. From current evidence, it does not appear likely that PAS alone has much effect on phenytoin metabolism.

MANAGEMENT: PAS is generally used in combination with isoniazid, an agent known to enhance phenytoin blood levels. If PAS is used alone with phenytoin, no special precautions appear to be necessary.

Antacids[166–169]

MECHANISM: There is some evidence that antacids may impair the gastrointestinal absorption of phenytoin.

CLINICAL SIGNIFICANCE: Some studies have found that antacids impair the gastrointestinal absorption of phenytoin.[166,167] but this has not been substantiated by other reports.[168,169] If the interaction does occur, it is probably only under certain specific circumstances of dose, type of antacid, and proximity of the doses of antacid and phenytoin.

MANAGEMENT: Although most patients are likely to be unaffected, one should be alert for evidence of reduced phenytoin effect in the presence of antacid therapy.

Antidepressants, Tricyclic[86,178]

MECHANISM: Limited evidence indicates that imipramine may inhibit phenytoin metabolism.

CLINICAL SIGNIFICANCE: A preliminary study in three subjects found that amitriptyline did not affect phenytoin disposition.[86] However, two patients were subsequently described in whom imipramine, 75 mg daily, was associated with an increase in serum phenytoin.[178] In one of the patients discontinuation of valproic acid therapy may have contributed to the increase in serum phenytoin, but in both patients serum phenytoin levels decreased when the imipramine was discontinued. Additional study is needed to determine if this interaction is real.

MANAGEMENT: Until more is known, one should be alert for evidence of increased phenytoin effect if a tricyclic antidepressant is used concurrently.

DRUGS	DISCUSSION

Antihistamines[145]

MECHANISM: It has been proposed that chlorpheniramine may inhibit the metabolism of phenytoin, but this is conjecture.

CLINICAL SIGNIFICANCE: A patient developed phenytoin intoxication (plasma level over 60 mcg/ml) following concomitant administration of chlorpheniramine (12 mg/day) and phenytoin (300 mg/day).[145] A causal relationship between the chlorpheniramine administration and the toxic levels of phenytoin is possible but additional study is needed.

MANAGEMENT: It does not seem necessary to avoid concomitant use of phenytoin and chlorpheniramine. However, one should be alert for evidence of enhanced phenytoin plasma levels when antihistamines such as chlorpheniramine are given concurrently.

Barbiturates[2,12–15,47,51,52,54,56,71–77,118,130]

MECHANISM: Phenobarbital administration results in induction of hepatic microsomal enzymes, with resultant increase in phenytoin metabolism. However, phenobarbital also appears to competitively inhibit the metabolism of phenytoin. With normal doses of phenobarbital, the enzyme induction would occur, but the competitive inhibition would be negligible. Large doses of phenobarbital, and perhaps normal doses in patients with impaired liver function, may elevate serum phenytoin levels. A detailed description of these mechanisms has been published.[15]

CLINICAL SIGNIFICANCE: An increase in phenytoin blood levels to toxic concentrations following discontinuation of phenobarbital has been reported briefly in one case[71] and confirmed in other patients.[76] A number of studies have shown decreased phenytoin blood levels with concomitant phenobarbital administration. However, it has also been noted that phenytoin blood levels do not change in some patients, and may even increase in some. This is probably a function of differences in the relative influence of the two mechanisms just described, as well as a number of other variables. Patients with relatively "saturated" phenytoin-metabolizing enzymes appear most likely to manifest increased serum phenytoin levels following barbiturate administration. The ability of phenobarbital to induce the metabolism of phenytoin would depend on previous drug therapy. Other drugs may have already maximally induced the microsomal enzymes. The ability of phenobarbital to inhibit phenytoin competitively would depend on the dose of phenobarbital, with average doses having a minimal inhibiting effect. There is also clinical evidence to indicate that phenytoin may increase phenobarbital plasma levels,[76,130] but this increase may benefit some patients by increasing control of seizures. Finally, the combination of phenytoin and phenobarbital may be more likely to cause osteomalacia than either agent alone.[14]

MANAGEMENT: Epileptic patients who manifest decreases in phenytoin blood levels due to phenobarbital administration do not appear to be adversely affected clinically, and no action is required. Some patients receiving phenytoin as an antiarrhythmic might manifest clinically significant decreases in serum phenytoin, but this remains to be shown. Large doses of phenobarbital should probably be avoided in patients with high blood levels of phenytoin, especially if signs of intoxication are present. Patients maintained on phenytoin and a barbiturate should be observed for signs of phenytoin intoxication if the barbiturate therapy is stopped.

Benzodiazepines[3,50,55,69,70,87,131–133]

MECHANISM: It has been proposed that benzodiazepines such as diazepam (Valium), chlordiazepoxide (Librium), and nitrazepam alter phenytoin metabolism. Also phenytoin may enhance the metabolism of benzodiazepines.[133]

CLINICAL SIGNIFICANCE: Data from one study indicate that patients receiving phenytoin with either diazepam or chlordiazepoxide may have higher phenytoin blood levels than patients on phenytoin therapy without either of the other drugs.[3] Others have also noted high phenytoin plasma levels when diazepam or chlordiazepoxide[50] is given concomitantly. Finally, a case of phenytoin toxicity has been reported in which a drug similar to diazepam, nitrazepam, might have contributed to the high phenytoin plasma levels.[70] However, at least two studies have indicated that benzodiazepines may actually *decrease* serum phenytoin levels.[131,132] In summary, benzodiazepines do not appear to have any consistent effect on serum phenytoin levels. Also, the increased disposition of diazepam in the presence of phenytoin or phenobarbital[133] would not appear to present important clinical difficulties.

MANAGEMENT: It would not appear necessary to avoid benzodiazepines in patients receiving phenytoin, but one should be alert for signs of altered phenytoin levels when benzodiazepines are started or stopped.

Chloramphenicol (Chloromycetin)[17,57,82,119,183–188]

MECHANISM: Chloramphenicol appears to inhibit the metabolism of phenytoin by affecting microsomal enzyme activity in the liver.

CLINICAL SIGNIFICANCE: Numerous case reports and clinical studies have shown that chloramphenicol can considerably increase plasma phenytoin levels; phenytoin toxicity may occur.[57,82,119,183–186] It has also been proposed that phenytoin may decrease[187] or increase[188] serum chloramphenicol levels; additional study is needed to resolve this.

MANAGEMENT: If possible, avoid chloramphenicol use in patients receiving phenytoin. Patients who do receive both phenytoin and chloramphenicol should be watched closely for signs of phenytoin toxicity. Anticonvulsant dosage should be decreased if necessary.

PHENYTOIN INTERACTIONS (CONT.)

DRUGS	DISCUSSION

Corticosteroids[18-23,48,90,91,99,100,134,189]

MECHANISM: Phenytoin enhances the metabolism of corticosteroids due to enzyme induction.

CLINICAL SIGNIFICANCE: It is well documented that phenytoin interferes with dexamethasone suppression tests. It seems likely that phenytoin also impairs the therapeutic response to dexamethasone.[99] In a study of methylprednisolone disposition in normal subjects, phenytoin (300 mg/day for 3 weeks) was found to produce a considerable decrease in methylprednisolone half-life.[91] A similar effect of phenytoin on prednisolone half-life was reported in another study involving normal subjects.[134] It has also been noted that patients receiving anticonvulsants have a higher incidence of graft failure following renal allografts,[100] presumably because the anticonvulsants increase the metabolism of the corticosteroids and thus reduce their immunosuppressive effect. Indeed, kidney transplant patients on anticonvulsants have been shown to have higher plasma clearance of both bound and unbound prednisolone than similar patients not on anticonvulsants.[189] In summary, phenytoin (especially in combination with phenobarbital) has the ability to reduce the therapeutic effect of several commonly used corticosteroids such as dexamethasone, prednisolone, prednisone, and methylprednisolone.

MANAGEMENT: When corticosteroids are required in patients receiving anticonvulsants such as phenytoin and phenobarbital, one should be especially alert for inadequate therapeutic response to the corticosteroid. Theoretically, an adequate response could be obtained by increasing the corticosteroid dose. Also, interpret dexamethasone suppression tests with care in patients receiving phenytoin.

Cyclophosphamide (Cytoxan)[142]

MECHANISM: Enzyme-inducing agents such as phenytoin theoretically could enhance the formation of alkylating metabolites of cyclophosphamide.

CLINICAL SIGNIFICANCE: Although some limited clinical evidence indicates that enzyme inducers may increase peak plasma levels of alkylating metabolites of cyclophosphamide, this might be counteracted by a more rapid disposition of such metabolites.[142] Thus, the clinical significance of concomitant use of phenytoin and cyclophosphamide remains unknown.

MANAGEMENT: Not known (see Clinical Significance).

Diazoxide (Hyperstat)[115,135]

MECHANISM: The limited evidence available to date indicates that diazoxide enhances phenytoin metabolism.

CLINICAL SIGNIFICANCE: Three children receiving phenytoin and diazoxide concomitantly developed very low serum phenytoin levels (in

PHENYTOIN INTERACTIONS (CONT.)

two cases phenytoin was undetectable).[115,135] Urinary excretion of the major metabolite of phenytoin (HPPH) was measured in one patient and found to be considerably increased during diazoxide administration.[135] In another patient, phenytoin half-life was only 3.5 hours during chronic diazoxide therapy, which is considerably shorter than normal.[115] Based on these three cases, it does appear that patients receiving concomitant phenytoin and diazoxide may develop subtherapeutic phenytoin levels.

MANAGEMENT: Patients receiving concomitant phenytoin and diazoxide should be monitored for signs of decreased phenytoin levels.

Digitalis Glycosides[24,25,110]

MECHANISM: Not established. Phenytoin appears to enhance the metabolism of digitoxin, probably by induction of hepatic microsomal enzymes.

CLINICAL SIGNIFICANCE: A preliminary study in one patient on digitoxin has shown decreased plasma digitoxin levels when phenytoin was given.[24] Study in more patients is needed to assess clinical significance.

MANAGEMENT: Until more is known about this interaction, patients receiving both digitoxin and phenytoin should be watched more closely for underdigitalization.

Disulfiram (Antabuse)[38–40,104,190]

MECHANISM: It appears that disulfiram inhibits the hepatic metabolism of phenytoin. Blood levels of phenytoin are increased, and urinary excretion of the major metabolite (HPPH) is decreased.

CLINICAL SIGNIFICANCE: Disulfiram (400 mg/day) has been shown to considerably increase serum phenytoin concentrations in several patients. The effect was rapid, with increases in serum phenytoin occurring within 4 hours of the administration of the first dose of disulfiram.[39] The effect was also prolonged, requiring about 3 weeks to ensure that phenytoin levels had returned to normal. Similar results have been obtained in normal volunteers given phenytoin before and after 4 days of disulfiram.[104] Also, a patient developed phenytoin toxicity (ataxia, nystagmus) and a serum phenytoin level of 39.5 μg/ml following initiation of disulfiram therapy.[190] Based on current evidence it seems likely that disulfiram would enhance phenytoin serum levels in most patients.

MANAGEMENT: Patients receiving phenytoin and disulfiram should be monitored for excessive phenytoin effect. Reduction of phenytoin dose may be necessary.

Dopamine (Intropin)[176,177]

MECHANISM: Not established.

PHENYTOIN INTERACTIONS (CONT.)

DRUGS	DISCUSSION

CLINICAL SIGNIFICANCE: Several patients requiring dopamine infusions to maintain blood pressure developed severe hypotension following intravenous phenytoin. This response was reproduced in dogs. However, certain predisposing factors appear to be required since not all patients receiving intravenous phenytoin and dopamine develop such reactions.

MANAGEMENT: In patients receiving intravenous dopamine, intravenous phenytoin should be administered only with careful monitoring of cardiovascular status.

Ethanol (Alcohol, Ethyl)[58,83]

MECHANISM: There is evidence that ethanol induces the production of hepatic microsomal enzymes, resulting in enhanced phenytoin metabolism.

CLINICAL SIGNIFICANCE: Alcoholics (while sober) have been shown to metabolize phenytoin more rapidly than control subjects. Theoretically, prolonged excessive ethanol ingestion could result in seizures in an epileptic controlled on a given dose of phenytoin. It is not known what effect smaller amounts of ethanol would have on phenytoin metabolism, but it would probably not be large. It should also be noted that alcohol withdrawal in a chronic alcoholic may result in seizures in nonepileptic patients, and phenytoin has been recommended in the treatment of such seizures.[83]

MANAGEMENT: Epileptics receiving phenytoin who drink heavily should be watched more closely for decreased anticonvulsant effect.

Fluroxene (Fluoromar)[26,27]

MECHANISM: It has been proposed that phenytoin may stimulate the metabolism of fluroxene, presumably to a product toxic to the liver.

CLINICAL SIGNIFICANCE: Reynolds and associates[26] have reported a case of an epileptic controlled on phenytoin and phenobarbital who developed hepatic necrosis following the use of fluroxene anesthesia. They proposed that the anticonvulsants may have increased the hepatotoxic potential of fluroxene, as has been shown experimentally for other anesthetics.

MANAGEMENT: This potential interaction should be considered in the selection of an anesthetic for a patient receiving phenytoin. However, the many other factors to be considered in such a selection would appear to be more important because of the small amount of documentation for this interaction.

Folic Acid (Folvite)[4,6–11,65,66,92–94,116,191–193]

MECHANISM:
1. Replacement of folic acid in folate-deficient patients receiving phenytoin may increase the metabolism of phenytoin with a resultant decrease in serum phenytoin levels.

PHENYTOIN INTERACTIONS (CONT.)

DRUGS	DISCUSSION

2. There is clinical and experimental evidence to suggest that at least some of the anticonvulsant effect of phenytoin is due to depletion of folate, the replacement of which may reverse some of the anticonvulsant activity of phenytoin.

CLINICAL SIGNIFICANCE: One case report has appeared in which folic acid administration in a patient on phenytoin therapy was followed by a decrease in serum phenytoin levels to subtherapeutic levels and an increase in fit frequency (Mechanism #1).[65] Decreases in serum phenytoin were also noted in three of four normal subjects when folic acid (10 mg/day) was added to phenytoin (300 mg/day).[92] Most patients, however, manifest relatively small decreases in serum phenytoin with folic acid therapy (e.g., not to subtherapeutic levels of phenytoin).[7,65,191] Available evidence indicates that the fall in serum phenytoin is greatest in those patients with higher initial serum phenytoin levels.[191] The ability of folic acid to directly antagonize the anticonvulsant effect of phenytoin (Mechanism #2) is not well established, but occasional patients stabilized on chronic phenytoin manifest decreased seizure control when folic acid is given. In one study, very small doses of folic acid (5 mg/week) corrected phenytoin-induced folate deficiency without affecting seizure control.[192] In summary, folic acid therapy in a patient receiving phenytoin has the potential for decreasing serum phenytoin levels to a clinically significant degree in an occasional patient. In addition, folic acid therapy has the potential for antagonizing the anticonvulsant effects of phenytoin, although the incidence of this problem clinically is not clear.

MANAGEMENT: When folic acid is given to patients receiving phenytoin, patients should be watched for decreased control of seizures (although most patients are probably not significantly affected).

Furosemide (Lasix)[101,136]

MECHANISM: Phenytoin appears to inhibit the gastrointestinal absorption of furosemide.[136] An additional inhibitory effect of phenytoin on the diuretic response to furosemide is possible.[101]

CLINICAL SIGNIFICANCE: Following the clinical observation that patients on anticonvulsant therapy responded poorly to diuretics, the diuretic response to furosemide was studied in a group of epileptics and normal subjects.[101] The diuretic response was significantly smaller and delayed in the 17 patients receiving anticonvulsants (phenytoin and phenobarbital, with some also receiving other anticonvulsants). A subsequent study in five normal subjects showed that phenytoin (300 mg/day for 10 days) reduced oral furosemide absorption by about 50% without affecting its serum clearance.[136]

MANAGEMENT: In patients receiving phenytoin, one should be alert for impaired diuretic response to furosemide; larger furosemide doses may be required. It is not known if separating the doses of the drugs would minimize the interaction.

PHENYTOIN INTERACTIONS (CONT.)

DRUGS	DISCUSSION

Glucagon[137]

MECHANISM: Phenytoin appears to inhibit the stimulant effect of glucagon on insulin release by the islet cells.

CLINICAL SIGNIFICANCE: Phenytoin reportedly may result in false negative results in the glucagon stimulation test for insulinoma.[137]

MANAGEMENT: It has been recommended that drugs which can affect insulin release (e.g., phenytoin, diazoxide, thiazides, tolbutamide) should be withdrawn several weeks prior to glucagon stimulation tests.[137] However, this may be difficult in the case of phenytoin.

Halothane (Fluothane)[59]

MECHANISM: Halothane may produce hepatotoxicity, with resultant impairment of hepatic metabolism of phenytoin.

CLINICAL SIGNIFICANCE: A single case has been reported in which a patient developed phenytoin toxicity following exposure to halothane. The patient had been satisfactorily stabilized on a set dose of phenytoin, and it appeared that the halothane-induced hepatic dysfunction was responsible for the elevated phenytoin plasma levels.

MANAGEMENT: Halothane and other hepatotoxic drugs should be given cautiously to patients receiving phenytoin.

Influenza vaccine[170]

MECHANISM: Not established.

CLINICAL SIGNIFICANCE: In seven patients stabilized on phenytoin, influenza vaccination was associated with a slight decrease in plasma phenytoin levels.[170] It seems unlikely that the effect would be of sufficient magnitude to impair the anticonvulsant effect of phenytoin in most patients.

MANAGEMENT: No special precautions appear necessary.

Isoniazid (INH)[41-43,60,61,78,194]

MECHANISM: Isoniazid inhibits the hepatic metabolism of phenytoin. Blood levels of phenytoin are increased and urinary excretion of its major metabolite is decreased.

CLINICAL SIGNIFICANCE: Well documented. Administration of INH alone as well as in combination with aminosalicylic acid (PAS) in patients receiving phenytoin has been shown to result in signs of phenytoin intoxication. Epidemiologic data also indicate that toxic central nervous system effects are considerably more common in patients receiving isoniazid and phenytoin than in those receiving phenytoin in the absence of isoniazid.[194] This interaction is probably most important in patients who are "slow" metabolizers of INH, and in those receiving both INH and PAS. In both cases, INH blood levels tend to be higher.

DRUGS	DISCUSSION

MANAGEMENT: Patients receiving both INH and phenytoin should be watched closely for signs of phenytoin toxicity. Anticonvulsant dosage should be decreased if necessary. Patients who develop peripheral neuropathy while they are receiving INH are more likely to be "slow" metabolizers and thus would be more likely to manifest this interaction.

Levodopa (Dopar, Larodopa)[108]

MECHANISM: Not established.

CLINICAL SIGNIFICANCE: In five patients with parkinsonism and levodopa-induced dyskinesias, phenytoin administration alleviated the levodopa dyskinesias but also inhibited the therapeutic effect of levodopa in controlling the parkinsonism.[108] Four of the five patients were receiving levodopa-carbidopa (e.g., Sinemet), so it is clear that carbidopa does not prevent this interaction.

MANAGEMENT: Although this interaction is based on limited evidence, it would be prudent to avoid phenytoin in parkinsonian patients receiving levodopa. If the combination is used, a larger dose of levodopa may be required.

Lithium Carbonate[148-150]

MECHANISM: Not established.

CLINICAL SIGNIFICANCE: A few cases of possible phenytoin-enhanced lithium toxicity have been reported.[148-150] However, it was not clearly established that a lithium-phenytoin interaction was responsible for the effects. The patients developed ataxia,[148] tremor with gastrointestinal symptoms,[149] and tremor with polyuria and increased thirst.[150]

MANAGEMENT: Until more information is available, one should be alert for evidence of lithium toxicity if phenytoin is given concurrently.

Loxapine (Loxitane)[138]

MECHANISM: It is proposed that loxapine stimulates phenytoin metabolism.

CLINICAL SIGNIFICANCE: A case has been reported where loxapine administration was associated with relatively low serum phenytoin levels, and discontinuation of the loxapine was followed by a considerable increase in serum phenytoin.[138] More study is needed to assess clinical significance.

MANAGEMENT: Concomitant use need not be avoided, but it would be prudent to monitor for altered serum phenytoin if loxapine is started or stopped.

DRUGS	DISCUSSION

Meperidene (Demerol)[161]

MECHANISM: Phenytoin appears to enhance the hepatic metabolism of meperidine.

CLINICAL SIGNIFICANCE: The pharmacokinetics of meperidine (50 mg IV and 100 mg orally) was studied in four normal subjects, before and after the administration of phenytoin (1 gm followed by 300 mg daily for 9 days).[161] Phenytoin enhanced the systemic clearance of meperidine and reduced meperidine's half-life and bioavailability. The area under the blood concentration-time curve for normeperidine was considerably increased in the presence of phenytoin. The elevated blood normeperidine levels in the presence of phenytoin probably result from a phenytoin-induced increase in N-demethylation of meperidine to normeperidine by hepatic microsomal enzymes. However, the degree to which phenytoin would reduce the clinical analgesic efficacy of meperidine or increase toxicity due to increased normeperidine levels is not established.

MANAGEMENT: Until more information is available one should be alert for evidence of reduced analgesic efficacy and/or increased toxicity when meperidine is used in patients receiving phenytoin. Since oral meperidine produces more normeperidine than equianalgesic intravenous doses of meperidine, it has been suggested that parenteral meperidine would be preferable to oral administration in patients receiving phenytoin.[161] However, this has not been tested clinically.

Methadone[139,195]

MECHANISM: Phenytoin may enhance the metabolism of methadone by hepatic microsomal enzymes.

CLINICAL SIGNIFICANCE: A methadone-treated patient has been described who developed signs and symptoms of methadone withdrawal after a few days of phenytoin therapy.[139] There was a remission of the signs and symptoms when the phenytoin was stopped, and a reappearance when the patient was challenged with phenytoin. In a study of five patients on methadone maintenance, phenytoin therapy resulted in withdrawal symptoms within 3 or 4 days.[195] These findings are consistent with the known ability of another enzyme inducer, rifampin, to reduce the effect of methadone.

MANAGEMENT: Enzyme inducers such as phenytoin would be best avoided in patients controlled on methadone. If this is not possible, one should be alert for the possible necessity of changing methadone dosage if phenytoin therapy is started or stopped.

Methylphenidate (Ritalin)[49,80,81,106,143]

MECHANISM: It has been proposed that methylphenidate inhibits the metabolism of phenytoin,[49] but there is question as to the significance of this effect.

CLINICAL SIGNIFICANCE: One patient in whom this interaction report-edly occurred was receiving a relatively large dose of phenytoin.[49] In another patient, increasing plasma phenytoin levels followed the administration of methylphenidate on one occasion but not on another.[80] It is interesting that the increasing phenytoin levels oc-curred following discontinuation of amphetamine therapy.[80] Animal studies have indicated that amphetamine impairs gastrointestinal phenytoin absorption.[143] Another study of the phenytoin-methyl-phenidate interaction in 11 patients did not show any effect on phen-ytoin plasma levels.[81] One clinician cites experience with more than 100 patients who received concomitant phenytoin and methyl-phenidate without any obvious complications.[106] It may be that this interaction is manifest only in those patients who are receiving doses of phenytoin large enough to nearly saturate the hepatic enzymes re-sponsible for its metabolism or in patients with some other predispos-ing factors.

MANAGEMENT: No special precautions appear necessary, but it should be kept in mind that certain susceptible patients might manifest ele-vated serum phenytoin levels.

Metyrapone (Metopirone)[28,29]

MECHANISM: Phenytoin probably enhances the metabolism of orally administered metyrapone on its first pass through the liver. An inhib-itory effect of phenytoin on the gastrointestinal absorption of metyrapone is also possible, but does not appear as likely as enhanced metyrapone metabolism.

CLINICAL SIGNIFICANCE: Oral metyrapone administration in patients receiving chronic phenytoin therapy results in inadequate metyrapone blood levels[28] and invalidates the metyrapone test.[28,29] Doubling the metyrapone dose or giving the metyrapone intravenously circum-vented the interfering effect of phenytoin with normal plasma ACTH and corticosteroid responses.[28]

MANAGEMENT: It should be realized that the standard oral metyrapone test will be invalid in patients receiving chronic pheny-toin therapy. Doubling the oral metyrapone dose in such patients may result in valid results.[28]

Nitrofurantoin (Furadantin)[171]

MECHANISM: Not established.

CLINICAL SIGNIFICANCE: A patient on chronic phenytoin therapy de-veloped a fall in plasma phenytoin concentration and seizures follow-ing initiation of nitrofurantoin therapy.[171] The nitrofurantoin ap-peared to be responsible for the change in phenytoin levels in this patient, but it is not known how commonly it would occur in other persons.

DRUGS	DISCUSSION

MANAGEMENT: Monitor for altered phenytoin response if nitrofurantoin is initiated or discontinued.

Phenothiazines[50,55,87,196]

MECHANISM: Phenothiazines presumably inhibit phenytoin metabolism.

CLINICAL SIGNIFICANCE: Kutt and McDowell[50] report that they found rare clinical cases of chlorpromazine and prochlorperazine-induced inhibition of phenytoin metabolism. Also, two cases of phenytoin intoxication possibly caused by thioridazine have been reported.[196] Others have found that phenothiazines tend to be associated with *decreased* phenytoin serum levels.[87] More study in patients receiving these drugs is needed to assess clinical significance.

MANAGEMENT: No special precautions appear necessary, but one should be alert for signs of altered phenytoin serum levels if phenothiazines are started or stopped.

Phenylbutazone (Butazolidin)[30,37,44,57,68,113,197]

MECHANISM: It has been proposed that phenylbutazone and its metabolite oxyphenbutazone compete with phenytoin for hepatic metabolism.[30] In addition, in-vitro studies have shown that phenylbutazone can displace phenytoin from plasma protein binding.[68]

CLINICAL SIGNIFICANCE: In a study of 14 pairs of healthy twins, phenylbutazone was shown to increase the half-life of intravenously administered phenytoin,[30] which lends support to earlier undocumented statements that a significant interaction occurs between phenylbutazone and phenytoin.[37,44,57] In a subsequent study of six patients stabilized on phenytoin, phenylbutazone decreased serum phenytoin after 2 days, followed by increasing serum phenytoin over the next 12 days.[197] One patient developed evidence of phenytoin toxicity.

MANAGEMENT: Patients receiving both phenylbutazone and phenytoin should be watched more closely for signs of phenytoin intoxication. Serum phenytoin determinations may be useful, but one should be aware that a given total phenytoin concentration may represent a higher than expected free serum phenytoin level.

Phenyramidol[45]

MECHANISM: It appears that phenyramidol inhibits the hepatic metabolism of phenytoin.

CLINICAL SIGNIFICANCE: In one study, the mean half-life of phenytoin increased from 25 hours to 55 hours in five subjects who were also given phenyramidol. However, phenyramidol is no longer commercially available in the United States.

PHENYTOIN INTERACTIONS (CONT.)

DRUGS	DISCUSSION

MANAGEMENT: If the drugs were to be given concomitantly, it is quite likely that the dose of phenytoin would have to be decreased.

Primidone (Mysoline)[2,31,32,69,118,121]

MECHANISM: A considerable amount of primidone is converted to phenobarbital in man. The addition of phenytoin to primidone therapy increases the phenobarbital blood levels found, probably by stimulating the conversion of primidone to phenobarbital. A contributing effect might be phenytoin-induced competitive inhibition of phenobarbital metabolism.

CLINICAL SIGNIFICANCE: It has been found that serum phenobarbital levels are considerably higher in patients receiving primidone plus phenytoin than in patients receiving primidone alone.[31,118] In another study[2] serum phenobarbital levels were found to be consistently higher in patients receiving primidone plus phenytoin than in patients receiving phenobarbital plus phenytoin. Finally, an infant has been described who developed extremely high *phenobarbital* levels (202 μg/ml) following the use of phenytoin and primidone in "recommended" doses.[32] Although the preceding reports offer good evidence that phenytoin promotes the formation of phenobarbital from primidone, this may be a favorable interaction in most epileptics treated with the combination of phenytoin and primidone, with only an occasional susceptible patient being adversely affected.

MANAGEMENT: No special precautions appear to be necessary with the concomitant use of phenytoin and primidone, although one should keep in mind that relatively high levels of phenobarbital can be generated. The finding of clearly supratherapeutic levels of phenobarbital in patients receiving phenytoin, primidone, and phenobarbital[31] raises the question of the propriety of adding phenobarbital to a regimen of phenytoin and primidone.

Pyridoxine (Vitamin B$_6$)[96]

MECHANISM: It is proposed that pyridoxine administration may enhance the activity of phenytoin-metabolizing enzymes in the liver.

CLINICAL SIGNIFICANCE: Preliminary study in epileptic patients indicated that pyridoxine (200 mg/day for 4 weeks) was associated with decreased phenytoin serum levels.[96] Although phenytoin levels were reduced to about one-half in several patients, other patients did not appear to be affected by pyridoxine therapy. It is not known if pyridoxine doses smaller than 200 mg/day would have any effect on serum phenytoin.

MANAGEMENT: No special precautions appear necessary with small doses of pyridoxine (as in multivitamins) in patients receiving phenytoin. Monitoring for altered serum phenytoin is probably warranted if large doses of pyridoxine are used.

PHENYTOIN INTERACTIONS (CONT.)

DRUGS	DISCUSSION

Salicylates[67,68,102,113,122,198–200]

MECHANISM: Salicylates appear to displace phenytoin from plasma protein binding.

CLINICAL SIGNIFICANCE: Large doses of aspirin have been shown to reduce total serum phenytoin concentration without much effect on free serum phenytoin levels. This should be considered when interpreting serum phenytoin levels in the presence of salicylate therapy. It is possible that salicylates could occasionally produce phenytoin toxicity in predisposed individuals (e.g., those with high preexisting phenytoin levels and/or low albumin levels). Low doses of salicylate (e.g., less than 2 g/day) probably have minimal effects on phenytoin disposition.[200]

MANAGEMENT: One should consider the effect of large salicylate doses on total serum phenytoin levels (see Clinical Significance). Large doses of salicylates should be administered with some caution to patients on phenytoin therapy, especially if they appear prone to phenytoin toxicity.

Sulfonamides[33,37,44,57,68,109,172]

MECHANISM: Sulfamethizole (Thiosulfil) and sulfaphenazole may inhibit the metabolism of phenytoin.[33,57,109] Sulfisoxazole (Gantrisin) has been shown to displace phenytoin from plasma protein binding in vitro.[68]

CLINICAL SIGNIFICANCE: Following the observation of phenytoin intoxication in a patient receiving concomitant sulfamethizole, the half-life of phenytoin was determined in six patients before and after sulfamethizole administration (4 g/day for 7 days). The phenytoin half-life increased from an average of 11.3 h before to 20.5 h after sulfamethizole treatment.[33] This study was subsequently described in more detail and involving two additional subjects with essentially the same results.[109] Sulfaphenazole has apparently also been noted to inhibit phenytoin metabolism in patients[37,57] but descriptions of the magnitude and incidence of this interaction have not appeared. The ability of sulfisoxazole to inhibit the in-vitro plasma protein binding of phenytoin[68] has not yet been shown to be significant clinically. Siersbaek-Nielsen and associates[33] reportedly found no inhibition of phenytoin metabolism by sulfisoxazole, sulfadimethoxine, or sulfamethoxypyridazine. Thus, on the basis of current evidence, sulfamethizole and sulfaphenazole are the only sulfonamides likely to affect phenytoin metabolism. Little is known about the remaining sulfonamides.

MANAGEMENT: When using sulfamethizole or sulfaphenazole in patients receiving phenytoin, one should be alert for excessive phenytoin effect.

PHENYTOIN INTERACTIONS (CONT.)

DRUGS	DISCUSSION

Sulthiame (Ospolot)[34,35,46,69,95]

MECHANISM: It has been proposed that sulthiame inhibits the metabolism of phenytoin by the liver.

CLINICAL SIGNIFICANCE: This interaction is fairly well documented. One study in eight patients has shown that sulthiame administration can considerably increase phenytoin blood levels and prolong its half-life.[46] Another group found that eight of 20 patients receiving phenytoin plus sulthiame had serum phenytoin levels in the toxic range, while only 15 of 116 patients receiving phenytoin without sulthiame had such levels.[95] Also, Kariks and associates[69] mentions five patients with high serum phenytoin levels, presumably due to interaction with sulthiame.

MANAGEMENT: Patients receiving both drugs should be watched for signs of phenytoin intoxication, and phenytoin dosage should be reduced if necessary.

Tetracyclines[5,36,98]

MECHANISM: Phenytoin probably stimulates doxycycline (Vibramycin) metabolism.[5]

CLINICAL SIGNIFICANCE: The half-life of doxycycline was found to be shorter in seven patients on chronic phenytoin therapy (mean, 7.2 hours) than in nine control patients (mean, 15.1 hours).[5] A subsequent study by the same group gave similar results.[98] The effect of this shortened half-life on the clinical antibacterial effect of doxycycline has not been assessed, but the magnitude of the differences in half-life certainly indicates that this would be a possibility. Chlortetracycline, demeclocycline, methacycline, oxytetracycline do *not* appear to be affected by phenytoin administration.[98]

MANAGEMENT: When phenytoin is used concomitantly with doxycycline, attention should be directed to ensuring adequate doxycycline serum levels.

Theophylline[159,160]

MECHANISM: Phenytoin probably enhances hepatic theophylline metabolism.

CLINICAL SIGNIFICANCE: In one case report, a patient on long-term phenytoin (Dilantin) therapy (400 mg/day) did not respond adequately to large doses of sustained-release theophylline (Theo-Dur). Subsequently, ten healthy subjects were given aminophylline (5.6 mg/kg body weight IV over 30 minutes) with and without phenytoin pretreatment (300 to 400 mg daily for 10 to 15 days). The theophylline half-life was shorter (5.2 versus 10.1 hours) and theophylline clearance was higher (75.5 versus 43.7 ml/hour/kg body weight) following phenytoin therapy in the ten subjects. In the above patient, the theophylline half-life was 3.75 hours while on phenytoin and 6.3 hours

DRUGS	DISCUSSION

1 month after phenytoin was discontinued. However, the phenytoin was replaced by valproic acid (Depakene), and the potential ability of valproic acid to act as an enzyme inhibitor was apparently not considered. The magnitude of the changes in the theophylline disposition following phenytoin appear large enough to reduce the therapeutic response to theophylline. Furthermore, a preliminary report in 14 volunteers indicated that theophylline may reduce phenytoin serum levels somewhat.[160] Thus, combined therapy may result in lowered serum concentrations of both theophylline and phenytoin.

MANAGEMENT: One should be alert for the need to adjust theophylline dosage if phenytoin therapy is initiated or discontinued. In patients on chronic phenytoin therapy, initiation of theophylline therapy may require larger than expected theophylline doses.

Thyroid Hormones[53,201]

MECHANISM: Phenytoin appears to enhance the metabolism of thyroid hormones and may also displace thyroxine from plasma protein binding.

CLINICAL SIGNIFICANCE: In patients without an intact pituitary-thyroid axis, phenytoin-induced increases in the metabolism of thyroid hormones may increase thyroid replacement dose requirements. This has been reported in one case.[201] Other enzyme inducers might produce a similar effect. Also, a case has been reported in which a patient with atrial flutter on thyroid replacement therapy developed supraventricular tachycardia when he was given intravenous phenytoin.[53] The tachycardia may have been due to displacement of thyroxine to sites of action by the phenytoin.

MANAGEMENT: In patients on thyroid replacement, initiation or discontinuation of phenytoin therapy may alter thyroid dose requirements. Also, patients requiring thyroid replacement therapy should be given intravenous phenytoin with caution, especially if they also have a cardiac disease.

Trimethoprim[172]

MECHANISM: Trimethoprim appears to inhibit the hepatic metabolism of phenytoin.

CLINICAL SIGNIFICANCE: In seven subjects given phenytoin (100 mg IV) with and without pretreatment with trimethoprim (320 mg daily for 7 days), the trimethoprim increased phenytoin half-life by about 50%.[172] Phenytoin half-life was similarly prolonged by trimethoprim-sulfamethoxazole (Bactrim, Septra), but sulfamethoxazole alone produced only a small increase in phenytoin half-life.

MANAGEMENT: Monitor for phenytoin toxicity (e.g., nystagmus, ataxia, mental impairment) if trimethoprim is given concurrently. Serum phenytoin determinations would be useful if the interaction is suspected.

PHENYTOIN INTERACTIONS (CONT.)

Valproate (Depakene)[123,124,126,140,202–206]

MECHANISM: There is evidence to indicate that valproate may displace phenytoin from plasma protein binding,[126] and phenytoin may stimulate valproic acid metabolism.

CLINICAL SIGNIFICANCE: In patients receiving phenytoin, administration of valproic acid lowers total plasma phenytoin levels by approximately 30% during the first several weeks of valproic acid therapy. However, total serum phenytoin levels usually return to pre-valproic acid levels after a few more weeks of continuous valproic acid therapy. During the time that serum phenytoin levels are depressed there is a concomitant rise in the percent of serum phenytoin present in the unbound form. Thus, the concentration of the free or active form of phenytoin in the serum is usually not appreciably changed in the presence of valproic acid. Although the half-life of phenytoin tends to be shortened during the first several weeks of valproic acid therapy, a prolongation of phenytoin half-life has been noted after several more weeks on valproic acid. The effect of phenytoin on valproic acid levels has also been studied, and it was found that serum valproic acid levels tend to be lower in patients who are receiving phenytoin concurrently than in patients receiving valproic acid alone. Some patients have developed an increase in seizure frequency when valproic acid was added to phenytoin therapy, but this is uncommon; the relationship of this clinical observation to this drug interaction is unclear. Conversely, an occasional patient with serum phenytoin levels close to the toxic range might develop phenytoin toxicity as a result of the displacement of phenytoin from plasma protein binding sites by valproic acid. The clinical importance of the lowered serum valproic acid levels due to phenytoin is not clear, but serum valproic acid measurements may be useful in detecting patients who need increased doses of valproic acid.

MANAGEMENT: Most patients receiving phenytoin do not require an alteration in the dose of phenytoin when valproic acid therapy is initiated since the free serum concentration of phenytoin is not changed. The decreased total serum phenytoin levels should therefore not prompt an increase in phenytoin dose unless dictated by lack of epilepsy control.

PRIMIDONE (MYSOLINE) INTERACTIONS

| DRUGS | DISCUSSION |

Acetazolamide (Diamox)[114]

MECHANISM: Preliminary evidence indicates that acetazolamide reduces the gastrointestinal absorption of primidone.[114]

CLINICAL SIGNIFICANCE: A patient receiving primidone and acetazolamide developed decreasing anticonvulsant control, and undetectable levels of primidone and phenobarbital.[114] Subsequent study in this

DRUGS	DISCUSSION

patient showed that primidone was absorbed in the absence of acetazolamide. In two other patients given primidone with and without acetazolamide, absorption of primidone appeared to be delayed in one patient, and not affected in the other. In summary, it appears that acetazolamide may have a tendency to inhibit gastrointestinal absorption of primidone, but only in certain patients.

MANAGEMENT: It does not seem necessary to avoid concomitant use. However, until this interaction is better described, patients receiving primidone and acetazolamide should be monitored for decreased primidone effect.

Barbiturates[2,31,32,105]

MECHANISM: A considerable portion of primidone is converted to phenobarbital in the body. Thus, concomitant administration of primidone and phenobarbital may result in excessive serum phenobarbital levels.

CLINICAL SIGNIFICANCE: Excessive serum levels of phenobarbital have been found in patients receiving primidone plus phenobarbital[105] or primidone plus phenobarbital and phenytoin.[31] Thus, some workers have questioned the propriety of adding phenobarbital to a regimen which already includes primidone. This would be especially true in patients also receiving phenytoin since it seems to promote the conversion of primidone to phenobarbital.[2,31,32]

MANAGEMENT: For most patients, it is illogical to use primidone and phenobarbital concomitantly. If the combination is used, the patient should be monitored for excessive phenobarbital serum levels.

Clorazepate (Tranxene)[117]

MECHANISM: Not established.

CLINICAL SIGNIFICANCE: Several patients receiving primidone and clorazepate developed personality changes including depression, irritability, and aggressive behavior.[117] It was proposed that a drug interaction between primidone and clorazepate may have contributed to these findings, but little supporting evidence was given.

MANAGEMENT: No special precautions appear necessary at this point.

Isoniazid (INH)[141]

MECHANISM: Preliminary evidence indicates that isoniazid inhibits the metabolism of primidone to its metabolites, phenobarbital and phenylethylmalonamide.

CLINICAL SIGNIFICANCE: In a patient taking primidone and isoniazid, it was noted that serum primidone levels were high and serum phenobarbital levels were lower than expected.[141] Subsequent study in this patient with and without isoniazid indicated that isoniazid inhibited

PRIMIDONE (MYSOLINE) INTERACTIONS (CONT.)

DRUGS	DISCUSSION

primidone metabolism. More study is needed to determine the incidence of this interaction in patients receiving both drugs.

MANAGEMENT: Although concomitant use need not be avoided, patients should be monitored for altered primidone disposition.

Valproate (Depakene)[140]

MECHANISM: Not established.

CLINICAL SIGNIFICANCE: Addition of valproate therapy in patients receiving primidone reportedly may result in initial increases in serum primidone followed by a return to normal with continued valproate therapy.[140] More study is needed.

MANAGEMENT: Patients receiving primidone should be watched for signs of altered primidone disposition if valproate is given concomitantly.

VALPROIC ACID INTERACTIONS

DRUGS	DISCUSSION

Barbiturates[173–175]

MECHANISM: Valproic acid inhibits the hepatic metabolism of phenobarbital.

CLINICAL SIGNIFICANCE: Well documented. Several studies have shown that phenobarbital elimination is substantially reduced in the presence of valproic acid.[173–175] The magnitude of the interaction is large enough to cause phenobarbital toxicity (e.g., excessive sedation) in some patients.

MANAGEMENT: Monitor for excessive phenobarbital effect (using plasma levels if possible) if valproic acid is given concurrently. Reductions in phenobarbital dosage may be necessary for many patients.

Benzodiazepines[162–164]

MECHANISM: Valproic acid appears to inhibit the hepatic metabolism of diazepam.

CLINICAL SIGNIFICANCE: Six healthy subjects received diazepam (Valium) (10 mg IV) with and without valproic acid (1.5 g orally).[162] Serum diazepam levels were higher in the presence of valproic acid, but the possibility of enhanced diazepam effect was not studied. Also, the combined use of clonazepam (Clonopin) and valproic acid has been associated with absence seizures,[163,164] although the role drug interaction in this phenomenon is not established.

MANAGEMENT: One should be alert for increased benzodiazepine effect in the presence of valproic acid. If absence seizures increase with combined clonazepam and valproic acid, an alternative anticonvulsant regimen should be instituted.

References

1. HOOPER WD, et al: Plasma protein binding of diphenylhydantoin. Effects of sex hormones, renal and hepatic disease. Clin Pharmacol Ther 15:276, 1974.
2. GALLAGHER BB, et al: Primidone, diphenylhydantoin and phenobarbital. Aspects of acute and chronic toxicity. Neurology 23:145, 1973.
3. VAJDA FJE, et al: Interaction between phenytoin and the benzodiazepines (Letter). Br Med J 1:346, 1971.
4. REYNOLDS EH: Anticonvulsants, folic acid, and epilepsy. Lancet 1:1376, 1973.
5. PENTTILA O, et al: Interaction between doxycycline and some antiepileptic drugs. Br Med J 2:470, 1974.
6. SMITH DB, RACUSEN LC: Folate metabolism and the anticonvulsant efficacy of phenobarbital. Arch Neurol 28:18, 1973.
7. JENSEN ON, OLESEN OV: Subnormal serum folate due to anticonvulsive therapy. A double-blind study of the effect of folic acid treatment in patients with drug-induced subnormal serum folates. Arch Neurol 22:181, 1970.
8. NORRIS JW, PRATT RF: A controlled study of folic acid in epilepsy. Neurology 21:659, 1971.
9. SPAANS F: No effect of folic acid supplement on CSF folate and serum vitamin B in patients on anticonvulsants. Epilpsia 11:403, 1970.
10. RALSTON AJ, et al: Effects of folic acid on fit—frequency and behavior of epileptics on anticonvulsants. Lancet 1:867, 1970.
11. SCOTT RB, et al: Reduced absorption of vitamin B_{12} in two patients with folic acid deficiency. Ann Intern Med 69:111, 1968.
12. GARRETTSON LK, DAYTON PG: Disappearance of phenobarbital and diphenylhydantoin from serum of children. Clin Pharmacol Ther 11:674, 1970.
13. BUCHANAN RA, ALLEN RJ: Diphenylhydantoin and phenobarbital blood levels of epileptic children. Neurology 21:866, 1971.
14. HAHN TJ, et al: Effect of chronic anticonvulsant therapy on serum 25-hydroxy calciferol levels in adults. N Engl J Med 287:900, 1972.
15. HANSTEN PD: Interactions between anticonvulsant drugs: primidone, diphenylhydantoin and phenobarbital. Northwest Med J 1:17 (Oct.), 1974.
16. CHRISTIANSEN J, DAM M: Influence of phenobarbital and diphenylhydantoin of plasma carbamazepine levels in patients with epilepsy. Acta Neurol Scand 49:543, 1973.
17. PRATER MS: Diphenylhydantoin metabolism (Letter). Hosp Pharm 9:158, 1974.
18. REYNOLDS JW, MIRKIN BL: Urinary corticosteroid and diphenylhydantoin metabolite patterns in neonates exposed to anticonvulsant drugs in utero. Clin Pharmacol Ther 14:891, 1973.
19. WERK EE, et al: Interference in the effect of dexamethasone by diphenylhydantoin. N Engl J Med 281:32, 1969.
20. JUBIZ W, et al: Effect of diphenylhydantoin on the metabolism of

References (CONT.)

dexamethasone. Mechanism of the abnormal dexamethasone suppression in humans. N Engl J Med 283:11, 1970.

21. WERK EE Jr, et al: Cortisol production in epileptic patients treated with diphenylhydantoin. Clin Pharmacol Ther 12:698, 1971.

22. BECKER B, et al: Diphenylhydantoin and dexamethasone-induced changes of plasma cortisol: comparison of patients with and without glaucoma. J Clin Endocrinol Metab 32:669, 1971.

23. HAQUE N, et al: Studies on dexamethasone metabolism in man: effect of diphenylhydantoin, J Clin Endocrinol Metab 34:44, 1972.

24. SOLOMON HM, et al: Interactions between digitoxin and other drugs *in vitro* and *in vivo*. Ann NY Acad Sci 179:362, 1971.

25. SOLOMON HM, ABRAMS WB: Interactions between digitoxin and other drugs in man. Am Heart J 83:277, 1972.

26. REYNOLDS ES, et al: Massive hepatic necrosis after fluroxene anesthesia—a case of drug interaction? N Engl J Med 286:530, 1972.

27. STENGER, RJ: Enhanced hepatotoxicity of fluroxene (Letter). N Engl J Med 286:1005, 1972.

28. MEIKLE AW, et al: Effect of diphenylhydantoin on the metabolism of metyrapone and release of ACTH in man. J Clin Endocrinol Metab 29:1553, 1969.

29. WERK EE Jr, et al: Failure of metyrapone to inhibit 11-hydroxylation of 11-deoxycortisol during drug therapy. J Clin Endocrinol Metab 27:1358, 1967.

30. ANDREASEN PB, et al: Diphenylhydantoin half life in man and its inhibition by phenylbutazone: the role of genetic factors. Acta Med Scand 193:561, 1973.

31. FINCHAM RW, et al: The influence of diphenylhydantoin on primidone metabolism. Arch Neurol 30:259, 1974.

32. WILSON JT, WILKINSON GR: Chronic and severe phenobarbital intoxication in a child treated with primidone and diphenylhydantoin. J Pediatr 83:484, 1973.

33. SIERSBAEK-NIELSEN K, et al: Sulfamethizole-induced inhibition of diphenylhydantoin and tolbutamide metabolism in man (Abstract). Clin Pharmacol Ther 14:148, 1973.

34. RICHENS A, HOUGHTON GW: Phenytoin intoxication caused by sulthiame (Letter). Lancet 2:1442, 1973.

35. MORSELLI PL, et al: Effect of sulthiame on blood and brain levels of diphenylhydantoin in the rat. Biochem Pharmacol 19:1846, 1970.

36. NEUVONEN PJ, PENTTILA O: Interaction between doxycycline and barbiturates. Br Med J 1:535, 1974.

37. HANSEN JM, et al: Dicumarol-induced diphenylhydantoin intoxication. Lancet 2:265, 1966.

38. OLESEN OV: The influence of disulfiram and calcium carbimide on the serum diphenylhydantoin. Arch Neurol 16:642, 1967.

39. OLESEN OV: Disulfiram (Antabuse) as inhibitor of phenytoin metabolism. Acta Pharmacol Toxicol 24:317, 1966.

40. KIORBOE E: Phenytoin intoxication during treatment with Antabuse (disulfiram). Epilepsia, 7:246, 1966.

41. MURRAY FJ: Outbreak of unexpected reactions among epileptics taking isoniazid. Am Rev Respir Dis 86:729, 1962.

42. KUTT H, et al: Depression of parahydroxylation of diphenylhydantoin by antituberculosis chemotherapy. Neurology 16:594, 1966.

References (CONT.)

43. KUTT H, et al: Inhibition of diphenylhydantoin metabolism in rats and rat liver microsomes by antitubercular drugs. Neurology 18:706, 1968.
44. LUCAS BG: "Dilantin" overdosage (Letter). Med J Aust 2:639, 1968.
45. SOLOMON HM, SCHROGIE JJ: The effect of phenyramidol on the metabolism of diphenylhydantoin. Clin Pharmacol Ther 8:554, 1967.
46. HANSEN JM, et al: Sulthiame (Ospolot) as inhibitor of diphenylhydantoin metabolism. Epilepsia 9:17, 1968.
47. CUCINELL SA, et al: Drug interactions in man. I. Lowering effect of phenobarbital on plasma levels of bishydroxycoumarin (Dicumarol) and diphenylhydantoin (Dilantin). Clin Pharmacol Ther 6:420, 1965.
48. WERK EE Jr, et al: Effect of diphenylhydantoin on cortisol metabolism in man. J Clin Invest 43:1824, 1964.
49. GARRETSON LK, et al: Methylphenidate interaction with bond anticonvulsants and ethyl biscoumacetate. JAMA 207:2053, 1969.
50. KUTT H, McDOWELL F: Management of epilepsy with diphenylhydantoin sodium. JAMA 203:969, 1968.
51. KUTT H, et al: The effect of phenobarbital on plasma diphenylhydantoin level and metabolism in man and in rat liver microsomes. Neurology 19:611, 1969.
52. BUCHANAN RA, et al: The effect of phenobarbital on diphenylhydantoin metabolism in children. Pediatrics 43:114, 1969.
53. FULOP M, et al: Possible diphenylhydantoin-induced arrhythmia in hypothyroidism. JAMA 196:454, 1966.
54. KUTT H, et al: The effect of phenobarbital upon diphenylhydantoin metabolism in man (Abstract). Neurology 15:274, 1965.
55. KUTT H, VEREBELY K: Metabolism of diphenylhydantoin by rat liver microsomes. I. Characteristics of the reaction. Biochem Pharmacol 19:675, 1970.
56. KOKENGE R, et al: Neurological sequelae following Dilantin overdose in a patient and in experimental animals. Neurology 15:823, 1965.
57. CHRISTENSEN LK, SKOVSTED L: Inhibition of drug metabolism by chloramphenicol. Lancet 2:1397, 1969.
58. KATER RMH, et al: Increased rate of clearance of drugs from the circulation of alcoholics. Am J Med Sci 258:35, 1969.
59. KARLIN JM, KUTT H: Acute diphenylhydantoin intoxication following halothane anesthesia. J Pediatr 76:941, 1970.
60. KUTT, H, et al: Diphenylhydantoin intoxication. A complication of isoniazid therapy. Am Rev Respir Dis 101:377, 1970.
61. BRENNAN RW, et al: Diphenylhydantoin intoxication attendant to slow inactivation of isoniazid. Neurology 20:687, 1970.
62. ESPIR M, et al: Epilepsy and oral contraception. Br Med J 1:294, 1969.
63. McARTHUR J: Oral contraceptives and epilepsy (Notes and Comments). Br Med J 3:162, 1967.
64. DALLOS V, HEATHFIELD K: Iatrogenic epilepsy due to antidepressant drugs. Br Med J 4:80, 1969.
65. BAYLIS EM, et al: Influence of folic acid on blood-phenytoin levels. Lancet 1:62, 1971.
66. HOUBEN PFM, et al: Anticonvulsant drugs and folic acid in young mentally retarded epileptic patients. Epilepsia 12:235, 1971.
67. TOAKLEY JG: "Dilantin" overdosage (Letter). Med J Aust 2:640, 1968.
68. LUNDE PKM, et al: Plasma protein binding of diphenylhydantoin in

References (CONT.)

man. Interaction with other drugs and the effect of temperature and plasma dilution. Clin Pharmacol Ther 11:846, 1970.

69. KARIKS, J, et al: Serum folic acid and phenytoin levels in permanently hospitalized epileptic patients receiving anticonvulsant drug therapy. Med J Aust 2:368, 1971.

70. TREASURE T, TOSELAND PA: Hyperglycaemia due to phenytoin toxicity. Arch Dis Child 46:563, 1971.

71. TUDHOPE GR: Advances in medicine. Practitioner 203:405, 1969.

72. DIAMOND WD, BUCHANAN RA: A clinical study of the effect of phenobarbital on diphenylhydantoin plasma levels. J Clin Pharmacol 10:306, 1970.

73. SOTANIEMI E, et al: The clinical significance of microsomal enzyme induction in the therapy of epileptic patients. Ann Clin Res 2:223, 1970.

74. BOOKER HE, et al: Concurrent administration of phenobarbital and diphenylhydantoin: lack of an interference effect. Neurology 21:383, 1971.

75. BUCHTHAL F, SVENSMARK O: Serum concentrations of diphenylhydantoin (phenytoin) and phenobarbital and their relation to therapeutic and toxic effects. Psychiatr Neurol Neurochir 74:117, 1971.

76. MORSELLI PL, et al: Interaction between phenobarbital and diphenylhydantoin in animals and in epileptic patients. Ann NY Acad Sci 179:88, 1971.

77. RIZZO M, et al: Further observations on the interactions between phenobarbital and diphenylhydantoin during chronic treatment in the rat. Biochem Pharmacol 21:449, 1972.

78. ENGEL J, et al: Phenytoin encephalopathy? (Letter). Lancet 2:824, 1971.

79. HANSEN JM, et al: Carbamazepine-induced acceleration of diphenylhydantoin and warfarin metabolism in man. Clin Pharmacol Ther 12:539, 1971.

80. MIRKIN BL, WRIGHT F: Drug interactions: effect of methylphenidate on the disposition of diphenylhydantoin in man. Neurology 21:1123, 1971.

81. KUPFERBERG HJ, et al: Effect of methylphenidate on plasma anticonvulsant levels. Clin Pharmacol Ther 13:201, 1972.

82. BALLEK RE, et al: Inhibition of diphenylhydantoin metabolism by chloramphenicol (Letter). Lancet 1:150, 1973.

83. FINER MJ: Diphenylhydantoin in alcohol withdrawal (Letter). JAMA 217:211, 1971.

84. PINEDA MR, et al: The use of a tricyclic antidepressant in epilepsy. Dis Nerv Syst 35:323, 1974.

85. PEHITA, et al: Imipramine and seizures. Am J Psychiatry 132:5, 1975.

86. POND SM, et al: Effects of tricyclic antidepressants on drug metabolism. Clin Pharmacol Ther 18:191, 1975.

87. SIRIS JH, et al: Anticonvulsant drug-serum levels in psychiatric patients with seizure disorders. NY State J Med 74:1554, 1974.

88. CEREGHINO JJ, et al: The efficacy of carbamazepine combinations in epilepsy. Clin Pharmacol Ther 18:733, 1975.

89. KENYON IE: Unplanned pregnancy in an epileptic. Br Med J 1:686, 1972.

90. KOBBERLING J, MUHLEN AVZ: The influence of diphenylhydantoin and

References (CONT.)

carbamazepine on the circadian rhythm of free urinary corticoids and on the suppressibility of the basal and the "impulsive" activity by dexamethasone. Acta Endocrinol 72:308, 1973.

91. STJERNHOLM MR, KATZ FH: Effects of diphenylhydantoin, phenobarbital, and diazepam on the metabolism of methylprednisolone and its sodium succinate. J Clin Endocrinal Metab 41:887, 1975.

92. GLAZKO AJ: Antiepileptic drugs: biotransformation, metabolism, and serum half-life. Epilepsia 16:367, 1975.

93. REYNOLDS EH: Folate metabolism and anticonvulsant therapy. Proc R Soc Med 67:68, 1974.

94. CH'IEN LT, KRUMDIECK CL, et al: Harmful effect of megadoses of vitamins: electroencephalogram abnormalities and seizures induced by intravenous folate in drug-treated epileptics. Am J Clin Nutr 28:51, 1975.

95. HOUGHTON GW, RICHENS A: Phenytoin intoxication induced by sulthiame in epileptic patients. J Neurol Neurosurg Psychiatr 37:275, 1974.

96. HANSSON O, SILLANPAA M: Pyridoxine and serum concentrations of phenytoin and phenobarbitone (Letter). Lancet 1:256, 1976.

97. MATSUDA I, et al: Renal tubular acidosis and skeletal demineralization in patients on long-term anticonvulsant therapy. J Pediatr 87:202, 1975.

98. NEUVONEN PJ, et al: Effect of antiepileptic drugs on the elimination of various tetracycline derivatives. Eur J Clin Pharmacol 9:147, 1975.

99. BOYLAN JJ, et al: Phenytoin interference with dexamethasone (Letter). JAMA 235:803, 1976.

100. WASSNER SJ, et al: The adverse effect of anticonvulsant therapy on renal allograft survival. J Pediatr 88:134, 1976.

101. AHMAD S: Renal insensitivity to frusemide caused by chronic anticonvulsant therapy. Br Med J 3:657, 1974.

102. ODAR-CEDERLÖF I, BORGA O: Impaired plasma protein binding of phenytoin in uremia and displacement effect of salicylic acid. Clin Pharmacol Ther 20:36, 1976.

103. JANZ D, SCHMIDT D: Anti-epileptic drugs and failure of oral contraceptives (Letter). Lancet 1:1113, 1974.

104. SVENDSEN TL, et al: The influence of disulfiram on the half-life and metabolic clearance rate of diphenylhydantoin and tolbutamide in man. Eur J Clin Pharmacol 9:439, 1976.

105. GRIFFIN GD, et al: Primidone-phenobarbital intoxication. Drug Ther 60:76, 1976.

106. OETTINGER L: Interaction of methylphenidate and diphenylhydantoin (Questions and Answers). Drug Ther 5:107, 1976.

107. LAENGNER H, DETERING K: Antiepileptic drugs and failure of oral contraceptives (Letter). Lancet 2:600, 1974.

108. MENDEZ JS, et al: Diphenylhydantoin blocking of levadopa effects. Arch Neurol 32:44, 1975.

109. LUMHOLTZ B, et al: Sulfamethizole-induced inhibition of diphenylhydantoin, tolbutamide, and warfarin metabolism. Clin Pharmacol Ther 17:731, 1975.

110. BINNION PF, DASGUPTA R: Tritiated digoxin metabolism after prior treatment with propranolol or diphenylhydantoin sodium. Int J Clin Pharmacol 12:96, 1975.

145

References (CONT.)

111. ROBERTSON YR, JOHNSON ES: Interactions between oral contraceptives and other drugs: A review. Curr Med Res Opin 3:647, 1976.
112. RANE A, et al: Kinetics of carbamazepine and its 10,11-epoxide metabolite in children. Clin Pharmacol Ther 19:276, 1976.
113. LUNDE PKM: Plasma protein binding of diphenylhydantoin in man. Acta Pharmacol Toxicol 29:152, 1971.
114. SYVERSEN GB, et al: Acetazolamide-induced interference with primidone absorption. Arch Neurol 34:80, 1977.
115. PETRO DJ, et al: Diazoxide-diphenylhydantoin interaction (Letter). J Pediatr 89:331, 1976.
116. STRAUSS RG, BERNSTEIN R: Folic acid and dilantin antagonism in pregnancy. Obstet Gynecol 44:345, 1974.
117. FELDMAN RG: Chlorazepate in temporal lobe epilepsy (Letter). JAMA 236:2603, 1976.
118. CALLAGHAN N, et al: The effect of anticonvulsant drugs which induce liver enzymes on derived and ingested phenobarbitone levels. Acta Neurol Scand 56:1, 1977.
119. ROSE JQ, et al: Intoxication caused by interaction of chloramphenicol and phenytoin. JAMA 237:2630, 1977.
120. JOHANNESSEN SI, et al: Lack of effect of clonazepam on serum levels of diphenylhydantoin, phenobarbital and carbamazepine. Acta Neurol Scand 55:506, 1977.
121. WINDORFER A: Drug interaction during anticonvulsive therapy (Abstract). Int J Clin Pharmacol 14:236, 1976.
122. EHRNEBO M, ODAR-CEDERLOF I: Distribution of pentobarbital and diphenylhydantoin between plasma and cells in blood: effect of salicylic acid, temperature and total drug concentration. Eur J Clin Pharmacol 11:37, 1977.
123. BARDY A, et al: Valproate may lower serum-phenytoin (Letter). Lancet 2:1297, 1976.
124. PATSALOS PN, LASCELLES PT: Valproate may lower serum-phenytoin (Letter). Lancet 1:50, 1977.
125. DRAVET C, et al: Interaction between carbamazepine and triacetyloleandomycin (Letter). Lancet 2:810, 1977.
126. PATSALOS PN, LASCELLES PT: Effect of sodium valproate on plasma protein binding of diphenylhydantoin. J Neurol Neurosurg Psychiatr 40:570, 1977.
127. DAM M, CHRISTIANSEN J: Interaction of propoxyphene with carbamazepine (Letter). Lancet 2:509, 1977.
128. MALLETTE LE: Anticonvulsants, acetazolamide, and osteomalacia (Letter). N Engl J Med 293:668, 1975.
129. MALLETTE LE: Acetazolamide-accelerated anticonvulsant osteomalacia. Arch Intern Med 137:1013, 1977.
130. LAMBIE DG, et al: Therapeutic and pharmacokinetic effects of increasing phenytoin in chronic epileptics on multiple drug therapy. Lancet 2:386, 1976.
131. HOUGHTON GW, RICHENS A: The effect of benzodiazepines and pheneturide on phenytoin metabolism in man. Br J Clin Pharmacol 1:P344, 1974.
132. SIRIS JH, et al: Anticonvulsant drug-serum levels in psychiatric patients with seizure disorders. Effects of certain psychotropic drugs. NY State J Med 74:1554, 1974.

References (CONT.)

133. HEPNER GW, et al: Disposition of aminopyrine, antipyrine, diazepam and indocyanine green in patients with liver disease or on anticonvulsant drug therapy: diazepam breath test and correlations in drug elimination. J Lab Clin Med 90:440, 1977.

134. PETEREIT, LB, MEIKLE AW: Effectiveness of prednisolone during phenytoin therapy. Clin Pharmacol Ther 22:912, 1977.

135. ROE TF, et al: Drug interaction-diazoxide and diphenylhydantoin. J Pediatr 87:480, 1975.

136. FINE A, et al: Malabsorption of frusemide caused by phenytoin. Br Med J 4:1061, 1977.

137. KUMAR D, et al: Diagnostic use of glucagon-induced insulin response. Studies in patients with insulinoma or other hypoglycemic conditions. Ann Intern Med 80:697, 1974.

138. RYAN GM, MATTHEWS PA: Phenytoin metabolism stimulated by loxapine (Letter). Drug Intell Clin Pharm 11:428, 1977.

139. FINELLI PF: Phenytoin and methadone tolerance (Letter). N Engl J Med 294:227, 1976.

140. WINDORFER A, et al: Elevation of diphenylhydantoin and primidone serum concentration by addition of dipropylacetate, a new anticonvulsant drug. Acta Paediatr Scand 64:771, 1975.

141. SUTTON G, KUPFERBERG HJ: Isoniazid as an inhibitor of primidone metabolism. Neurology 25:1179, 1975.

142. BAGLEY CM, et al: Clinical pharmacology of cyclophosphamide. Cancer Res 33:226, 1973.

143. FREY HH, KAMPMANN, E: Interaction of amphetamine with anticonvulsant drugs. II. Effect of amphetamine on the absorption of anticonvulsant drugs. Acta Pharmacol Toxicol 24:310, 1966.

144. LEVY RH, et al: Pharmacokinetics of carbamazepine in normal man. Clin Pharmacol Ther 17:657, 1977.

145. PUGH RNH, et al: Interaction of phenytoin with chlorpheniramine (Letter). Br J Clin Pharmacol 2:174, 1975.

146. WONG YY, et al: Effect of erythromycin on carbamazepine kinetics. Clin Pharmacol Ther 33:460, 1983.

147. MESDJIAN E, et al: Carbamazepine intoxication due to triacetyloleandomycin administration in epileptic patients. Epilepsia 21:489, 1980.

148. SALEM RB, et al: Drug Intell Clin Pharm 14:621, 1980.

149. SPIERS J, HIRSCH SR: Severe lithium toxicity within normal serum concentrations. Br Med J 1:815, 1978.

150. MACCALLUM WAG: Interaction of lithium and phenytoin. Br Med J 280:610, 1980.

151. GHOSE K. Effect of carbamazepine in polyuria associated with lithium therapy. Pharmacopsychiatria 11:241, 1978.

152. AYD FJ. Int Drug Ther Newslett 17:10, 1982.

153. LIPINSKI JF, POPE HG JR: Possible synergistic action between carbamazepine and lithium carbonate in the treatment of three acutely manic patients. Am J Psychiatry 139:948, 1982.

154. BLOCK SH: Carbamazepine-isoniazid interaction. Pediatrics 69:494, 1982.

155. VALSALAN VC, COOPER GL: Carbamazepine intoxication caused with isoniazid. Br Med J 285:261, 1982.

156. WRIGHT JM, et al: Isoniazid-induced carbamazepine toxicity and vice versa. Med Intell 307:1325, 1982.

References (CONT.)

157. PERUCCA E, RICHENS A: Paracetamol disposition in normal subjects and in patients treated with antiepileptic drugs. Br J Clin Pharmacol 7:201, 1971.
158. NEUVONEN PJ, et al: Antipyretic analgesics in patients on antiepileptic drug therapy. Eur J Clin Pharmacol 15:263, 1979.
159. MARQUIS JF, et al: Phenytoin-theophylline interaction. N Engl J Med 307:1189, 1982.
160. TAYLOR JW et al. The interaction of phenytoin and theophylline. Drug Intell Clin Pharm 14:638, 1980.
161. POND SM, KRETSCHMAR KM: Effect of phenytoin on meperdine clearance and normeperidine formation. Clin Pharmacol Ther 30:680, 1981.
162. DHILLON SA, RICHENS A: Valproic acid and diazepam interaction in vivo. Br J Clin Pharmacol 13:553, 1982.
163. JEAVONS PM, et al: Treatment of generalized epilepsies of childhood and adolescence with sodium valproate ('epilim'). Dev Med Child Neurol 19:9, 1977.
164. BROWNE TR: Interaction between clonazepam and sodium valproate. N Engl J Med 300:678, 1979.
165. YOKOCHI K, et al: Ther Drug Monit 4:353, 1982.
166. KULSHRESTHA VK, et al: Interaction between phenytoin and antacids. Br J Clin Pharmacol 6:177, 1978.
167. GARNETT WR, et al: Bioavailability of phenytoin administered with antacids. Therap Drug Monit 1:435, 1979.
168. O'BRIEN, WM, et al: Failure of antacids to alter the pharmacokinetics of phenytoin. Br J Clin Pharmacol 6:276, 1978.
169. CHAPRON DJ, et al: Effect of calcium and antacids on phenytoin bioavailability. Arch Neurol 36:436, 1979.
170. SAWCHUK RJ, et al: Effect of influenza vaccination on plasma phenytoin concentration. Ther Drug Monit 1:285, 1979.
171. HEIPERTZ R, et al: J Neurol 218:297, 1978.
172. HANSEN JM, et al: The effect of different sulfonamides on phenytoin metabolism in man. Acta Med Scand Suppl 624:106, 1979.
173. WILDER BJ, et al: Valproic acid: interaction with other anticonvulsant drugs. Neurology 28:892, 1978.
174. PATEL IH, et al: Phenobarbital-valproic acid interaction. Clin Pharmacol Ther 27:515, 1980.
175. BRUNI J, et al: Valproic acid and plasma levels of phenobarbital. Neurology 30:94, 1980.
176. BIVINS BA, et al: Dopamine-phenytoin interaction. Arch Surg 113:245, 1978.
177. HANSTEN PD: Personal observations. 1983.
178. PERUCCA E, RICHENS A: Interaction between phenytoin and imipramine. Br J Clin Pharmacol 4:485, 1977.
179. COULAM CB, ANNEGERS JF: Do anticonvulsants reduce the efficacy of oral contraceptives? Epilepsia 20:519, 1979.
180. HANSEN BS, et al: Influence of dextropropoxyphene on steady state serum levels and protein binding of three anti-epileptic drugs in man. Acta Neurol Scand 61:357, 1980.
181. KUBACKA RT, FERRANTE JA: Carbamazepine-propoxyphene interaction. Clin Pharm 2:104, 1983.
182. MESDJIAN E, et al: Carbamazepine intoxication due to triacetylolean-

References (CONT.)

domycin administration in epileptic patients. Epilepsia 21:489, 1980.
183. KOUP JR, et al. Interaction of chloramphenicol with phenytoin and phenobarbital. Case report. Clin Pharmacol Ther 24:571, 1978.
184. SALTIEL MS, STEPHENS NM: Phenytoin-chloramphenicol interaction. Drug Intell Clin Pharm 14:221, 1980.
185. GREENLAW CW: Chloramphenicol-phenytoin drug interaction. Drug Intell Clin Pharm 13:609, 1979.
186. HARPER JM, et al: Phenytoin-chloramphenicol interaction: a retrospective study. Drug Intell Clin Pharm 13:425, 1979.
187. POWELL DA, et al: Interactions among chloramphenicol, phenytoin, and phenobarbital in a pediatric patient. J Pediatr 98:1001, 1981.
188. KRASINSKI K, et al: Pharmacologic interactions among chloramphenicol, phenytoin and phenobarbital. Pediatr Infect Dis 1:232, 1982.
189. GAMBERTOGLIO JG: Corticosteroids and anticonvulsants. Drug Interactions Newsletter 3:55, 1983.
190. TAYLOR JW, et al: Mathematical analysis of a phenytoin-disulfiram interaction. Am J Hosp Pharm 38:93, 1981.
191. FURLANUT M, et al: Effects of folic acid on phenytoin kinetics in healthy subjects. Clin Pharmacol Ther 24:294, 1978.
192. INOUE F: Clinical implications of anticonvulsant-induced folate deficiency. Clin Pharm 1:372, 1982.
193. MACCOSBE PE, TOOMEY K: Interaction of phenytoin and folic acid. Clin Pharm 2:362, 1983.
194. MILLER RR, et al: Clinical importance of the interaction of phenytoin and isoniazid. Chest 75:356, 1979.
195. TONG TG, et al: Phenytoin-induced methadone withdrawal. Ann Intern Med 94:349, 1981.
196. VINCENT FM: Phenothiazine-induced phenytoin intoxication. Ann Intern Med 93:56, 1980.
197. NEURONEN PJ, et al: Antipyretic analgesics in patients on antiepileptic drug therapy. Eur J Clin Pharmacol 15:263, 1979.
198. PAXTON JW: Effects of aspirin on salivary and serum phenytoin kinetics in healthy subjects. Clin Pharmacol Ther 27:170, 1980.
199. FRASER GD, et al: Displacement of phenytoin from plasma binding sites of salicylate. Clin Pharmacol Ther 27:165, 1980.
200. LEONARD RF, et al: Phenytoin-salicylate interaction. Clin Pharmacol Ther 29:56, 1981.
201. BLACKSHEAR JL, et al: Thyroxine replacement requirements in hypothyroid patients receiving phenytoin. Ann Intern Med 99:341, 1983.
202. REUNANEN MI, et al: Low serum valproic acid concentrations in epileptic patients on combination therapy. Curr Ther Res 28:456, 1980.
203. DAHLQVIST R, et al: Decreased plasma protein binding of phenytoin in patients on valproic acid. Br J Clin Pharmacol 8:547, 1979.
204. SANSOM LN, et al: Interaction between phenytoin and valproate. Med J Aust 2:212, 1980.
205. MONKS A, RICHENS A: Effect of single doses of sodium valproate on serum phenytoin levels and protein binding in epileptic patients. Clin Pharmacol Ther 27:89, 1980.
206. BRUNI J, et al: Interactions of valproic acid with phenytoin. Neurology 30:1233, 1980.

149

CHAPTER 4

Antidiabetic Drug Interactions

ANTIDIABETIC DRUG INTERACTIONS

DRUGS	DISCUSSION

Acetazolamide (Diamox)[32]

MECHANISM: Not established.

CLINICAL SIGNIFICANCE: Acetazolamide reportedly can produce considerable increases in blood glucose in prediabetics and diabetics on oral hypoglycemic therapy while having little effect in normal subjects.[32] Confirmation of these findings is needed.

MANAGEMENT: Although evidence for an interaction is very scanty, patients receiving oral hypoglycemics should be watched for changes in antidiabetic drug requirements if acetazolamide is added.

Allopurinol (Zyloprim)[3]

MECHANISM: It has been proposed that allopurinol or its metabolites might compete with chlorpropamide for renal tubular secretion.[3]

CLINICAL SIGNIFICANCE: A preliminary report briefly described seven patients who received concomitant therapy with allopurinol and chlorpropamide.[3] Two of these patients had a markedly prolonged chlorpropamide half-life (over 200 hours). In two other patients the half-life appeared to be slightly prolonged. The remaining three patients had only been on allopurinol for 1 to 2 days and had chlorpropamide half-lives within the normal limits. Thus, these data suggest an interaction between allopurinol and chlorpropamide resulting in increased chlorpropamide effect. Additional studies are needed to define more clearly the incidence and magnitude of this reaction.

MANAGEMENT: Although evidence for an interaction is preliminary, patients receiving chlorpropamide (and possibly other sulfonylureas) who subsequently receive allopurinol should be watched for excessive hypoglycemic activity.

Ammonium Chloride[113]

MECHANISM: Large doses of ammonium chloride acidify the urine, thus decreasing the ionization of chlorpropamide (Diabinese) and decreasing its urinary excretion.

ANTIDIABETIC DRUG INTERACTIONS (CONT.)

DRUGS	DISCUSSION

CLINICAL SIGNIFICANCE: In six healthy subjects given chlorpropamide (250 mg orally) pretreatment with ammonium chloride (urine pH, 4.7 to 5.5) increased chlorpropamide half-life from 50 to 69 hours.[113] The extent to which ammonium chloride-induced acidification of the urine would enhance the hypoglycemic effect of chorpropamide is not established, but it may be clinically important in some patients. Patients whose urine was alkaline prior to the ammonium chloride (e.g., due to a vegetarian diet) would be likely to have a greater reduction in urine pH and thus a greater increase in serum chlorpropamide levels.

MANAGEMENT: One should be alert for evidence of enhanced chlorpropamide effect if ammonium chloride is used concurrently.

Anabolic Steroids[10,11,20,47]

MECHANISM: First, anabolic steroids alone may decrease blood glucose in some diabetic patients. Normal patients do not appear to be so affected. Also, it has been proposed that anabolic steroids may inhibit the metabolism of oral hypoglycemic agents.[10,11]

CLINICAL SIGNIFICANCE: Methandrostenolone (Dianabol) has been shown to enhance the hypoglycemic response to tolbutamide while nandrolone (Durabolin) and methenolone acetate did not have this effect.[47] Also, it has been noted clinically that anabolic steroids may decrease insulin requirements in diabetics and may restore sensitivity in the insulin-resistant patient.[20] Thus, in general, one would expect an enhanced hypoglycemic response to antidiabetic drugs in the presence of anabolic steroid therapy although most specific combinations of anabolic steroids and antidiabetic drugs have not been tested.

MANAGEMENT: If anabolic steroids are added to antidiabetic drug therapy, the patient should be monitored more closely for evidence of hypoglycemia. Attention should be given to possible changes in antidiabetic dosage requirements.

Calcium Channel Blockers[114-117]

MECHANISM: Calcium channel blockers may have intrinsic effects on carbohydrate metabolism.

CLINICAL SIGNIFICANCE: After a patient was observed to have reduced serum glucose following the discontinuation of nifedipine, six healthy subjects were given an oral glucose tolerance test (OGTT) before and after nifedipine (20 mg every 8 hours for 3 days).[115] Nifedipine was associated with a considerable decrease in glucose tolerance. In another study, ten nondiabetics and ten "chemical" diabetics received an OGTT before and after nifedipine (10 mg three times daily for 10 days).[114] Nifedipine further reduced glucose tolerance in the patients with chemical diabetes, but paradoxically improved glucose tolerance in the healthy subjects. In another study, nifedipine (20 mg during an OGTT) reduced glucose tolerance in both normal persons and patients with non-insulin-dependent diabetes mellitus (NIDDM).[116]

151

DRUGS	DISCUSSION

Thus, the preponderance of evidence indicates that nifedipine tends to reduce glucose tolerance in patients with NIDDM. Conversely, available evidence indicates that both oral and intravenous verapamil improve glucose tolerance in patients with NIDDM.[117] Thus in patients with NIDDM, nifedipine might be expected to increase antidiabetic drug requirements, while verapamil may have the opposite effect. Little information is available regarding the effect of verapamil or nifedipine on insulin dosage requirements in insulin-dependent diabetics, but one should be alert for the possibility of poor diabetic control. Little is known regarding the effect of diltiazem on glucose tolerance.

MANAGEMENT: One should alert for evidence of altered antidiabetic drug requirements if calcium blockers are initiated or discontinued.

Chloramphenicol (Chloromycetin)[3,48,65,106]

MECHANISM: Chloramphenicol inhibits hepatic microsomal enzyme activity, resulting in impaired tolbutamide metabolism.[48] Preliminary evidence indicates that the half-life of chlorpropamide is also prolonged by concomitant chloramphenicol administration.[65]

CLINICAL SIGNIFICANCE: Chloramphenicol administration (2 g/day for about 10 days) has resulted in nearly a threefold increase in the half-life of tolbutamide.[48] A case is also reported in which this interaction appeared to be responsible for an episode of severe hypoglycemia. In another study, chloramphenicol produced about a twofold increase in morning tolbutamide levels in eight diabetic patients.[106] Similarly, in another study chloramphenicol (1.5 to 3 g/day) prolonged the half-life of chlorpropamide in five patients.[65] Their half-lives were 40, 60, 82, 116, and 146 hours as compared to the normal range of 30 to 36 hours. A subsequent report adds a sixth patient on concomitant chloramphenicol and chlorpropamide therapy who had a chlorpropamide half-life of slightly over 100 hours.[3] The effect of chloramphenicol on other oral hypoglycemic agents is not established, but one should be alert for evidence of enhanced hypoglycemic effects.

MANAGEMENT: Current evidence indicates that a patient on tolbutamide who receives chloramphenicol will have an enhanced hypoglycemic response to tolbutamide. Reduction of tolbutamide enhanced hypoglycemic response to tolbutamide. Reduction of tolbutamide dosage is likely to be necessary in some patients. Although the interaction with chlorpropamide is less well documented, the same precautions should be taken if chloramphenicol is given concomitantly.

Clofibrate (Atromid-S)[3,91,94,95,97,99,102]

MECHANISM: The mechanism for the purported increase in the hypoglycemic effect of sulfonylureas caused by clofibrate is not established. Proposed mechanisms include (1) displacement of sulfonylureas from plasma protein binding, (2) decreased insulin resistance,[94] and (3) competition between clofibrate and chlorpropamide for renal tubular secretion.[3] The mechanism for the inhibitory effect of glibenclamide (a sulfonylurea) on clofibrate-induced antidiuresis in patients with diabetes insipidus is not established.[95]

CLINICAL SIGNIFICANCE: Although some have failed to detect an effect of clofibrate on the hypoglycemic response to sulfonylureas in diabetics,[97,102] others have noted enhanced hypoglycemia.[91,94,99] Also, a study in five subjects given clofibrate plus chlorpropamide indicated that clofibrate may prolong chlorpropamide half-life somewhat.[3] In two patients with pituitary diabetes insipidus, glibenclamide inhibited clofibrate-induced antidiuresis.[95] In summary, certain diabetic patients appear to develop enhanced hypoglycemia when clofibrate is given concomitantly with sulfonylureas, while others are not so affected. Low serum albumin may predispose patients to the enhanced hypoglycemia.[91]

MANAGEMENT: It does not appear necessary to avoid concomitant use of clofibrate and sulfonylureas, but patients so treated should be monitored more closely for hypoglycemia. This caution would apply especially to patients stabilized on a sulfonylurea in whom clofibrate is started or stopped.

Clonidine (Catapres)[108]

MECHANISM: The increased production of catecholamines in response to insulin-induced hypoglycemia is apparently inhibited by pretreatment with clonidine.[108]

CLINICAL SIGNIFICANCE: A group of hypertensive and normal subjects were given a single dose of insulin before and during treatment with clonidine.[108] Clonidine suppressed the marked increase in catecholamine production which normally follows insulin hypoglycemia and also reduced the signs and symptoms of hypoglycemia.

MANAGEMENT: Patients receiving antidiabetic drugs and clonidine should be aware that clonidine may suppress the signs and symptoms of hypoglycemia.

Colestipol (Colestid)[109]

MECHANISM: Not established.

CLINICAL SIGNIFICANCE: In a trial of the use of colestipol in the treatment of hypercholesterolemia it was found that patients receiving combined sulfonylurea and phenformin did not respond to colestipol therapy.[109] Conversely colestipol did appear to be effective in two patients receiving insulin.

MANAGEMENT: Too little information is available to recommend avoiding concomitant use of oral hypoglycemic agents and colestipol. However, in patients receiving oral hypoglycemics who fail to respond to colestipol, the antidiabetic drugs should be considered a potential cause.

ANTIDIABETIC DRUG INTERACTIONS (CONT.)

Contraceptives, Oral[63,64,86]

MECHANISM: Oral contraceptives have been noted to impair glucose tolerance. This tendency depends upon a number of factors such as type of steroid, type of patients, and duration of administration.

CLINICAL SIGNIFICANCE: It has been stated that oral contraceptives might occasionally increase insulin reqirements, but the effect would probably not be large. However, Reder and Tulgan[63] have described a patient receiving acetohexamide in whom an oral contraceptive (norethylnodrel, 2.5 mg with mestranol 0.1 mg) appeared to result in the loss of control of diabetes. It was not conclusively established that the oral contraceptive was responsible, however. In another study of patients with prostatic cancer given diethylstilbestrol (DES), two of 28 patients with normal glucose tolerance developed prediabetic values on DES and one of two other prediabetics became diabetic during DES.[86] However three patients with diabetes *prior* to DES developed a *fall* in fasting blood glucose during the first 10 days of DES therapy. Thus, the effects of oral contraceptives or estrogens on glucose tolerance are complex with the outcome depending on the type of patient, dose of drug, etc.

MANAGEMENT: It has been suggested that diabetic patients try to use methods of contraception other than oral agents.[63] If this is not practical, the patient should be watched more closely for altered diabetic control.

Corticosteroids[84,85]

MECHANISM: Corticosteroids have intrinsic hyperglycemic activity.

CLINICAL SIGNIFICANCE: The hyperglycemic effect of corticosteroids is well documented, and occurs regularly in patients receiving pharmacologic doses of corticosteroids.

MANAGEMENT: One should be alert for evidence of altered diabetic control if corticosteroids are initiated, discontinued, or changed in dosage.

Dextrothyroxine (Choloxin)[26,58]

MECHANISM: The mechanism is probably an intrinsic metabolic effect of dextrothyroxine, although an effect on the action of antidiabetic drugs cannot be excluded at this time.

CLINICAL SIGNIFICANCE: Some diabetic patients have manifested an increase in blood glucose and antidiabetic therapy requirements following dextrothyroxine administration.[26,58]

MANAGEMENT: Patients receiving both dextrothyroxine and an antidiabetic drug should be watched for possible decreased diabetic control.

ANTIDIABETIC DRUG INTERACTIONS (CONT.)

DRUGS	DISCUSSION

Disulfiram (Antabuse)[89]

MECHANISM: None.

CLINICAL SIGNIFICANCE: A study in ten normal subjects demonstrated no effect of disulfiram on tolbutamide half-life or metabolic clearance rate[89]. The effect of disulfiram on other sulfonylureas or insulin was not studied.

MANAGEMENT: None required.

Epinephrine (Adrenalin)[62]

MECHANISM: Epinephrine may increase blood glucose by inhibiting glucose uptake by peripheral tissues and by promoting glycogenolysis.

CLINICAL SIGNIFICANCE: The hyperglycemic effect of epinephrine administration may necessitate an increase in insulin or oral hypoglycemic dosage.

MANAGEMENT: Epinephrine and, to a lesser extent, other adrenergic agents should be used cautiously in diabetic patients.

Ethanol (Alcohol, Ethyl)[8,9,24,30,39,40–46,66–69,81–83,88,96]

MECHANISM:
1. Ethanol may exhibit intrinsic hypoglycemic activity although hyperglycemia has also been noted.
2. Chlorpropamide and, to a lesser extent, other sulfonylureas may provoke an "Antabuse reaction" to ethanol with flushing, headache, etc.[40,88,96]
3. Prolonged heavy intake of ethanol has been shown to markedly decrease the half-life of tolbutamide.[41,42,69,83] Induction of hepatic microsomal enzymes is probably responsible for this effect. Acetohexamide is metabolized to a product with significant hypoglycemic activity. Thus, the effect of enzyme induction on acetohexamide disposition is not clear.
4. Ethanol ingestion may contribute to lactic acidosis in patients receiving phenformin.[*44,45,66–68]
5. Ethanol may inhibit the antidiuretic effect of chlorpropamide used to treat diabetes insipidus.[82]

CLINICAL SIGNIFICANCE: Acute ingestion of ethanol by patients on any antidiabetic agent carries the risk of severe hypoglycemia due to the hypoglycemic effect of ethanol, especially in fasting patients.[24,30,46,81] The increased tolbutamide metabolism in alcoholics and heavy drinkers probably decreases its hypoglycemic effect, although the intrinsic hypoglycemic activity of ethanol may counteract this somewhat. Also, the intoxicated diabetic may have difficulty in properly self-administering his antidiabetic medication. A case has been reported in which a diabetic apparently took an overdose of chlorpropamide while in-

*Phenformin is no longer generally available in the United States.

155

ANTIDIABETIC DRUG INTERACTIONS (CONT.)

DRUGS	DISCUSSION

toxicated, and the resultant hypoglycemia was probably enhanced by the ethanol.[39] Finally, two patients receiving chlorpropamide for diabetes insipidus developed polyuria and polydipsia following ethanol intake, presumably due to ethanol-induced inhibition of chlorpropamide-induced antidiuresis.[82]

MANAGEMENT: Since an "Antabuse reaction" may occur following ethanol ingestion in patients receiving sulfonylureas, they should be informed of this possibility when therapy is initiated. Ingestion of moderate to large amounts of ethanol should probably be avoided in patients on antidiabetic drugs due to possible adverse effects on diabetic control. However, smaller amounts of alcohol, especially if taken with a meal, would not seem likely to cause difficulty.

Fenfluramine (Pondamin)[12,110]

MECHANISM: Fenfluramine appears to increase the uptake of glucose by skeletal muscle.

CLINICAL SIGNIFICANCE: Initial experiments indicate that fenfluramine has intrinsic hypoglycemic activity and may be most effective in this regard when given immediately before a meal.[12] It appears to lower postprandial blood glucose levels in diabetics maintained on insulin, tolbutamide, or diet alone. Fenfluramine may prove useful as an antidiabetic drug,[110] but its potential hypoglycemic activity should be kept in mind when it is used as an anorectic agent.

MANAGEMENT: Diabetic patients maintained on insulin or sulfonylureas should watch for altered hypoglycemic activity when fenfluramine is started or stopped.

Glucagon[13,14]

MECHANISM: Glucagon has hyperglycemic activity that may antagonize the hypoglycemic effect of antidiabetic agents.

CLINICAL SIGNIFICANCE: The hyperglycemic effect of glucagon must be considered in diabetic patients receiving glucagon for its positive inotropic action. Although some investigators[13] have detected little effect on blood glucose in patients receiving glucagon for heart failure, others[14] have noted a hyperglycemic effect. One diabetic on insulin developed "marked" hyperglycemia.[14] The hyperglycemic response to glucagon may be dependent on dose, method of administration, etc.

MANAGEMENT: Diabetic patients receiving glucagon for its positive inotropic action should be watched more closely for signs of decreased diabetic control.

Guanethidine (Ismelin)[25,31,70]

MECHANISM: Guanethidine has been shown to possess antidiabetic activity, but the mechanism has not been established. It is possible that depletion of tissue catecholamines may be involved.

ANTIDIABETIC DRUG INTERACTIONS (CONT.)

CLINICAL SIGNIFICANCE: One patient has been described in whom a considerable increase in insulin requirements followed the termination of guanethidine therapy.[25] Subsequent study in three diabetics showed guanethidine to considerably improve glucose tolerance tests in these patients.[31]

MANAGEMENT: Patients on any antidiabetic drug should be watched more closely for altered hypoglycemic effect if guanethidine therapy is started or stopped.

Halofenate[102,104]

MECHANISM: Not established. It is proposed that halofenate displaces sulfonylureas from plasma protein binding.

CLINICAL SIGNIFICANCE: Six of nine diabetics receiving sulfonylureas required a reduction in antidiabetic drug dosage when halofenate was added.[102] Accordingly, halofenate enhanced tolbutamide serum levels and serum glucose decreases in twelve normal subjects.[102] Others have noted a similar enhancement of oral hypoglycemic response with halofenate, which may be a beneficial response in some patients by allowing better control of the diabetes.[104] The enhanced hypoglycemic response appears to take several weeks to develop fully.[102]

MANAGEMENT: Concomitant use of halofenate and oral hypoglycemics need not be avoided; some patients apparently benefit from the combination. However, one should be alert for the possible necessity of altered dose requirements for the hypoglycemic agents.

Marijuana[76,77,120,121]

MECHANISM: Not established.

CLINICAL SIGNIFICANCE: Preliminary evidence has been presented that marijuana may impair glucose tolerance,[77] Also, a case has occurred in which a juvenile diabetic developed a threefold increase in insulin requirements following the use of amphetamines and marijuana.[76] Whether either drug was responsible for the effect on insulin requirements in this case was not determined. In another case, diabetic ketoacidosis followed the oral ingestion of large amounts of marijuana in a 21-year-old man.[120] In a study of six subjects, tetrahydrocannabinol (6 mg IV) impaired glucose tolerance.[121]

MANAGEMENT: No special precautions appear necessary, but physicians should be aware that marijuana might affect glucose tolerance.

Monoamine Oxidase Inhibitors (MAOI)[15,16,34,35,71,98]

MECHANISM: It has been proposed that MAOI interfere with the compensatory adrenergic response to hypoglycemia.[15] However, subsequent studies have failed to confirm this mechanism.[31,35] Tranylcypromine (Parnate) has been shown to stimulate insulin secretion in animals, probably because of beta-adrenergic stimulation.[34]

CLINICAL SIGNIFICANCE: Clinically, MAOI have been shown to enhance and/or prolong the hypoglycemic response to both insulin and sulfonylurea hypoglycemics. This may be of sufficient magnitude to produce unexpected hypoglycemic episodes if the effect is not anticipated. However, some patients may be expected to benefit from the enhanced hypoglycemic response.

MANAGEMENT: MAOI should be administrated with caution to patients also receiving antidiabetic drugs; excessive hypoglycemia may occur.

Phenothiazines[27,28,33,111]

MECHANISM: It has been proposed that phenothiazines might activate adrenergic mechanisms.

CLINICAL SIGNIFICANCE: Arneson[33] records five diabetics controlled on insulin in whom the disease became unstable during chlorpromazine therapy. The effect appears to be dose related; chlorpromazine doses less than 100 mg/day appear less likely to affect glucose tolerance.[28,111] Little information is available on the effect of phenothiazines other than chlorpromazine on glucose tolerance.

MANAGEMENT: Patients receiving antidiabetic agents should probably watch for decreased diabetic control if large doses of chlorpromazine are added to the regimen.

Phenylbutazone (Butazolidin)[1,4,18,23,38,49,56,72,73,101,112]

MECHANISM: Phenylbutazone administration has been shown to prolong the half-life of the active metabolite of acetohexamide (hydroxyhexamide).[23] The authors postulate that this is due to inhibition of urinary hydroxyhexamide excretion. The half-life of acetohexamide itself was not affected. The increased serum tolbutamide levels following phenylbutazone administration are presumably due to inhibition of carboxylation of tolbutamide.[18,112] Displacement of tolbutamide from plasma protein binding by phenylbutazone may also be involved in the enhanced hypoglycemic effect of tolbutamide.

CLINICAL SIGNIFICANCE: Enhanced hypoglycemic responses to acetohexamide and tolbutamide should be anticipated following phenylbutazone administration. Theoretical considerations and isolated reports indicate that other sulfonylurea hypolycemics would be similarly affected. The case of a patient with a fatal hypoglycemic coma from tolbutamide[38] and two cases of patients with hypoglycemia from acetohexamide[23,101] have been reported in which phenylbutazone may have contributed to the reactions. Four additional cases have been reported by three separate groups[1,4,72] in which severe hypoglycemia developed apparently due to combined tolbutamide-

ANTIDIABETIC DRUG INTERACTIONS (CONT.)

DRUGS	DISCUSSION

phenylbutazone therapy. Studies in normal volunteers support the clinical findings in that phenylbutazone and oxyphenbutazone considerably prolong tolbutamide half-life.[112] A single case has appeared in which phenylbutazone appeared to *antagonize* the hypoglycemic effect of tolbutamide.[73] Phenylbutazone reportedly also potentiates the action of insulin,[56] but the clinical significance of this cannot be determined without more information. It is not known whether other sulfonylureas are affected by phenylbutazone.

MANAGEMENT: Patients receiving sulfonylureas should be watched more closely for signs of hypoglycemia if phenylbutazone or oxyphenbutazone is also given. Alteration in sulfonylurea dose may be necessary if phenylbutazone or oxyphenbutazone is started or stopped.

Phenyramidol[19]

MECHANISM: Phenyramidol is known to inhibit the metabolism of several drugs. The ability of phenyramidol to increase the half-life of tolbutamide is probably related to this property.

CLINICAL SIGNIFICANCE: The more than twofold increase in tolbutamide half-life and the resultant elevation of tolbutamide plasma levels can be expected to enhance the hypoglycemic response to tolbutamide. It should be noted that phenyramidol is no longer commercially available in the United States.

MANAGEMENT: A reduction in tolbutamide dosage is likely to be necessary if phenyramidol is also given.

Potassium Salts[50-52]

MECHANISM: Not established. However, potassium *loss* is known to impair glucose tolerance,[51] and replacement of potassium in uremic patients with a potassium deficit improves their glucose tolerance.[52]

CLINICAL SIGNIFICANCE: Potentiation of the hypoglycemic effect of acetohexamide was observed in eight of 11 patients given potassium chloride (30 ml of 25% solution daily for 1 week).[50] However, no mention was made of the potassium status of these patients prior to potassium chloride therapy. The clinical significance of the interaction must await further study.

MANAGEMENT: The effect of potassium is not likely to be large enough to warrant any precautionary measures.

Probenecid (Benemid)[3,17,21]

MECHANISM: It has been proposed that probenecid may inhibit the renal tubular secretion of chlorpropamide.[3]

CLINICAL SIGNIFICANCE: In six patients receiving probenecid (1 to 2 g/day) the average half-life of chlorpropamide was found to be 50 hours,[3] and it was concluded that probenecid may have the ability to

ANTIDIABETIC DRUG INTERACTIONS (CONT.)

enhance the effect of chlorpropamide. An earlier report[17] indicated that probenecid increased the half-life of tolbutamide, but a later study failed to confirm this finding.[21] Thus, probenecid possibly increases the effect of chlorpropamide and probably has little effect on tolbutamide. The effect of probenecid on other antidiabetic drugs is unknown.

MANAGEMENT: Patients maintained on chlorpropamide should probably watch more closely for signs of excessive hypoglycemic response if probenecid is added to the regimen.

Rifampin (Rifadin, Rimactane)[87,93,103]

MECHANISM: Rifampin appears to stimulate the metabolism of tolbutamide by hepatic microsomal enzymes.

CLINICAL SIGNIFICANCE: Rifampin has been shown to enhance considerably the disposition of tolbutamide in patients with tuberculosis,[93] patients with cirrhosis or cholestasis,[103] and normal volunteers.[87] Due to the magnitude of the decreases in tolbutamide half-life, one would expect to see impaired hypoglycemic response to rifampin. Little is known concerning the effect of rifampin on antidiabetic drugs other than tolbutamide.

MANAGEMENT: When rifampin and tolbutamide are used concomitantly one should be alert for diminished hypoglycemic activity of tolbutamide.

Salicylates[1,3,17,29,37,53,54]

MECHANISM: Large doses of salicylates may have an intrinsic effect on carbohydrate metabolism which tends to decrease the hyperglycemia of diabetics. In-vitro studies have shown sodium salicylate to displace tolbutamide and chlorpropamide from plasma protein binding, thus increasing unbound (active) sulfonylurea.[53] It has also been proposed that salicylates might interfere with the renal tubular secretion of chlorpropamide,[17] which is consistent with the contention that tubular secretion is an important mechanism of chlorpropamide elimination.[3] In one patient, chlorpropamide appeared to enhance the blood level of salicylate.[17] Thus, it is possible that chlorpropamide-induced increases in salicylate blood level enhance the intrinsic hypoglycemic activity of the salicylate.

CLINICAL SIGNIFICANCE: Salicylate administration has been shown to enhance the hypoglycemic response to chlorpropamide, and in some cases this effect has been seen at serum salicylate levels of 10 mg/dl or lower.[17] Cases have been reported in which aspirin appeared to have contributed to hypoglycemic coma in patients receiving sulfonylureas.[29,54] Based on current evidence, it appears that chlorpropamide is more likely to be affected by salicylates than other sulfonylureas. In summary, large doses of salicylate might enhance the hypoglycemic effect of sulfonylureas or insulin through an intrinsic

ANTIDIABETIC DRUG INTERACTIONS (CONT.)

DRUGS	DISCUSSION

hypoglycemic effect of the salicylate. Small doses of salicylates as used for analgesia probably have minimal effects on antidiabetic drugs with the possible exception of chlorpropamide.

MANAGEMENT: One should be alert for evidence of altered response to oral hypoglycemics if salicylate therapy is started or stopped.

Smoking[118,119]

MECHANISM: Smoking may result in release of endogenous substances that antagonise the hypoglycemic effect of insulin.

CLINICAL SIGNIFICANCE: Diabetic patients who smoke heavily may have insulin requirements almost one-third higher than non-smokers.[118] This may be at least partly due to the increased catecholamine and corticosteroid release caused by smoking. Smoking has also been shown to reduce the rate of insulin absorption following subcutaneous injection, probably as a result of smoking-induced peripheral vasoconstriction.[119] Thus, smoking should be considered as one of the factors that can affect insulin requirements as well as the time course of insulin action.

MANAGEMENT: Patients should be informed that a change in smoking habits may change the response to insulin.

Sulfinpyrazone (Anturane)[5,56]

MECHANISM: See Clinical Significance.

CLINICAL SIGNIFICANCE: Since the structurally related drug, phenylbutazone, may potentiate the effect of sulfonylureas, the manufacturers of sulfinpyrazone suggest caution in concomitant sulfinpyrazone and sulfonylurea administration. However, clinical studies involving these drugs are needed to determine the specific clinical significance. One patient has been briefly mentioned who developed hypoglycemia while on insulin and sulfinpyrazone.[5] Whether sulfinpyrazone was responsible was apparently not established.

MANAGEMENT: Pending the availability of more information on this interaction, some caution should be exercised with sulfinpyrazone administration in patients receiving sulfonylureas or insulin.

Sulfonamides[6,18,22,37,55,74,92]

MECHANISM: More than one mechanism may be involved. It has been proposed that sulfaphenazole[18] and sulfamethizole (Thiosulfil)[6] inhibit the carboxylation of tolbutamide. Displacement of tolbutamide from plasma protein binding may also be partially involved in the potentiation by sulfaphenazole.

CLINICAL SIGNIFICANCE: The ability of sulfaphenazole to enhance the hypoglycemic effect of tolbutamide is fairly well documented. Serum levels of tolbutamide are increased considerably, as is the half-life.[18]

Preliminary evidence in two patients[6] indicates that sulfamethizole also has the ability to prolong tolbutamide half-life. Sulfadiazine and sulfadimethoxine do not appear to have this effect. Sulfamethazine appeared to result in severe hypoglycemia in a patient maintained on chlorpropamide.[55] Sulfisoxazole (Gantrisin) has been reported to potentiate the effect of tolbutamide in two patients, and severe hypoglycemia resulted. However, one of the patients also received chloramphenicol and it is likely that this contributed to the interaction.[22] More study is needed to confirm this effect of sulfisoxazole on tolbutamide; it may be that the effect is only seen when blood levels of sulfisoxazole are high and when precipitating factors are present (e.g., old age, uremia, etc.). A single case has been reported in which sulfisoxazole appeared to enhance the effect of chlorpropamide, so that hypoglycemic coma resulted.[74] Sulfonamides have not been reported to affect the response to insulin.

MANAGEMENT: Concomitant sulfonylurea and sulfonamide administration should be undertaken with the realization that enhanced hypoglycemic effects may occur. The following is a guide to the degree of caution to be observed with the various combinations.
    Known Interactions
    1. Tolbutamide plus sulfaphenzole (Sulfabid)
    Possible Interactions
    1. Chlorpropamide plus sulfisoxazole (Gantrisin)
    2. Chlorpropamide plus sulfamethazine
    3. Tolbutamide plus sulfisoxazole (Gantrisin)
    4. Tolbutamide plus sulfamethizole (Thiosulfil)
    Probably No Interaction
    1. Tolbutamide plus sulfadiazine
    2. Tolbutamide plus sulfadiamethoxine
    Not Enough Information (Interaction may or may not occur)
    1. Any other combination of a sulfonylurea and a sulfonamide

Sulindac (Clinoril)[105]

MECHANISM: None.

CLINICAL SIGNIFICANCE: Twelve diabetics stabilized on tolbutamide were given sulindac (400 mg/day for 1 week).[105] No significant changes were noted in tolbutamide plasma levels or half-life.

MANAGEMENT: No special precautions appear necessary.

Tetracyclines[78,79,100]

MECHANISM: Not established. Animal studies indicate that oxytetracycline enhances the hypoglycemic effect of insulin.[79]

CLINICAL SIGNIFICANCE: Two cases have been reported in which oxytetracycline appeared to reduce insulin requirements considerably,[78] and in another patient the hypoglycemic effect of tolbutamide increased following tolbutamide administration.[79] Although only a few

DRUGS	DISCUSSION

such cases have been reported, studies in man using oxytetracycline alone and animal studies support a hypoglycemic action of oxytetracycline. There is also some preliminary clinical information indicating that tetracycline may contribute to lactic acidosis in patients receiving phenformin.[100]

MANAGEMENT: When oxytetracycline is used in a patient receiving antidiabetic drugs, the physician and patient should be alert for signs of hypoglycemia. Adjustment of antidiabetic drug dosage may be necessary.

Thiazide Diuretics[2,7,36,59-61,75,80]

MECHANISM:
1. The diabetogenic effect of thiazide diuretics may be partially due to potassium depletion. It has also been proposed that thiazides may inhibit insulin secretion,[75] but not all evidence supports such a view.[80]
2. Thiazides and chlorpropamide can both produce hyponatremia probably by different mechanisms.[7]

CLINICAL SIGNIFICANCE: Thiazides tend to elevate blood glucose in diabetics and prediabetics and thus may antagonize the hypoglycemic effect of antidiabetic drugs.[59-61] However, in most patients this effect does not cause significant clinical problems. It has also been noted in some patients that combined therapy with chlorpropamide (Diabenese) and a thiazide diuretic may result in hyponatremia of a degree not seen with the use of either agent alone.[7] Another patient (with diabetes, hypertension, and congestive heart failure) has been briefly described who was resistant to "ordinary diuretic treatment" while receiving chlorpropamide, but responded when the chlorpropamide was replaced by glibenclamide.[2]

MANAGEMENT: One should watch for decreased diabetic control when thiazide therapy is started in a patient receiving any diabetic drug. When chlorpropamide is used with a thiazide, one should be alert for hyponatremia or thiazide reistance in addition to decreased diabetic control.

Thyroid Hormones[57]

MECHANISM: Not established.

CLINICAL SIGNIFICANCE: Initiating thyroid replacement therapy may cause increases in insulin or oral hypoglycemic requirements. The effects seen are poorly understood and depend on a variety of factors, such as the dose and type of thyroid preparations, endocrine status of the patient, etc.

MANAGEMENT: Patients receiving insulin or oral hypoglycemics should probably be watched more closely during initiation of thyroid replacement therapy.

ANTIDIABETIC DRUG INTERACTIONS (CONT.)

DRUGS	DISCUSSION

Trimethoprim/Sulfamethoxazole (Bactrim, Septra, Co-trimoxazole)[90]

MECHANISM: Not established.

CLINICAL SIGNIFICANCE: A group of 18 diabetics were given trimethoprim/sulfamethoxazole (TMP/SMX) for 14 days. Blood glucose and insulin levels measured before, during, and after TMP/SMX indicated a possible enhanced hypoglycemic response in one patient receiving a sulfonylurea (specific drug not stated),[90] but not in seven other patients receiving "oral hypoglycemics." TMP/SMX had no consistent effect in diabetics receiving insulin or in diabetics on diet alone. It seems likely that if the enhanced hypoglycemic response in the one patient on a sulfonylurea was due to drug interaction, the sulfamethoxazole was responsible rather than the trimethoprim.

MANAGEMENT: Although there is little evidence of interaction, patients on sulfonylureas should be monitored more closely if TMP/SMX is given concomitantly.

References

1. ANON: Therapeutic conferences. Drug interaction. Br Med J 1:389, 1971.
2. RAVINA A: Antidiuretic action of chlorpropamide (Letter). Lancet 2:203, 1973.
3. PETITPIERRE B, et al: Behavior of chlorpropamide in renal insufficiency and under the effect of associated drug therapy. Int J Clin Pharmacol Ther Toxicol 6:120, 1972.
4. TANNENBAUM H, et al: Phenylbutazone-tolbutamide drug interaction (Letter). N Engl J Med 290:344, 1974.
5. KAEGL A, et al: Arteriovenous-shunt thrombosis. Prevention by sulfinpyrazone. N Engl J Med 290:304, 1974
6. SIERSBAEK-NIELSEN K, et al: Sulfamethizone-induced inhibition of diphenylhydantoin and tolbutamide metabolism in man (Abstract). Clin Pharmacol Ther 14:148, 1973.
7. FICHMAN MP, et al: Diuretic-induced hyponatremia. Ann Intern Med 75:853, 1971.
8. PODGAINY H, BRESSLER R: Biochemical basis of the sulfonylurea-induced antabuse syndrome. Diabetes 17:679, 1968.
9. SHAH MN, et al: Comparison of blood clearance of ethanol and tolbutamide and the activity of hepatic ethanol-oxidizing and drug metabolizing enyzmes in chronic alcoholic subjects. Am J Clin Nutr 25:135, 1972.
10. SOTANIEMI EA, et al: Drug metabolism and androgen control therapy in prostatic cancer. Clin Pharmacol Ther 14:413, 1973.
11. KONTTURI M, SOTANIEMI E: Estrogen induced metabolic changes during treatment of prostatic cancer. Scand J Lab Clin Invest 25:45 (Supplement 113), 1970.
12. TURTLE JR, BURGESS JA: Hypoglycemic action of fenfluramine in diabetes mellitus. Diabetes 22:858, 1973.

References (CONT.)

13. BROGAN E, et al: Glucagon therapy in heart failure. Lancet 1:482, 1969.
14. NORD HJ, et al: Treatment of congestive heart failure with glucagon. Ann Intern Med 72:649, 1970.
15. COOPER AJ, ASHCROFT G: Modification of insulin and sulfonylurea hypoglycemia by monoamine-oxidase inhibitor drugs. Diabetes 16:272,1967.
16. COOPER AJ, ASHCROFT G: Potentiation of insulin hypoglycaemia by MAOI antidepressant drugs. Lancet 1:407, 1966.
17. STOWERS JM, et al: Clinical and pharmacological comparison of chlorpropamide and other sulfonylureas. Ann NY Acad Sci 74:689, 1959.
18. CHRISTENSEN LK, et al: Sulfaphenazole-induced hypoglycemic attacks in tolbutamide-treated diabetics. Lancet 2:1298, 1963.
19. SOLOMON HM, SCHROGIE JJ: Effect of phenyramidol and bishydroxycoumarin on the metabolism of tolbutamide in human subjects. Metabolism 16:1029, 1967.
20. SACHS BA, WOLFMAN L: Effect of oxandrolone on plasma lipids and lipoproteins of patients with disorders of lipid metabolism. Metabolism 17:400, 1968.
21. BROOK R, et al: Failure of probenecid to inhibit the rate of metabolism of tolbutamide in man. Clin Pharmacol Ther 9:314, 1968.
22. SOELDNER JS, STEINKE J: Hypoglycemia in tolbutamide-treated diabetes JAMA 193:398, 1965.
23. FIELD JB, et al: Potentiation of acetohexamide hypoglycemia by phenylbutazone N Engl J Med 277:889, 1967.
24. ARKY RA, et al: Irreversible hypoglycemia, a complication of alcohol and insulin. JAMA 206:575, 1968.
25. GUPTA KK, LILLICRAP CA: Guanethidine and diabetes (Letter). Br Med J 2:697, 1968.
26. ANON: Sodium dextrothyroxine (Choloxin). Med Let Drugs Ther 9:103, 1967.
27. JORI A, CARRARA MC: On the mechanism of the hyperglycemic effect of chlorpromazine. J Pharm Pharmacol 18:623, 1966.
28. THONNARD-NEUMANN E: Phenothiazines and diabetes in hospitalized women. Am J Psychiatry 124:978, 1968.
29. PEASTON MJT, FINNEGAN P: A case of combined poisoning with chlorpropamide, actylsalicylic acid and paracetamol. Br J Clin Pract 22:30, 1968.
30. Editorial: Alcohol and hypoglycemic coma. JAMA 206:639, 1968.
31. GUPTA KK: Guanethidine and glucose tolerance in diabetics (Letter). Br Med J 3:679, 1968.
32. KURZ M: Diamox und Manifestierung von Diabetes Mellitus, Wien Med Wochenschr 118:239, 1968. (From de Haen, Drugs in Use, Acetazolamide, U0239/31.).
33. ARNESON G: Phenothiazine derivatives and glucose metabolism. J Neuropsychiatry 5:181, 1964.
34. BRESSLER R, et al: Tranylcypromine: a potent insulin secretagogue and hypoglycemic agent. Diabetes 17:617, 1968.
35. ADNITT PI: Hypoglycemic action of monoamine oxidase inhibitors (MAOI's). Diabetes 17:628, 1968.
36. JOHNSON B, et al: Effect of tolbutamide on hypotensive and oliguric drugs (Abstract). Clin Res 17:248, 1969.

References (CONT.)

37. BERGMAN H: Hypoglycemic coma during sulfonylurea therapy. Acta Med Scand 177:287, 1965.
38. SLADE IH, IOSEFA RN: Fatal hypoglycemic coma from the use of tolbutamide in elderly patients: report of two cases. J Am Geriatr Soc 15:948, 1967.
39. PRYOR DS: Hypoglycaemic effect of chlorpropamide. Med J Aust 2:539, 1960.
40. FITZGERALD MG, et al: Alcohol sensitivity in diabetics receiving chlorpropamide. Diabetes 2:40, 1962.
41. KATER RMH, et al: Increased rate of tolbutamide metabolism in alcoholic patients. JAMA 207:363, 1969.
42. KATER RMH, et al: Increased rate of clearance of drugs from the circulation of alcoholics. Am J Med Sci 258:35, 1969.
43. NELSON E: Zero order oxidation of tolbutamide in vivo. Nature 193:76, 1962.
44. JOHNSON HK, WATERHOUSE C: Relationship of alcohol and hyperlactatemia in diabetic subjects treated with phenformin. Am J Med 45:98, 1968.
45. DAVIDSON MB, et al: Phenformin, hypoglycemia and lactic acidosis. N Engl J Med 275:886, 1966.
46. MOSS JM: Cocktails and diabetes (Information Please). Gen Pract 40:129, 1969.
47. LANDON J, et al: The effect of anabolic steroids on blood sugar and plasma insulin levels in man. Metabolism 12:924, 1963.
48. CHRISTENSEN LK, SKOVSTED L: Inhibition of drug metabolism by chloramphenicol. Lancet 2:1397, 1969.
49. DALGAS M, et al: Hypoglycemic episodes induced by phenylbutazone in diabetic patients treated with chlorpropamide. Ugeskr Laeger 127:834, 1965.
50. GERSHBERG H, HECHT A: Antidiabetic effect of acetohexamide. Effect of potassium supplements. NY J Med 69:1287, 1969.
51. CONN JW: Hypertension, the potassium ion and impaired carbohydrate tolerance. N Engl J Med 273:1135, 1965.
52. SPERGEL G, et al: The effect of potassium on the impaired glucose tolerance in chronic uremia. Metabolism 16:581, 1967.
53. WISHINSKY H, et al: Protein interactions of sulfonylurea compounds. Diabetes (Supplement) 2:18, 1962.
54. CHERNER R, et al: Prolonged tolbutamide-induced hypoglycemia. JAMA 185:883, 1963.
55. DALL JLC, et al: Hypoglycaemia due to chlorpropamide. Scott Med J 12:403, 1967.
56. Anturane®. Product Information, Geigy Pharmaceuticals, 1978.
57. REFETOFF S: Thyroid hormone therapy. Med Clin North Am 59:1147, 1975.
58. Council on Drugs: Evaluation of a hypocholesterolemic agent. Dextrothyroxine sodium (Choloxin). JAMA 208:1014, 1969.
59. HICKMAN JW, KIRTLEY WR: Five years' experience with Dymelor. J Indiana Med Assoc 61:1114, 1968.
60. MALIMS JM: Diuretics in diabetes mellitus (Notes and Queries). Practitioner 201:529, 1968.
61. TRANQUADA RE: Diuretic for diabetic patient taking an oral hypoglycemic agent (Questions and Answers). JAMA 206:1580, 1968.

References (CONT.)

62. MIDDLETON E, FINKE SR: Metabolic response to epinephrine in bronchial asthma. J Allergy, 42:288, 1968.
63. REDER JA, TULGAN H: Impairment of diabetic control by norethynodrel with mestranol. NY J Med 67:1073, 1967.
64. SPELLACY WN, et al: Growth hormone alterations by a sequential-type oral contraceptive. Obstet Gynecol 33:506, 1969.
65. PETITPIERRE B, FABRE J: Chlorpropamide and chloramphenicol (Letter). Lancet 1:789, 1970.
66. SHIRRIFFS GG, BEWSHER PD: Hypothermia, abdominal pain, and lactic acidosis in phenformin-treated diabetic. Br Med J 3:506, 1970.
67. KREISBERG RA, et al: Hyperlacticacidemia in man: ethanol-phenformin synergism. J Clin Endocrinol 34:29, 1972.
68. LACHER J, LASAGNA L: Phenformin and lactic acidosis. Clin Pharmacol Ther 7:477, 1966.
69. CARULLI N, et al: Alcohol-drugs interaction in man: alcohol and tolbutamide. Eur J Clin Invest 1:421, 1971.
70. GUPTA KK: The anti-diabetic action of guanethidine. Postgrad Med J 45:455, 1969.
71. BARRETT AM: Modification of the hypoglycaemic response to tolbutamide and insulin by mebanazine, an inhibitor of monoamine oxidase. J Pharm Pharmacol 17:19, 1965.
72. HARRIS EL: Adverse reactions to oral antidiabetic agents. Br Med J 3:29, 1971.
73. OWUSU SK, OCRAN K: Paradoxical behaviour of phenylbutazone in African diabetics (Letter). Lancet 1:440, 1972.
74. TUCKER HSG, HIRSCH JI: Sulfonamide-sulfonylurea interaction (Letter). N Engl J Med 286:110, 1972.
75. LEVINE R: Mechanisms of insulin secretion. N Engl J Med 283:522, 1970.
76. LOCKHART JG: Effects of "speed" and "pot" on the juvenile diabetic (Questions and Answers). JAMA 214:2065, 1970.
77. PODOLSKY S, et al: Effect of marijuana on the glucose-tolerance test. Ann NY Acad Sci 191:54, 1971.
78. MILLER JB: Hypoglycaemic effect of oxytetracycline (Letter). Br Med J 2:1007, 1966.
79. HIATT N, BONORRIS G: Insulin response in pancreatectomized dogs treated with oxytetracycline. Diabetes 19:307, 1970.
80. REMENCHIK AP, et al: Insulin secretion by hypertensive patients receiving hydrochlorothiazide (Abstract). JAMA 212:869, 1970.
81. BARUH S, et al: Fasting hypoglycemia. Med Clin North Am 57:1441, 1973.
82. YAMAMOTO LT: Diabetes insipidus and drinking alcohol (Letter). N Engl J Med 294:55, 1976.
83. SOTANIEMI EA, et al: Half-life of intravenous tolbutamide in the serum of patients in medical wards. Ann Clin Res 6:146, 1974.
84. BEAUDRY C, LAPLANTE L: Treatment of renal failure from diabetic nephropathy with cadaveric homograft. Can Med Assoc J 108:887, 1973.
85. HUNDER GG, et al: Daily and alternate-day corticosteroid regimens in treatment of giant cell arteritis. Comparison in a prospective study. Ann Intern Med 82:613, 1975.
86. SOTANIEMI EA, et al: Effect of diethylstilbestrol on blood glucose of prostatic cancer patients. Invest Urol 10:438, 1973.

References (CONT.)

87. ZILLY W, et al: Induction of drug metabolism in man after rifampicin treatment measured by increased hexobarbital and tolbutamide clearance. Eur J Clin Pharmacol 9:219, 1975.

88. ASAAD MM, CLARKE DE: Studies on the biochemical aspects of the "disulfiram-like" reaction induced by oral hypoglycemics. Eur Pharmacol 35:301, 1976.

89. SVENDSEN TL, et al: The influence of disulfiram on the half-life and metabolic clearance rate of diphenylhydantoin and tolbutamide in man. Eur J Clin Pharmacol 9:439, 1976.

90. MIHIC M, et al: Effect of trimethoprim-sulfamethoxazole on blood insulin and glucose concentrations of diabetics. Can Med Assoc J 112:805, 1975.

91. DAUBRESSE JC, et al: Potentiation of hypoglycemic effect of sulfonylureas by clofribrate (Letter). N Engl J Med 294:613, 1976.

92. LUMHOLTZ G, et al: Sulfamethizole-induced inhibition of diphenylhydantoin, tolbutamide, and warfarin metabolism. Clin Pharmacol Ther 17:731, 1975.

93. SYVALAHTI E, et al: Effect of tuberculostatic agents on the response of serum growth hormone and immunoreactive insulin to intravenous tolbutamide, and on the half-life of tolbutamide. Int J Clin Pharmacol 13:83, 1976.

94. FERRARI C, et al: Potentiation of hypoglycemic response to intravenous tolbutamide by clofibrate. N Engl J Med 294:613, 1976.

95. RADO JP, SZENDE L: Inhibition of clofibrate-induced antidiuresis by glybenclamide in patients with pituitary diabetes insipidus. J Clin Pharmacol 14:290, 1974.

96. WARDLE EN, RICHARDSON GO: Alcohol and glibenclamide. Br Med J 3:309, 1971.

97. ALBERT M, STANSELL MJ: Vascular symptomatic relief during administration of ethylchlorophenoxyisobutyrate (clofibrate). Metabolism 18:635, 1969.

98. WICKSTROM L, PETTERSSON K: Treatment of diabetics with monoamine-oxidase inhibitors. Lancet 2:995, 1964.

99. DAUBRESSE JC, et al: Clofibrate and diabetes control in patients treated with oral hypoglycaemic agents. Br J Clin Pharmacol 7:599, 1979.

100. PHILIPS PJ, et al: Phenformin, tetracycline and lactic acidosis (Letter). Ann Intern Med 86:111, 1977.

101. METZ R: Bulletin of the Mason Clinic (Case Notes). 30:38, 1976.

102. JAIN AK, et al: Potentiation of hypoglycemic effect of sulfonylureas by halofenate. N Engl J Med 293:1283, 1975.

103. ZILLY W, et al: Stimulation of drug metabolism by rifampicin in patients with cirrhosis or cholestasis measured by increased hexobarbital and tolbutamide clearance. Eur J Clin Pharmacol 11:287, 1977.

104. KUDZMA DJ, et al: Potentiation of hypoglycemic effect of chlorpropamide and phenformin by halofenate. Diabetes 26:291, 1977.

105. RYAN JR, et al: On the question of an interaction between sulindac and tolbutamide in the control of diabetes. Clin Pharmacol Ther 21:231, 1977.

106. BRUNOVA E, et al: Interaction of tolbutamide and chloramphenicol in diabetic patients. Int J Clin Pharmacol 15:7, 1977.

References (CONT.)

107. SANDERS M, BREIDAHL H: The effect of an anorectic agent (mazindol) on control of obese diabetics. Med J Aust 2:576, 1976.
108. HEDELAND H, et al: The effect of insulin induced hypoglycaemia on plasma renin activity and urinary catecholamines before and following clonidine (catapresan) in man. Acta Endocrinol 71:321, 1972.
109. BANDISODE MS, BOSHELL BR: Hypocholesterolemic activity of colestipol in diabetes. Curr Ther Res 18:276, 1975.
110. KESSON CM, IRELAND JT: Phenformin compared with fenfluramine in the treatment of obese diabetic patients. Practitioner 216:577, 1976.
111. ERLE G, et al: Effect of chlorpromazine on blood glucose and plasma insulin in man. Eur J Clin Pharmacol 11:15, 1977.
112. POND SM, et al: Mechanisms of inhibition of tolbutamide metabolism: phenylbutazone, oxyphenbutazone, sulfaphenazole. Clin Pharmacol Ther 22:573, 1977.
113. NEUVONEN PJ, KARKKAINEN S: Effects of charcoal, sodium bicarbonate, and ammonium chloride on chlorpropamide kinetics. Clin Pharmacol Ther 33:386, 1983.
114. GIUGLIANO D, et al: Impairment of insulin secretion in man by nifedipine. Eur J Clin Pharmacol 18:395, 1980.
115. CHARLES S, et al: Hyperglycaemic effect of nifedipine. Br Med J 283:19, 1981.
116. FERLITO S, et al: Effect of nifedipine on blood sugar, insulin and glucagon levels after an oral glucose load. Panminerva Med 23:75, 1981.
117. ANDERSON DEH, ROJDMARK S: Improvement of glucose tolerance by verapamil in patients with non-insulin-dependent diabetes mellitus. Acta Med Scand 210:27, 1981.
118. MADSBAD S, et al: Influence of smoking on insulin requirement and metabolic status in diabetes mellitus. Diabetes Care 3:41, 1980.
119. KLEMP P, et al: Smoking reduces insulin absorption from subcutaneous tissue. Br Med J 284:237, 1982.
120. HUGHES JE, et al: Marihuana and the diabetic coma. JAMA 214:1113, 1970.
121. HOLLISTER LE, REAVEN GM: Delta-9-tetrahydrocannabinol and glucose tolerance. Clin Pharmacol Ther 16:297, 1974.

Chapter 5

Antihypertensive Drug Interactions

BETHANIDINE INTERACTIONS

DRUGS	DISCUSSION

Antidepressants, Tricyclic[2-5,97]

MECHANISM: Tricyclic antidepressants probably inhibit the uptake of bethanidine into its site of action in the adrenergic neuron.

CLINICAL SIGNIFICANCE: Desipramine has been shown to markedly antagonize the antihypertensive effect of bethanidine in several patients.[3,5] Amitriptyline and imipramine have also been shown to reduce the antihypertensive response to bethanidine in several patients.[97] The antagonism occurs fairly rapidly (within a few hours) and lasts for several days following discontinuation of the desipramine.

MANAGEMENT: Tricyclic antidepressants should probably be avoided in patients receiving bethanidine. If tricyclics are to be used, consideration might be given to selecting an antihypertensive agent *other* than bethanidine, guanethidine, or debrisoquin.

Diethylpropion (Tenuate)[63]

MECHANISM: None.

CLINICAL SIGNIFICANCE: In 32 obese hypertensive patients receiving various antihypertensives (including bethanidine in some patients), diethylpropion therapy reportedly did not interfere with the antihypertensive response.[63] More study is needed to confirm these findings.

MANAGEMENT: No special precautions appear necessary.

Doxepin (Adapin, Sinequan)[2]

MECHANISM: Not established. Doxepin may inhibit the uptake of bethanidine to its site of action in the adrenergic neuron.

CLINICAL SIGNIFICANCE: In a preliminary report, Oates and associates[2] found that doxepin can antagonize the antihypertensive effect of bethanidine, but the effect was apparently not marked and developed slowly. Desipramine is apparently a stronger antagonist of bethanidine than doxepin, even at doxepin doses of 300 mg/day.[2]

MANAGEMENT: Doxepin should probably be used with caution in patients receiving bethanidine, but it appears to be preferable to the

BETHANIDINE INTERACTIONS (CONT.)

DRUGS	DISCUSSION

tricyclic antidepressants with regard to the magnitude of the interaction with bethanidine.

Ephedrine[1,5,8]

MECHANISM: Not established.

CLINICAL SIGNIFICANCE: A patient maintained on bethanidine therapy has been described who developed severe headache, visual disturbances and distortion of hearing whenever ephedrine was taken.[8] These symptoms were thought to be due to loss of control of hypertension. One would expect ephedrine to antagonize bethanidine on theoretical grounds, but few conclusions can be drawn from a single case.

MANAGEMENT: Even in the absence of more clinical documentation of this interaction, it would appear wise to avoid ephedrine use in patients receiving bethanidine if possible. If ephedrine is used, the blood pressure should be monitored closely to detect any loss of antihypertensive effect of bethanidine.

Phenylpropanolamine (Propadrine)[9]

MECHANISM: Not established.

CLINICAL SIGNIFICANCE: One hypertensive patient was started on a combination product containing phenylpropanolamine, chlorpheniramine maleate, and isopropamide after being controlled on bethanidine therapy. The blood pressure rose considerably after the first dose of the cold capsule and was not controlled again until the cold capsule was stopped and the bethanidine replaced with methyldopa. It seems likely that the phenylpropanolamine was responsible for the loss of blood pressure control.

MANAGEMENT: Although admittedly based on limited clinical evidence, it would seem prudent to avoid phenylpropanolamine use in patients receiving bethanidine. If phenylpropanolamine is used, the blood pressure should be monitored closely to detect any interaction.

CAPTOPRIL INTERACTIONS

DRUGS	DISCUSSION

Indomethacin (Indocin)[90-92]

MECHANISM: The ability of indomethacin to inhibit prostaglandin synthesis is probably responsible for the inhibition of the antihypertensive response to captopril.

CLINICAL SIGNIFICANCE: Several studies have shown that indomethacin (75 to 150 mg/day) inhibits the antihypertensive response to captopril.[90-92] The magnitude of the inhibition is generally large enough to adversely affect the patient. It is likely that other prostaglandin

CAPTOPRIL INTERACTIONS (CONT.)

DRUGS	DISCUSSION

inhibitors (e.g., nonsteroidal anti-inflammatory drugs) would also reduce the antihypertensive response to captopril, but little clinical information is available.

MANAGEMENT: Patients receiving captopril and indomethacin should be monitored carefully for reduced antihypertensive response. Since indomethacin may inhibit the response to other antihypertensives, substituting another antihypertensive drug for captopril may not circumvent the problem.

Probenecid (Benemid)[93]

MECHANISM: Not established.

CLINICAL SIGNIFICANCE: Study in healthy subjects indicates that probenecid moderately increases serum captopril levels.[93] The magnitude of the increases might be sufficient to increase the antihypertensive response to captopril in some patients, but this has not been established.

MANAGEMENT: Monitor for enhanced hypotensive response to captopril and lower captopril dose if necessary.

Salicylates[92]

MECHANISM: The ability of salicylates to inhibit prostaglandin synthesis is probably responsible for the inhibition of antihypertensive response to captopril.

CLINICAL SIGNIFICANCE: In a study of eight hypertensive patients, aspirin (600 mg every 6 hours) reduced the hypotensive response to a single dose of captopril (25 to 100 mg) in half of the patients.[92] Additional study is needed to assess the clinical significance of this interaction in patients on chronic captopril therapy. Occasional doses of salicylates probably have little negative effect on captopril therapy.

MANAGEMENT: If more than occasional doses of salicylates are used in a patient on captopril, blood pressure should be monitored to detect impaired control. Acetaminophen is not known to affect captopril response and thus may be a suitable alternative.

CLONIDINE (CATAPRES) INTERACTIONS

DRUGS	DISCUSSION

Antidepressants, Tricyclic[81,104]

MECHANISM: Not established.

CLINICAL SIGNIFICANCE: Four of five hypertensive patients on chronic clonidine therapy developed a rise in blood pressure when desipramine was also taken (75 mg/day for 2 weeks) but not during placebo.[81] The magnitude of the increases in blood pressure was suffi-

CLONIDINE (CATAPRES) INTERACTIONS (CONT.)

cient to have a potential adverse clinical effect. A hypertensive crisis also occurred in a 77-year-old woman stabilized on clonidine who then received imipramine.[104]

MANAGEMENT: If possible, concomitant use of clonidine and tricyclic antidepressants should be avoided. Since tricyclic antidepressants also appear to interact with guanethidine, bethanidine, and debrisoquin, they would not be suitable alternatives. Methyldopa appears to be reasonably safe when used with tricyclic antidepressants, but little is known about the combined use of tricyclics with the remaining antihypertensives.

Levodopa (Dopar, Larodopa)[76,98]

MECHANISM: It is proposed that clonidine may inhibit the anti-parkinson activity of levodopa by stimulating central alpha-adrenergic receptors.

CLINICAL SIGNIFICANCE: In seven patients with parkinsonism (five on piribedil, two on levodopa plus carbidopa) administration of clonidine was associated with an exacerbation of the parkinsonism.[76] Patients who were receiving anticholinergics in addition to the levodopa or piribedil seemed to be less affected by the clonidine administration. The interaction was not seen in another study of ten patients.[98]

MANAGEMENT: Until more information is available, one should be alert for evidence of reduced antiparkinson effect of levodopa if clonidine is given concurrently.

Nicotinic Acid (Niacin)[82]

MECHANISM: Clonidine is thought to inhibit nicotinic acid-induced vasodilation, thus inhibiting the skin flushing commonly seen with the latter drug.

CLINICAL SIGNIFICANCE: In a group of patients with hyperlipidemia, clonidine appeared to be more effective than placebo in inhibiting the flushing caused by a derivative of nicotinic acid, pentaerythritol tetranicotinate.[82]

MANAGEMENT: None. Favorable interaction.

Nitroprusside (Nipride)[73]

MECHANISM: Clonidine and nitroprusside appear to have additive hypotensive effects.

CLINICAL SIGNIFICANCE: Three patients have been described in whom simultaneous discontinuation of nitroprusside and initiation of clonidine was associated with severe hypotensive reactions.[73] More study is needed to better define the consequences of such combined use.

CLONIDINE (CATAPRES) INTERACTIONS (CONT.)

DRUGS	DISCUSSION

MANAGEMENT: Clonidine should be used cautiously in patients receiving nitroprusside or very recently receiving it.

Piribedil[76]

MECHANISM: It is proposed that clonidine may inhibit the anti-parkinson activity of piribedil by stimulating central alpha-adrenergic receptors.

CLINICAL SIGNIFICANCE: In five patients with parkinsonism, administration of clonidine was associated with an exacerbation of the parkinsonism.[76] Patients who were receiving anticholinergics in addition to the piribedil seemed to be less affected by the clonidine administration.

MANAGEMENT: Patients receiving piribedil for parkinsonism should be monitored for reduced antiparkinson effect if clonidine is given concurrently.

DEBRISOQUIN INTERACTIONS

DRUGS	DISCUSSION

Antidepressants, Tricyclic[5,97]

MECHANISM: Tricyclic antidepressants probably inhibit the uptake of debrisoquin into its site of action in the adrenergic neuron.

CLINICAL SIGNIFICANCE: Two patients receiving debrisoquin manifested reversal of its antihypertensive effect when desipramine was given.[5] In another patient amitriptyline reduced the antihypertensive response to debrisoquin.[97] These reports, combined with theoretical considerations, indicate that the interaction is probably real.

MANAGEMENT: Although the amount of clinical evidence on this interaction is not large, it would be prudent to avoid the use of tricyclic antidepressants in patients receiving debrisoquin. If tricyclics are used in such a patient, the blood pressure should be monitored closely and debrisoquin dosage increased as needed.

Phenylephrine (Neo-Synephrine)[10,61]

MECHANISM: It is possible that the monoamine oxidase (MAO) inhibitory activity of debrisoquin[61] is sufficient to result in a hypertensive reaction from phenylephrine (an MAO substrate). Other factors may be involved.

CLINICAL SIGNIFICANCE: One patient controlled on debrisoquin for 6 months was given phenylephrine (50 mg orally).[10] Within 20 minutes his blood pressure was about 210/180 mm Hg, and was lowered by phentolamine (5 mg intravenously) to 172/100 mm Hg. It seems likely that drug interaction was responsible for this effect.

DEBRISOQUINE INTERACTIONS (CONT.)

DRUGS	DISCUSSION

MANAGEMENT: Although based on limited clinical evidence, the severity of the possible interaction dictates caution in the use of phenylephrine therapy in patients receiving debrisoquin.

DIAZOXIDE INTERACTIONS

DRUGS	DISCUSSION

Cisplatin (Platinol)[89]

MECHANISM: It has been proposed that potent hypotensive agents may increase the nephrotoxic effect of cisplatin.

CLINICAL SIGNIFICANCE: A 58-year-old man with normal renal function developed severe hypertension 3 hours after receiving intravenous cisplatin 70 mg/m^2 body surface area.[89] The patient suffered severe nausea and vomiting, and the blood pressure increased to 248/140 mm Hg. Treatment with furosemide (Lasix) 40 mg IV, hydralazine (Apresoline) 10 mg IM, diazoxide (Hyperstat) 300 mg IV, and propranolol (Inderal) 20 mg bid for 2 days decreased the blood pressure while maintaining a urine output of at least 150 ml/hour. At no time during treatment was the blood pressure less than 110/70 mm Hg. Nine days after this dose of cisplatin, the patient's renal function decreased as evidenced by an elevated serum urea nitrogen. On two subsequent occasions, the use of cisplatin in the same dose again precipitated severe nausea, vomiting, and blood pressure elevation; however, antihypertensive therapy was not initiated and the renal function did not deteriorate. Although cisplatin or aggressive antihypertensive therapy can decrease renal function, this patient's renal dysfunction probably can be best explained by an interaction of these drugs. The renal function did not decrease after two subsequent cisplatin infusions, and the antihypertensive therapy did not result in a hypotensive overshoot. Therefore, it is possible that aggressive antihypertensive treatment may have altered renal hemodynamics in a way that would promote cisplatin nephrotoxicity.

MANAGEMENT: Potent antihypertensive agents should be used with caution in patients receiving cisplatin.

Hydralazine (Apresoline)[72,79,83]

MECHANISM: Diazoxide and hydralazine may exhibit additive hypotensive effects.

CLINICAL SIGNIFICANCE: Several cases have been reported of severe hypotensive reactions in patients receiving diazoxide and hydralazine, usually within an hour or two of each other.[72,79,83]

MANAGEMENT: Concomitant use of diazoxide and hydralazine should be undertaken with caution, and with adequate monitoring for excessive hypotension.

DIAZOXIDE INTERACTIONS (CONT.)

DRUGS	DISCUSSION

Phenothiazines[69]

MECHANISM: Not established.

CLINICAL SIGNIFICANCE: A 2-year-old boy on chronic diazoxide and thiazide therapy for hypoglycemia developed severe hyperglycemia following a single 30-mg dose of chlorpromazine.[69] It was proposed that the chlorpromazine, acting in concert with the diazoxide and thiazide, was responsible for the hyperglycemia.

MANAGEMENT: Until this potential interaction is better described, chlorpromazine and other phenothiazines should be used with caution in patients receiving diazoxide in treatment of hypoglycemia.

Thiazides[11-13]

MECHANISM: It has been proposed that diazoxide may compete with the diuretic thiazides for plasma protein binding.[11] However, other factors may be involved.[12]

CLINICAL SIGNIFICANCE: The concomitant use of diazoxide and thiazide diuretics has been shown to result in an enhanced hyperglycemic activity in a number of patients.

MANAGEMENT: This effect should be kept in mind when thiazide diuretics are used to treat diazoxide-induced sodium retention.

GUANETHIDINE INTERACTIONS

DRUGS	DISCUSSION

Amphetamines[4,6,15,24,46]

MECHANISM: Amphetamines antagonize the adrenergic neuron blockage produced by guanethidine, probably by displacing guanethidine from adrenergic neurons and inhibiting its uptake by adrenergic neurons. It has also been proposed that amphetamines may have a direct effect on vasoconstrictor receptors.[15]

CLINICAL SIGNIFICANCE: This interaction has been described in several hypertensive patients and is likely to be clinically significant. The effect has been noted with both dextroamphetamine and methamphetamine, and is pronounced enough to interfere considerably with hypertensive control.

MANAGEMENT: Since there are few clear-cut medical indications for amphetamines, their use in patients receiving guanethidine would not appear difficult to avoid.

Antidepressants, Tricyclic[3-5,15,24,31-35,45,47,49-51]

MECHANISM: Tricyclic antidepressants inhibit the uptake of guanethidine into the adrenergic neuron, resulting in an inhibition of the antihypertensive effect. The ability of tricyclic antidepressants to inhibit uptake of norepinephrine may also be involved.

CLINICAL SIGNIFICANCE: This interaction is well documented. It is especially important in patients with moderate to severe hypertension, the group most likely to receive guanethidine. Early reports indicate that doxepin (Adapin, Sinequan) is less potent as an antagonist to the antihypertensive effect of guanethidine than the tricyclic antidepressants. Confirmation of this information is needed. One case has appeared in which an interaction between guanethidine and imipramine was implicated in producing cardiac standstill and death.[49] However, a causal relationship was not established.

MANAGEMENT: Satisfactory control of hypertension can sometimes be achieved by dosage adjustment, but it would be preferable to avoid the combination. Maproteline (Ludiomil) may be less likely to interact with guanethidine than tricyclic antidepressants. Methyldopa may be less likely to interact with tricyclic antidepressants, but more information is needed.

Cocaine[6]

MECHANISM: Not established.

CLINICAL SIGNIFICANCE: Animal studies reportedly indicate that cocaine may antagonize the antihypertensive effect of guanethidine.[6] Studies in humans are needed to confirm these findings.

MANAGEMENT: Although clinical evidence is lacking, the possibility of interaction should be realized.

Diethylpropion (Tenurate, Tepanil)[6,63]

MECHANISM: Not established.

CLINICAL SIGNIFICANCE: In 32 obese hypertensive patients receiving various antihypertensives (including guanethidine in some patients) diethylpropion therapy reportedly did not interfere with the antihypertensive response.[63] Earlier animal studies had indicated that diethylpropion may inhibit the antihypertensive response to guanethidine.[6] More study is needed.

MANAGEMENT: No special precautions appear to be necessary, but one should be aware of the possibility of interaction.

Doxepin (Adapin, Sinequan)[2]

MECHANISM: Doxepin may inhibit the uptake of guanethidine to its site of action in the adrenergic neuron.

CLINICAL SIGNIFICANCE: Preliminary study indicates that doxepin (300 mg/day) can antagonize the antihypertensive effect of guanethidine, but even at this dose the antagonism is less than that produced

GUANETHIDINE INTERACTIONS (CONT.)

DRUGS	DISCUSSION

by tricyclic antidepressants.[2] Based on this preliminary evidence, doxepin appears to be preferable to tricyclic antidepressants in patients receiving guanethidine.

MANAGEMENT: One should watch for decreased antihypertensive efficacy when guanethidine and greater than 200 mg/day of doxepin are used concomitantly.

Ephedrine[1,6,24]

MECHANISM: Ephedrine probably acts much the same as the amphetamines in antagonizing the adrenergic neuron blockade produced by guanethidine.

CLINICAL SIGNIFICANCE: This interaction has been described in several hypertensive patients and is likely to be clinically significant. Although the effect is not as large as seen with amphetamines, it would be sufficient to interfere with control of hypertension.

MANAGEMENT: If ephedrine must be used in the patient receiving guanethidine, the patient should be watched closely for decreased control of hypertension. An increased dose of guanethidine or avoiding the use of ephedrine may be necessary in certain cases.

Ethanol (Alcohol, Ethyl)[22]

MECHANISM: Ethanol produces vasodilatation, which may enhance the orthostatic hypotension of guanethidine.

CLINICAL SIGNIFICANCE: Although case reports describing this interaction are lacking, it probably does occur.

MANAGEMENT: Patients receiving guanethidine should be cautioned about this effect. If the patient is prone to orthostatic hypotension, he would be wise to limit his ethanol intake.

Haloperidol (Haldol)[64]

MECHANISM: Not established. Haloperidol might inhibit the uptake of guanethidine into sites of action in the adrenergic neuron in a manner similar to that of tricyclic antidepressants.

CLINICAL SIGNIFICANCE: In three hypertensive patients stabilized on guanethidine, haloperidol (6 to 9 mg/day) was associated with an increase in mean blood pressure of about 15 to 20 mm Hg.[64]

MANAGEMENT: Until more is known about this possible interaction, patients receiving guanethidine and haloperidol should be watched more closely for decreased antihypertensive response. It has been proposed that increasing the guanethidine dose may overcome the interaction.[64] Another alternative would be changing to another antihypertensive (e.g., methyldopa) that may be less likely to interact.

GUANETHIDINE INTERACTIONS (CONT.)

Levarterenol (Norepinephrine)[27,28]

MECHANISM: The response to norepinephrine in guanethidine-treated patients is enhanced. Possible mechanisms include increased sensitivity of the adrenergic receptor to norepinephrine and inhibition of norepinephrine uptake (and thus inactivation) by the adrenergic neuron.

CLINICAL SIGNIFICANCE: The increased pressor effect of norepinephrine in patients receiving guanethidine is well documented and of sufficient magnitude to be clinically significant. In addition, there appears to be an increased tendency for cardiac arrhythmias to occur in guanethidine-treated patients who are given norepinephrine.

MANAGEMENT: In patients receiving guanethidine, norepinephrine should be avoided if possible. If norepinephrine is necessary, use conservative doses and monitor blood pressure carefully.

Levodopa (Dopar, Larodopa)[53,54]

MECHANISM: Not established. However, some possible mechanisms of interaction have been proposed.[54]

CLINICAL SIGNIFICANCE: Not established. The hypotensive effect of guanethidine appeared to be enhanced by levodopa in two patients, but a causal relationship was not established.[53]

MANAGEMENT: Although evidence for interaction is scanty at the present time, it may be wise to watch patients on guanethidine therapy more closely for excessive hypotensive effects if levodopa is added to the therapy.

Maprotiline (Ludiomil)[94,95]

MECHANISM: Not established.

CLINICAL SIGNIFICANCE: Isolated cases of inhibition of the antihypertensive response to drugs have been reported following treatment with maprotiline.[94,95] Although data are scanty, it appears that the tetracyclic maprotiline is less likely to interfere with guanethidine-like drugs than tricyclic antidepressants such as imipramine, desipramine, and amitriptyline.

MANAGEMENT: Monitor for altered antihypertensive response to guanethidine if maprotiline is initiated or discontinued.

Methotrimeprazine (Levoprome)[23]

MECHANISM: Orthostatic hypotension is one of the major side effects of methotrimeprazine therapy. Additive effects would be seen with concomitant guanethidine therapy.

CLINICAL SIGNIFICANCE: The orthostatic hypotension following methotrimeprazine is well documented and is likely to be quite significant in the patient receiving guanethidine.

GUANETHIDINE INTERACTIONS (CONT.)

DRUGS	DISCUSSION

MANAGEMENT: If possible, methotrimeprazine should not be used in patients receiving guanethidine.

Methylphenidate (Ritalin)[6,24–26]

MECHANISM: Methylphenidate, like the amphetamines, probably antagonizes the adrenergic neuron blockade produced by guanethidine.

CLINICAL SIGNIFICANCE: The inhibition of the hypotensive effect of guanethidine is not as large as that from amphetamines, but it would be sufficient to interfere with the control of hypertension. In one report, a patient receiving both methylphenidate and guanethidine developed ventricular tachycardia, apparently as a result of drug interaction.[25]

MANAGEMENT: In view of the possibility of both decreased control of hypertension and the development of ventricular tachycardia, administration of methylphenidate to patients receiving guanethidine should be avoided if possible.

Mianserin[74,99]

MECHANISM: None described.

CLINICAL SIGNIFICANCE: Limited clinical evidence indicates that mianserin does not affect the antihypertensive response to guanethidine.[99] These findings are consistent with pharmacologic study of concomitant administration of guanethidine and mianserin to the eye indicating that mianserin may not antagonize the peripheral effects of guanethidine as the tricyclic antidepressants do.[74]

MANAGEMENT: No special precautions appear necessary.

Monoamine Oxidase Inhibitors (MAOI)[6,24,44,46,52]

MECHANISM: MAOI reportedly antagonize the antihypertensive effect of guanethidine,[6,24,52] possibly by counteracting guanethidine-induced neuronal catecholamine depletion. In a patient receiving an MAOI, the initial release of norepinephrine following guanethidine therapy may produce a greater response due to MAOI-induced increased norepinephrine stores.[44]

CLINICAL SIGNIFICANCE: In one preliminary study nialamide (Niamid) appeared to reverse somewhat the hypotensive effect of guanethidine in four of five patients. The reversal was not as marked as with amphetamines. More study is needed to determine the magnitude and significance of this interaction.

MANAGEMENT: Pending the availability of further information, patients receiving guanethidine should be watched for decreased control of hypertension if an MAOI is administered. Patients receiving MAOI therapy might be watched for excessive sympathomimetic activity on initiation of guanethidine therapy.

GUANETHIDINE INTERACTIONS (CONT.)

DRUGS	DISCUSSION

Phenothiazines[6,15,16,40,47,48,64]

MECHANISM: Chlorpromazine (Thorazine) appears to inhibit the uptake of guanethidine into the adrenergic neuron in a manner similar to the tricyclic antidepressants. Animal and in-vitro studies indicate that chlorpromazine may be more effective than phenothiazines such as perphenazine (Trilafon) or trifluoperazine (Stelazine) in inhibiting norepinephrine uptake. Thus, the possibility exists that guanethidine may be antagonized more by some phenothiazines than others.

CLINICAL SIGNIFICANCE: In several patients receiving guanethidine, chlorpromazine administration has been associated with considerable increases in mean blood pressure.[40,48,64] In all patients the dose of chlorpromazine was 100 mg per day or more; it is not known whether smaller doses of chlorpromazine would have a similar effect. The antagonism of guanethidine did not appear immediately; several days were usually required.

MANAGEMENT: Hypertensive patients receiving guanethidine should be monitored more closely during phenothiazine therapy. If guanethidine antagonism is noted, increasing guanethidine dose or substituting another antihypertensive agent (e.g., methyldopa) might be appropriate. However, it should be remembered that the intrinsic hypotensive effect of phenothiazines might *enhance* the effect of antihypertensives other than guanethidine.

Phenylephrine (Neo-Synephrine)[14,29,30]

MECHANISM: Phenylephrine, like norepinephrine, is a direct-acting sympathomimetic and is probably more active in patients receiving guanethidine because of the increased sensitivity of the receptor.

CLINICAL SIGNIFICANCE: A marked increase in the pupillary response to phenylephrine eye drops has been noted following guanethidine eye drops[14,29] and chronic oral guanethidine therapy.[30] It appears likely that the cardiovascular response to phenylephrine would be similarly enhanced, but clinical studies are not available to support this possibility.

MANAGEMENT: Patients receiving guanethidine should be given phenylephrine eye drops only with caution. The effects of nasally or systemically administered phenylephrine might also be expected to be enhanced pending further information.

Thiothixene (Navane)[64]

MECHANISM: Not established. Thiothixene might inhibit the uptake of guanethidine into sites of action in a manner similar to that of tricyclic antidepressants.

CLINICAL SIGNIFICANCE: In a hypertensive patient stabilized on guanethidine, thiothixene (60 mg/day) was associated with an increase in mean blood pressure of 30 mm Hg.[64] Study in additional patients is needed to assess clinical significance.

GUANETHIDINE INTERACTIONS (CONT.)

DRUGS	DISCUSSION

MANAGEMENT: Although evidence for an interaction is scanty at present, patients on guanethidine therapy might be watched more closely for decreased antihypertensive response if thioxanthines are also given.

MECAMYLAMINE INTERACTIONS

DRUGS	DISCUSSION

Sodium Bicarbonate[77]

MECHANISM: Sodium bicarbonate alkalinizes the urine, thus increasing the renal tubular reabsorption of mecamylamine.

CLINICAL SIGNIFICANCE: Maintaining urinary pH at 7.5 or above with sodium bicarbonate markedly reduced urinary excretion of mecamylamine in patients with hypertension.[77] It seems likely that other drugs that can alkalinize the urine such as acetazolamide (Diamox) would have a similar effect.

MANAGEMENT: Urinary alkalinizers should probably be avoided during mecamylamine therapy. If the combination is used, one should be alert for excessive or prolonged hypotension.

METHYLDOPA INTERACTIONS

DRUGS	DISCUSSION

Amphetamines[28]

MECHANISM: Amphetamines act indirectly by displacing norepinephrine to sites of action, with resultant increase in sympathetic activity and decrease in antihypertensive effect of methyldopa.

CLINICAL SIGNIFICANCE: This interaction is based primarily on theoretical considerations and animal studies, but it seems possible that it could occur in humans.

MANAGEMENT: Amphetamines should be given cautiously to patients receiving methyldopa, with the realization that decreased control of hypertension may occur.

Antidepressants, Tricyclic[5,42,58,62,65,66]

MECHANISM: Not established.

CLINICAL SIGNIFICANCE: A hypertensive patient controlled on methyldopa therapy developed worsening of the hypertension when amitriptyline was also given. Animal studies have indicated that tricyclic antidepressants may block hypotensive responses to methyldopa.[58,65,66] However, others have found that desipramine (75 mg/day) did not antagonize the hypotensive effect of methyldopa in three

METHYLDOPA INTERACTIONS (CONT.)

patients.[5] It may be that most patients on methyldopa are not adversely affected by tricyclic antidepressants, with certain predisposed patients manifesting decreased control of hypertension.

MANAGEMENT: Concomitant methyldopa and tricyclic antidepressant therapy should be undertaken with some caution, although most patients are probably not adversely affected.

Barbiturates[17,59,60]

MECHANISM: None established.

CLINICAL SIGNIFICANCE: Although Kaldor and associates[59] presented evidence to indicate that phenobarbital may reduce methyldopa blood levels. Kristensen and associates could not confirm these findings using a more specific assay for methyldopa.[17,60]

MANAGEMENT: No special precautions appear to be necessary.

Diethylpropion (Tenuate, Tepanil)[63]

MECHANISM: None.

CLINICAL SIGNIFICANCE: In 32 obese hypertensive patients (some of whom were receiving methyldopa) administration of diethylpropion reportedly did not interfere with antihypertensive response.[63] More study is needed to confirm these preliminary findings.

MANAGEMENT: No special precautions appear necessary.

Ephedrine[36]

MECHANISM: Methyldopa appears to reduce the amount of norepinephrine available for release due to the presence of alpha-methylnorepinephrine as a "false" neurotransmitter. Most of the sympathomimetic activity of ephedrine is due to an indirect effect resulting in release of norepinephrine. Thus, ephedrine would be expected to be less active in methyldopa-treated patients.

CLINICAL SIGNIFICANCE: Clinically, the only descriptions of this interaction have been concerned with the eye, where methyldopa treatment decreased the mydriasis of topical ephedrine. Presumably, methyldopa would also inhibit somewhat the effect of systemically administered ephedrine.

MANAGEMENT: Pending the availability of further information, ephedrine may be expected to be somewhat less effective in patients receiving methyldopa, and patients should be managed accordingly.

Haloperidol (Haldol)[68,100]

MECHANISM: Not established. A combined inhibitory effect on dopamine in the central nervous system has been proposed.[68]

METHYLDOPA INTERACTIONS (CONT.)

DRUGS	DISCUSSION

CLINICAL SIGNIFICANCE: Two patients on chronic methyldopa therapy developed dementia (e.g., slowed mentation, disorientation, etc.) within 1 week of starting haloperidol therapy.[68] Symptoms cleared within 72 hours when haloperidol was discontinued. A similar case was subsequently reported.[100] The symptoms appeared to be due to drug interaction in these three patients, but more information is needed to assess incidence and severity of this reaction.

MANAGEMENT: One should be alert for adverse psychiatric symptoms if concomitant therapy with haloperidol and methyldopa is begun.

Levarterenol (Norepinephrine)[28,84]

MECHANISM: Not established.

CLINICAL SIGNIFICANCE: Levarterenol (1 to 8 μg by rapid IV injection) was administered to ten hypertensive patients before and after methyldopa therapy.[84] A slight increase in the pressor response to levarterenol was seen following methyldopa, and the duration of the pressor response was considerably prolonged.

MANAGEMENT: In patients receiving methyldopa, norepinephrine should be administered cautiously, beginning with small doses.

Levodopa (Dopar, Larodopa)[18–20,37,38,41,54–57,78,88]

MECHANISM: The mechanism for the reported inhibitory effect of methyldopa on the therapeutic response to levodopa has not been established. Methyldopa has been reported to both cause[88] and relieve parkinsonism. It is possible that methyldopa replaces dopamine with a "false" neurotransmitter, thus antagonizing the effect of levodopa. Also, the hypotension seen when levodopa is given alone may be additive with that produced by methyldopa. Carbidopa (without levodopa) has been shown to produce a small decrease in supine diastolic pressure of patients maintained on methyldopa.[78]

CLINICAL SIGNIFICANCE: Although methyldopa reportedly inhibits the response to levodopa,[37,57] several researchers have intentionally used this combination to advantage, especially in patients with fluctuating response to levodopa.[19,20,55,56] Patient variation, dose of drugs, and other factors probably determine the outcome of combined therapy. The possible additive hypotensive effect of methyldopa and levodopa should also be kept in mind.[18]

MANAGEMENT: Although there appears to be little danger in giving methyldopa to patients receiving levodopa, the possibility that this combination might adversely affect response to levodopa in selected patients must still be considered.

Lithium Carbonate (Eskalith, Lithane, Lithonate)[71,85,101,102]

MECHANISM: Not established.

CLINICAL SIGNIFICANCE: Two patients stabilized on lithium carbonate therapy developed signs of lithium toxicity when methyldopa was added to their therapy.[71,85] Another patient receiving methyldopa developed signs of lithium intoxication after 2 days of lithium therapy.[101] Three healthy subjects also developed adverse effects when methyldopa was added to lithium therapy.[102] In all of the above cases the serum lithium levels were within the therapeutic range.

MANAGEMENT: Avoid concurrent use if possible. If the combination is used, monitor for evidence of lithium intoxication. Plasma lithium levels may not be useful in detecting this interaction since they may be in the therapeutic range.

Methotrimeprazine (Levoprome)[23]

MECHANISM: Orthostatic hypotension and a general decrease in blood pressure are seen fairly frequently in patients receiving methotrimeprazine. Additive effects may be seen with concomitant methyldopa therapy.

CLINICAL SIGNIFICANCE: The hypotensive effect of methotrimeprazine is well documented and is likely to be significant in the patient receiving methyldopa.

MANAGEMENT: If possible, methotrimeprazine should not be used in patients receiving methyldopa.

Monoamine Oxidase Inhibitors (MAOI)[39,43,103]

MECHANISM: Not established.

CLINICAL SIGNIFICANCE: A single case report, supported by animal studies, has appeared describing this interaction. This patient developed hallucinations while receiving both methyldopa and pargyline (Eutonyl), although it was not unequivocally established that drug interaction was responsible.[39] Further, others have reported the combination to be safe.[103]

MANAGEMENT: Although based on limited clinical evidence, methyldopa and MAOI should be given concomitantly only with caution.

Phenothiazines[21,86]

MECHANISM: It has been proposed that phenothiazines can block the reuptake of the methyldopa metabolite, alpha-methyl-norepinephrine, into the adrenergic neuron, resulting in a paradoxical hypertensive response to methyldopa.[21,86]

CLINICAL SIGNIFICANCE: A 23-year-old woman with systemic lupus erythematosus and renal disease developed an increasing blood pressure when methyldopa was added to her trifluoperazine (Stelazine) therapy.[21] This response was felt to be due to excess alpha-methyl-norepinephrine due to both phenothiazine-induced inhibition of up-

METHYLDOPA INTERACTIONS (CONT.)

DRUGS	DISCUSSION

take and diminished excretion as a result of the renal disease. It should be noted that hypertensive reactions had been previously noted with methyldopa administration in a patient not receiving phenothiazines.[86]

MANAGEMENT: Although this interaction is based on limited clinical evidence, it would be wise to monitor blood pressure closely in patients receiving concomitant methyldopa and phenothiazines.

PRAZOSIN INTERACTIONS

DRUGS	DISCUSSION

Indomethacin (Indocin)[96]

MECHANISM: Indomethacin-induced inhibition of prostaglandin synthesis may be involved.

CLINICAL SIGNIFICANCE: Indomethacin pretreatment may have inhibited the hypotensive effect of a single 5-mg dose of prazosin in four of nine healthy subjects.[96] The effect of chronic therapy with both drugs is not known.

MANAGEMENT: Monitor for reduced hypotensive response to prazosin (or other antihypertensive agents) if indomethacin (or other non-steroidal anti-inflammatory agents) is given concurrently.

RESERPINE INTERACTIONS

DRUGS	DISCUSSION

Diethylpropion (Tenuate, Tepanil)[63]

MECHANISM: None.

CLINICAL SIGNIFICANCE: In 32 obese hypertensive patients (some of whom were receiving reserpine) administration of diethylpropion reportedly did not interfere with antihypertensive response.[63] More study is needed to confirm these preliminary findings.

MANAGEMENT: No special precautions appear necessary.

Digitalis Glycosides[87]

MECHANISM: Not established. It is possible that reserpine-induced release of catecholamines may be involved.

CLINICAL SIGNIFICANCE: The concomitant use of reserpine and digitalis glycosides reportedly may predispose the patient to the development of cardiac arrhythmias. Three possible examples of this interaction have been reported.[87] The arrhythmias seen were atrial tachycardia, ventricular bigeminy and tachycardia, and atrial fibrillation. It should be noted that reserpine and digitalis are frequently

DRUGS	DISCUSSION

given together with no apparent ill effects. If release of catecholamines by reserpine is the mechanism involved, it is likely that the greatest chance of interaction would be in administering large doses of reserpine to already digitalized patients.

MANAGEMENT: No action is likely to be necessary, but the possibility should be realized in the arrhythmia-prone patient.

Ephedrine[36]

MECHANISM: Reserpine administration results in depletion of norepinephrine from the adrenergic neuron. Much of the sympathomimetic activity of ephedrine is due to an indirect effect resulting in release of norepinephrine. Thus, ephedrine would be expected to be less active in reserpine-treated patients.

CLINICAL SIGNIFICANCE: Clinically, reserpine treatment has been shown to decrease the mydriasis of topical ephedrine, and it was thought that reserpine could also inhibit somewhat the effect of systemically-administered ephedrine. However, more clinical information is needed.

MANAGEMENT: Pending accumulation of further information, it might be well to watch patients receiving both ephedrine and reserpine for any unusual effects.

Levodopa (Dopar, Larodopa)[7,37,54]

MECHANISM: Not established. Reserpine has been reported to cause parkinsonism, perhaps by depleting the brain of dopamine. Dopamine depletion would be in direct opposition to the effects of levodopa in relieving parkinsonism.

CLINICAL SIGNIFICANCE: Clinical descriptions of the inhibitory effect of reserpine on the response to levodopa are lacking, but Cotzias[37] reports that it does occur. Theoretical considerations also tend to support the existence of the interaction.

MANAGEMENT: Pending the availability of further information, reserpine should probably be avoided in patients receiving levodopa.

Methotrimeprazine (Levoprome)[23]

MECHANISM: Orthostatic hypotension and a general decrease in blood pressure are seen fairly frequently in patients receiving methotrimeprazine. Additive effects may be seen with concomitant reserpine therapy.

CLINICAL SIGNIFICANCE: The hypotensive effect of methotrimeprazine is well documented. Since it is an analgesic and is generally used intermittently, control of hypertension with reserpine may be erratic.

RESERPINE INTERACTIONS (CONT.)

DRUGS	DISCUSSION

MANAGEMENT: If possible, methotrimeprazine should be avoided in patients receiving any antihypertensive.

Monoamine Oxidase Inhibitors (MAOI)[44]

MECHANISM: MAOI result in accumulation of norepinephrine in storage sites within the adrenergic neuron. If reserpine is subsequently given, the reserpine-induced release of norepinephrine results in an exaggerated response due to the increased quantity of neurotransmitter present at the adrenergic receptor. Other factors may also be involved.

CLINICAL SIGNIFICANCE: Excitation and hypertension reportedly may occur if reserpine is given to a patient receiving an MAOI, but clinical reports describing this interaction are lacking. If the patient receives the reserpine for several days and then is given an MAOI, theoretically this interaction would not occur, but again, study in humans is lacking.

MANAGEMENT: Although more clinical information is needed to clarify this interaction, it would probably be wise to avoid concomitant use of MAOI and reserpine. It should be remembered that the effects of both MAOI and reserpine may persist many days after the drug has been essentially cleared from the body.

References

1. STARR KJ, PETRIE JC: Drug interactions in patients on long-term oral anticoagulant and antihypertensive adrenergic neuron-blocking drugs. Br Med J 4:133, 1972.
2. OATES JA, et al: Effect of doxepin on the norepinephrine pump. A preliminary report. Psychosomatics 10:12, 1969.
3. MITCHELL JR, et al: Antagonism of the antihypertensive action of guanethidine sulfate by desipramine hydrochloride. JAMA 202:973, 1967.
4. FEAGIN OT, et al: Uptake and release by guanethidine and bethanidine by the adrenergic neuron (Abstract). J Clin Invest 48:23a, 1969.
5. MITCHELL, JR, et al: Guanethidine and related agents. III. Antagonism by drugs which inhibit the norepinephrine pump in man. J Clin Invest 49:1596, 1970.
6. DAY MD, RAND MJ: Antagonism of guanethidine and bretylium by various agents (Letter). Lancet 2:1282, 1962.
7. BIANCHINE JR, SUNYAPRIDAKUL L: Interactions between levodopa and other drugs: significance in the treatment of parkinson's disease. Drugs 6:364, 1973.
8. ANON: Therapeutic conferences. Drug interaction. Br. Med J 1:389, 1971.
9. MISAGE JR, McDONALD RH: Antagonism of hypotensive action of bethanidine by "common cold" remedy. Br Med J 4:347, 1970.
10. AMINU J, et al: Interaction between debrisoquine and phenylephrine (Letter). Lancet 2:935, 1970.

References (CONT.)

11. SELLERS EM, KOCH-WESER J: Protein binding and vascular activity of diazoxide. N Engl J Med 281:1141, 1969.
12. SELTZER HS, ALLEN EW: Hyperglycemia and inhibition of insulin secretion during administration of diazoxide and trichlormethiazide in man. Diabetes 18:19, 1969.
13. WOLFF F: Diazoxide misunderstood (Letter). N Engl J Med 286:612, 1972.
14. JABLONSKI J: Guanethidine (Ismelin) as an adjuvant in pharmacological mydriasis. Ophthalmologica 168:27, 1974.
15. OBER KF, WANG RIH: Drug interactions with guanethidine. Clin Pharmacol Ther 14:190, 1973.
16. TUCK D, et al: Drug interactions: effect of chlorpromazine on the uptake of monoamines into adrenergic neurons in man (Letter). Lancet 2:492, 1972.
17. KRISTENSEN M, et al: Barbiturates and methyldopa metabolism (Letter). Br Med J 1:49, 1973.
18. GIBBERD FB, SMALL E: Interaction between levodopa and methyldopa. Br. Med J 2:90, 1973.
19. FERMAGLICH J, CHASE TN: Methyldopa or methyldopa-hydrazine as levodopa synergists (Letter). Lancet 1:1261, 1973.
20. MONES RJ: Evaluation of alpha methyl dopa and alpha methyl dopa hydrazine with L-dopa therapy. NY State J Med 74:47, 1974.
21. WESTERVELT FB Jr, ATUK NO: Methyldopa-induced hypertension (Letter). JAMA 227:557, 1974.
22. MEYERS FH, et al: Review of Medical Pharmacology, 3rd Ed., Lange Medical Publications, Los Altos, California, 1972, pp. 103–104.
23. Levoprome. Product Information, Lederle Laboratories, 1966.
24. GULATI OD, et al: Antagonism of adrenergic neuron blockade in hypertensive subjects. Clin Pharmacol Ther 7:510, 1966.
25. DESHMANKAR BS, LEWIS JA: Ventricular tachycardia associated with the administration of methylphenidate during guanethidine therapy. Can Med Assoc J 97:1166, 1967.
26. Ritalin. Product Information. Summit, New Jersey, CIBA Pharmaceutical Co., 1984.
27. MUELHEIMS GH, et al: Increased sensitivity of the heart to catecholamine-induced arrhythmias following guanethidine. Clin Pharmacol Ther 6:757, 1965.
28. DOLLERY CT: Physiological and pharmacological interactions of antihypertensive drugs. Proc R Soc Med 58:983, 1965.
29. SNEDDON JM, TURNER P: The interactions of local guanethidine and sympathomimetic amines in the human eye. Arch Ophthamol 81:622, 1969.
30. COOPER B: Neo-synephrine (10%) eye drops (Letter). Med J Aust 2:420, 1968.
31. MITCHELL JR, et al: Antagonism of the antihypertensive action of guanethidine sulfate by desipramine hydrochloride. JAMA 202:973, 1967.
32. STONE CA, et al: Antagonism of certain effects of catecholamine-depleting agents by antidepressant and related drugs. J Pharmacol Exp Ther 144:196, 1964.
33. LEISHMAN AWD, et al: Antagonism of guanethidine by imipramine. Lancet 1:112, 1963.

References (CONT.)

34. OATES JA, et al: Effect of doxepin on the norepinephrine pump. A preliminary report. Psychosomatics 10:12, 1969.
35. PITTS NE: The clinical evaluation of doxepin. A new psychotherapeutic agent. Psychosomatics 10:164, 1969.
36. SNEDDON JM, TURNER P: Ephedrine mydriasis in hypertension and the response to treatment. Clin Pharmacol Ther 10:64, 1969.
37. COTZIAS GC, et al: L-Dopa in Parkinson's syndrome (Letter). N Engl J Med 281:272, 1969.
38. SPIERS ASD, et al: Miosis during L-Dopa therapy. Br Med J 2:639, 1970.
39. PAYKEL ES: Hallucinosis on combined methyldopa and pargyline. Br Med J 1:803, 1966.
40. FDA Reports of Suspected Adverse Reactions to Drugs. 1970, No. 700201-056-00101.
41. YAHR MD, et al: Treatment of parkinsonism with levodopa. Arch Neurol 21:343, 1969.
42. WHITE AG: Methyldopa and amitriptyline. Lancet 2:441, 1965.
43. VAN ROSSUM JM: Potential dangers of monoamineoxidase inhibitors and alphamethyldopa. Lancet 1:950, 1963.
44. GOLDBERG LI: Monoamine oxidase inhibitors. Adverse reactions and possible mechanisms. JAMA 190:456, 1964.
45. MEYER JF, et al: Insidious and prolonged antagonism of guanethidine by amitriptyline. JAMA 213:1487, 1970.
46. STARKE K: Interactions of guanethidine and indirect-acting sympathomimetic amines. Arch Int Pharmacodyn Ther 195:309, 1972.
47. LAHTI RA, MAICKEL RP: The tricyclic antidepressants—inhibition of norepinephrine uptake as related to potentiation of norepinephrine and clinical efficacy. Biochem Pharmacol 20:482, 1971.
48. FANN WE, et al: Chlorpromazine reversal of the antihypertensive action of guanethidine (Letter). Lancet 2:436, 1971.
49. WILLIAMS RB, JR, SHERTER C: Cardiac complications of tricyclic antidepressant therapy. Ann Intern Med 74:395, 1971.
50. BOSTON COLLABORATIVE DRUG SURVEILLANCE PROGRAM: Adverse reactions to the tricyclic antidepressant drugs. Lancet 1:529, 1972.
51. MITCHELL JR, OATES JA: Guanethidine and related agents. I. Mechanism of the selective blockade of adrenergic neurons and its antagonism by drugs. J Pharmacol Exp Ther 172:100, 1970.
52. ESBENSHADE JH, JR, et al: A long-term evaluation of pargyline hydrochloride in hypertension. Am J Med Sci 251: 119, 1966.
53. HUNTER KR, et al: Use of levodopa with other drugs. Lancet 2:1283, 1970.
54. MORGAN JP, BIANCHINE JR: The clinical pharmacology of levodopa. Rational Drug Ther 5:1(Jan.) 1971.
55. SWEET RD, et al: Methyldopa as an adjunct to levodopa treatment of Parkinson's disease. Clin Pharmacol Ther 13:23, 1972.
56. FERMAGLICH J, O'DOHERTY DS: Second generation of L-Dopa therapy (Abstract). Neurology 21:408, 1971.
57. KOFMAN O: Treatment of Parkinson's disease with L-Dopa: A current appraisal. Can Med Assoc J 104:483, 1971.
58. KALE AK, SATOSKAR RS: Modification of the central hypotensive ef-

References (CONT.)

fect of alphamethyldopa by reserpine, imipramine and tranylcypromine. Eur J Pharmacol 9:120, 1970.

59. KALDOR A, et al: Enhancement of methyldopa metabolism with barbiturate. Br Med J 3:518, 1971.

60. KRISTENSEN M, et al: Plasma concentration of alfamethyldopa and its main metabolite, methyldopa-O-sulfate during long-term treatment with alfamethyldopa, with special reference to possible interaction with other drugs given simultaneously (Abstract). Clin Pharmacol Ther 14:139, 1973.

61. PETTINGER WA, et al: Debrisoquin, a selective inhibitor of intraneuronal monoamine oxidase in man. Clin Pharmacol Ther 10:667, 1969.

62. JEFFERSON JW: A review of the cardiovascular effects and toxicity of tricyclic antidepressants. Psychosom Med 37:160, 1975.

63. SEEDAT YK, REDDY J: Diethylpropion hydrochloride (tenuate dospin) in the treatment of obese hypertensive patients (Letter). S Afr Med J 48:569, 1974.

64. JANOWSKY DS, et al: Antagonism of guanethidine by chlorpromazine. Am J Psychiatry 130:808, 1973.

65. VANSPANNING HW, VANZWIETEN PA: The interaction between α-methyl-dopa and tricyclic antidepressants. Int J Clin Pharmacol Biopharm 11:65, 1975.

66. VANZWIETEN PA: Interaction between centrally acting hypotensive drugs and tricyclic antidepressants. Arch Int Pharmacodyn Ther 214:12, 1975.

67. PETRICK RJ: More on hypertension, depression, and drug interactions (Letter). Drug Therapy 5:7, (Aug.) 1975.

68. THORNTON WE: Dementia induced by methyldopa with haloperidol. N Engl J Med 294:1222, 1976.

69. AYNSLEY-GREEN A, ILLIG R: Enhancement by chlorpromazine of hyperglycemic action of diazoxide (Letter). Lancet 2:658, 1975.

70. PITTS NE: The clinical evaluation of doxepin—a new psychotherapeutic agent. Psychosomatics 10:164, 1969.

71. O'REGAN JB: Adverse interactions of lithium carbonate and methyldopa (Letter). Can Med Assoc J 115:385, 1976.

72. HENRICH WL, et al: Hypotensive sequelae of diazoxide and hydralazine therapy. JAMA 237:264, 1977.

73. COHEN IM, et al: Danger in nitroprusside therapy (Letter). Ann Intern Med 85:205, 1976.

74. GHOSE K, et al: Autonomic actions and interactions of mianserin hydrochloride (org. GB 94) and amitriptyline in patients with depressive illness. Psychopharmacology 49:201, 1976.

75. JOHNSON RA: Adverse neonatal reaction to maternal administration of intravenous chlormethiazole and diazoxide. Br Med J 1:943, 1976.

76. SHOULSON I, CHASE TN: Clonidine and the anti-parkinsonian response to L-dopa or piribedil. Neuropharmacology 15:25, 1976.

77. ALLANBY KD, TROUNCE JR: Excretion of mecamylamine after intravenous and oral administration. Br. Med J 2:1219, 1957.

78. KERSTING F, et al: Clinical and cardiovascular effects of alpha methyldopa in combination with decarboxylase inhibitors. Clin Pharmacol Ther 21:547, 1977.

References (CONT.)

79. MIZROCH S, YURASEK M: Hypotension and bradycardia following diazoxide and hydralazine therapy (Letter). JAMA 237:2471, 1977.
80. MELANDER A, et al: Enhancement of hydralazine bioavailability by food. Clin Pharmacol Ther 22:104, 1977.
81. BRIANT RH, et al: Interaction between clonidine and desipramine in man. Br Med J 1:522, 1973.
82. SIGROTH K: Effect of clonidine on nicotinic-acid flushing (Letter). Lancet 2:58, 1974.
83. ROMBERG GP, LORDON RE: Hypotensive sequelae of diazoxide and hydralazine therapy (Letter). JAMA 238:1025, 1977.
84. DOLLERY CT, et al: Haemodynamic studies with methyldopa: effect on cardiac output and response to pressor amines. Br Heart J 25:670, 1963.
85. BYRD GJ: Methyldopa and lithium carbonate: suspected interaction (Letter). JAMA 233:320, 1975.
86. LEVINE RJ, STRAUCH BS: Hypertensive responses to methyldopa. N Engl J Med 275:946, 1966.
87. DICK H, et al: Reserpine-digitalis toxicity. Arch Intern Med 109:503, 1962.
88. STRANG RR: Parkinsonism occurring during methyldopa therapy. Can Med Assoc J 95:928, 1966.
89. MARKMAN M, TRUMP DL: Nephrotoxicity with cisplatin and antihypertensive medications. Ann Intern Med 96:257, 1982.
90. FUJITA T, et al: Effect of indomethacin on antihypertensive action of captopril in hypertensive patients. Clin Exp Hypertens 3:939, 1981.
91. OGIHARA T, et al: Hormonal responses to long-term converting enzyme inhibition in hypertensive patients. Clin Pharmacol Ther 30:328, 1981.
92. MOORE TJ, et al: Contribution of prostoglandins to the antihypertensive action of captopril in essential hypertension. Hypertension 3:168, 1981.
93. SINGHVI SM, et al: Renal handling of captopril: effect of probenecid. Clin Pharmacol 32:182, 1982.
94. SMITH AJ, BANT WP.: Interaction between postganglionic sympathetic blocking drugs and antidepressants. J Int Med Res 3(Supplement 2):55, 1975.
95. BRIANT RH, GEORGE CF: The assessment of potential drug interaction with a new tricyclic antidepressant drug. Br J Clin Pharmacol 1:113, 1974.
96. RUBIN P, et al: Studies on the clinical pharmacology of prazosin. II. The influence of indomethacin and of propranolol on the action and disposition of prazosin. Br J Clin Pharmacol 10:33, 1980.
97. SKINNER C, et al: Antagonism of the hypotensive action of bethanidine and debrisoquine by tricyclic antidepressants. Lancet 2:564, 1969.
98. TARSY D, et al: Clonidine in parkinson disease. Arch Neurol 32:134, 1975.
99. BURGESS CD, et al: Cardiovascular responses to mianserin hydrochloride: A comparison with tricyclic antidepressant drugs. Br J Clin Pharmacol 5:215, 1978.

References (CONT.)

100. NADEL I, WALLACH M: Drug interaction between haloperidol and methyldopa. Br J Psychiatr 135:484, 1979.
101. OSANLOO E, DEGLIN JH: Interaction of lithium and methyldopa. Ann Intern Med 92:433, 1980.
102. WALKER N, et al: Lithium-methyldopa interactions in normal subjects. Drug Intell Clin Pharm 14:638, 1980.
103. HERTING RL: Monoamine oxidase inhibitors. Lancet 1:1324, 1965.
104. HUI KK: Hypertensive crisis induced by interaction of clonidine with imipramine. J Am Geriatr Soc 31:164, 1983.

CHAPTER 6

Anti-infective Drug Interactions

AMANTADINE (SYMMETREL) INTERACTIONS

DRUGS	DISCUSSION

Anticholinergics[48,118,162]

MECHANISM: Not established.

CLINICAL SIGNIFICANCE: It has been observed that in patients who are receiving close to the maximum tolerable doses of anticholinergic drugs such as trihexyphenidyl (Artane) and benztropine (Cogentin), amantadine may potentiate anticholinergic side effects. Confusion and hallucinations that are characteristic of excessive anticholinergic activity have been reported.

MANAGEMENT: Although more information is needed, it would be wise to consider reducing high-dose anticholinergic therapy before administering amantadine.

AMINOGLYCOSIDE INTERACTIONS

DRUGS	DISCUSSION

Amphotericin B (Fungizone)[246]

MECHANISM: It is proposed that amphotericin B and gentamicin exhibit synergistic nephrotoxicity.

CLINICAL SIGNIFICANCE: In four patients receiving gentamicin, the addition of amphotericin B was associated with deterioration of renal function.[246] Since neither drug was being used in a dose likely to be nephrotoxic, it was assumed that synergistic nephrotoxicity occurred. Additional study will be required to establish such a relationship.

MANAGEMENT: Patients on combined therapy with amphotericin B and an aminoglycoside should be monitored closely for deterioration of renal function.

Extended Spectrum Penicillins: Azlocillin (Azlin), Carbenicillin (Geopen, Pyopen), Mezlocillin (Mezlin), Piperacillin (Piperacil), Ticarcillin (Ticar)[6,7,131-135,163,205,284,286,333,363]

MECHANISM: Both carbenicillin and ticarcillin (and probably also the related penicillins listed above) chemically inactivate aminoglycosides such as gentamicin or tobramycin.

194

AMINOGLYCOSIDE INTERACTIONS (CONT.)

CLINICAL SIGNIFICANCE: There is good evidence for the in-vitro inactivation of gentamicin or tobramycin by carbenicillin or ticarcillin, but it is not likely that such inactivation takes place in vivo in patients with normal renal function. In patients with severe renal impairment there is now clinical evidence that carbenicillin or ticarcillin may inactivate gentamicin or tobramycin in vivo.[205,284,286,363] The available data indicate that the inactivation of gentamicin by carbenicillin in patients with renal failure is sufficient to reduce the antimicrobial efficacy of gentamicin. There is some evidence that amikacin and netilmicin may be less likely to interact with extended spectrum penicillins, but one should use the same precautions as with other combinations. One should also consider the possibility that aminoglycoside serum assays could be affected by penicillin therapy, especially if there is a delay in performing the assay.

MANAGEMENT: Extended spectrum penicillins and aminoglycosides should not be mixed together before infusion, but in most patients, in-vivo antagonism does not appear to be a problem. In patients with renal failure, if the combination cannot be avoided, serum gentamicin levels should be monitored for evidence of interaction and doses adjusted accordingly.

Cephalosporins[3,6,12–17,127,164–168,180–182,192,193,224,226–229,241]

MECHANISM: It appears that gentamicin and cephalothin have additive nephrotoxic effects in some predisposed patients.

CLINICAL SIGNIFICANCE: Several reports have appeared describing nephrotoxicity when gentamicin was combined with cephaloridine or cephalothin.[3,12,13,15,127,164–168,192,193,224,226,228,229] These case reports seem to indicate that the combined use of cephalosporins and gentamicin can increase the chance of nephrotoxicity over the use of either drug alone. Factors which probably predispose patients to developing nephrotoxicity with this combination include preexisting renal disease, large doses of one or both drugs, and old age. The combination of cephalosporins with aminoglycosides other than gentamicin might also be expected to result in an increased chance of nephrotoxicity, but not as much clinical evidence is available to support this. In patients with normal renal function prior to therapy the combined use of aminoglycosides and cephalosporins probably does not constitute an excessive risk, especially when one considers the severity of the infections usually involved. However, in patients with preexisting renal disease the possibility of further deterioration of renal impairment must be considered when choosing the antibiotic therapy.

MANAGEMENT: In a patient with preexisting renal disease the combined use of an aminoglycoside and a cephalothin should be undertaken with caution, with careful selection of doses, and with close monitoring of renal function. If another appropriate antibiotic regimen can be determined for such a patient, it may be prudent to avoid the aminoglycoside-cephalosporin combination. In a patient with

AMINOGLYCOSIDE INTERACTIONS (CONT.)

normal renal function proper dosing and monitoring of the drugs should seldom result in nephrotoxicity.

Clindamycin (Cleocin)[236]

MECHANISM: It is proposed that clindamycin may enhance the likelihood of gentamicin nephrotoxicity.

CLINICAL SIGNIFICANCE: Three patients have been described in whom the administration of clindamycin appeared to predispose to gentamicin nephrotoxicity.[236] All had normal renal function prior to therapy and improved rapidly when the antibiotics were discontinued. Confirmation of these preliminary results is needed.

MANAGEMENT: Until this potential interaction is better described, patients on combined therapy should be monitored closely for signs of renal impairment.

Digitalis Glycosides[213]

MECHANISM: Neomycin and possibly other orally administered aminoglycosides appear to inhibit the gastrointestinal absorption of digoxin. However, oral aminoglycosides might also reduce the inactivation of digoxin by bacteria in the gastrointestinal tract, thus counteracting the reduction in digoxin absorption. This latter mechanism occurs in only 10% or less of patients, while the inhibition of absorption is likely to occur more regularly.

CLINICAL SIGNIFICANCE: In a study involving normal subjects, digoxin was given alone and with oral neomycin (1 to 3 g).[213] Both single dose and multiple dose studies demonstrated that digoxin absorption (both rate and amount) was considerably lower when neomycin was administered concomitantly. Impaired digoxin absorption was also noted when the neomycin was given 3 or 6 hours prior to the digoxin. The magnitude of the decreases in serum digoxin appear such that adverse clinical consequences might occur.

MANAGEMENT: Based on available information, spacing the doses of digoxin and neomycin to avoid mixing in the gut may not circumvent this interaction. Thus, it would be prudent to monitor serum digoxin levels if neomycin is started or stopped in a patient stabilized on digoxin.

Dimenhydrinate (Dramamine)[88]

MECHANISM: The symptoms of the possible ototoxicity of the aminoglycoside antibiotics reportedly may be masked by concomitant dimenhydrinate administration.

CLINICAL SIGNIFICANCE: Clinical examples of this interaction are lacking, but the possible adverse effects are serious enough to warrant consideration of this interaction.

AMINOGLYCOSIDE INTERACTIONS (CONT.)

MANAGEMENT: If dimenhydrinate or a similar drug is given concomitantly with one of the aminoglycoside antibiotics, the vigilance toward detecting ototoxicity should be increased.

Ethacrynic Acid (Edecrin)[18,87,89–92,136]

MECHANISM: Ethacrynic acid can produce ototoxicity that may add to or potentiate the ototoxicity of aminoglycoside antibiotics.

CLINICAL SIGNIFICANCE: A number of cases have been reported wherein ethacrynic acid appeared to enhance the ototoxicity of agents such as kanamycin, neomycin, gentamicin, and streptomycin. The presence of impaired renal function markedly enhances the danger of ototoxicity from any of these agents. Experimental evidence indicates that administration of ethacrynic acid following discontinuation of kanamycin might also increase the ototoxic effect.[18] Furosemide (Lasix) and bumetanide (Bumex) probably also enhance the ototoxicity of aminoglycosides. It is not established whether or not they are safer than ethacrynic acid, but theoretically they would be.

MANAGEMENT: Ethacrynic acid should be used only with extreme caution in patients receiving aminoglycoside antibiotics, and the patient should be monitored for evidence of ototoxicity.

5-Fluorouracil[285]

MECHANISM: Neomycin may decrease the rate of absorption of orally administered 5-fluorouracil (5-FU).

CLINICAL SIGNIFICANCE: In a group of 12 patients with adenocarcinoma, pretreatment with oral neomycin (2 g/day for 1 week) appeared to delay the absorption of 5-FU during the first few hours. However, in only one case was 5-FU absorption affected sufficiently so that clinical consequences might be possible.

MANAGEMENT: If 5-FU is given orally, neomycin should be considered a potential interfering factor. There is little information indicating whether separating doses of the two drugs would minimize any effect of 5-FU absorption, but it does not seem likely.

Methotrexate[240]

MECHANISM: Oral aminoglycosides may reduce absorption of oral methotrexate.

CLINICAL SIGNIFICANCE: Absorption of methotrexate was determined in 10 patients with bronchogenic carcinoma before and after administration of a group of oral antibiotics (paromomycin, polymyxin B, nystatin, and vancomycin).[240] Administration of the antibiotics was associated with a mean decrease in absorption of methotrexate from a control of 69% to 44%. Paromomycin probably accounted for some of

DRUGS	DISCUSSION

this decrease, but it is not possible to determine the relative contribution of the various antibiotics used.

MANAGEMENT: In patients receiving oral methotrexate, one should be alert for evidence of decreased therapeutic response if oral aminoglycosides are also given.

Methoxyflurane (Penthrane)[19-21]

MECHANISM: Aminoglycoside antibiotics and methoxyflurane may have additive or synergistic nephrotoxic effects.

CLINICAL SIGNIFICANCE: Several cases of nephrotoxicity have appeared following the administration of kanamycin or gentamicin to patients who had recently received methoxyflurane. The nephrotoxicity seems to appear at lower doses of the drugs than those at which one would ordinarily expect to see renal impairment. More study is needed.

MANAGEMENT: Current evidence indicates that nephrotoxic antibiotics such as aminoglycosides should be given only if they are truly necessary to patients who have recently received methoxyflurane.

Penicillin V (Compocillin, Pen-Vee, V-Cillin)[86]

MECHANISM: Oral neomycin has been shown to decrease the absorption of penicillin V, presumably due to the production of a malabsorption syndrome.

CLINICAL SIGNIFICANCE: In one study of five volunteers, neomycin (3.0 g four times a day) reduced serum concentrations of penicillin V by over 50% compared to control values. It is possible that penicillin G would be similarly affected.

MANAGEMENT: Patients receiving oral neomycin who also require a penicillin should probably be given the penicillin parenterally. An alternative might be doubling the dose of oral penicillin, but the efficacy of such a procedure has not been tested.

Neuromuscular Blocking Agents[82-84,137,138,191]

MECHANISM: Kanamycin, tobramycin, gentamicin, neomycin, and streptomycin have all been shown to produce a neuromuscular blockade that may enhance the blockade of skeletal muscle relaxants.

CLINICAL SIGNIFICANCE: Well documented. A number of cases have been reported in which aminoglycoside antibiotics produced respiratory paralysis, both alone and in combination with surgical neuromuscular blocking agents. This may occur following administration of the antibiotic by a variety of routes (e.g., intramuscular, intravenous, intraperitoneal, intrapleural, beneath skin flaps, etc.).

AMINOGLYCOSIDE INTERACTIONS (CONT.)

DRUGS	DISCUSSION

MANAGEMENT: Aminoglycoside antibiotics should be administered with extreme caution during surgery or in the postoperative period, as the effect of surgical neuromuscular blocking agents may be enhanced. Treatment with anticholinesterase agents or calcium has been associated with improvement in some cases.

Vitamin B_{12} (Cyanocobalamin)[85,93]

MECHANISM: The gastrointestinal absorption of vitamin B_{12} can be considerably decreased by oral neomycin. Colchicine administration appears to increase neomycin-induced malabsorption of vitamin B_{12}.

CLINICAL SIGNIFICANCE: Not established. It is likely that prolonged administration of large doses of neomycin would be necessary before pernicious anemia would be apparent. Further, since most vitamin B_{12} is given parenterally, few patients are likely to be at risk. However, Schilling tests may be affected.

MANAGEMENT: No special precautions appear necessary.

Combined Use of Two or More Aminoglycoside Antibiotics[87]

MECHANISM: The combined or sequential use of aminoglycoside antibiotics increases the chance of ototoxicity and nephrotoxicity.

CLINICAL SIGNIFICANCE: Cases of patients have been reported in which additive toxicity of this nature has been suspected. The severity of the possible interaction enhances its clinical significance.

MANAGEMENT: Due to the similarities of antimicrobial spectra among the aminoglycoside antibiotics, concomitant use is not likely to occur frequently. If it does, the patient should be watched quite closely for ototoxicity and nephrotoxicity.

AMINOSALICYLIC ACID (PAS) INTERACTIONS

DRUGS	DISCUSSION

Ammonium Chloride[52]

MECHANISM: Ammonium chloride tends to render the urine acidic, thereby increasing the possibility of aminosalicylic acid (PAS) crystalluria.

CLINICAL SIGNIFICANCE: Doses of ammonium chloride large enough to increase urine acidity probably can be expected to increase the chance of crystalluria, although specific examples of this interaction have not appeared. Using the sodium salt of PAS apparently decreases the chance of crystalluria considerably.

MANAGEMENT: Acidifying doses of ammonium chloride should probably be avoided in patients receiving PAS in the free-acid form.

AMINOSALICYLIC ACID (PAS) INTERACTIONS (CONT.)

DRUGS	DISCUSSION

Digitalis glycosides[329]

MECHANISM: Aminosalicylic acid may reduce the absorption of digoxin, possibly by affecting the function of intestinal absorbing cells.

CLINICAL SIGNIFICANCE: Ten healthy subjects were given digoxin (0.75 mg orally) with and without pretreatment with aminosalicylic acid (2 g four times daily for 2 weeks).[329] Bioavailability of digoxin (as measured by cumulative urinary digoxin excretion) was reduced by 20% following aminosalicylic acid. It is not known whether this interaction would be seen under more typical clinical conditions (e.g., actual patients receiving smaller digoxin doses chronically). Further, a 20% reduction in digoxin absorption may not be clinically important in many patients.

MANAGEMENT: Monitor for reduced digoxin response in patients also receiving aminosalicylic acid. If the mechanism is impaired function of absorbing cells, separating the doses of the drugs may not circumvent the interaction.

Diphenhydramine (Benadryl)[22]

MECHANISM: Diphenhydramine appears to impair the gastrointestinal absorption of aminosalicylic acid (PAS), possibly because of the effect of diphenhydramine on gastrointestinal motility.

CLINICAL SIGNIFICANCE: Studies in rats and normal subjects have shown that pretreatment with parenteral diphenhydramine lowers plasma levels of orally administered aminosalicylic acid.[22] Although the decreases in PAS blood levels were not large, the total amount of PAS absorbed did appear to be decreased. Thus, it is possible that this interaction could become significant under the conditions of multiple dosing of PAS. The effect of other antihistamines and anticholinergics on PAS absorption is not known, but the possibility should be considered.

MANAGEMENT: In patients receiving both PAS and diphenhydramine, an effort should probably be made to administer the PAS when the pharmacologic effect of the diphenhydramine is at a minimum.

Ethanol (Alcohol, Ethyl)[204]

MECHANISM: Not established.

CLINICAL SIGNIFICANCE: In a group of patients receiving aminosalicylic acid for hyperlipidemia (types IIa and IIb), the three patients who ingested ethanol developed a diminished hypolipidemic response.

MANAGEMENT: Patients receiving aminosalicylic acid for hyperlipidemia should probably limit their intake of ethanol.

AMINOSALICYLIC ACID (PAS) INTERACTIONS (CONT.)

Isoniazid (INH)[52]

MECHANISM: Aminosalicylic acid reduces the acetylation of isoniazid and results in increased INH blood levels.

CLINICAL SIGNIFICANCE: This interaction is generally considered beneficial rather than harmful. The incidence of excessive blood levels of isoniazid due to aminosalicylic acid therapy is probably quite low.

MANAGEMENT: No special precautions are required.

Para-aminobenzoic Acid (PABA)[52]

MECHANISM: Aminosalicylic acid appears to act on tubercle bacilli in a manner similar to that of sulfonamides on other organisms (by competing with PABA). Thus, the administration of PABA may be expected to inhibit the antimicrobial activity of PAS.

CLINICAL SIGNIFICANCE: Not established. Alone, PABA is used only rarely today, but it is combined with aspirin in a number of proprietary analgesic mixtures. Since aminosalicylic acid is almost never used alone in the treatment of tuberculosis, inhibition of its effect by a PABA-containing analgesic is not likely to be noticed by the clinician.

MANAGEMENT: Based on available information, it would appear prudent to avoid PABA administration in patients receiving PAS. This should not be difficult since the medical indications for the systemic use of PABA are not well established.

Probenecid (Benemid)[58,59]

MECHANISM: Probenecid probably inhibits the renal excretion of aminosalicyclic acid (PAS).

CLINICAL SIGNIFICANCE: Probenecid administration can enhance the blood levels of PAS up to two- or fourfold. It may be expected that normal doses of PAS would result in PAS toxicity if probenecid were also given.

MANAGEMENT: Patients receiving PAS should be given probenecid with caution. It is likely that the dose of PAS could be reduced without impairing the therapeutic effect.

Pyrazinamide[56,57]

MECHANISM: Aminosalicylic acid may delay or somewhat inhibit the hyperuricemia produced by pyrazinamide in some patients.

CLINICAL SIGNIFICANCE: The inhibition of pyrazinamide-induced hyperuricemia by PAS does not appear to be marked. Other measures may be necessary to control the hyperuricemia.

MANAGEMENT: None required.

AMINOSALICYLIC ACID (PAS) INTERACTIONS (CONT.)

DRUGS	DISCUSSION

Rifampin (Rifadin) (Rimactane)[123,196]

MECHANISM: Aminosalicylic acid may impair gastrointestinal absorption of rifampin,[123] apparently due to bentonite present in the PAS granules.[196]

CLINICAL SIGNIFICANCE: Preliminary study in 30 patients indicated that when PAS granules and rifampin are given together, serum rifampin levels are considerably reduced when compared to rifampin given alone.[123] Subsequent study in six volunteers indicated that the inhibition of rifampin absorption is due to the bentonite present in the PAS granules, and not PAS itself.[196]

MANAGEMENT: It would be prudent to space doses of these agents 8 to 12 hours apart from each other if possible.[123] The use of PAS preparations that do not contain bentonite (or a similar substance) should avoid the interaction.

Salicylates[52,55]

MECHANISM: Not established. Aminosalicylic acid is not similar to the salicylates pharmacologically and apparently does not produce salicylism. An effect of salicylates on the renal excretion or plasma protein binding of PAS may be involved.

CLINICAL SIGNIFICANCE: Isolated cases have occurred in which treatment of patients with apparent PAS toxicity with aspirin resulted in further increase in toxic symptoms. However, more study is needed to assess the clinical significance.

MANAGEMENT: The limited evidence available to date indicates that salicylates should probably not be given to any patient with suspected PAS toxicity, or to patients who may be prone to PAS toxicity.

Vitamin B_{12} (Cyanocobalamin)[23,24,53,54]

MECHANISM: Not established. The decreased vitamin B_{12} absorption induced by aminosalicylic acid may be due to the mild malabsorption syndrome that occurs in some patients treated with PAS.

CLINICAL SIGNIFICANCE: Not established. It is likely that prolonged administration of large doses of PAS would be necessary before pernicious anemia would be apparent. Further, most vitamin B_{12} is given parenterally, so few patients are likely to be at risk. Schilling tests may be affected.

MANAGEMENT: No special precautions appear necessary.

AMPHOTERICIN B (FUNGIZONE) INTERACTIONS

DRUGS	DISCUSSION

Corticosteroids[119,120]

MECHANISM: Corticosteroids may enhance the potassium depletion caused by amphotericin B.[119] The possibility also exists that amphotericin B decreases adrenocortical responsiveness to corticotropin.[120]

DRUGS	DISCUSSION

CLINICAL SIGNIFICANCE: One report described four cases in which the concomitant use of amphotericin B and hydrocortisone was followed by cardiac enlargement and congestive heart failure.[119] These adverse effects were thought to be due to the excessive hypokalemia and salt retention, with the hypokalemia primarily a result of amphotericin B therapy, and salt retention primarily due to the corticosteroid therapy.

MANAGEMENT: Patients receiving amphotericin B and corticosteroids should be monitored closely for electrolyte abnormalities and signs of cardiac dysfunction. The propensity of corticosteroids to decrease resistance to infection should also be kept in mind.

Digitalis Glycosides[49-51]

MECHANISM: The hypokalemia that may occur following systemic amphotericin B therapy may facilitate the development of digitalis toxicity.

CLINICAL SIGNIFICANCE: Hypokalemia following amphotericin B is not infrequent and may be severe.

MANAGEMENT: The course of patients on digitalis who require amphotericin B therapy should be followed quite closely. Any potassium deficit that develops should be treated promptly.

Miconazole[221]

MECHANISM: Not established.

CLINICAL SIGNIFICANCE: Preliminary studies in vitro and in a few patients indicate that systemic use of both amphotericin B and miconazole may result in antagonistic rather than additive antifungal effects.[221] More study is needed.

MANAGEMENT: Until this potential interaction is better described, one should be alert for signs of antagonistic antifungal activity with combined use.

Skeletal Muscle Relaxants (Surgical)[49-51]

MECHANISM: The hypokalemia that may occur following amphotericin B therapy may enhance the effect of curariform drugs.

CLINICAL SIGNIFICANCE: Hypokalemia due to amphotericin B is well documented and is likely to be of sufficient magnitude to enhance the response to skeletal muscle relaxants.

MANAGEMENT: The potassium balance of patients on amphotericin B should be checked carefully before use of skeletal muscle relaxants.

CEPHALOSPORIN INTERACTIONS

DRUGS	DISCUSSION

Colistin (Coly-Mycin)[62]

MECHANISM: Not established.

DRUGS	DISCUSSION

CLINICAL SIGNIFICANCE: In a study of adverse reactions to colistin, it was found that concomitant cephalothin (Keflin) administration was associated with an increase in the incidence of renal toxicity. Although this is only preliminary information, the severity of the possible adverse reactions increases the clinical significance of this possible interaction.

MANAGEMENT: Although evidence is still scanty, renal function should probably be monitored closely in patients receiving both colistin and cephalothin.

Ethanol (Alcohol, ethyl)[299-308]

MECHANISM: Some cephalosporins result in disulfiram-like reactions, possibly producing acetaldehyde accumulation.

CLINICAL SIGNIFICANCE: Cefamandole (Mandol), cefoperazone (Cefobid), and moxalactam (Moxam) have resulted in disulfiram-like reactions (e.g., flushing, nausea, headache, tachycardia) following the ingestion of alcohol. The reactions have been mild in most cases, but in a few patients the reactions have been severe, necessitating the use of fluids and dopamine to correct hypotension. The reaction closely resembles the disulfiram-alcohol reaction with respect to onset, symptoms, and severity.

MANAGEMENT: Ethanol should be avoided in patients receiving cefamandole, cefoperazone, or moxalactam, and within 2 or 3 days of stopping the cephalosporin.

Furosemide (Lasix)[3,25,125,126,214]

MECHANISM: Furosemide (and perhaps also ethacrynic acid) may enhance the nephrotoxicity of certain cephalosporins. The basic mechanism is not known.

CLINICAL SIGNIFICANCE: Several reports have described patients receiving furosemide plus cephaloridine* or cephalothin who developed nephrotoxicity,[3,25,126] and it appears likely that furosemide enhanced the nephrotoxic potential of the cephalosporins in these patients. Animal studies support this clinical evidence and also implicate ethacrynic acid as a potentiator of cephaloridine nephrotoxicity.[125] Recently, oral furosemide (80 mg daily) was shown to increase the half-life of cephaloridine by about 25% in 14 patients.[214] In summary, there is good evidence that combined use of furosemide and cephaloridine may result in enhanced nephrotoxicity, but only limited evidence that furosemide plus cephalothin would do so. There is little evidence of difficulty with the combined use of furosemide and other cephalosporins.

MANAGEMENT: No special precautions appear necessary, but one should consider the possibility that the combination of furosemide

*Cephaloridine is not available for general use in the United States.

CEPHALOSPORIN INTERACTIONS (CONT.)

DRUGS	DISCUSSION

and cephalothin might be nephrotoxic in predisposed patients (e.g., those with preexisting renal impairment).

Probenecid (Benemid)[60,61,124,194,195,235,254,255]

MECHANISM: Probenecid inhibits the renal excretion of cephalosporins.

CLINICAL SIGNIFICANCE: Probenecid has been shown to reduce the renal clearance of most cephalosporins. Plasma levels of cephalothin are affected to a greater extent than cephaloridine, presumably because renal tubular excretion is more important in the elimination of cephalothin.

MANAGEMENT: The prescriber should be aware that cephalosporin blood levels will be higher than normal, but special precautions are usually not required.

CHLORAMPHENICOL CHLOROMYCETIN INTERACTIONS

DRUGS	DISCUSSION

Acetaminophen (Datril, Tylenol)[315,334]

MECHANISM: Not established.

CLINICAL SIGNIFICANCE: Following an observation of prolonged chloramphenicol half-life during concurrent acetaminophen therapy in children, six adults were given chloramphenicol (1.0 g intravenously) followed by acetaminophen (100 mg intravenously) 2 hours later.[315] The chloramphenicol half-life was 3.25 hours prior to the acetaminophen and increased to 15 hours following acetaminophen administration. However, the possibility that acetaminophen may interfere with the chloramphenicol assay was apparently not ruled out. Also, a subsequent study in 26 children did not find the interaction.[334]

MANAGEMENT: Until this interaction is resolved, one should be alert for evidence of excessive chloramphenicol plasma levels in patients receiving acetaminophen.

Barbiturates[321,322]

MECHANISM: Barbiturates may enhance chloramphenicol metabolism, and chloramphenicol may inhibit barbiturate metabolism.

CLINICAL SIGNIFICANCE: Chloramphenicol appeared to enhance serum phenobarbital levels in one patient,[321] whereas serum chloramphenicol concentrations have been lower than expected in patients receiving phenobarbital.[322] Although these findings are consistent with the known properties of the drugs, determination of the incidence and magnitude of these interactions must await additional studies.

MANAGEMENT: In patients receiving barbiturates (and possibly other enzyme inducers) one should be alert for evidence of reduced chloramphenicol effect. Serum chloramphenicol determinations may be useful when the interaction is suspected. Increased chloramphenicol dosage may be needed in some patients. One should also be alert for evidence of increased effect of phenobarbital (and possibly other barbiturates) when chloramphenicol is given concurrently. Reduced barbiturate dosage may be required.

Cyclophosphamide (Cytoxan)[199]

MECHANISM: Chloramphenicol presumably slows the metabolism of cyclophosphamide.

CLINICAL SIGNIFICANCE: The metabolism of cyclophosphamide was studied in four patients before and after they were given oral chloramphenicol (2 g/day for 12 days).[199] Cyclophosphamide half-life was considerably prolonged following treatment with chloramphenicol, and the rate of production of cyclophosphamide metabolites appeared to be reduced. Since cyclophosphamide metabolites are thought to be active therapeutically, rather than the parent drug, chloramphenicol could theoretically reduce the activity of cyclophosphamide. Clinical studies are needed to confirm this.

MANAGEMENT: It does not seem necessary to avoid concomitant use, but one should be alert for altered cyclophosphamide response in patients receiving chloramphenicol.

Ethanol (Alcohol, Ethyl)[51]

MECHANISM: Chloramphenicol reportedly inhibits aldehyde dehydrogenase to some extent and results in accumulation of acetaldehyde following ethanol ingestion.

CLINICAL SIGNIFICANCE: Not established. The magnitude of this effect was not stated, nor was clinical evidence presented.

MANAGEMENT: Too little evidence is available to make a statement on management.

Folic Acid (Folvite)[67]

MECHANISM: Not established. However, chloramphenicol is known to interfere with erythrocyte maturation in a considerable number of patients treated with the drug (not related to the aplastic anemia, which is quite rare).

CLINICAL SIGNIFICANCE: A patient with a folic acid deficiency has been described in whom chloramphenicol antagonized the response to folic acid therapy. Study in more patients is needed to assess clinical significance.

MANAGEMENT: Pending the accumulation of further information, the hematologic response to folic acid in patients with folic acid deficiency should be followed closely if chloramphenicol is also given.

CHLORAMPHENICOL CHLOROMYCETIN
INTERACTIONS (CONT.)

DRUGS	DISCUSSION

Iron Preparations[63]

MECHANISM: Not established. However, chloramphenicol is known to interfere with erythrocyte maturation in a considerable number of patients treated with the drug (not related to aplastic anemia, which is quite rare).

CLINICAL SIGNIFICANCE: Chloramphenicol administration may inhibit the response to iron therapy in patients with iron-deficiency anemia.

MANAGEMENT: Patients with iron-deficiency anemia who are receiving iron therapy would probably do better if chloramphenicol were not administered.

Penicillins[2,26,64-66]

MECHANISM: A bacteriostatic drug such as chloramphenicol presumably may interfere with the action of a bactericidal agent such as penicillin. Since penicillin acts by inhibiting cell wall synthesis, agents that inhibit protein synthesis (e.g., chloramphenicol) could theoretically mask the bactericidal effect of penicillin.

CLINICAL SIGNIFICANCE: It has been pointed out that antibiotic antagonism may occur only under specific conditions of dose, order of therapy, etc., and it probably plays a minor role in clinical medicine.[65,66] In fact, De Ritis and associates[26] found chloramphenicol plus ampicillin to be superior to chloramphenicol alone in the treatment of typhoid. However, potential chloramphenicol-induced antagonism of penicillin effect in diseases such as meningitis has not been adequately studied in humans and remains a possibility.

MANAGEMENT: Although some workers would strictly avoid the combination of chloramphenicol and penicillins,[2] it is probably sufficient to observe the following points when the combination is felt to be necessary.
 1. Be sure that adequate amounts of each agent are being given.
 2. If possible, begin administration of the penicillin a few hours or longer before the chloramphenicol.

Vitamin B_{12} (Cyanocobalamin)[63]

MECHANISM: Not established. However, chloramphenicol is known to interfere with erythrocyte maturation in a considerable number of patients treated with the drug (not related to the aplastic anemia, which is quite rare).

CLINICAL SIGNIFICANCE: Patients with pernicious anemia have been said to respond poorly to vitamin B_{12} therapy if chloramphenicol is given concomitantly.

MANAGEMENT: In patients with pernicious anemia, the hematologic response to vitamin B_{12} should be followed closely if chloramphenicol is also given. Chloramphenicol is the drug of choice for few conditions, and it should not be difficult to find an alternative antibiotic if one becomes necessary.

CHLOROQUINE INTERACTIONS

DRUGS	DISCUSSION

Antacids, Oral[320]

MECHANISM: Magnesium trisilicate appears to reduce the gastrointestinal absorption of chloroquine.

CLINICAL SIGNIFICANCE: In six healthy subjects, magnesium trisilicate (1 g) reduced the area under the chloroquine plasma concentration time curve by 18%.[320] It is not established whether the magnitude of this reduction would be sufficient to reduce the therapeutic effect of chloroquine. Also, the effect of antacids other than magnesium trisilicate on chloroquine absorption is not established.

MANAGEMENT: Separate doses of antacids from chloroquine as much as possible, and be alert for evidence of reduced chloroquine response.

Kaolin-pectin (Kaopectate)[320]

MECHANISM: Kaolin appears to reduce the gastrointestinal absorption of chloroquine.

CLINICAL SIGNIFICANCE: Chloroquine (1.0 g orally) was given with and without concurrent administration of kaolin (1.0 g orally in six healthy subjects.[320] Kaolin reduced the area under the chloroquine plasma concentration time curve by about 30%. The effect of kaolin on the absorption of hydroxychloroquine (Plaquenil) was not studied, but one might expect it to be similarly affected by kaolin.

MANAGEMENT: Separate doses of kaolin-containing products from chloroquine as much as possible, and be alert for evidence of reduced chloroquine response.

CLINDAMYCIN (CLEOCIN) INTERACTIONS

DRUGS	DISCUSSION

Erythromcyin[4]

MECHANISM: It has been stated that clindamycin and erythromycin compete for the "same ribosomal binding site."[4]

CLINICAL SIGNIFICANCE: This antagonism is apparently based on in-vitro studies, with little supporting clinical evidence.

MANAGEMENT: Until more information is available, it would probably be advisable to avoid concomitant use of these drugs if possible. Even

CLINDAMYCIN (CLEOCIN) INTERACTIONS (CONT.)

DRUGS	DISCUSSION

disregarding the possibility of interaction, there should be very few cases where concomitant use would be indicated.

Skeletal Muscle Relaxants (Surgical)[206,203,231]

MECHANISM: Clindamycin may have some neuromuscular blocking activity.

CLINICAL SIGNIFICANCE: In-vitro studies have indicated that clindamycin may have neuromuscular blocking activity and may enhance the effect of neuromuscular blockers.[206,231] Only isolated clinical examples of such an effect of clindamycin have been reported.[230]

MANAGEMENT: In patients receiving clindamycin and neuromuscular blockers concomitantly, one should be alert for prolongation of neuromuscular blockade.

CYLOSERINE (SEROMYCIN) INTERACTIONS

DRUGS	DISCUSSION

Isoniazid (INH)[293]

MECHANISM: It is proposed that cycloserine and isoniazid have a combined toxic action on the central nervous system.

CLINICAL SIGNIFICANCE: In a study of 11 subjects given cycloserine with and without isoniazid, central nervous system effects (dizziness or drowsiness) occurred in 9 of 11 on combined therapy.[293] With cycloserine alone, only one of the 11 subjects developed such symptoms.

MANAGEMENT: Patients receiving both cycloserine and isoniazid should be monitored more closely for signs of central nervous system toxicity, especially if performing tasks requiring alertness.

ERYTHROMYCIN INTERACTIONS

DRUGS	DISCUSSION

Digitalis Glycosides[318,319]

MECHANISM: Approximately 10% of patients treated with digoxin excrete substantial amounts (40% or more of the total urinary excretion of digoxin and its metabolites) of cardioinactive digoxin metabolites in their urine. The bacterial flora of the intestine are involved in this process, and the administration of antibiotics, by altering the bacterial flora, arrests the process and results in higher serum levels of digoxin.

CLINICAL SIGNIFICANCE: Three subjects who were known to respond to digoxin therapy by excreting substantial amounts of cardioinactive dogoxin reduction products in their urine were given digoxin

DRUGS	DISCUSSION

(0.25 mg, two tablets daily) for 22 to 29 days (two subjects received Lanoxin; the other subject received a generic preparation of poor bioavailability).[318] After 10 to 17 days, enteric-coated erythromcyin base (1 to 2 gm/day) or tetracycline (500 mg every 6 hours) was administered concomitantly for 5 days. In all three subjects, urinary excretion of cardioinactive digoxin metabolites fell dramatically within 48 hours of antibiotic administration. As the urinary excretion of carioinactive metabolites decreased, steady-state serum digoxin levels increased, and in two of the subjects (both of whom received erythromycin), the serum digoxin levels approximately doubled after the course of antibiotic therapy.

The clinical significance of this interaction remains to be determined. Although this potential problem is limited to a minority of patients, and although the increase in serum digoxin is greatest with digoxin products of poor bioavailability, this interaction could result in digoxin toxicity.[318,319] Furthermore, antibiotic therapy prior to digitalization may temporarily decrease digoxin requirements; return of the original flora would result in underdigitalization. The effect of antibiotics on the bacterial flora that inactivate digoxin appears to persist for at least 9 weeks and may persist in some for several months.[318]

MANAGEMENT: In the one patient in ten who metabolizes substantial amounts of digoxin in the gut, concomitant antibiotic therapy may increase serum digoxin concentrations. One should be alert for the possibility that antibiotic therapy may increase the response to digoxin. Reduce digoxin dosage as needed.

Lincomycin (Lincocin)[4,71]

MECHANISM: Not established.

CLINICAL SIGNIFICANCE: Not established. There is reportedly some evidence to indicate an antagonism between lincomycin and erythromycin.[71] This antagonism is apparently based on in-vitro studies, with little supporting clinical evidence.

MANAGEMENT: Although clinical evidence appears to be scanty, it has been recommended that erythromycin and lincomycin not be used concomitantly.[4] Even disregarding the possibility of interaction, there should be very few cases where concomitant use would be indicated.

Penicillins[2,5,65,66,179,238]

MECHANISM: Erythromycins are bacteriostatic antibiotics that presumably may interfere with the action of a bactericidal agent such as penicillin. Since penicillin acts by inhibiting cell wall synthesis, agents that inhibit protein synthesis (e.g., erythromycin) could theoretically mask the bactericidal effect of penicillin.

CLINICAL SIGNIFICANCE: It has been pointed out that antibiotic antagonism may occur only under specific conditions of dose, order of ther-

DRUGS	DISCUSSION

apy, etc., and probably plays a minor role in clinical medicine.[65,66,179] It has been stated that clinical evidence exists for erythromycin-penicillin antagonism in patients with group A hemolytic streptococcal pharyngitis. However, Kabins[5] has pointed out that erythromycin is bactericidal against streptococci when high doses are used and thus may act synergistically with penicillins under these conditions. Others have used erythromycin plus ampicillin in the treatment of pulmonary nocardiosis with apparently favorable bacteriologic and clinical results.[238] Thus, the possibility of antagonism exists, but it has not been sufficiently documented in clinical studies.

MANAGEMENT: Combination therapy with antibiotics should be used only when necessary. Since penicillin and erythromycin have similar spectra, indications for their concomitant use should be rare. If a penicillin is used with erythromycin, it would be prudent to observe the following points:
1. Be sure that adequate amounts of each agent are given; antagonism is most likely when barely sufficient amounts of each agent are given.
2. Begin administration of the penicillin at least a few hours before the erythromycin.

Theophylline[287,335-343]

MECHANISM: Erythromycin appears to inhibit the metabolism of theophylline.

CLINICAL SIGNIFICANCE: Several clinical studies and case reports have shown that erythromycin reduces theophylline clearance and increases serum theophylline levels.[287,335-340] The effect usually occurs only after at least several days of erythromycin therapy. Although other studies failed to find the interaction,[341-343] in some cases this may have been due to short duration of erythromycin therapy or a possible inhibitory effect of smoking on the interaction. It appears that any salt of erythromycin is capable of increasing serum theophylline levels, but the effect may be larger with those erythromycin salts which yield higher erythromycin serum levels. Also preliminary information indicates that serum erythromycin levels may be lower in the presence of theophylline,[340] but more information is needed to assess the likelihood that clinically important decreases in serum erythromycin will be produced.

MANAGEMENT: Patients who are receiving large doses of theophylline or who are otherwise at increased risk for theophylline toxicity should be closely monitored when erythromycin therapy is initiated. Although some clinicians suggest lowering the dose of theophylline by 25% when erythromycin is initiated, such a precaution may excessively complicate the management of low risk patients (i.e., those likely to have a low serum theophylline concentration). One should be aware that a reduction in erythromycin serum concentrations by theophylline may also be observed.

ETHIONAMIDE (TRECATOR) INTERACTIONS

DRUGS	DISCUSSION

Ethanol (Alcohol, Ethyl)[72]

MECHANISM: Not established.

CLINICAL SIGNIFICANCE: A case has been reported in which ethanol may have contributed to the psychotoxic reaction in an ethionamide-treated patient. More study is needed to assess clinical significance.

MANAGEMENT: Pending the availability of further information, it may be wise to advise patients on ethionamide therapy to avoid excessive ethanol ingestion.

FURAZOLIDONE (FUROXONE) INTERACTIONS

DRUGS	DISCUSSION

Amphetamines[73,74]

MECHANISM: Furazolidone appears to inhibit monoamine oxidase, thus increasing the pressor effect of indirect acting sympathomimetics such as amphetamines.

CLINICAL SIGNIFICANCE: The pressor response to dextro-amphetamine was increased in nine hypertensive patients after administration of furazolidone (400 to 800 mg/day).[73] The effect was apparently seen only after several days of furazolidone administration. One would expect an enhanced response to other sympathomimetics with indirect activity (e.g., phenylpropanolamine, ephedrine, etc.), but this has apparently not been studied.

MANAGEMENT: Patients receiving furazolidone should probably avoid taking amphetamines. Medical indications for amphetamines are infrequent enough so that this should not be difficult.

Antidepressants, Tricyclic[128]

MECHANISM: Not established.

CLINICAL SIGNIFICANCE: Not established. A single case has appeared in which a patient receiving amitriptyline (Elavil) developed a toxic psychosis soon after furazolidone therapy was begun. Other drugs were being taken, however, and it was not established that drug interaction was responsible.

MANAGEMENT: Pending further information, furazolidone and tricyclic antidepressants should be administered together with caution.

Ethanol (Alcohol, Ethyl)[51,75]

MECHANISM: It is possible that furazolidone may inhibit aldehyde dehydrogenase and result in accumulation of acetaldehyde following ethanol ingestion.

FURAZOLIDONE (FUROXONE) INTERACTIONS (CONT.)

DRUGS	DISCUSSION

CLINICAL SIGNIFICANCE: A disulfiram-like reaction reportedly may occur following ethanol ingestion in patients receiving furazolidone. The incidence of this reaction is not known.

MANAGEMENT: Patients on furazolidone should be warned that a disulfiram-like reaction (flushing, nausea, sweating, etc.) may occur following enthanol ingestion.

GRISEOFULVIN INTERACTIONS

DRUGS	DISCUSSION

Barbiturates[76-78]

MECHANISM: Earlier reports indicated that phenobarbital may increase the metabolism of griseofulvin by hepatic microsomal enzyme induction. However, more recent evidence from pharmacokinetic studies has shown that phenobarbital impairs the absorption of griseofulvin.

CLINICAL SIGNIFICANCE: Although decreased plasma levels of griseofulvin are well documented, the effect of these decreases on therapeutic response has not been established. A single case of possible impaired therapeutic response to griseofulvin was cited by Riegelman and associates,[76] but more study is needed to assess the clinical significance of this interaction.

MANAGEMENT: Pending further information, it would be preferable to avoid giving phenobarbital to patients receiving griseofulvin. If concomitant therapy is desired, Riegelman and associates[76] suggest that divided doses (e.g., three times a day) of griseofulvin may be absorbed better than larger doses taken less often. Whether an increase in the daily griseofulvin dose is warranted requires further study.

Food[247-249]

MECHANISM: Dissolution of griseofulvin is probably enhanced in the presence of a fatty meal, thus enhancing gastrointestinal absorption.

CLINICAL SIGNIFICANCE: A study in which ten subjects were fed a high fat meal (bacon, eggs, cream, and butter) and given 1.0 g of griseofulvin demonstrated that fat in the gut can increase the absorption of the drug.[247] Serum levels of griseofulvin following the high fat intake were shown to be approximately double the level when compared with the fasting state.[247] Subsequent study using microcrystalline griseofulvin yielded similar results.[248] These findings might be used to advantage in patients whose clinical resistance is due to inadequate gastrointestinal absorption.[247]

MANAGEMENT: In select patients for whom increased absorption of griseofulvin yielding higher serum levels is indicated, administration of the drug with a high fat meal may prove beneficial.[247]

HYDROXYCHLOROQUINE (PLAQUENIL) INTERACTIONS

DRUGS	DISCUSSION

Digoxin (Lanoxin)[309]

MECHANISM: Not established.

CLINICAL SIGNIFICANCE: Two patients aged 65 and 68 years on chronic digoxin (0.25 mg/day) developed increased serum digoxin levels of 2.4 and 2.3 mg/ml after hydroxychloroquine was given for rheumatoid arthritis. Serum digoxin levels decreased to 0.7 and 0.6 mg/ml after discontinuation of hydroxychloroquine, which supports the contention that the elevated levels were caused by hydroxychloroquine. The patients did not develop symptoms of digitalis toxicity.

MANAGEMENT: One should be alert for evidence of altered digoxin effect if hydroxychloroquine is initiated or discontinued in a patient receiving digoxin. Digoxin dosage may need to be altered.

ISONIAZID (INH) INTERACTIONS

DRUGS	DISCUSSION

Antacids, Oral[27]

MECHANISM: Aluminum hydroxide gel (Amphojel) and, to a lesser extent, magaldrate (Riopan) appear to inhibit the gastrointestinal absorption of isoniazid. It has been proposed that this effect may be due to a delay in gastric emptying caused by the aluminum in the antacids.[27]

CLINICAL SIGNIFICANCE: In a study of 11 patients with tuberculosis, aluminum hydroxide gel decreased the rate and amount of isoniazid absorbed as measured by the plasma drug concentration-time curve.[27] The effect of magaldrate on isoniazid blood levels was less marked. Curiously, one alcoholic patient demonstrated a marked *increase* in isoniazid plasma levels when aluminum hydroxide or magaldrate was given.

MANAGEMENT: On the basis of current evidence, the simultaneous administration of doses of isoniazid and aluminum-containing antacids should probably be avoided. Giving the isoniazid at least an hour before the antacid would appear to minimize any effect of this interaction.

Benzodiazepines[313,314]

MECHANISM: Isoniazid probably inhibits the hepatic metabolism of diazepam.

CLINICAL SIGNIFICANCE: In nine healthy subjects single 5.0- or 7.5-mg intravenous doses of diazepam (Valium) were administered with and without pretreatment with isoniazid (180mg/day).[313] Isonazid prolonged the diazepam plasma half-life from 34 to 45 hours and reduced diazepam clearance from 0.54 to 0.40 ml/minute/kg body weight. Diazepam disposition was also studied in seven patients receiving triple

ISONIAZID (INH) INTERACTIONS (CONT.)

DRUGS	DISCUSSION

therapy with isonazid, refampin (Rifadin), and ethambutol (Myambutol) and compared to healthy controls matches for age and sex. Diazepam half-life was *shorter* in the patients than in the controls, probably because the enzyme-inducing effect of rifampin more than offset the enzyme inhibition of isonazid. However, the fact that the tuberculosis patients were compared to healthy controls raises the possibility that part of the difference in diazepam disposition was due to factors other than drug interaction. Preliminary evidence indicates that triazolam (Halcion) metabolism may be reduced by isoniazid.[314]

MANAGEMENT: One should be alert for evidence of altered diazepam (and possibly triazolam) effect if isoniazid is initiated or discontinued.

Corticosteroids[311,312]

MECHANISM: Not established. Enhanced hepatic isoniazid metabolism and/or enhanced renal excretion of isoniazid may be involved. Also, isoniazid may reduce the hepatic metabolism of corticosteroids.

CLINICAL SIGNIFICANCE: In 26 patients given 10 mg/kg body weight of INH with and without concomitant prednisolone (20 mg),[311] prednisolone therapy was associated with a 25% decrease in plasma isoniazid levels in slow INH acetylators and a 40% decrease in rapid INH acetylators. Plasma concentrations were not reduced by prednisolone in the presence of rifampin. In another study, there was evidence of INH-induced reduction in the hepatic microsomal oxidation of endogeneous cortisol,[312] raising the possibility that exogenous corticosteroids might be similarly affected. The clinical significance of these interactions is not established.

MANAGEMENT: In patients receiving concurrent isoniazid and corticosteroids, one should be alert for evidence of reduced isoniazid effect and enhanced corticosteroid effect. Dosage adjustment of one or both drugs may be necessary.

Disulfiram (Antabuse)[79,80,129,160]

MECHANISM: It has been proposed[160] that the disulfiram and isoniazid inhibit two of the three known metabolic pathways for dopamine. Disulfiram inhibits beta-hydroxylase, while isoniazid may inhibit monoamine oxidase. Whittington and Grey hypothesize that this inhibition results in increased metabolism of dopamine by catechol-0-methyltransferase, and the resultant methylated metabolites of dopamine are responsible for the adverse mental changes and coordination problems.[160] Another possible factor is that both monoamine oxidase (possibly inhibited by INH) and aldehyde dehydrogenase (inhibited by disulfiram) are involved in the conversion of norepinephrine to 3,4-dihydroxymandelic acid. Thus, one might speculate that inhibition of both of these enzymes could increase levels of norepinephrine.

CLINICAL SIGNIFICANCE: Seven possible clinical examples of this interaction have been presented.[160] Patients on concomitant isoniazid and

DRUGS	DISCUSSION

disulfiram therapy developed changes in effect and behavior as well as coordination difficulties. Although drug interaction does seem likely to be involved in the adverse reactions, no definite conclusions can be drawn from the data presented. Some of the patients received relatively large doses of INH, and other drugs were also being given. One case has been presented in which a patient receiving INH, disulfiram, and rifampin did not manifest signs of interaction.[129]

MANAGEMENT: Enough evidence has been presented to warrant caution in the concomitant use of INH and disulfiram. It would be wise in most cases to avoid the use of disulfiram in patients receiving INH until more information is known about the interaction.

Ethanol[51,122]

MECHANISM: Chronic alcoholics reportedly metabolize isoniazid more rapidly than nonalcoholics.

CLINICAL SIGNIFICANCE: Not established. It is possible that alcoholics would respond less well to isoniazid therapy. Also, ethanol intolerance reportedly may occur in patients receiving INH.[122]

MANAGEMENT: Too little information is available to determine management.

Food[266,294,344]

MECHANISM: The mechanism for inhibition of isoniazid absorption by food is not established. The reaction to cheese may be due to inhibition of monoamine oxidase by isoniazid.

CLINICAL SIGNIFICANCE: A study in nine healthy male volunteers demonstrated that the peak serum concentrations and the total amount of INH absorbed were decreased when the compound was taken with food as compared with the fasting state.[266] The decreases were considerable in many cases, indicating that the therapeutic response to INH could be impaired. Also, a patient receiving isoniazid developed a reaction (flushing, chills, headache) each time she ingested Swiss cheese, but no reactions occurred after isoniazid was stopped.[294] In a similar case cheese produced flushing, chills, tachycardia, and hypertension in a patient on INH, but not when the INH was discontinued.[344]

MANAGEMENT: For optimal absorption, isoniazid should be given on an empty stomach.[266] Also one should be alert for "cheese reactions" in patients on INH.

Laxatives[217]

MECHANISM: Laxative-induced diarrhea may result in inhibition of gastrointestinal absorption of isoniazid.

CLINICAL SIGNIFICANCE: Isoniazid serum levels and urinary excretion were studied in 11 normal subjects with and without diarrhea in-

DRUGS	DISCUSSION

duced by sodium sulfate or castor oil.[217] The sodium sulfate was associated with a delay in isoniazid absorption, and possibly a reduction in amount of isoniazid absorbed. Castor oil had little effect on isoniazid blood levels during the first 90 minutes, but was associated with decreased urinary excretion of isoniazid during the first 4 hours.

MANAGEMENT: No special precautions appear necessary, but excessive laxative use might be considered a possible cause of failure to respond to isoniazid.

Meperidine (Demerol)[80,81]

MECHANISM: Not established. Meperidine is known to interact with monoamine oxidase (MAO) inhibitors. The possible MAO inhibition of INH may thus be involved.

CLINICAL SIGNIFICANCE: The concomitant use of meperidine and INH reportedly increases adverse effects. Clinical descriptions of this interaction are lacking.

MANAGEMENT: Too little information is available to determine management.

Pyrazinamide[210]

MECHANISM: Not established.

CLINICAL SIGNIFICANCE: Pyrazinamide administration has been associated with reduced serum levels of acetyl isoniazid, especially in slow isoniazid acetylators.[210] The clinical significance of this finding is not clear, but probably is not large.

MANAGEMENT: No special precautions appear necessary.

Rifampin (Rifadin) (Rimactane)[130,210,215,222,288,295,345,346,348]

MECHANISM: It has been proposed that enzyme inducers may enhance the conversion of isoniazid to hepatotoxic metabolites,[288] and rifampin is known to induce microsomal enzymes.

CLINICAL SIGNIFICANCE: There is some clinical evidence to indicate that the combined use of INH and rifampin may result in hepatotoxicity, especially in patients with previous liver impairment.[130,215,222,296,345,346,348] However, this association has been questioned because the actual incidence of hepatotoxicity in patients receiving the combination is low. It seems clear that the vast majority of patients receiving INH and rifampin do not develop clinically evident synergistic hepatotoxicity. Indeed, combined use of these two agents is recommended as the initial treatment of choice for uncomplicated pulmonary tuberculosis.[347] However, it is also possible that some patients may be predisposed to this synergistic hepatotoxicity. Predisposed patients may include those receiving large doses of INH, those who have recently undergone general anesthesia, those with preexisting liver disease, and women.[348]

ISONIAZID (INH) INTERACTIONS (CONT.)

DRUGS	DISCUSSION

MANAGEMENT: One should be alert for evidence of hepatotoxicity in patients receiving isoniazid and rifampin, alone and especially in combination.

Sympathomimetics[80]

MECHANISM: Not established. The possible monoamine oxidase inhibition of isoniazid[80] may be involved.

CLINICAL SIGNIFICANCE: Not established. Sympathomimetics reportedly enhance the side effects of INH but there appears to be little supporting evidence.

MANAGEMENT: On the basis of current evidence, no specific precautions appear to be necessary, but the possibility of increased side effects should be realized.

KETOCONAZOLE INTERACTIONS

DRUGS	DISCUSSION

Antacids[330]

MECHANISM: Antacids possibly reduce the gastrointestinal absorption of ketoconazole by increasing the pH of the gut.

CLINICAL SIGNIFICANCE: Evidence from a few subjects indicates that antacids considerably reduce ketoconazole plasma levels.[330] More data are needed to assess the incidence and magnitude of this purported interaction.

MANAGEMENT: Until more is known about this interaction, it would be prudent to administer ketoconazole 2 or more hours prior to antacids.

Cimetidine (Tagamet)[330]

MECHANISM: Cimetidine possibly reduces the gastrointestinal absorption of ketoconazole by increasing the pH of the gut.

CLINICAL SIGNIFICANCE: Evidence from a few subjects indicates that cimetidine considerably reduces ketoconazole plasma levels.[330] More data are needed to assess the incidence and magnitude of this purported interaction.

MANAGEMENT: Until more is known about this interaction, one should be alert for evidence of reduced ketoconazole effect. Increase ketoconazole dose if needed.

LINCOMYCIN (LINCOCIN) INTERACTIONS

DRUGS	DISCUSSION

Food[97,98,279-283]

MECHANISM: Not established.

DRUGS	DISCUSSION

CLINICAL SIGNIFICANCE: Single dose studies in healthy subjects have demonstrated that gastrointestinal absorption of lincomycin after food ingestion is poor and erratic, with significant delays and decreases in absorption.[280–282] Average serum concentrations when taken with food appear to be about one-half the serum concentrations when taken in the fasting state. Diet foods or drinks with sodium cyclamate have been shown to decrease significantly the serum levels of the antibiotic.[279] Serum levels of oral lincomycin when taken with 8 oz. of Diet-Rite cola reduced serum concentrations of lincomycin 62% to 85% when the cola contained sodium cyclamate as the artificial sweetener. This may be of clinical significance in countries where cyclamates are still available.

MANAGEMENT: For optimal absorption nothing should be given by mouth except water for a period of 1 to 2 hours before and after oral lincomycin.[283]

Kaolin-pectin (Kaopectate)[94–96]

MECHANISM: Kaolin-pectin mixtures inhibit the absorption of orally administered lincomycin.

CLINICAL SIGNIFICANCE: Well documented. If Kaopectate and lincomycin are given at the same time, resultant serum concentrations of lincomycin are about one-tenth of those seen with lincomycin alone. When Kaopectate is given 2 hours after lincomycin, serum lincomycin is approximately one-half that of lincomycin alone. Kaopectate administered 2 hours before lincomycin administration does not significantly affect serum lincomycin concentration. It should also be remembered that food impairs lincomycin absorption; lincomycin should be given on an empty stomach (e.g., 1 hour before or 2 hours after meals).

MANAGEMENT: It would be preferable to use some form of diarrhea control other than Kaopectate in patients receiving oral lincomycin. If they are used concomitantly, the Kaopectate should be given at least 2 hours before or 3 to 4 hours after the lincomycin. This would make dosing difficult if the lincomycin were given every 6 hours, especially since lincomycin should be given on an empty stomach.

METHENAMINE COMPOUND INTERACTIONS

DRUGS	DISCUSSION

Acetazolamide (Diamox)[99]

MECHANISM: Acetazolamide tends to render the urine alkaline. During therapy with methenamine compounds, the urine must be kept at about pH 5.5 or lower to effect proper conversion of methenamine to free formaldehyde in the urine.

CLINICAL SIGNIFICANCE: Acetazolamide is an effective urinary alkalinizer and would be expected to antagonize the effect of methenamine compounds.

DRUGS	DISCUSSION

MANAGEMENT: If the urine cannot be kept at about pH 5.5 or lower during the use of acetazolamide, methenamine compounds should not be used.

Sodium Bicarbonate[99]

MECHANISM: Sodium bicarbonate tends to render the urine alkaline. During therapy with methenamine compounds, the urine must be kept at about pH 5.5 or lower to effect proper conversion of methenamine to free formaldehyde in the urine.

CLINICAL SIGNIFICANCE: Large doses of sodium bicarbonate can effectively alkalinize the urine and would be expected to inhibit the effect of methenamine compounds.

MANAGEMENT: If the urine cannot be kept at about pH 5.5 or lower during the use of sodium bicarbonate, methenamine compounds should not be used.

Sulfonamides[99]

MECHANISM:
1. With some sulfonamides the danger of crystalluria is enhanced in the presence of an acid urine. Methenamine requires a urine pH of about 5.5 or less in order to be active.
2. The concomitant administration of methenamine compounds and sulfamethizole (Thiosulfil) frequently results in formation of a precipitate in the urine. Methenamine and sulfathiazole reportedly result in a similar effect.

CLINICAL SIGNIFICANCE: Sulfonamides such as sulfadiazine, sulfapyridine, and sulfamerazine are more likely to result in crystalluria in an acid urine. This has been well documented in the past, but rarely occurs now since more soluble agents such as sulfisoxazole (Gantrisin) are more widely used. The propriety of using sulfathiazole or sulfamethizole with methenamine compounds has been questioned,[99] and Mesulfin (sulfamethizole plus methenamine mandelate) has been withdrawn from the market.

MANAGEMENT:
1. Methenamine compounds should not be used with sulfonamides that may precipitate in an acid urine.
2. Although the precipitate formed in the urine with concomitant use of sulfamethizole or sulfathiazole and a methenamine may not have proved harmful to date, there appears to be no advantage of these combinations over other forms of therapy. If a methenamine product and a sulfonamide are to be used together, it would be preferable to use a sulfonamide that does not result in a precipitate in the urine.

METRONIDAZOLE (FLAGYL) INTERACTIONS

DRUGS	DISCUSSION

Barbiturates[331]

MECHANISM: Barbiturates may enhance the hepatic metabolism of metronidazole.

CLINICAL SIGNIFICANCE: A woman with vaginal trichomoniasis failed to respond to metronidazole while on phenobarbital (100 mg daily), but did respond when the dose of metronidazole was doubled (to 500 mg daily for 7 days).[331] Pharmacokinetic studies in this patient indicated that she eliminated metronidazole very rapidly. More study is needed.

MANAGEMENT: Until more information is available, one should be aware that patients on barbiturates (or other enzyme inducers) may require larger doses of metronidazole.

Disulfiram (Antabuse)[103,104,170]

MECHANISM: Not established. A combined inhibition of aldehyde dehydrogenase or some other enzyme may be involved.

CLINICAL SIGNIFICANCE: Preliminary reports describe patients with psychotic episodes and confusional states that may have been due to combined metronidazole-disulfiram therapy. Although these reports involved only a few patients, it seems likely that the interaction is clinically significant.

MANAGEMENT: Until this potential interaction is better described, it would be wise to avoid concomitant use of metronidazole and disulfiram.

Ethanol (Alcohol, Ethyl)[28,100–102,209]

MECHANISM: Metronidazole presumably acts in a manner similar to that of disulfiram by inhibiting the activity of aldehyde dehydrogenase.

CLINICAL SIGNIFICANCE: Both "Antabuse reactions" and a decreased desire to drink have been reported in some patients receiving metronidazole. However, the relative lack of clinical reports indicates that adverse reactions to alcohol in patients receiving metronidazole must be uncommon. The place of metronidazole in the treatment of alcoholism has not been established, but most well-controlled clinical studies have demonstrated only minor beneficial effects.

MANAGEMENT: Patients receiving metronidazole should be warned about the possibility of reactions following ethanol ingestion.

NALIDIXIC ACID (NEGGRAM) INTERACTIONS

DRUGS	DISCUSSION

Antacids (Oral)[139]

MECHANISM: It has been proposed that antacids would increase the proportion of ionized nalidixic acid and therapy would decrease its absorption.

NALIDIXIC ACID (NEGGRAM) INTERACTIONS (CONT.)

DRUGS	DISCUSSION

CLINICAL SIGNIFICANCE: Clinical studies must be performed to assess the clinical significance of this interaction. Factors other than ionization may be involved (e.g., dissolution rate). Further, a *delay* in absorption does not necessarily mean a *decrease* in absorption, and under the conditions of multiple dosing, delayed absorption may or may not have a significant clinical effect. Finally, preliminary evidence has been presented that suggests that sodium bicarbonate might actually *increase* nalidixic acid absorption.[139]

MANAGEMENT: No special precautions appear to be necessary.

Nitrofurantoin (Furadantin)[105]

MECHANISM: Not established.

CLINICAL SIGNIFICANCE: Not established. Some preliminary in-vitro evidence indicates that nitrofurantoin may antagonize the effect of nalidixic acid. Clinical studies are needed to assess significance.

MANAGEMENT: Pending accumulation of further information it may be wise to avoid concomitant nitrofurantoin-nalidixic acid therapy.

Probenecid (Benemid)[208]

MECHANISM: Not established. It is possible that probenecid reduces the renal excretion of nalidixic acid.

CLINICAL SIGNIFICANCE: Extremely high serum nalidixic acid concentrations were noted in a patient who had apparently taken an overdose of a number of drugs, including nalidixic acid and probenecid.[208] Subsequent study in two normal subjects indicated that probenecid can considerably increase serum nalidixic acid levels.

MANAGEMENT: Until this potential interaction is better described, one should be alert for altered toxicity or efficacy of nalidixic acid if probenecid is taken concurrently.

NITROFURANTOIN (FURADANTIN) INTERACTIONS

DRUGS	DISCUSSION

Antacids (Oral)[51,55,185]

MECHANISM: It has been proposed that antacids would increase the proportion of ionized nitrofurantoin, thereby decreasing its absorption. However, it seems doubtful that such an effect occurs.

CLINICAL SIGNIFICANCE: Not established. At least one study in six subjects indicates that aluminum hydroxide gel does not affect nitrofurantoin absorption as measured by cumulative urinary excretion.

MANAGEMENT: No special precautions appear necessary.

DRUGS	DISCUSSION

Anticholinergics[188]

MECHANISM: It is proposed that anticholinergics may enhance nitrofurantoin bioavailability by slowing gastrointestinal motility, thus allowing increased dissolution of nitrofurantoin prior to its arrival in the small intestine where absorption occurs.

CLINICAL SIGNIFICANCE: Six healthy subjects were given nitrofurantoin (Macrodantin, 100 mg) with or without pretreatment with propantheline (30 mg orally).[188] Cumulative urinary excretion of nitrofurantoin was 17.1 mg on nitrofurantoin alone and 28.7 mg with propantheline pretreatment. The clinical significance of these findings is not obvious, but one might expect an increase in both therapeutic efficacy and dose-related adverse effects.

MANAGEMENT: No special precautions appear necessary.

Food[242–245]

MECHANISM: It has been suggested that since food delays gastric emptying, a greater amount of nitrofurantoin may be dissolved in the gastric fluids before being absorbed in the duodenum.[242]

CLINICAL SIGNIFICANCE: In two studies, each involving four healthy male volunteers, it was demonstrated that food in the gastrointestinal tract decreased the *rate* of nitrofurantoin absorption from both the microcrystalline and macrocrystalline forms, but increased the *bioavailability*. Food increased by approximately 2 hours the duration of therapeutic urinary concentrations of oral nitrofurantoin.[242,244]

MANAGEMENT: Nitrofurantoin may be given with milk or food to minimize gastrointestinal irritation.[245] An additional benefit of administering the drug with food would be the enhancement of the bioavailability of nitrofurantoin.

Oxolinic Acid (Utibid)[200]

MECHANISM: Not established.

CLINICAL SIGNIFICANCE: Nitrofurantoin appears to inhibit the in-vitro antibacterial effect of oxolinic acid, as noted in disc sensitivity testing. This inhibitory effect apparently applies to most non-lactose fermenting organisms,[200] but it is not known whether it occurs with the concomitant therapeutic use of both drugs.

MANAGEMENT: Until it is determined whether this interaction occurs during therapy with both drugs, one should be alert for evidence of decreased response to oxolinic acid if nitrofurantoin is used concomitantly.

PENICILLIN INTERACTIONS

DRUGS	DISCUSSION

Allopurinol (Zyloprim)[29-31]

MECHANISM: Not established.

CLINICAL SIGNIFICANCE: In an epidemiologic study of adverse drug reactions, an association between ampicillin rashes and allopurinol administration was detected.[29] Analysis of the data indicated that either allopurinol or hyperuricemia seemed to predispose patients receiving ampicillin to the development of rashes. More study is needed to determine whether the allopurinol itself is producing this effect.

MANAGEMENT: No special precautions appear necessary at this point, but prescribers should be aware of the possibility of interaction.

Antacids (Oral)

MECHANISM: Some have proposed that antacids would increase the proportion of ionized penicillin G, thereby decreasing its absorption.

CLINICAL SIGNIFICANCE: This is probably of little clinical significance. Penicillin G is acid-labile and frequently has a buffer incorporated into the oral dosage form. Thus, although antacids may increase the proportion of ionized penicillin, they also protect the penicillin from inactivation by gastric secretions.

MANAGEMENT: No special precautions appear to be necessary.

Contraceptives, Oral[201,349-354,361,362]

MECHANISM: Ampicillin may interrupt the enterohepatic circulation of estrogen by reducing the bacterial hydrolysis of conjugated estrogen in the gut.

CLINICAL SIGNIFICANCE: Ampicillin has been associated with a reduction in urinary excretion of endogenous estrogens and isolated cases of menstrual irregularities and unplanned pregnancies in patients receiving oral contraceptives. However, in another study oral ampicillin did not appear to interfere with the ability of an oral contraceptive (containing 50 mcg of estrogen) to suppress ovulation.[354] However, this study involved only 11 subjects observed for 2 months. In another study in 13 women on oral contraceptives, ampicillin lowered plasma ethinylestradiol in only two women.[362] Even if ampicillin increased ovulation severalfold in patients on oral contraceptives, ovulation would still be quite rare. Thus, a large number of patients would be required to document the interaction. Enough evidence has accumulated so that the interaction cannot be ignored even though the incidence of problems remains unknown.

MANAGEMENT: Since ampicillin is often given in relatively short courses, it may be best for the patient to continue the oral contraceptive and use supplementary contraception during cycles in which ampicillin is used. The patient should be told that spotting or breakthrough bleeding may be an indication that the interaction is occurring. Although the use of an alternative antibiotic with less effect on

DRUGS	DISCUSSION

bowel flora would theoretically be preferable, this has not been established. Whether intravenous ampicillin or amoxicillin (Amoxil) would be less likely to interact due to reduced effect on intestinal flora is also unknown.

Ethanol (Alcohol, Ethyl)[232]

MECHANISM: None known.

CLINICAL SIGNIFICANCE: Ingestion of alcohol reportedly enhances the degradation of "all penicillins" but no supporting clinical evidence is given.

MANAGEMENT: No special precautions appear necessary.

Food[250–253,260,261,275,276]

MECHANISM: Not established.

CLINICAL SIGNIFICANCE:

Ampicillin: Several single dose studies have indicated that the absorption of ampicillin is decreased when administered with food.[251–253] In a study of eight healthy male volunteers given single 250-mg doses of ampicillin on 4 separate days, food decreased the plasma concentrations of the drug.[251] Neuvonen and associates[252] reported that in eight healthy female subjects given a single dose of 500 mg of ampicillin food caused a delay in peak serum concentrations. Urinary excretion data indicated that total absorption of ampicillin was reduced by about one-third when administered with food. Welling and associates[253] reported that in nonfasted subjects peak antibiotic levels in the serum were reduced by about 50% when ampicillin was administered immediately following a standardized meal. In summary, total absorption and peak levels of ampicillin may be decreased somewhat by food, but it does not seem likely that this is a frequent cause of therapeutic failure.

Nafcillin (Unipen): A single dose study employing 1.0-g doses of nafcillin in healthy subjects indicated the absorption of nafcillin when administered immediately after a meal was delayed and decreased when compared with a dose given under fasting conditions. Both peak serum levels and total urinary recovery of active drug were somewhat reduced by food.

Amoxicillin (Amoxil, Larotid, Polymox): Food does not appear to significantly influence the absorption of amoxicillin. The levels of antibiotic have been shown to rise more slowly when amoxicillin is taken with food, yet peak concentrations do not appear to be affected.[261]

Oxacillin (Prostaphilin, Bactocill): A single dose study employing 1.0-g doses of oral oxacillin immediately following a meal indicated that peak levels of the antibiotic are considerably lower and achieved later than when the same dose is given in a fasting state or given 4 hours after a meal.[275]

PENICILLIN INTERACTIONS (CONT.)

DRUGS	DISCUSSION

Penicillin G: Penicillin G is more rapidly destroyed in the presence of acid, and higher blood levels are achieved when it is given on an empty stomach.

MANAGEMENT: For optimal absorption most penicillins should be dosed away from meals. However, this precaution probably does not apply to amoxicillin.

Indomethacin (Indocin)[142]

MECHANISM: It is proposed that indomethacin may compete with penicillin G for renal tubular secretion.

CLINICAL SIGNIFICANCE: Indomethacin has been associated with a slight increase in the half-life of penicillin G.[142] This interaction should be favorable in most cases.

MANAGEMENT: No special precautions appear necessary.

Methotrexate[316,317]

MECHANISM: Large doses of penicillins may interfere with the active renal tubular secretion of methotrexate.

CLINICAL SIGNIFICANCE: A patient receiving high-dose methotrexate with folinic acid rescue developed considerably elevated serum methotrexate levels following carbenicillin administration (30 g daily).[316] This effect has also been observed by others but no details have been given.[317] Elevated methotrexate serum might also be seen with other penicillins, especially those given in large doses, but little clinical information is available.

MANAGEMENT: One should be alert for evidence of enhanced methotrexate effect if large doses of carbenicillin or other penicillins are given.

Salicylates[142]

MECHANISM: It is proposed that salicylates may compete with penicillin G for renal tubular secretion.

CLINICAL SIGNIFICANCE: Aspirin (3 g/day for 5 to 7 days) has been shown to prolong the half-life of penicillin G in 11 patients, from a mean of 44.5 minutes to 72.4 minutes.[142] This interaction should be favorable in most cases.

MANAGEMENT: No special precautions appear necessary.

Sulfinpyrazone (Anturane)[142]

MECHANISM: Sulfinpyrazone probably inhibits the renal tubular secretion of penicillin G in a manner similar to that of probenecid.

DRUGS	DISCUSSION

CLINICAL SIGNIFICANCE: Sulfinpyrazone (600 mg/day for 5 to 7 days) has been shown to prolong the half-life of pencillin G in eight patients, from a mean of 42.6 minutes to 70.3 minutes.[142] This effect was somewhat less than with probenecids, which prolonged penicillin half-life from a mean of 40.4 minutes to 104.3 minutes in 22 patients.

MANAGEMENT: No special precautions appear necessary.

Sulfonamides[141,142]

MECHANISM: Some sulfonamides appear to inhibit the gastrointestinal absorption of oxacillin.

CLINICAL SIGNIFICANCE: In one study sulfamethoxypyridazine and sulfaethidole given in conjunction with oxacillin resulted in decreased oxacillin serum levels and diminished urinary recovery of oxacillin.[141] However, the doses of both the oxacillin and the sulfonamides were higher than normal, and the significance of these findings for patients on multiple dosing schedules with standard doses has not been established. In another study, preliminary evidence was presented that sulfaphenazole (but not sulfamethizole or sulfamethoxypyridazine) prolonged the half-life of penicillin G.[142]

MANAGEMENT: Until more is known about the oxacillin interaction, it might be prudent to avoid combined oral therapy with oxacillin and either sulfamethoxypyridazine or sulfaethidole.

Tetracyclines[2,5,65,66,179,355,356]

MECHANISM: Tetracyclines are bacteriostatic antibiotics that presumably may interfere with a bactericidal agent such as penicillin. Since penicillin acts by inhibiting cell wall synthesis, agents such as tetracycline, which inhibit protein synthesis, could mask the bactericidal effect of penicillin.

CLINICAL SIGNIFICANCE: It has been pointed out that antibiotic antagonism may occur only under specific conditions of dose, order of therapy, etc., and probably plays a minor role in clinical medicine. However, the following possible clinical examples of tetracycline antagonism of penicillin have occurred.
1. Chlortetracycline and penicillin in patients with pneumococcal meningitis.
2. Tetracycline and penicillin in patients with Group A hemolytic streptococcal pharyngitis.
It should be noted that manufacturer's product information may contain warnings against using tetracyclines and penicillins concomitantly. This could have medico-legal implications, should a patient experience difficulty while on such a combination.

MANAGEMENT: If a penicillin is used with a tetracycline, it would be prudent to observe the following points when possible:

PENICILLIN INTERACTIONS (CONT.)

DRUGS	DISCUSSION

1. Be sure that adequate amounts of each agent are given; antagonism is most likely when barely sufficient amounts of each agent are given.
2. Begin administration of the penicillin at least a few hours before the administration of tetracycline.

PIPERAZINE INTERACTIONS

DRUGS	DISCUSSION

Phenothiazines[106,107]

MECHANISM: It has been proposed that piperazine results in exaggeration of phenothiazine-induced extrapyramidal effects.

CLINICAL SIGNIFICANCE: One case has been reported in which a child recently treated with piperazine developed convulsions when he was treated with chlorpromazine. Subsequent animal studies of the interaction using large doses of chlorpromazine (10 mg/kg body weight intravenously) produced similar reactions.[106] However, these reactions could not be confirmed by another investigator.[107] Thus, it remains uncertain whether drug interaction was responsible for the convulsions seen in the one patient reported. Obviously, much more study is needed to assess the clinical significance of this interaction.

MANAGEMENT: Until more is known about this interaction, concomitant therapy with piperazine and a phenothiazine should be undertaken cautiously.

POLYMYXIN INTERACTIONS

DRUGS	DISCUSSION

Skeletal Muscle Relaxants (Surgical)[62,68–70,82,171]

MECHANISM: Both polymyxin B and colistin can produce a neuromuscular blockade that may enhance the blockade of skeletal muscle relaxants.

CLINICAL SIGNIFICANCE: Well documented. A number of cases have been reported in which patients receiving a polymyxin experienced respiratory paralysis, both when taken alone and in combination with surgical neuromuscular blocking agents. It has been proposed that this neuromuscular blockade may be enhanced by either an intracellular potassium deficit or a low serum ionized calcium concentration.

MANAGEMENT: Polymyxins should be administered with caution during surgery or in the postoperative period as the effect of surgical neuromuscular blocking agents may be enhanced. Intravenous calcium has been helpful in some cases, but not in others. Edrophonium has generally been found to be of little benefit.

PYRIMETHAMINE INTERACTIONS

DRUGS	DISCUSSION

Folic Acid (Folvite)[140,172]

MECHANISM: Pyrimethamine interferes with folic acid metabolism in the parasite, and folic acid administration would theoretically inhibit the antimicrobial effect.

CLINICAL SIGNIFICANCE: Folic acid administration reportedly interferes with the action of pyrimethamine against toxoplasmosis. However, malarial parasites apparently cannot use preformed folic acid, and the antimalarial effect of pyrimethamine should not be affected by folic acid administration. In patients with leukemia who receive pyrimethamine in treatment of *Pneumocystis carinii* infections, the addition of folic acid reportedly can produce a worsening of the leukemic condition.[172]

MANAGEMENT: Pending the availability of further information, folic acid should not be administered to patients receiving pyrimethamine for treatment of toxoplasmosis or leukemia.

Quinine[108]

MECHANISM: Pyrimethamine may displace quinine from plasma protein binding and results in excessive free quinine in the blood.

CLINICAL SIGNIFICANCE: This interaction may be important, but more information is needed to assess the clinical significance.

MANAGEMENT: Pending availability of further information, pyrimethamine should not be given to patients receiving quinine. If the drugs must be given together, consideration should be given to a reduction in the quinine dosage.

QUINACRINE INTERACTIONS

DRUGS	DISCUSSION

Ethanol (Alcohol, Ethyl)[51]

MECHANISM: Quinacrine reportedly inhibits aldehyde dehydrogenase to some extent and results in accumulation of acetaldehyde following ethanol ingestion.

CLINICAL SIGNIFICANCE: Not established. If aldehyde dehydrogenase were sufficiently inhibited, an "Antabuse reaction" might occur, but clinical evidence is lacking.

MANAGEMENT: Too little information is known to make a statement on management.

QUININE INTERACTIONS

DRUGS	DISCUSSION

Acetazolamide (Diamox)[290]

MECHANISM: The urinary alkalinization produced by acetazolamide may increase the proportion of quinine present in the un-ionized form, thus promoting renal tubular reabsorption of the quinine.

CLINICAL SIGNIFICANCE: Alkalinization of the urine has been shown to reduce the urinary output of quinine from 17.4% of the administered dose (with acid urine) to 8.9% (with alkaline urine).[290] The increased quinine blood level that one would expect to accompany the decreased urinary excretion could increase both the therapeutic efficacy of quinine as well as its dose-related adverse effects.

MANAGEMENT: No special precautions appear necessary.

Heparin[109]

MECHANISM: Quinine, a basic molecule, reportedly may react with the strongly acidic groups in the heparin molecule.

CLINICAL SIGNIFICANCE: Not established. The anticoagulant activity of heparin is reportedly impaired, but the magnitude and incidence of this interaction cannot be determined from available data.

MANAGEMENT: Since so little is known of the clinical significance, it should not be necessary to avoid concomitant use at this time.

Sodium Bicarbonate[290]

MECHANISM: The urinary alkalinization produced by sodium bicarbonate may increase the proportion of quinine present in the un-ionized form, thus promoting renal tubular reabsorption of the quinine.

CLINICAL SIGNIFICANCE: Alkalinization of the urine has been shown to reduce the urinary output of quinine from 17.4% of the administered dose (with acid urine) to 8.9% (with alkaline urine).[290] The increased quinine blood level that one would expect to accompany the decreased urinary excretion could increase both the therapeutic efficacy of quinine and its dose-related adverse effects.

MANAGEMENT: No special precautions appear necessary.

RIFAMPIN INTERACTIONS

DRUGS	DISCUSSION

Barbiturates[184,225,234,291,292]

MECHANISM: Rifampin appears to stimulate the hepatic metabolism of hexobarbital.

CLINICAL SIGNIFICANCE: The half-life of hexobarbital has been shown to be considerably shortened in the presence of rifampin, both in healthy subjects[184,291] and in patients with hepatic disease.[225] The ef-

RIFAMPIN INTERACTIONS (CONT.)

fect of rifampin administration on the disposition of other barbiturates has not been established, but it is possible that they are similarly affected by rifampin.

MANAGEMENT: It would not seem necessary to avoid concomitant use of rifampin and barbiturates, but rifampin should be considered a potential cause in patients failing to respond to barbiturates.

Benzodiazepines[313]

MECHANISM: Rifampin probably enhances the hepatic metabolism of diazepam (Valium).

CLINICAL SIGNIFICANCE: Diazepam disposition was studied in seven patients receiving isoniazid, rifampin, and ethambutol, and compared with healthy controls matched for sex and age. Diazepam plasma half-life was markedly shorter in the patients than in the healthy controls (14 versus 58 hours). Thus, the enzyme-inducing effect of rifampin apparently more than offset the ability of isoniazid to inhibit diazepam metabolism. The patients also appeared to eliminate desmethyldiazepam more rapidly than controls, so rifampin may also reduce the effect of those benzodiazepines which are metabolized to desmethyldiazepam such as halazepam (Paxipam), clorazepate (Tranxene), and prazepam (Centrax).

MANAGEMENT: One should be alert for evidence of reduced diazepam effect if rifampin is given concurrently. The response to halazepam, clorazepate, and prazepam may also be reduced by rifampin.

Clofibrate (Atromid)[323]

MECHANISM: Rifampin appears to enhance the hepatic metabolism of clofibrate.

CLINICAL SIGNIFICANCE: In five healthy subjects rifampin (600 mg/day for 7 days) reduced by 40% the steady state plasma levels of the active metabolite of clofibrate.[323] The degree to which this reduces the therapeutic response to clofibrate is not established. It seems unlikely that short-term rifampin therapy would significantly reduce the therapeutic response to cloribrate.

MANAGEMENT: If rifampin therapy is prolonged, one should monitor serum lipid levels to detect inhibition of clofibrate effect. Increase clofibrate dose if necessary.

Contraceptives, Oral[32,33,161,190,201,218,220]

MECHANISM: Rifampin probably enhances the metabolism of estrogens, thus reducing the effectiveness of oral contraceptives. (Especially those with low hormonal content). This is consistent with the effect of rifampin on other drugs such as warfarin.

CLINICAL SIGNIFICANCE: Preliminary information from one group indicates that women on oral contraceptives may have menstrual irreg-

231

DRUGS	DISCUSSION

ularities and an increased incidence of unplanned pregnancies if rifampin is also given.[33] Five pregnancies occurred in 88 women who took rifampin in addition to oral contraceptives. Most of the women had menstrual irregularities (e.g., breakthrough bleeding, spotting, etc.). Another report describes a woman who became pregnant twice while taking oral contraceptives and rifampin.[220] Also, amenorrhea has occurred in a patient on long-term oral contraceptive treatment who was subsequently given rifampin.[218] One should remember that the enzyme-inducing effect of rifampin may last for weeks after rifampin is discontinued.

MANAGEMENT: Patients receiving rifampin should probably use contraceptive methods other than oral contraceptives. If the combination is used, it would be prudent to use additional contraceptive methods during and for several weeks after rifampin administration.

Corticosteroids[187,202,203,218,357]

MECHANISM: Rifampin appears to stimulate the metabolism of corticosteroids.

CLINICAL SIGNIFICANCE: In patients with Addison's disease, rifampin administration has been associated with increased requirements for replacement therapy with cortisone.[187,203] Accordingly, the half-life of cortisol was decreased in one patient.[203] In another study, urinary 6-β-hydroxycortisol excretion was measured following administration of hydrocortisone (20 mg orally) in patients receiving antituberculosis therapy with or without rifampin.[202] Patients on rifampin had markedly higher urinary excretion rates of 6-β-hydroxycortisol. In a child with nephrotic syndrome, rifampin appeared to inhibit the therapeutic response to prednisolone.[357] Finally, rifampin administration was associated with decreasing renal allograft function in three patients, presumably due to enhanced metabolism of administered corticosteroids.[218] In summary, rifampin appears to produce a clinically significant reduction in the effect of administered corticosteroids in some patients.

MANAGEMENT: It does not seem necessary to avoid concomitant use of corticosteroids and rifampin, but one should be alert for evidence of reduced corticosteroid effect. It may be necessary to increase the dose of corticosteroids, and some have suggested that doubling the dose may be necessary in some cases.[218]

Digitalis[234,358,359]

MECHANISM: Rifampin appears to enhance the hepatic metabolism of digitoxin, presumably by induction of hepatic microsomal enzymes.

CLINICAL SIGNIFICANCE: A preliminary description of a study in six normal volunteers indicated that the half-life of digitoxin (1 mg IV) was considerably reduced by pretreatment with rifampin (1.2 g orally for 8 days).[234] The magnitude of the decrease in digitoxin half-life (288

RIFAMPIN INTERACTIONS (CONT.)

hours to 76 hours) would appear to be sufficient to produce a clinically significant decrease in serum digitoxin levels. Indeed, case reports of rifampin-induced reductions in serum digitoxin have appeared.[358,359]

MANAGEMENT: In patients receiving rifampin, digoxin may be preferable to digitoxin since digoxin is less likely to be affected by enzyme induction. If rifampin and digitoxin are used concomitantly, one should be alert for possible increased digitoxin requirements.

Halothane (Fluothane)[34]

MECHANISM: It has been proposed that the use of rifampin following halothane anesthesia may result in hepatotoxicity.

CLINICAL SIGNIFICANCE: A single case has been reported of a patient who was started on rifampin and isoniazid therapy immediately following halothane anesthesia and who subsequently developed nearly fatal hepatotoxicity.[34] It was presumed that this reaction was due to the combined effects of halothane and rifampin, but more study is needed to establish such an interaction.

MANAGEMENT: Although very little clinical evidence is available, the severity of the possible interaction would indicate that rifampin should probably not be given immediately before or after halothane anesthesia.

Narcotic Analgesics[207,237]

MECHANISM: Available evidence indicates that rifampin stimulates the hepatic metabolism of methadone. However, the evidence is not totally consistent, and other mechanisms may also be involved.

CLINICAL SIGNIFICANCE: Of 30 patients on methadone maintenance given rifampin (600 to 900 mg/day) 21 developed evidence of narcotic withdrawal.[207] Subsequent study in six of these patients showed that plasma methadone levels were considerably lower in the presence of rifampin. In another case, symptoms of methadone withdrawal occurred 5 days after rifampin was started (450 mg/day).[237] The interval between initiation of rifampin and symptoms of withdrawal is quite variable, but withdrawal usually occurs within the first week in patients with severe symptoms.

MANAGEMENT: One should be alert for evidence of methadone withdrawal when methadone-treated patients are started on rifampin. If methadone dosage is increased to offset the effect of rifampin, one should be alert for excessive methadone effect if the rifampin is discontinued.

Probenecid (Benemid)[35,173,174]

MECHANISM: Not established. It has been proposed that probenecid competes with rifampin for hepatic uptake resulting in higher rifampin blood levels.[35]

RIFAMPIN INTERACTIONS (CONT.)

DRUGS	DISCUSSION

CLINICAL SIGNIFICANCE: Although an initial study in normal subjects indicated that probenecid resulted in considerable increases in serum rifampin levels,[35] subsequent studies have indicated that this effect is not consistent.[173,174] It is possible that probenecid could increase the likelihood of dose-related adverse effects of rifampin in certain patients, but this has not been documented clinically. In some cases the increase in serum rifampin would be desirable.

MANAGEMENT: The increase in serum rifampin following probenecid does not appear to be predictable enough to warrant the use of probenecid for this purpose. In patients who do receive both drugs, one should be aware that occasionally patients develop increased serum rifampin levels.

SULFONAMIDE INTERACTIONS

DRUGS	DISCUSSION

Anesthetics, Local[121]

MECHANISM: Sulfonamides act by competitive inhibition of para-aminobenzoic acid (PABA) in the microorganism. Local anesthetics that are derivatives of PABA (e.g., benzocaine, procaine, tetracaine, butacaine, etc.) reportedly may antagonize the antibacterial activity of sulfonamides.

CLINICAL SIGNIFICANCE: Local infections reportedly have occurred in areas of procaine infiltration in the presence of adequate sulfonamide therapy. Clinical reports of the interaction in humans appear to be infrequent.

MANAGEMENT: Pending availability of further information, it would be wise to use local anesthetics that are not PABA derivatives in patients receiving antibacterial sulfonamides. Examples of non-PABA derivative local anesthetics would be dibucaine, lidocaine, diperodon, etc.

Antacids, Oral[37]

MECHANISM: It is proposed that antacids would increase the proportion of ionized sulfonamide, thereby decreasing its absorption.

CLINICAL SIGNIFICANCE: Clinical studies must be performed to assess the clinical significance of this interaction. Factors other than ionization may be involved (e.g., dissolution rate). Further, a *delay* in absorption does not necessarily mean a *decrease* in absorption, and under the conditions of multiple dosing, delayed absorption may or may not have a significant clinical effect.

MANAGEMENT: No special precautions appear necessary.

Barbiturates[36,143,144,212]

A. Sulfisoxazole (Gantrisin) plus thiopental.[143,144]

SULFONAMIDE INTERACTIONS (CONT.)

DRUGS	DISCUSSION

MECHANISM: It has been proposed that sulfisoxazole (Gantrisin) competes with thiopental (Pentothal) for plasma protein binding.

CLINICAL SIGNIFICANCE: In one study involving 48 patients, intravenous sulfisoxazole reduced the amount of thiopental required for anesthesia and shortened the awakening time.[144] It is not known whether chronic oral doses of sulfisoxazole would have a similar effect. Nor is it known whether other sulfonamides or other barbiturates would be involved in similar interactions.

MANAGEMENT: Until more is known about this interaction, physicians should be aware that patients receiving sulfisoxazole might require less thiopental for anesthesia.

B. Sulfasalazine (Azulfidine) plus phenobarbital.[36]

MECHANISM: Oral sulfasalazine is partially absorbed in the small intestine, and most of the remaining drug is cleaved in the colon by bacterial action to form sulfapyridine and 5-aminosalicyclic acid. It has been proposed that phenobarbital may increase biliary excretion of sulfasalazine, thus decreasing urinary excretion of the drug.[36] Also, the hydroxylation of sulfapyridine was increased and the acetylation of sulfapyridine was decreased following phenobarbital administration.[36]

CLINICAL SIGNIFICANCE: In a study of 26 healthy subjects and 19 patients with colitis,[36] phenobarbital affected serum and/or urine levels of sulfasalazine and some of its metabolites (see preceding Mechanism discussion). None of the observed changes seem likely to affect the therapeutic effect of sulfasalazine or increase its toxicity.

MANAGEMENT: No special precautions appear to be necessary.

C. Sulfisoxazole (Gantrisin) or sulfisomidine plus phenobarbital.[212]

MECHANISM: None. (See Clinical Significance.)

CLINICAL SIGNIFICANCE: A study conducted in children reportedly demonstrated that phenobarbital did not affect the disposition of sulfisoxazole or sulfisomidine.[212]

MANAGEMENT: No special precautions appear to be necessary.

Cyclophosphamide (Cytoxan)[199]

MECHANISM: Not established.

CLINICAL SIGNIFICANCE: The metabolism of cyclophosphamide was studied in seven patients before and after sulfaphenazole treatment (2 g/day for 9 to 14 days).[199] No consistent effect was seen, with prolonged cyclophosphamide half-life in two patients, no change in three patients, and shortened half-life in two patients. Study in additional patients is needed to resolve the clinical significance of these findings (if any).

235

SULFONAMIDE INTERACTIONS (CONT.)

DRUGS	DISCUSSION

MANAGEMENT: Until this tentative interaction is better described, one should be alert for altered cyclophosphamide effect if sulfaphenazole is also given.

Digitalis[239]

MECHANISM: Sulfasalazine appears to reduce the bioavailability of concomitantly administered digoxin, but the mechanism responsible for this reduction is not clear.

CLINICAL SIGNIFICANCE: Following the clinical observation of low serum digoxin levels in a patient receiving sulfasalazine, ten normal subjects were given digoxin elixir (0.5 mg) with and without pretreatment with sulfasalazine.[239] Sulfasalazine was associated with reduced serum digoxin levels and lower cumulative urinary digoxin excretion. These reductions were moderate, but of sufficient magnitude to have a potential effect on the therapeutic response to digoxin. Subjects receiving larger doses of sulfasalazine appeared to manifest larger decreases in digoxin bioavailability, while some receiving only 2 g/day of sulfasalazine were not affected.

MANAGEMENT: It does not seem necessary to avoid concomitant use of digoxin and sulfasalazine, but patients so treated should be monitored more carefully for evidence of altered digoxin effect. Based on the response of one patient,[239] separation of the doses of digoxin and sulfasalazine did not circumvent the interaction. It has been suggested that digitoxin may be less likely to interact with sulfasalazine, and may be preferable in sulfasalazine-treated patients.[239]

Ethanol (Alcohol, Ethyl)[113]

MECHANISM: Not established.

CLINICAL SIGNIFICANCE: Sulfonamides reportedly increase the adverse effects of ethanol and further impair driving ability. However, no supporting clinical data are given so that the clinical significance cannot be assessed.

MANAGEMENT: No statement on management can be made with the information available.

Laxatives[217]

MECHANISM: Laxative-induced diarrhea may affect the absorption rate of sulfisoxazole (Gantrisin).

CLINICAL SIGNIFICANCE: Sulfisoxazole serum levels and urinary excretion were studied in normal subjects with and without diarrhea induced by sodium sulfate or castor oil.[217] Although the absorption rate of sulfisoxazole was slowed somewhat by the cathartics, total urinary excretion over 24 hours was not significantly affected.

MANAGEMENT: No special precautions appear to be necessary.

SULFONAMIDE INTERACTIONS (CONT.)

DRUGS	DISCUSSION

Methotrexate[157-159]

MECHANISM: In-vitro studies have shown that certain sulfonamides are capable of displacing methotrexate from plasma protein binding, thus increasing free methotrexate concentrations. Studies in humans have shown sulfisoxazole (Gantrisin) infusions to decrease plasma protein-bound methotrexate by about one-fourth. Sulfisoxazole may also have a minor inhibitory effect on the renal tubular secretion of methotrexate.

CLINICAL SIGNIFICANCE: Clinical reports of combined toxicity have not appeared. However, it is possible that sulfisoxazole could enhance methotrexate toxicity due to protein displacement. Other less highly bound sulfonamides could have a similar, but less pronounced, effect. It has also been cautioned that other types of sulfonamides (e.g., sulfonylurea hypoglycemics, thiazide diuretics) could also displace methotrexate from plasma protein binding.[157]

MANAGEMENT: Due to the possible consequences of increasing free methotrexate in the serum, sulfonamides should be given only with caution to patients receiving methotrexate.

Mineral Oil[111,112]

MECHANISM: Mineral oil reportedly interferes with the action of the nonabsorbable sulfonamides, succinylsulfathiazole and phthalysulfathiazole. This is presumably due to a mechanical effect of the mineral oil in preventing mixing of the sulfonamide in the feces.

CLINICAL SIGNIFICANCE: The interaction is reasonable from a theoretical standpoint, but clinical reports of this interaction appear to be lacking. Further, these sulfonamides have been withdrawn from the market in the United States.

MANAGEMENT: Pending availability of further information, mineral oil should probably be avoided in patients receiving nonabsorbable sulfonamides.

Para-aminobenzoic Acid (PABA)[112]

MECHANISM: Sulfonamides act by competitive inhibition of PABA in the microorganism. PABA administration in sufficient doses thus antagonizes the antibacterial effect of the sulfonamides.

CLINICAL SIGNIFICANCE: Well documented. It should be remembered that PABA is combined with aspirin in a number of proprietary analgesic mixtures.

MANAGEMENT: PABA should not be administered to patients receiving antibacterial sulfonamides.

SULFONAMIDE INTERACTIONS (CONT.)

DRUGS	DISCUSSION

Paraldehyde[114]

MECHANISM: The increased acetate levels that may follow paraldehyde administration reportedly may increase the danger of sulfonamide crystalluria.

CLINICAL SIGNIFICANCE: Not established. Clinical examples of this interaction are lacking. The commonly used sulfonamides today (e.g., sulfisoxazole) are quite soluble, and crystalluria is seldom a problem.

MANAGEMENT: The less soluble sulfonamides (e.g., sulfadiazine, sulfapyridine, sulfamerazine) should probably be given with caution in conjunction with paraldehyde.

Sulfinpyrazone (Anturane)[110]

MECHANISM: Sulfinpyrazone may displace some sulfonamides from plasma protein binding, resulting in more active (free) drug in the plasma. An effect on the renal excretion may also be involved. Probenecid (Benemid) may have a similar effect.

CLINICAL SIGNIFICANCE: Not established. The actions of sulfadiazine and sulfisoxazole are reportedly enhanced by concomitant sulfinpyrazone administration.

MANAGEMENT: No special precautions appear to be necessary.

TETRACYCLINE INTERACTIONS

DRUGS	DISCUSSION

Antacids (Containing divalent or trivalent cations)[39,117,146,175–177,183,271]

MECHANISM: Antacids containing divalent or trivalent cations (e.g., aluminum, calcium, magnesium) impair the absorption of orally administered tetracyclines. This effect has been attributed to chelation of the cation by the tetracycline. However, an effect on dissolution of the tetracycline may also be involved.

CLINICAL SIGNIFICANCE: This interaction is well documented and well known; yet one study has indicated that over 5% of patients receiving tetracycline also receive such antacids.[146] The simultaneous administration of a tetracycline and these antacids may considerably decrease serum tetracycline levels.

MANAGEMENT: Tetracyclines should not be administered within an hour or two of the administration of antacids containing aluminum, magnesium, or calcium.

Barbiturates[40]

MECHANISM: Barbiturates presumably enhance the hepatic metabolism of doxycycline (Vibramycin).

TETRACYCLINE INTERACTIONS (CONT.)

CLINICAL SIGNIFICANCE: In each of five hospitalized patients, doxycycline half-life was decreased following administration of phenobarbital (150 mg daily for 10 days).[40] The mean half-life before phenobarbital was 15.3 hours and 11.1 hours after. Five additional patients on chronic barbiturate therapy had even shorter doxycycline half-lives (mean, 7.7 hours). Thus it is possible that the antibacterial efficacy of doxycycline could be decreased by concomitant administration of an enzyme inducer such as phenobarbital.

MANAGEMENT: If barbiturates (and probably other enzyme inducers) cannot be avoided in the patient receiving doxycycline, it would be desirable to monitor closely the clinical response to doxycycline.

Carbamazepine (Tegretol)[41]

MECHANISM: Carbamazepine appears to stimulate hepatic doxycycline (Vibramycin) metabolism.[41]

CLINICAL SIGNIFICANCE: Penttila and associates[41] found the half-life of doxycycline to be shorter in five patients on chronic carbamazepine therapy (mean, 8.4 hours) than in nine control patients (mean, 15.1 hours). The effect of this shortened half-life on the clinical antibacterial effect of doxycycline has not been assessed, but the magnitude of the differences in half-life certainly indicates that this would be a possibility. The effect of carbamazepine on other tetracyclines has not been established.

MANAGEMENT: When carbamazepine is used concomitantly with doxycycline, it would be desirable to monitor closely the clinical response to doxycycline.

Contraceptives, Oral[332]

MECHANISM: Not established. It is possible that tetracycline interferes with the enterohepatic circulation of estrogens by reducing bacterial hydrolysis of conjugated estrogen in the intestine.

CLINICAL SIGNIFICANCE: A woman on an oral contraceptive containing 30 mcg of estrogen became pregnant after a 5-day course of tetracycline.[332] Another woman on oral contraceptives developed breakthrough bleeding while on tetracycline. In addition, isolated cases of unwanted pregnancy following combined use of oral contraceptives and tetracyclines have been reported to the British Committee on the Safety of Medicines.

MANAGEMENT: Although evidence of interaction is scanty, it would be prudent for women on oral contraceptives to use additional forms of contraception during tetracycline therapy.

Corticosteroids[42]

MECHANISM: Prolonged tetracycline therapy may favor the emergence of organisms that are resistant to tetracycline. The corticosteroid-

TETRACYCLINE INTERACTIONS (CONT.)

induced decrease in resistance to infection may enable these organisms to produce a serious infection. Other broad-spectrum antibiotics might produce a similar effect.

CLINICAL SIGNIFICANCE: In one case report a patient received concomitant tetracycline and corticosteroid therapy for acne and subsequently developed a severe proteus infection.[42] The combination tetracycline-corticosteroid therapy was felt to be responsible for the infection.

MANAGEMENT: Prolonged concomitant therapy with corticosteroids and tetracycline (or other antibiotics) should be undertaken with caution. The possibility of severe superinfection should be considered.

Diuretics[154,155]

MECHANISM: Not established. Both tetracyclines and diuretics have independently been reported to produce elevated blood urea nitrogen (BUN) levels, with the tetracycline effect probably due to its antianabolic action.

CLINICAL SIGNIFICANCE: Analysis of data from an epidemiologic study has revealed that concomitant therapy with tetracycline and diuretics tends to result in elevated BUN levels.[154] The clinical consequences of this effect were not detailed in the report, but it is reasonable to assume that this effect would be undesirable in patients with previous renal impairment. The specific diuretics involved were not enumerated.

MANAGEMENT: It has been recommended that tetracyclines be avoided in patients receiving diuretics.[155] This would probably be most important in patients with renal malfunction. However, until more is known about the clinical consequences of the interaction and the diuretics involved, it would not seem too difficult to select alternative antibiotics to tetracycline in such patients.

Ethanol (Alcohol, Ethyl)[233]

MECHANISM: Chronic ingestion of large amounts of ethanol may result in induction of hepatic microsomal enzymes. Since doxycycline is metabolized by the liver, its metabolism may be enhanced in alcoholic patients.

CLINICAL SIGNIFICANCE: Tetracycline and doxycycline were administered to six alcoholics and six healthy subjects to determine differences in disposition.[233] The half-life of doxycycline was shorter in the alcoholics (10.5 hours) than in the healthy subjects (14.7 hours), while the half-life of tetracycline was the same in both groups.

MANAGEMENT: When a tetracycline is needed in an alcoholic patient, in may be preferable to use an agent other than doxycycline. If doxycycline is used one should be alert for diminished doxycycline effect.

TETRACYCLINE INTERACTIONS (CONT.)

DRUGS	DISCUSSION

Food (Milk and Dairy Products)[117,183,197,270-273]

MECHANISM: It is proposed that cations such as calcium and magnesium in food chelate with tetracyclines, thus impairing absorption of the drug. Other factors are probably also involved.

CLINICAL SIGNIFICANCE: It is well established that milk and dairy products can reduce absorption of tetracyclines. Ingestion of 240 ml to 300 ml of milk with various tetracyclines (tetracycline, oxytetracycline, methacycline, demeclocycline) has been shown to reduce serum concentrations, usually by about 50% or more.[117,270,271] Food and dairy products seem to have minimal effect on doxycycline absorption.[270,271] Also, minocycline is reportedly not significantly affected by food or dairy products.[197] In healthy volunteers serum levels of tetracycline were reduced approximately 50% and serum levels of doxycycline were reduced approximately 20% by various test meals.[273] These results are consistent with previous data showing considerable reductions in serum levels of tetracycline and demeclocycline when given 30 minutes after breakfast.[272]

MANAGEMENT: For optimal absorption, tetracyclines should be administered as far apart as possible from milk and other dairy products high in cation content.

Heparin[43]

MECHANISM: Not established.

CLINICAL SIGNIFICANCE: Tetracycline reportedly may antagonize the anticoagulant effect of heparin somewhat,[43] but no substantiating evidence was presented.

MANAGEMENT: Too little is known of the clinical significance to make a statement on management.

Iron Preparations[38,44,45,145,151,183,270,274,360]

MECHANISM: Oral ferrous sulfate appears to impair the gastrointestinal absorption of various tetracyclines, possibly because of chelation or other type of binding in the gut.

CLINICAL SIGNIFICANCE: In one study, the absorption of tetracycline, oxytetracycline, methacycline, and doxycycline was decreased considerably in subjects by the concomitant oral administration of 200 mg of ferrous sulfate.[145] The absorption of methacycline and doxycycline was decreased to a greater degree than the other two agents. A subsequent preliminary study[44] reportedly found evidence that enteric-coated ferrous sulfate is less likely to interfere with doxycycline absorption. However, Mattila and associates[38] did find decreased doxycycline serum levels with enteric-coated ferrous sulfate, although the effect was less than with sugar-coated ferrous sulfate. Because doxycycline undergoes enterohepatic circulation, iron may bind doxycycline even if the latter is given parenterally.[360]

TETRACYCLINE INTERACTIONS (CONT.)

MANAGEMENT: On the basis of current evidence, iron preparations should not be administered simultaneously with oral tetracyclines. If they both need to be given to a patient, the results of Mattila and associates[38] indicate that the ferrous sulfate should be administered 3 hours before or 2 hours after tetracycline to minimize the interaction. Separation of doses may not circumvent the interaction if doxycycline is the tetracycline being used.

Lithium Carbonate[310]

MECHANISM: Not established. It has been proposed that tetracycline-induced renal impairment may reduce urinary lithium excretion.

CLINICAL SIGNIFICANCE: A patient developed elevated plasma lithium levels (2175 mEg/L) following initiation of tetracycline therapy (750 mg/day).[310] More study is needed.

MANAGEMENT: One should be alert for evidence of lithium toxicity if a tetracycline is started. Plasma lithium determinations should be performed if evidence of toxicity occurs, and the lithium dose should be reduced as needed.

Methoxyflurane (Penthrane)[20,45–47,115,116,149,150,152,153,211]

MECHANISM: Not established. A combined nephrotoxic action appears to be involved.

CLINICAL SIGNIFICANCE: Five of seven patients who received tetracycline in addition to methoxyflurane anesthesia developed signs of nephrotoxicity (increasing blood urea nitrogen and serum creatinine).[115] Three of the patients died. A number of additional cases have appeared in which the combined use of methoxyflurane and tetracycline seemed to cause renal damage.[45,46,149] Methoxyflurane is known to have some nephrotoxic potential,[150] and tetracycline is known to be dangerous in patients with renal malfunction. The two drugs together appear to be a dangerous combination, although certainly more information is needed to establish unequivocally the relationship of drug interaction to renal failure. Kanamycin and gentamycin have also reportedly been implicated in the production of similar nephrotoxic effects in patients who receive methoxyflurane.[153]

MANAGEMENT: Although this interaction is based on preliminary reports, the severity of the possible reaction warrants great caution in administering tetracycline (and perhaps other nephrotoxic antibiotics) to patients who soon will or have recently undergone methoxyflurane anesthesia.

Sodium Bicarbonate[147,148,156,175,176,296]

MECHANISM: Not established.

TETRACYCLINE INTERACTIONS (CONT.)

DRUGS	DISCUSSION

CLINICAL SIGNIFICANCE: Preliminary study in eight subjects indicated that oral tetracycline absorption is decreased substantially by concomitant administration of 2 g of sodium bicarbonate.[148] However, subsequent study indicates that this reduction in absorption does not occur when using tetracycline with good bioavailability.[296]

MANAGEMENT: No special precautions appear to be necessary.

Zinc[198,216,219]

MECHANISM: Zinc appears to impair gastrointestinal absorption of tetracycline, possibly by chelation.

CLINICAL SIGNIFICANCE: Zinc sulfate administration (200 to 220 mg) is associated with decreases in both serum tetracycline levels[198,219] and total urinary excretion of tetracycline.[216] The magnitude of the decreases appears large enough to impair the therapeutic response to tetracycline. Doxycycline (Vibramycin) absorption was not significantly affected by concomitant zinc,[198] but other tetracyclines were not studied.

MANAGEMENT: In patients receiving both tetracycline and zinc sulfate, the doses of the two drugs should be separated as much as possible to minimize mixing in the gastrointestinal tract.

TROLEANDOMYCIN INTERACTIONS

DRUGS	DISCUSSION

Corticosteroids[324,326,328]

MECHANISM: Troleandomycin (TAO) probably inhibits the hepatic metabolism of methylprednisolone, and possibly some other corticosteroids.

CLINICAL SIGNIFICANCE: TAO has been shown to considerably reduce the elimination and dosage requirement of methylprednisolone.[324,328] Although prednisolone disposition was not affected by TAO in three steroid-dependent asthmatics, in the presence of phenobarbital TAO did reduce prednisolone elimination somewhat.[326] Animal studies indicate that TAO may enhance betamethasone effect but not hydrocortisone.[328] In summary, TAO markedly enhanced methylprednisolone effects, and may enhance prednisolone effect in some patients (e.g., those on enzyme inducers). Little is known regarding the effect of TAO on other corticosteroids in humans.

MANAGEMENT: A considerable reduction in methylprednisolone dosage requirement is likely in the presence of TAO. Patients on other corticosteroids should also be monitored for the need to adjust corticosteroid dose if TAO is started or stopped.

TROLEANDOMYCIN INTERACTIONS (CONT.)

DRUGS	DISCUSSION

Theophylline[189,223]

MECHANISM: Not established. Troleandomycin may impair the hepatic disposition of theophylline.

CLINICAL SIGNIFICANCE: Theophylline elimination was measured before and after troleandomycin (250 mg/day for at least 10 days) in eight patients with chronic asthma.[223] Troleandomycin was associated with a 50% decrease in the clearance of theophylline from serum, with corresponding increases in serum theophylline levels.

MANAGEMENT: One should be alert for alteration in serum theophylline levels when troleandomycin is started or stopped. Serum theophylline determinations may be useful in deciding whether a dosage adjustment is necessary.

References

1. BUSUTTIL AA, et al: Possible cephaloridine nephrotoxicity in a neonate (Letter). Lancet 1:264, 1973.
2. GARROD LP: Causes of failure in antibiotic treatment. Br Med J 4:441, 1972.
3. KLEINKNECHT D, et al: Nephrotoxicity of cephaloridine (Letter). Ann Intern Med 80:421, 1974.
4. ANON: AMA Drug Evaluations. 2nd Ed. Acton, Massachusetts, Publishing Sciences Group, 1973, p. 533.
5. KABINS SA: Interactions among antibiotics and other drugs. JAMA 219:206, 1972.
6. KLASTERSKY J, et al: Gram-negative infections in cancer. Study of empiric therapy comparing carbenicillin-cephalothin with and without gentamicin. JAMA 227:45, 1974.
7. RIFF LJ, JACKSON GG: Laboratory and clinical conditions for gentamicin inactivation by carbenicillin. Arch Intern Med 130:887, 1972.
8. LEVISON ME, KAYE D: Carbenicillin plus gentamicin (Letter). Lancet 2:45, 1971.
9. RIFF L, JACKSON GG: Gentamicin plus carbenicillin (Letter). Lancet 1:592, 1971.
10. McLAUGHLIN JE, REEVES DS: Gentamicin plus carbenicillin (Letter). Lancet 1:864, 1971.
11. EYKYN S, et al: Gentamicin plus carbenicillin (Letter). Lancet 1:545, 1971.
12. KLEINKNECHT D, et al: Acute renal failure after high doses of gentamicin and cephalothin (Letter). Lancet 1:1129, 1973.
13. BOBROW SN: Anuria and acute tubular necrosis associated with gentamicin and cephalothin. JAMA 222:1546, 1972.
14. NOONE P, et al: Renal failure in combined gentamicin and cephalothin therapy (Letter). Br Med J 2:776, 1973.
15. BAILEY RR: Renal failure in combined gentamicin and cephalothin therapy (Letter). Br Med J 2:776, 1973.
16. NOONE P, et al: Acute renal failure after high doses of gentamicin and cephalothin (Letter). Lancet 1:1387, 1973.

References (CONT.)

17. BURLAND WL, et al: Combining cephaloridine and streptomycin for the treatment and prophylaxis of neonatal infections. Postgrad Med J 46 (Supplement):85, 1970.

18. PRAZMA J, et al: Ethacrynic acid ototoxicity potentiation by kanamycin. Ann Otol Rhinol Laryngol 83:111, 1974.

19. CHURCHILL D: Persisting renal insufficiency after methoxyflurane anesthesia. Report of two cases and review of literature. Am J Med 56:575, 1974.

20. COUSINS MJ, MAZZE RI: Tetracycline, methoxyflurane anaesthesia, and renal dysfunction (Letter). Lancet 1:751, 1972.

21. FRASCINO JA: Tetracycline, methoxyflurane anaesthesia, and renal dysfunction (Letter). Lancet 1:1127, 1972.

22. LAVIGNE J-G, MARCHAND C: Inhibition of the gastrointestinal absorption of p-aminosalicylate (PAS) in rats and humans by diphenhydramine. Clin Pharmacol Ther 14:404, 1973.

23. PALVA IP, et al: Drug-induced malabsorption of vitamin B_{12}, V. Intestinal pH and absorption of vitamin B_{12} during treatment with para-aminosalicylic acid. Scand J Haematol 9:5, 1972.

24. HALSTED CH, MCINTYRE PA: Intestinal malabsorption caused by aminosalicylic acid therapy. Arch Intern Med 130:935, 1972.

25. SIMPSON IJ: Nephrotoxicity and acute renal failure associated with cephalothin and cephaloridine. N Z Med J 74:312, 1971.

26. DE RITIS F, et al: Chloramphenicol combined with ampicillin in treatment of typhoid. Br Med J 4:17, 1972.

27. HURWITZ A, SCHLOZMAN DL: Effects of antacids on gastrointestinal absorption of isoniazid in rat and man. Am Rev Respir Dis 109:41, 1974.

28. TAYLOR JT: Metronidazole—a new agent for combined somatic and psychic therapy of alcoholism. Los Angeles Neurol Soc Bull 29:158, 1964.

29. Boston Collaborative Drug Surveillance Program: Excess of ampicillin rashes associated with allopurinol or hyperuricemia. N Engl J Med 286:505, 1972.

30. BRAUNER GJ: Ampicillin rashes (Letter). N Engl J Med 286:1217, 1972.

31. SCHWARTZ HA: Ampicillin rashes (Letter). N Engl J Med 286:1217, 1972.

32. COHN HD: Rifampicin and the pill (Letter). JAMA 228:828, 1974.

33. NOCKE-FINCK L, et al: Effects of rifampicin on menstrual cycle and on estrogen excretion in patients taking oral contraceptives. Dtsch Med Wochenschr 98:1521, 1973 (Abstract: JAMA 226:378, 1973).

34. MOST JA, MARKLE GB IV: A nearly fatal hepatotoxic reaction to rifampin after halothane anesthesia. Am J Surg 127:593, 1974.

35. KENWRIGHT S, LEVI AJ: Impairment of hepatic uptake of rifamycin antibiotics by probenecid, and its therapeutic implications. Lancet 2:1401, 1973.

36. SCHRODER H, et al: Metabolism of salicylazosulfapyridine in healthy subjects and in patients with ulcerative colitis. Effects of colectomy and of phenobarbital. Clin Pharmacol Ther 14:802, 1973.

37. HURWITZ A: The effects of antacids on gastrointestinal drug absorption. II. Effect of sulfadiazine and quinine. J Pharmacol Exp Ther 179:485, 1971.

References (CONT.)

38. MATTILA MJ, et al: Interference of iron preparations and milk with the absorption of tetracyclines, in: Exerpta Medica International Congress Series No. 254. Amsterdam, Exerpta Medica, 1972, pp. 128–133.
39. Vibramycin. Product Information. New York, Pfizer Laboratories, 1974.
40. NEUVONEN PJ, PENTTILA O: Interaction between doxycycline and barbiturates. Br Med J 1:535, 1974.
41. PENTTILA O, et al: Interaction between doxycycline and some antiepileptic drugs. Br Med J 2:470, 1974.
42. PAVER K: Complications from combined oral tetracycline and oral corticoid therapy in acne vulgaris. Med J Aust 1:1059, 1970.
43. LEVINE WG: Anticoagulants: heparin and oral anticoagulants. In Goodman LS, Gilman A (Eds): The Pharmacological Basis of Therapeutics. 4th Ed. New York, Macmillan, 1970, pp. 1445–1463.
44. BATEMAN FJA: Effects of tetracyclines (Letter). Br Med J 4:802, 1970.
45. CHURCHILL D, et al: Persisting renal insufficiency after methoxyflurane anesthesia. Report of two cases and review of literature. Am J Med 56:575, 1974.
46. DRYDEN GE: Incidence of tubular degeneration with microlithiasis following methoxyflurane compared with other anesthetic agents. Anesth Analg 53:383, 1974.
47. STOELTING RK, GIBBS PS: Effect of tetracycline therapy on renal function after methoxyflurane anesthesia. Anesth Analg 52:431, 1973.
48. SCHWAB RS, et al: Amantadine in the treatment of Parkinson's disease. JAMA 208:1168, 1969.
49. MILLER RP, BATES JH: Amphotericin B toxicity. A follow-up report of 53 patients. Ann Intern Med 71:1089, 1969.
50. CUSHARD WG, et al: Blastomycosis of bone. Treatment with intramedullary amphotericin B. J Bone Joint Surg 51A:704, 1969.
51. AZARNOFF DL, HURWITZ A: Drug interactions. Pharmacol Physicians 4:1 (Feb.), 1970.
52. WEINSTEIN L: Antimicrobial Agents, In Goodman LS, Gilman A (Eds): The Pharmacological Basis of Therapeutics. 4th Ed. New York, Macmillan, 1970, pp. 1320–1324.
53. HEINIVAARA O, PALVA IP: Malabsorption of vitamin B_{12} during treatment with para-aminosalicylic acid: a preliminary report. Acta Med Scand 175:469, 1964.
54. LEVINE RA: Steatorrhea induced by para-aminosalicylic acid. Ann Intern Med 68:1265, 1968.
55. ANON: Drug interactions that can affect your patients. Patient Care 1:32 (Nov.), 1967.
56. SHAPIRO M, HYDE L: Hyperuricemia due to pyrazinamide. Am J Med 23:596, 1957.
57. CULLEN JH, et al: Studies of hyperuricemia produced by pyrazinamide. Am J Med 23:587, 1957.
58. BOGER WP, PITTS FW: Influence of p-(Di-N-propylsulfamyl)-benzoic acid. "Benemid," on para-aminosalicylic acid (PAS) plasma concentrations. Am Rev Tuberc 61:862, 1950.
59. CARR DT, et al: Concentration of PAS and tuberculostatic potency of serum after administration of PAS with and without Benemid. Proc Staff Meet Mayo Clin 27:209, 1952.

References (CONT.)

60. TUANO SB, et al: Cephaloridine versus cephalothin: relation of the kidney to blood level differences after parenteral administration. Antimicrob Agents Chemother—1966, pp. 101–106, 1967.
61. ANON: Evaluation of a new antibacterial agent. Cephaloridine (Loridine). JAMA 206:1289, 1968.
62. KOCH-WESER J, et al: Adverse effects of sodium colistimethate. Manifestations and specific reaction rates during 317 courses of therapy. Ann Intern Med 72:857, 1970.
63. SAIDI P, et al: Effect of chloramphenicol on erythropoiesis. J Lab Clin Med 57:247, 1961.
64. WALLACE JF, et al: Studies on the pathogenesis of meningitis. VI. Antagonism between penicillin and chloramphenicol in experimental pneumococcal meningitis. J Lab Clin Med 70:408, 1967.
65. JAWETZ E: The use of combinations of antimicrobial drugs. Ann Rev Pharmacol 8:151, 1968.
66. MILLS J, JAWETZ E: Clinical use of antimicrobials. In BG Katzung: Basic and Clinical Pharmacology. Los Altos, California, Lange Medical Publications, 1982, pp. 538–552.
67. JIJI RM, et al: Chloramphenicol and its sulfamoyl analogue. Report of reversible erythropoietic toxicity in healthy volunteers. Arch Intern Med 111:70, 1963.
68. POHLMANN G: Respiratory arrest associated with intravenous administration of polymyxin B sulfate. JAMA 196:181, 1966.
69. PARISI AF, KAPLAN MH: Apnea during treatment with sodium colistimethate. JAMA 194:298, 1965.
70. LEVINE RA, et al: Polymyxin B-induced respiratory paralysis reversed by intravenous calcium chloride. J Mt Sinai Hosp 36:380, 1969.
71. ANON: A second look at lincomycin (Lincocin). Med Lett 11:107, 1969.
72. LANSDOWN FS, et al: Psychotoxic reaction during ethionamide therapy. Am Rev Respir Dis 95:1053, 1967.
73. PETTINGER WA, et al: Inhibition of monoamine oxidase in man by furazolidone. Clin Pharmacol Ther 9:442, 1968.
74. PETTINGER WA, et al: Monoamine-oxidase inhibition by furazolidone in man. Clin Res 14:258, 1966.
75. TODD RG (Ed): Extra Pharmacopoeia—Martindale. 25th Ed. London, The Pharmaceutical Press, 1967, pp. 844–845.
76. RIEGELMAN S, et al: Griseofulvin-phenobarbital interaction in man. JAMA 213:426, 1970.
77. BUSFIELD D, et al: An effect of phenobarbitone on blood levels of griseofulvin in man. Lancet 2:1042, 1963.
78. SYMCHOWICZ S, et al: A comparative study of griseofulvin-^{14}C metabolism in the rat and rabbit. Biochem Pharmacol 16:2405, 1967.
79. FRIEND DG, et al: The action of L-dihydroxyphenylalanine in patients receiving nialamide. Clin Pharmacol Ther 6:362, 1965.
80. VITEK V, RYSANEK K: Interaction of D-cycloserine with the action of some monoamine oxidase inhibitors. Biochem Pharmacol 14:1417, 1965.
81. Demerol. Product Information, Winthrop Laboratories, 1984.
82. PITTINGER CB, et al: Antibiotic-induced paralysis. Anesth Analg 49:487, 1970.
83. MCQUILLEN MP, et al: Myasthenic syndrome associated with antibiotics. Arch Neurol 18:402, 1968.

References (CONT.)

84. FOLDES FF, et al: Prolonged respiratory depression caused by drug combinations. JAMA 183:672, 1963.
85. FALOON WW, CHODOS RB: Vitamin B_{12} absorption studies using colchicine, neomycin and continuous 57Co B_{12} administration (Abstract). Gastroenterology 56:1251, 1969.
86. CHENG SH, WHITE A: Effect of orally administered neomycin on the absorption of penicillin V. N Engl J Med 267:1296, 1962.
87. JOHNSON AH, HAMILTON CH: Kanamycin ototoxicity—possible potentiation by other drugs. South Med J 63:511, 1970.
88. Physicians' Desk Reference. 23rd Ed. Oradell, New Jersey, Medical Economics, Inc., 1984, p. 1831.
89. MATHOG RH, KLEIN WJ Jr: Ototoxicity of ethacrynic acid and aminoglycoside antibiotics in uremia. N Engl J Med 280:1223, 1969.
90. MATZ GJ, NAUNTON RF: Ototoxic drugs and poor renal function (Letter). JAMA 206:2119, 1968.
91. PILLAY VKG, et al: Transient and permanent deafness following treatment with ethacrynic acid in renal failure. Lancet 1:77, 1969.
92. SCHWARTZ GH, et al: Ototoxicity induced by furosemide. N Engl J Med 282:1413, 1970.
93. JACOBSON ED, et al: An experimental malabsorption syndrome induced by neomycin. Am J Med 28:524, 1960.
94. WAGNER JG: Pharmacokinetics 1. Definitions, modeling and reasons for measuring blood levels and urinary excretion. Drug Intell 2:38, 1968.
95. McCALL CE, et al: Lincomycin: activity in vitro and absorption and excretion in normal young men. Am J Med Sci 254:144, 1967.
96. McGEHEE RF Jr, et al: Comparative studies of antibacterial activity in vitro and absorption and excretion of lincomycin and clindamycin. Am J Med Sci 256:279, 1968.
97. ANON: The safety of cyclamate—an artificial sweetener. Med Lett 11:85, 1969.
98. WAGNER JG: Aspects of pharmacokinetics and biopharmaceutics in relation to drug activity. Am J Pharm 141:5, 1969.
99. Mandelamine. Physicians' Desk Reference. 38th Ed. Oradell, New Jersey, Medical Economics Co., 1984, p. 1497.
100. ITIL TI, et al: Central effects of metronidazole. Psychiatric Research Report 24, American Psychiatric Association, March, 1968.
101. PENICK SB, et al: Metronidazole in the treatment of alcoholism. Am J Psychiatry 125:1063, 1969.
102. FDA Reports of Suspected Adverse Reactions to Drugs, 1970, No. 700301-064-01001.
103. ROTHSTEIN E, CLANCY DD: Toxicity of disulfiram combined with metronidazole. N Engl J Med 280:1006, 1969.
104. GOODHUE WW Jr: Disulfiram-metronidazole (well identified) toxicity. N Engl J Med 280:1482, 1969.
105. PIGUET D: In vitro inhibitive action of nitrofurantoin on the bacteriostatic activity of nalidixic acid. Ann Inst Pasteur 116:43, 1969 (Abst. International Pharmaceutical Abstracts No. 63873).
106. BOULOS BM, DAVIS LE: Hazard of simultaneous administration of phenothiazine and piperazine (Letter). N Engl J Med 280:1245, 1969.
107. ARMBRECHT BH: Reaction between piperazine and chlorpromazine (Letter). N Engl J Med 282:1490, 1970.

References (CONT.)

108. MORRELLI HF, MELMON KL: The clinician's approach to drug interactions. Calif Med 109:380, 1968.
109. GOODMAN LS, GILMAN A (Eds): The Pharmalogical Basis of Therapeutics. 4th Ed. New York, Macmillan, 1970, pp. 1446–1451.
110. ANTON AH: The effect of disease, drugs, and dilution on the binding of sulfonamides in human plasma. Clin Pharmacol Ther 9:561, 1968.
111. Sulfasuxidine. Product Information. West Point, Pennsylvania, Merck, Sharp and Dohme, 1965.
112. GOODMAN LS, GILMAN A (Eds.): The Pharmalogical Basis of Therapeutics. 4th Ed. New York, Macmillan, 1970, pp. 1177–1203.
113. SHEPHERD M: Psychotropic Drugs I. Interactions between centrally acting drugs in man: some general considerations. Proc R Soc Med 58:964, 1965.
114. HADDEN JW, METZNER RJ: Pseudoketosis and hyperacetaldehydemia in paraldehyde acidosis. Am J Med 47:642, 1969.
115. KUZUCU EY: Methoxyflurane, tetracycline, and renal failure. JAMA 211:1162, 1970.
116. SHILS ME: Some metabolic aspects of tetracycline. Clin Pharmacol Ther 3:321, 1962.
117. SCHEINER J, ALTEMEIER WA: Experimental study of factors inhibiting absorption and effective therapeutic levels of declomycin. Surg Gynecol Obstet 114:9, 1962.
118. PARKES JD, et al: Treatment of Parkinson's disease with amantadine and levodopa. A one-year study. Lancet 1:1083, 1971.
119. CHUNG D-K, KOENIG MG: Reversible cardiac enlargement during treatment with amphotericin B and hydrocortisone. Report of three cases. Am Rev Respir Dis 103:831, 1971.
120. GOODPASTURE HC, et al: Clinical correlations during amphotericin B therapy (Abstract). Ann Intern Med 76:872, 1972.
121. GOODMAN LS, GILMAN A (Eds): The Pharmalogical Basis of Therapeutics. 4th Ed. New York, Macmillan, 1970, pp. 382–383.
122. MEYLER L (Ed): Side Effects of Drugs. 4th Ed. Amsterdam, Exerpta Medica Foundation, 1964, pp. 137–141.
123. BOMAN G, et al: Drug interaction: decreased serum concentrations of rifampicin when given with P.A.S. (Letter). Lancet 1:800, 1971.
124. MEYERS BR, et al: Cephalexin-microbiological effects and pharmacologic parameters in man. Clin Pharmacol Ther 10:810, 1969.
125. DODDS MG, FOORD RD: Enhancement by potent diuretics of renal tubular necrosis induced by cephaloridine. Br J Pharmacol 40:227, 1970.
126. GABRIEL R, et al: Reversible encephalopathy and acute renal failure after cephaloridine. Br Med J 4:283, 1970.
127. OPITZ A, et al: Akute niereninsuffizienz nach gentamicin-cephalosporin-kombinations therapie. Med Welt 22:434, 1971.
128. ADERHOLD RM, MUNIZ CE: Acute psychosis with amitriptyline and furazolidone (Letter). JAMA 213:2080, 1970.
129. ROTHSTEIN E: Rifampin with disulfiram (Letter). JAMA 219:1216, 1972.
130. LAL S, et al: Effect of rifampicin and isoniazid on liver function. Br Med J 1:148, 1972.
131. WINTERS RE, et al: Combined use of gentamicin and carbenicillin. Ann Intern Med 75:925, 1971.

References (CONT.)

132. SCHIMPFF S, et al: Empiric therapy with carbenicillin and gentamicin for febrile patients with cancer and granulocytopenia. N Engl J Med 284:1061, 1971.
133. JACOBY GA: Carbenicillin and gentamicin (Editorial). N Engl J Med 284:1096, 1971.
134. MCLAUGHLIN JE, REEVES DS: Clinical and laboratory evidence for inactivation of gentamicin by carbenicillin. Lancet 1:261, 1971.
135. KONICKOVA L, PRAT V: Effect of carbenicillin, gentamicin, and their combination on experimental *Pseudomonas aeruginosa* urinary tract infection. J Clin Pathol 24:113, 1971.
136. MERIWETHER WD, et al: Deafness following standard intravenous dose of ethacrynic acid. JAMA 216:795, 1971.
137. WARNER WA, SANDERS E: Neuromuscular blockade associated with gentamicin therapy. JAMA 215:1153, 1971.
138. WRIGHT EA, MCQUILLEN MP: Antibiotic-induced neuromuscular blockade. Ann NY Acad Sci 183:358, 1971.
139. ADAM WR, DAWBORN JK: Plasma levels and urinary excretion of nalidixic acid in patients with renal failure. Aust NZ J Med 2:126, 1971.
140. TONG MJ, et al: Supplemental folates in the therapy of *Plasmodium falciparum* malaria. JAMA 214:2330, 1970.
141. KUNIN CM: Clinical pharmacology of the new penicillins II. Effect of drugs which interfere with binding to serum proteins. Clin Pharmacol Ther 7:180, 1966.
142. KAMPMANN J, et al: Effect of some drugs on penicillin half-life in blood. Clin Pharmacol Ther 13:516, 1972.
143. CSOGOR SI, PAPP J: Competition between sulphonamides and thiopental for the binding sites of plasma proteins. Arzneimmittelforsch 20:1925, 1970.
144. CSOGOR SI, KEREK SF: Enhancement of thiopentone anesthesia by sulpha furazole. Br J Anaesth 42:988, 1970.
145. NEUVONEN P, et al: Interference of iron with the absorption of tetracyclines in man. Br Med J 4:532, 1970.
146. ANON: Risk of drug interaction may exist in 1 of 13 prescriptions (Medical News). JAMA 220:1287, 1972.
147. ELLIOTT GR, ARMSTRONG MF: Sodium bicarbonate and oral tetracycline (Letter). Clin Pharmacol Ther 13:459, 1972.
148. BARR WH, et al: Decrease of tetracycline absorption in man by sodium bicarbonate. Clin Pharmacol Ther 12:779, 1971.
149. ALBERS DD, et al: Renal failure following prostatovesiculectomy related to methoxyflurane anesthesia and tetracycline complicated by candida infection. J Urol 106:348, 1971.
150. MAZZE RI, et al: Renal dysfunction associated with methoxyflurane anesthesia. A randomized, prospective clinical evaluation. JAMA 216:278, 1971.
151. GREENBERGER NJ: Absorption of tetracyclines: interference by iron (Editorial Notes). Ann Intern Med 74:792, 1971.
152. FRASCINO JA: Tetracycline, methoxyflurane anaesthesia and renal dysfunction (Letter). Lancet 1:1127, 1972.
153. COUSINS MJ, MAZZE RI: Tetracycline, methoxyflurane anaesthesia, and renal dysfunction (Letter). Lancet 1:751, 1972.
154. BOSTON COLLABORATIVE DRUG SURVEILLANCE PROGRAM: Tetracycline

References (CONT.)

and drug-attributed rises in blood urea nitrogen. JAMA 220:377, 1972.

155. TANNENBERG AM: Tetracycline and rises in urea nitrogen (Letter). JAMA 221:713, 1972.
156. JUHL RP, BLAUG SM: Factors affecting release of medicaments from hard gelatin capsules (Letter). J Pharm Sci 62:170, 1973.
157. Methotrexate. Physicians' Desk Reference. 38th Ed. Oradell, New Jersey, Medical Economics Co., 1984, pp. 1080–1083.
158. DIXON RL, et al: Plasma protein binding of methotrexate and its displacement by various drugs. Fed Proc 24:454, 1965.
159. LIEGLER DG, et al: The effect of organic acids on renal clearance of methotrexate in man. Clin Pharmacol Ther 10:849, 1969.
160. WHITTINGTON HG, GREY L: Possible interaction between disulfiram and isoniazid. Am J Psychiatry 125:1725, 1969.
161. ALTSCHULER SL, VALENTEEN JW: Amenorrhea following rifampin administration during oral contraceptive use. Obstet Gynecol 44:771, 1974.
162. POSTMA JU, TILBURG WV: Visual hallucinations and delirium during during treatment with amantadine (Symmetrel). J Am Geriatr Soc 23:212, 1975.
163. KLUGE RM, et al: The carbenicillin-gentamicin combination against pseudomonas aeruginosa. Correlation of effect with gentamicin sensitivity. Ann Intern Med 81:584, 1974.
164. GIUDICELLI C, et al: Insuffisance renale aigue due a l'association cephalotine-gentamycine. Lyon Med 231:1171, 1974.
165. ZAZGORNIK VJ, et al: Akutes nierenversagen bei kombinieter cephaloridin-gentamycin-therapie. Wein Med Wochenschr 85:839, 1973.
166. FILLASTRE JP, KLEINKNECHT D, et al: Acute renal failure associated with cephalosporin therapy. Am Heart J 89:809, 1975.
167. HARRISON WO, SILVERBLATT FJ, et al: Gentamycin nephrotoxicity: Failure of three cephalosporins to potentiate injury in rats. Antimicrob Agents Chemoth Aug. 1975, p. 209.
168. TOBIAS JS, WHITEHOUSE JM, et al: Severe renal dysfunction after tobramycin/cephalothin therapy (Letter). Lancet 1:425, 1976.
169. HOLTZMAN JL: Gentamicin and neuromuscular blockade (Letter). Ann Intern Med 84:55, 1976.
170. SCHER JM: Psychotic reaction to disulfiram (Letter). JAMA 201:1051, 1967.
171. FOGDALL RP, MILLER RD: Prolongation of a pancuronium-induced neuromuscular blockade by polymyxin B. Anesthesiology 40:84, 1974.
172. HELMER RE III: Hazard of folinic acid with pyrimethamine and sulfadiazine (Letter). Ann Intern Med 82:124, 1975.
173. ALLEN BW, ELLARD GA, et al: Probenecid and serum-rifampicin (Letter). Lancet 2:1309, 1975.
174. FALLON RJ, ALLAN GW, et al: Probenecid and rifampicin serum levels. Lancet 2:792, 1975.
175. JAFFE JM, et al: Effect of altered urinary pH on tetracycline and doxycycline excretion in humans. J Pharmacokinet Biopharm 1:267, 1973.
176. JAFFE JM, et al: Influence of repetitive dosing and altered urinary pH on doxycycline excretion in humans. J Pharm Sci 63:1256, 1974.

References (CONT.)

177. CHIN TF, et al: Drug diffusion and bioavailability: tetracycline metallic chelation. Am J Hosp Pharm 32:625, 1975.
178. SHAPIRO S, et al: Fatal drug reactions among medical impatients. JAMA 216:467, 1971.
179. JAWETZ E: Synergism and antagonism among antimicrobial drugs, a personal perspective. West J Med 123:87, 1975.
180. DELLINGER P, et al: Protective effect of cephalothin against gentamicin-induced nephrotoxicity in rats. Antimicrob Agents Chemother 9:172, 1976.
181. LUFT FC, et al: Nephrotoxicity of cephalosporin-gentamicin combinations in rats. Antimicrob Agents Chemother 9:831, 1976.
182. DELLINGER P, et al: Effect of cephalothin on renal cortical concentrations of gentamicin in rats. Antimicrob Agents Chemother 9:587, 1976.
183. NEUVONEN PJ: Interactions with the absorption of tetracyclines. Drugs 11:45, 1976.
184. ZILLY W, et al: Induction of drug metabolism in man after rifampicin treatment measured by increased hexobarbital and tolbutamide clearance. Eur J Clin Pharmacol 9:219, 1975.
185. JAFFE JM, et al: Nitrofurantoin-antacid interaction (Letter). Drug Intell Clin Pharm 10:419, 1976.
186. BOLT HM, et al: Rifampicin and oral contraception (Letter). Lancet 1:1280, 1974.
187. MAISEY DN, et al: Rifampicin and cortisone replacement therapy. Lancet 2:896, 1974.
188. JAFFE JM: Effect of propantheline on nitrofurantoin absorption (Letter). J Pharm Sci 64:1729, 1975.
189. WEINBERGER M, et al: Effect of triacetyloleandomycin (TAO) on the metabolism of theophylline (Abstract). Clin Pharmacol Ther 19:118, 1976.
190. BOLT HM, et al: Effect of rifampicin treatment on the metabolism of oestradiol and 17a-ethinyloestradiol by human liver microsomes. Eur J Clin Pharmacol 8:301, 1975.
191. LEVANEN J, NORDMAN R: Complete respiratory paralysis caused by a large dose of streptomycin and its treatment with calcium chloride. Ann Clin Res 7:47, 1975.
192. GILLETT P, et al: Tobramycin/cephalothin nephrotoxicity (Letter). Lancet 1:547, 1976.
193. CABANILLAS F, et al: Nephrotoxicity of combined cephalothin-gentamicin regimen. Arch Intern Med 135:850, 1975.
194. TUNE BM: Relationship between the transport and toxicity of cephalosporins in the kidney. J Infect Dis 132:189, 1975.
195. MISCHLER TW, et al: Influence of probenecid and food on the bioavailability of cephradine in normal male subjects. J Clin Pharmacol 14:604, 1974.
196. BOMAN G, et al: Mechanism of the inhibitory effect of PAS granules on the absorption of rifampicin: absorption of rifampicin by an excipient, bentonite. Eur J Clin Pharmacol 8:293, 1975.
197. Minocin. Physicians' Desk Reference. 37th Ed. Oradell, New Jersey, Medical Economics Co., 1983, pp. 1083–1085.
198. PENTTILA O, et al: Effect of zinc sulphate on the absorption of tetracycline and doxycycline in man. Eur J Clin Pharmacol 9:131, 1975.

References (CONT.)

199. Faber OK, et al: The effect of chloramphenicol and sulphaphenazole on the biotransformation of cyclophosphamide in man. Br J Clin Pharmacol 2:281, 1975.
200. Westwood GPC, Hooper WL: Antagonism of oxolinic acid by nitrofurantoin (Letter). Lancet 1:460, 1975.
201. Roberton YR, Johnson ES: Interactions between oral contraceptives and other drugs: a review. Curr Med Res Opin 3:647, 1976.
202. Yamada S, Iwai K: Induction of hepatic cortisol-6-hydoxylase by rifampicin. Lancet 2:366, 1976.
203. Edwards OM, et al: Changes in cortisol metabolism following rifampicin therapy. Lancet 2:549, 1974.
204. Kuo PT, et al: Combined para-aminosalicylic acid and dietary therapy in long term control of hypercholesterolemia and hypertriglyceridemia (types II_a and II_b hyperlipoproteinemia). Circulation 53:338, 1976.
205. Ervin FR, et al: Inactivation of gentamicin by penicillins in patients with renal failure. Antimicrob Agents Chemother 9:1004, 1976.
206. Becker LD, Miller RD: Clindamycin enhances a nondepolarizing neuromuscular blockade. Anesthesiology 45:84, 1976.
207. Kreek MJ, et al: Rifampin-induced methadone withdrawal. N Engl J Med 294:1104, 1976.
208. Rowe JW, et al: Severe metabolic acidosis associated with nalidixic acid overdose. Ann Intern Med 84:570, 1976.
209. Gupta NK, et al: Effect of metronidazole on liver alcohol dehydrogenase. Biochem Pharmacol 19:2805, 1970.
210. Venho VMK, Koskinen R: The effect of pyrazinamide, rifampicin and cycloserine on the blood levels and urinary excretion of isoniazid. Ann Clin Res 3:277, 1971.
211. Proctor EA, Barton FL: Polyuric acute renal failure after methoxyflurane and tetracycline. Br Med J 4:661, 1971.
212. Krauer B: Comparative investigations of elimination kinetics of two sulfonamides in children with and without phenobarbital administration. Schweiz Med Wochenschr 101:668, 1971 (Abstract JAMA 216:1888, 1971).
213. Lindenbaum J, et al: Inhibition of digoxin absorption by neomycin. Gastroenterology 71:399, 1976.
214. Norrby R, et al: Interaction between cephaloridine and furosemide in man. Scand J Infect Dis 8:209, 1976.
215. Pessayre D, et al: Isoniazid-rifampin fulminant hepatitis. A possible consequence of the enhancement of isoniazid hepatotoxicity by enzyme induction. Gastroenterology 72:284, 1977.
216. Mapp RK, McCarthy TJ: The effect of zinc sulphate and of bicitropeptide on tetracycline absorption. S Afr Med J (Oct.) 50:1829, 1976.
217. Mattila MJ, et al: Effect of sodium sulphate and castor oil on drug absorption from the human intestine. Ann Clin Res 6:19, 1974.
218. Buffington GA, et al: Interaction of rifampin and glucocorticoids. JAMA 236:1958, 1976.
219. Andersson KE, et al: Inhibition of tetracycline absorption by zinc. Eur J Clin Pharmacol 10:59, 1976.
220. Skolnick JL, et al: Rifampicin, oral contraceptives, and pregnancy. JAMA 236:1382, 1976.
221. Schacter LP, et al: Antagonism between miconazole and amphotericin B (Letter). Lancet 2:318, 1976.

References (CONT.)

222. SCHEUER PJ, et al: Rifampicin hepatitis. Lancet, 2:421, 1974.
223. WEINBERGER M, et al: Inhibition of theophylline clearance by trolean-domycin. J Allergy Clin Immunol 59(3):228, 1977.
224. HANSEN MM, KAABER K: Nephrotoxicity in combined cephalothin and gentamicin therapy. Acta Med Scand 201:463, 1977.
225. ZILLY W, et al: Stimulation of drug metabolism by rifampicin in patients with cirrhosis or cholestasis measured by increased hexobarbital and tolbutamide clearance. Eur J Clin Pharmacol 11:287, 1977.
226. TVEDEGAARD E: Interaction between gentamicin and cephalothin as cause of acute renal failure. Lancet 2:581, 1976.
227. KLASTERSKY J, et al: Empiric therapy for cancer patients: comparative study of ticarcillin-tobramycin, ticarcillin-cephalothin, and cephalothin-tobramycin. Antimicrob Agents Chemother 7:640, 1975.
228. SCHULTZE RG, et al: Possible nephrotoxicity of gentamicin. J Infect Dis 124(Supplement):S145, 1971.
229. FANNING WL, et al: Gentamicin- and cephalothin-associated rises in blood urea nitrogen. Antimicrob Agents Chemother 10:80, 1976.
230. AVERY D, FINN R: Succinylcholine—prolonged apnea associated with clindamycin and abnormal liver function tests. Dis Nerv Syst 38:473, 1977.
231. RUBBO JT, et al: Comparative neuromuscular effects of lincomycin and clindamycin. Anesth Analg 56:329, 1977.
232. KITTO W: Antibiotics and ingestion of alcohol (Questions and Answers). JAMA 193:411, 1965.
233. NEUVONEN PJ, et al: Effect of long-term alcohol consumption on the half-life of tetracycline and doxycycline in man. Int J Clin Pharmacol 14:303, 1976.
234. ZILLY W, et al: Pharmacokinetic interactions with rifampicin. Clin Pharmacokinet 2:61, 1977.
235. GRIFFITH RS, et al: Effect of probenecid on the blood levels and urinary excretion of cefamandole. Antimicrob Agents Chemother 11:809, 1977.
236. BUTKUS DE, et al: Renal failure following gentamicin in combination with clindamycin. Nephron 17:307, 1976.
237. BENDING MR, SKACEL PO: Rifampicin and methadone withdrawal (Letter). Lancet, 1:1211, 1977.
238. BACH MC, et al: Pulmonary nocardiosis: therapy with minocycline and with erythromycin plus ampicillin. JAMA 224:1378, 1973.
239. JUHL RP, et al: Effect of sulfasalazine on digoxin bioavailability. Clin Pharmacol Ther 20:387, 1976.
240. COHEN MH, et al: Effect of oral prophylactic broad spectrum nonabsorbable antibiotics on the gastrointestinal absorption of nutrients and methotrexate in small cell bronchogenic carcinoma patients. Cancer 38:1556, 1976.
241. NOONE P, et al: Experience in monitoring gentamicin therapy during treatment of serious gram-negative sepsis. Br Med J 1:477, 1974.
242. BATES TR, et al: Effect of food on nitrofurantoin absorption. Clin Pharmacol Ther 16:63, 1974.
243. BATES TR, et al: pH-dependent dissolution rate of nitrofurantoin from commercial suspensions, tablets, and capsules. J Pharm Sci 63:643, 1974.
244. ROSENBERG HA, BATES TR: The influence of food on nitrofurantoin bioavailability. Clin Pharmacol Ther 20:227, 1976.

References (CONT.)

245. Macrodantin. Physicians' Desk Reference. 31st Ed.,Oradell, New Jersey, Medical Economics Co., 1977, p. 799.
246. CHURCHILL DN, SEELY J: Nephrotoxicity associated with combined gentamicin-amphotericin B therapy. Nephron 19:176, 1977.
247. CROUNSE RG: Human pharmacology of griseofulvin: the effect of fat intake on gastrointestinal absorption. J Invest Dermatol 37:529, 1961.
248. CROUNSE RG: Effective use of griseofulvin. Arch Dermatol 87:176, 1963.
249. FULVICIN U/F. Physicians' Desk Reference, 32nd Ed. Oradell, New Jersey, Medical Economics Co., 1978, p. 1481.
250. KLEIN JO, et al: Ampicillin: Activity *in vitro* and absorption and excretion in normal young men. Am J Med Sci 245:544, 1963.
251. JORDAN MC, et al: Clinical pharmacology of pivampicillin as compared with ampicillin. Antimicrob Agents Chemother, 1970, p. 438.
252. NEUVONEN PJ, et al: Comparative effect of food on absorption of ampicillin and pivampicillin. J Int Med Res 5:71, 1977.
253. WELLING PG, et al: Bioavailability of ampicillin and amoxicillin in fasted and nonfasted subjects. J Pharm Sci 66:549, 1977.
254. GOWER PE, DASH CH: Cephalexin: Human studies of absorption and excretion of a new cephalosporin antibiotic. Br J Pharmacol 37:738, 1969.
255. BRAUN P, et al: Cephalexin and cephaloglycin activity in vitro and absorption and urinary excretion of single oral doses in normal young adults. Appl Microbiol 16:1684, 1968.
256. GRIFFITH RS, BLACK HR: Cephalexin: a new antibiotic. Clin Med (Nov.) 1968, p. 14.
257. MEYERS BR, et al: Cephalexin: Microbiological effects and pharmacologic parameters in man. Clin Pharmacol Ther 10:810, 1969.
258. HARVENGT C, et al: Cephradine absorption and excretion in fasting and nonfasting volunteers. J Clin Pharmacol 13:36, 1973.
259. MISCHLER TW, et al: Influence of probenecid and food on the bioavailability of cephradine in normal male subjects. J Clin Pharmacol (Nov.–Dec.) 14:604, 1974.
260. ZAROWNY D, et al: Pharmacokinetics of amoxicillin. Clin Pharmacol Ther 16:1046, 1974.
261. NEU HC: Session I: In vitro activity and human pharmacology of amoxicillin. J Infect Dis 129(Supplement):S123, 1974.
262. SEIGLER DI, et al: Effect of meals on rifampicin absorption (Letter). Lancet 2:197, 1974.
263. GILL GV: Rifampicin and breakfast (Letter). Lancet 2:1135, 1976.
264. VERBIST L, GYSELLEN A: Antituberculous activity of rifampicin in vitro and in vivo and the concentrations attained in human blood. Am Rev Respir Dis 98:923, 1968.
265. DANS PE, et al: Rifampin: Antibacterial activity in vitro and absorption and excretion in normal young men. Am J Med Sci 259:120, 1970.
266. MELANDER A, et al: Reduction of isoniazid bioavailability in normal men by concomitant intake of food. Acta Med Scand 200:93, 1976.
267. PETERSON OL, FINLAND M: The effect of food and alkali on the absorption and excretion of sulfonamide drugs after oral and duodenal administration. Am J Med Sci 204:581, 1942.

References (CONT.)

268. MacDonald H, et al: Effect of food on absorption of sulfonamides in man. Chemotherapia 12:282, 1967.
269. Melander A, et al: On the influence of concomitant food intake on sulfonamide bioavailability. Acta Med Scand 200:497, 1976.
270. Mattila MJ, et al: Interference of iron preparations and milk with the absorption of tetracyclines. Exerpta Medica International Congress Series No. 254: Toxicological Problems of Drug Combinations, 1972, p. 128.
271. Rosenblatt JE, et al: Comparison of in vitro activity and clinical pharmacology of doxycycline with other tetracyclines. Antimicrob Agents Chemother 1966, p. 134.
272. Kirby WM, et al: Comparison of two new tetracyclines with tetracycline and demethylchlortetracycline. Antimicrob Agents Chemother 1961, p. 286.
273. Welling PG, et al: Bioavailability of tetracycline and doxycycline in fasted and nonfasted subjects. Antimicrob Agents Chemother 1977, p. 462.
274. Neuvonen PJ, et al: Interference of iron with the absorption of tetracyclines in man. Br Med J 4:532, 1970.
275. Klein JO, et al: Laboratory studies of oxacillin. Parts I, II. Am J Med Sci 245:399, 1963.
276. Klein JO, et al: Nafcillin: antibacterial action in vitro and absorption and excretion in normal young men. Am J Med Sci 246:10, 1963.
277. Wagner JG, et al: Absorption, excretion and half-life of clindamycin in normal adult males. Am J Med Sci 256:25, 1968.
278. Waterman PM, Smith RB: Tobramycin-curare interaction. Anesth Analg 56:587, 1977.
279. DeHaan RM, et al: Clindamycin serum concentrations after administration of clindamycin palmitate with food. J Clin Pharmacol 12:205, 1972.
280. McCall CE, et al: Lincomycin: activity in vitro and absorption and excretion in normal young men. Am J Med Sci 254:144, 1967.
281. Kaplan K, et al: Microbiological, pharmacological and clinical studies of lincomycin. Am J Med Sci 250:137, 1965.
282. McGehee RF, et al: Comparative studies of antibacterial activity in vitro and absorption and excretion of lincomycin and clindamycin. Am J Med Sci 256:279, 1968.
283. Lincomycin. Physicians' Desk Reference. 31st Ed. Oradell, New Jersey, Medical Economics Co., 1977.
284. Weibert RT, Keane WF: Carbenicillin-gentamicin interaction in acute renal failure. Am J Hosp Pharm 34:1137, 1977.
285. Bruckner HW, Creasey WA: The administration of 5-fluorouracil by mouth. Cancer 33:14, 1974.
286. Davies M, et al: Interactions of carbenicillin and ticarcillin with gentamicin. Antimicrob Agents Chemother 7:431, 1975.
287. Kozak PP, et al: Administration of erythromycin to patients on theophylline (Letter). J Allergy Clin Immunol 60:149, 1977.
288. Mitchell JR, Potter WZ: Drug metabolism in the production of liver injury. Med Clin North Am 59:877, 1975.
289. Samuelson RJ, et al: Lincomycin-curare interaction. Anesth Analg 54:103, 1975.
290. Haag HB, et al: The effect of urinary pH on the elimination of quinine in man. J Pharmacol 79:136, 1943.

References (CONT.)

291. BREIMER DD, et al: Influence of rifampicin on drug metabolism: differences between hexobarbital and antipyrine. Clin Pharmacol Ther 21:470, 1977.
292. MIGUET JP, et al: Induction of hepatic microsomal enzymes after brief administration of rifampicin in man. Gastroenterology 72:924, 1977.
293. MATTILA MJ, et al: Serum levels, urinary excretion, and side-effects of cycloserine in the presence of isoniazid and p-aminosalicyclic acid. Scand J Respir Dis 50:291, 1969.
294. SMITH CK, DURACK DT: Isoniazid and reaction to cheese. Ann Intern Med 88:520, 1978.
295. LLORENS J, et al: Pharmacodynamic interference between rifampicin and isoniazid. Chemotherapy 24:97, 1978.
296. KRAMER PA, et al: Tetracycline absorption in elderly patients with achlorhydria. Clin Pharmacol Ther 23:467, 1978.
297. McGENNIS AJ: Lithium carbonate and tetracycline interaction. Br Med J 2:1183, 1978.
298. DOSSETOR J: Drug interactions with oral contraceptives (Letter). Br Med J 4:467, 1975.
299. McMAHON FG: Disulfiram-like reaction to a cephalosporin. JAMA 243:2397, 1980.
300. NEU HC, PRINCE AS: Interaction between moxalactam and alcohol. Lancet 1:1422, 1980.
301. FOSTER TS, et al: Disulfiram-like reaction associated with a parental cephalosporin. Am J Hosp Pharm 37:858, 1980.
302. PORTIER H, et al: Interaction between cephalosporins and alcohol. Lancet 2:263, 1980.
303. REEVES DS, DAVIES AJ: Antabuse effect with cephalosporins. Lancet 2:540, 1980.
304. DRYMMER S, et al: Antabuse-like effect of β-lactam antibiotics. N Engl J Med 303:1417, 1980.
305. BROWN KR, et al: Theophylline elixir, moxalactam, and a disulfiram reaction. Ann Intern Med 97:621, 1982.
306. WITT LG, WITT LD: Cephalosporins and ethanol. Drug Interactions Newslett 3:27, 1983.
307. ELENBAAS RM, et al: On the disulfiram-like activity of moxalactam. Clin Pharmacol Ther 32:347, 1982.
308. BUENING MK, et al: Disulfiram-like reaction to β-lactams. JAMA 245:2027, 1981.
309. LEDEN I: Digoxin-hydroxychloroquine interaction? Acta Med Scand 211:411, 1982.
310. McGENNIS AJ: Lithium carbonate and tetracycline interaction. Br Med J 1:1183, 1978.
311. SARMA GR, et al: Effect of prednisone and rifampin on isoniazid metabolism in slow and rapid inactivators of isoniazid. Antimicrob Agents Chemother 18:661, 1980.
312. BRODIE MJ, et al: Effect of isoniazid on Vitamin D metabolism and hepatic monooxygenase activity. Clin Pharmacol Ther 30:363, 1981.
313. OCHS HR, et al: Diazepam interaction with antituberculosis drugs. Clin Pharmacol Ther 29:671, 1981.
314. OCHS HR, et al: Interaction of triazolam with ethanol and isoniazid. Clin Pharmacol Ther 33:241, 1983.

References (CONT.)

315. BUCHANAN N, MOODLEY GP: Interaction between chloramphenicol and paracetamol. Br Med J 3:307, 1979.
316. GIBSON DL, et al: Midyear Clinical Meeting Abstracts. New Orleans, American Society of Hospital Pharmacists, December 6–10, 1981, p. 305.
317. BLEYER WA: The clinical pharmacology of methotrexate: new applications of an old drug. Cancer 41:36, 1978.
318. LINDENBAUM J, et al: Inactivation of digoxin by the gut flora: reversal by antibiotic therapy. N Engl J Med 305:789, 1981.
319. DOHERTY JE: A digoxin-antibiotic drug interaction. N Engl J Med 305:827, 1981.
320. MCELNAY JC, et al: In vitro experiments on chloroquine and pyrimethamine absorption in the presence of antacid constituents or kaolin. J Trop Med Hyg 85:153, 1982.
321. KOUP JR, et al: Interaction of chloramphenicol with phenytoin and phenobarbital. Case report. Clin Pharmacol Ther 24:571, 1978.
322. BLOXHAM RA, et al: Chloramphenicol and phenobarbitone. A drug interaction. Arch Dis Child 54:76, 1979.
323. HOUIN G, TILLEMENT JP: Clofibrate and enzymatic induction in man. Int J Clin Pharmacol 16:150, 1978.
324. SZEFLER SJ, et al: The effect of troleandomycin on methylprednisolone elimination. J Allergy Clin Immunol 66:447, 1980.
325. SZEFLER SJ, et al: Dose- and time-related effect of troleandomycin on methylprednisolone elimination. Clin Pharmacol Ther 32:166, 1982.
326. SZEFLER SJ, et al: Steroid-specific and anticonvulsant interaction aspects of troleandomycin-steroid therapy. J Allergy Clin Immunol 69:455, 1982.
327. ZEIGER RS, et al: Efficacy of troleandomycin in outpatients with severe, corticosteroid-dependent asthma. J Allergy Clin Immunol 66:438, 1980.
328. SELENKE W, et al: Nonantibiotic effects of macrolide antibiotics of the oleandomycin-erythromycin group with special reference to their "steroid-sparing" effects. J Allergy Clin Immunol 65:454, 1980.
329. BROWN DD, et al: Decreased bioavailability of digoxin due to hypocholesterolemic interventions. Circulation 58:164, 1978.
330. VAN DER MEER JWM, et al: J Antimicrob Chemother 6:552, 1980.
331. MEAD PB, et al: Possible alteration of metronidazole metabolism by phenobarbital. N Engl J Med 306:1490, 1982.
332. BACON JF, SHENFIELD GM: Pregnancy attributable to interaction between tetracycline and oral contraceptives. Br Med J 280:293, 1980.
333. HENDERSON JL, et al: In vitro inactivation of gentamicin, tobramycin, and netilmicin by carbenicillin, azlocillin, or mezlocillin. Am J Hosp Pharm 38:1167, 1981.
334. KEARNS GL, et al: Absence of a pharmacokinetic interaction between chloramphenicol and acetaminophen in children. (Abstract 707) Abstracts of the World Conference on Clinical Pharmacology in Therapeutics, Washington DC, July 31–Aug 5, 1983.
335. BRANIGAN TA, et al: The effect of erythromycin on the absorption and disposition kinetics of theophylline. Eur J Clin Pharmacol 21:115, 1981.
336. ZAROWITZ BJM, et al: Effect of erythromycin base on theophylline kinetics. Clin Pharmacol Ther 29:601, 1981.

References (CONT.)

337. RENTON KW, et al: Depression of theophylline elimination by erythromycin. Clin Pharmacol Ther 30:422, 1981.
338. LAFORCE CF, et al: Effect of erythromycin on theophylline clearance in asthmatic children. J Pediatr 99:153, 1981.
339. MAY DC, et al: The effects of erythromycin on theophylline elimination in normal males. J Clin Pharmacol 22:125, 1982.
340. ILIOPOULOU A, et al: Pharmacokinetics interaction between theophylline and erythromcyin. Br J Clin Pharmacol 14:495, 1982.
341. PFEIFER HJ, et al: Effects of three antibiotics on theophylline kinetics. Clin Pharmacol Ther 26:36, 1979.
342. MADDUX MS, et al: The effect of erythromycin on theophylline pharmacokinetics at steady state. Chest 81:563, 1982.
343. MELETHIL S, et al: Steady state urinary excretion of theophylline and its metabolites in the presence of erythromycin. Res Com Chem Pathol Pharmacol 35:341, 1982.
344. LEJONC JL, et al: Isoniazid and reaction to cheese. Ann Intern Med 91:793, 1979.
345. BISTRITZER T, et al: Isoniazid-rifampin-induced fulminant liver disease in an infant. J Pediatr 97:480, 1980.
346. LLORENS J, et al: Pharmacodynamic interference between rifampicin and isoniazid. Chemotherapy 24:97, 1978.
347. Drugs for Tuberculosis. Med Lett 24:17, 1982.
348. PESSAYRE D, et al: Isoniazid-rifampin fulminant hepatitis. Gastroenterology 72:284, 1977.
349. TRYBUCHOWSKI H: Effect of ampicillin on the urinary output of steroidal hormones in pregnant and non-pregnant women. Clin Chim Acta 45:9, 1973.
350. BOEHM FH, et al: The effect of ampicillin administration on urinary estriol and serum estradiol in the normal pregnant patient. Am J Obstet Gynecol 119:98, 1974.
351. SYBULSKI S, MAUGHAN GB: Effect of ampicillin administration on estradiol, estriol, and cortisol levels in maternal plasma and on estriol levels in urine. Am J Obstet Gynecol 124:379, 1976.
352. ADLERCREUTZ H, et al: Effect of ampicillin administration on plasma conjugated and unconjugated estrogen and progesterone levels in pregnancy. Am J Obstet Gynecol 128:266, 1977.
353. ORME ML, BACK DJ: Drug interactions with oral contraceptive steroids. Pharmacol Int 1:38, 1980.
354. FRIEDMAN CI, et al: The effect of ampicillin on oral contraceptive effectiveness. Obstet Gynecol 55:33, 1980.
355. LEPPER MH, DOWLING HF: Treatment of pneumococcic meningitis with penicillin compared with penicillin plus aureomycin: studies including observations on an apparent antagonism between penicillin and aureomycin. Arch Intern Med 88:489, 1951.
356. OLSSON RA, et al: Pneumococcal meningitis in the adult. Ann Intern Med 55:545, 1961.
357. VAN MARLE W, et al: Concurrent steroid and rifampicin therapy. Br Med J 1:1029, 1979.
358. BOMAN G, et al: Acute cardiac failure during treatment with digitoxin, an interaction with rifampicin. Br J Clin Pharmacol 10:89, 1980.

References (CONT.)

359. POOR DM, et al: Interaction of rifampin and digitoxin. Arch Intern Med 143:599, 1983.
360. NEUVONEN PJ, PENTTILA O: Effect of oral ferrous sulphate on the half-life of doxycycline in man. Eur J Clin Pharmacol 7:361, 1974.
361. DeSANO EA, HURLEY SC: Possible interactions of antihistamines and antibiotics with oral contraceptive effectiveness. Fertil Steril 37:853, 1982.
362. BACK DJ, et al: The effects of ampicillin on oral contraceptive steroids in women. Br J Clin Pharmacol 14:43, 1982.
363. MATZKE GR, et al: Effect of ticarcillin on gentamicin and tobramycin pharmacokinetics in a patient with end-stage renal disease. Pharmacotherapy 4:158, 1984.

CHAPTER 7

Antineoplastic Drug Interactions

ANTINEOPLASTIC AGENT (GENERAL) INTERACTIONS

DRUGS	DISCUSSION

Digitalis glycosides[39,43]

MECHANISM: Cytotoxic drugs appear to produce a reversible impairment of the intestinal mucosa, resulting in malabsorption of digoxin.

CLINICAL SIGNIFICANCE: Six patients with malignant lymphoma were given a single 0.8-mg dose of β-acetyl-digoxin (a digitalis glycoside derivative with onset and duration of action similar to digoxin) prior to and 25 hours after therapy with a variety of cytotoxic agents singly or in combination (cyclophosphamide, oncovin, procarbazine, prednisone).[39] Several plasma glycoside levels measured 0 to 8 hours thereafter indicated that the rate of absorption was delayed, and that the extent of absorption may have been decreased. Mean steady-state digoxin concentrations before and after similar chemotherapy in 15 cancer patients were 50% lower than those prior to chemotherapy. Digoxin levels began to fall 24 hours after therapy and reached their nadir at 48 hours. Digoxin levels returned to their original values 8 days following the last dose of cytotoxic agents. The renal excretion of digoxin was also decreased. The magnitude of these changes would appear sufficient to reduce the therapeutic effect of digoxin. Unlike digoxin, digitoxin absorption does not appear to be reduced by cytotoxic drugs.[43]

MANAGEMENT: One should be alert for evidence of reduced digoxin response during cytotoxic drug therapy. If oral doses of digoxin are increased to compensate for this effect, it is likely that reductions in digoxin dosage would be required if the cytotoxic drugs are stopped for more than a few days. The use of digitoxin instead of digoxin may lessen the likelihood of interaction with cytotoxic drugs.

AZATHIOPRINE (IMURAN) INTERACTIONS

DRUGS	DISCUSSION

Allopurinol (Zyloprim)[25,26]

MECHANISM: Azathioprine is first metabolized to 6-mercaptopurine (6-MP) and then to inactive products. The concomitant use of azathioprine and allopurinol impairs the conversion of 6-MP to inactive products by inhibiting xanthine oxidase. Thus, higher blood levels of 6-MP are likely to result.

AZATHIOPRINE (IMURAN) INTERACTIONS (CONT.)

DRUGS	DISCUSSION

CLINICAL SIGNIFICANCE: This interaction may well have been a major contributing factor to one death that was reported in some detail.[25] The increased blood levels of 6-MP may exert profound toxic effects on the bone marrow and other tissues.

MANAGEMENT: Allopurinol and azathioprine should never be given together without meticulous attention to adjusting the dosage of the azathioprine. Several authors have recommended that the azathioprine dose be reduced to one-fourth of the recommended dose.

CARMUSTINE (BiCNU) INTERACTIONS

DRUGS	DISCUSSION

Cimetidine (Tagamet)[47–51]

MECHANISM: Not established. Possibilities include additive effects on the bone marrow and/or cimetidine effects on carmustine metabolism.

CLINICAL SIGNIFICANCE: Patients receiving carmustine plus cimetidine appear to manifest a greater degree of bone marrow suppression than those receiving carmustine alone.[47,48] Cimetidine might also be expected to increase the myelosuppression of other cytotoxic drugs, and isolated reports indicate that chloramphenicol[49] and phenytoin[50,51] may be more myelosuppressive in the presence of cimetidine.

MANAGEMENT: Until more is known regarding the incidence and magnitude of this potential interaction, one should monitor carefully for evidence of excessive bone marrow suppression if cimetidine is used concurrently with carmustine or other myelosuppressive drugs.

CISPLATIN INTERACTIONS

DRUGS	DISCUSSION

Ethacrynic Acid (Edecrin)[41]

MECHANISM: Additive ototoxicity.

CLINICAL SIGNIFICANCE: Animal studies indicate that combined use of cisplatin and ethacrynic acid markedly enhances the likelihood of ototoxicity over either drug used alone.[41]

MANAGEMENT: Avoid concurrent use if possible. Furosemide appears to be less ototoxic than ethacrynic acid and might be less likely to cause ototoxicity when combined with cisplatin. If either ethacrynic acid or furosemide is used with cisplatin, the patient should be monitored carefully for ototoxicity.

CYCLOPHOSPHAMIDE (CYTOXAN) INTERACTIONS

DRUGS	DISCUSSION

Allopurinol (Zyloprim)[1,2,27,29,42]

MECHANISM: Not established.

CLINICAL SIGNIFICANCE: Preliminary epidemiologic information indicated that allopurinol might increase the frequency of bone marrow depression in patients receiving cyclophosphamide.[1] Of 58 patients receiving cyclophosphamide, bone marrow depression occurred in 57.7% of those also receiving allopurinol, and in 18.8% of patients not receiving allopurinol. In a subsequent study of 143 patients with malignant lymphoma, allopurinol did not appear to affect the bone marrow suppression of cytotoxic therapy.[42] In another study,[27] four patients who had been receiving allopurinol had a longer mean cyclophosphamide half-life than patients not receiving allopurinol, but the fraction of cyclophosphamide appearing as alkylating metabolites in the urine was the same in both groups. In summary, there is some clinical evidence that the effect of cyclophosphamide may be enhanced by allopurinol, but the clinical significant is not clear at this time.

MANAGEMENT: It has been proposed that the appropriateness of routine prophylactic use of allopurinol in patients receiving cytotoxic drugs be re-evaluated. When it is necessary to give allopurinol and cyclophosphamide concomitantly, one should be alert for evidence of excessive cyclophosphamide effect.

Barbiturates[3,27]

MECHANISM: It is proposed that barbiturates may promote the conversion of cyclophosphamide to active alkylating metabolites. However, the inactivation of these alkylating metabolites may also be enhanced.

CLINICAL SIGNIFICANCE: In a group of patients receiving cyclophosphamide, it was found that those receiving enzyme-inducing agents such as barbiturates developed higher peak plasma levels of alkylating metabolites of cyclophosphamide.[27] However, these patients also showed a more rapid decline in plasma levels of these metabolites. Thus, although it appears that barbiturates may alter cyclophosphamide disposition, the clinical effect of such altered disposition is not clear.

MANAGEMENT: Although little clinical evidence appears to be available, patients receiving both cyclophosphamide and a barbiturate should be watched for altered cyclophosphamide effect.

Corticosteroids[3,27,30]

MECHANISM: It has been proposed that corticosteroids may inhibit the hepatic microsomal enzymes that activate cyclophosphamide to its alkylating metabolites.

CLINICAL SIGNIFICANCE: Some have indicated that reduction of corticosteroid dosage in a patient also receiving cyclophosphamide may

CYCLOPHOSPHAMIDE (CYTOXAN)
INTERACTIONS (CONT.)

DRUGS	DISCUSSION

result in excessive cyclophosphamide effect,[3] but this has been refuted by others.[30] In one study, massive single doses of prednisolone did not appear to affect cyclophosphamide metabolism in several patients. Thus, more study is needed to resolve the clinical significance of this purported interaction.

MANAGEMENT: Until this potential interaction is better described, one should be alert for altered cyclophosphamide effect if corticosteroids are given concomitantly.

Succinylcholine (Anectine, Quelicin)[4,9,18,23,24]

MECHANISM: Cyclophosphamide may decrease pseudocholinesterase levels in the plasma, and succinylcholine is metabolized by pseudocholinesterase.

CLINICAL SIGNIFICANCE: Not established. Preliminary evidence from in-vitro studies and limited clinical observations indicate that prolonged apnea might occur following succinylcholine administration in some patients who also receive cyclophosphamide. The possibility may be higher in very ill patients who are receiving large intravenous doses of cyclophosphamide.

MANAGEMENT: It may be wise to administer succinylcholine with caution to patients also receiving cyclophosphamide (and probably other antineoplastics). Plasma pseudocholinesterase determinations may be desirable prior to succinylcholine administration. Avoidance of succinylcholine or cyclophosphamide has been recommended if the patient has significantly depressed pseudocholinesterase levels.[24]

DOXORUBICIN INTERACTIONS

DRUGS	DISCUSSION

Barbiturates[40]

MECHANISM: Not established.

CLINICAL SIGNIFICANCE: Preliminary clinical evidence indicates that barbiturates increase the plasma clearance of doxorubicin,[40] but more data are needed to assess the incidence and magnitude of this purported interaction.

MANAGEMENT: Monitor for altered doxorubicin effect if barbiturates are initiated or discontinued.

FLUOROURACIL INTERACTIONS

DRUGS	DISCUSSION

Methotrexate[33]

MECHANISM: In-vitro studies indicate that methotrexate may interfere with the effect of 5-fluorodeoxyuridine (FLD-URD) by inhibiting

FLUOROURACIL INTERACTIONS (CONT.)

DRUGS   DISCUSSION

the biosynthesis of a cofactor that is necessary for the antitumor activity of FLD-URD. Since 5-fluorouracil (5-FU) and FLD-URD reportedly have the same mechanism of action, it is proposed that methotrexate might inhibit the antitumor effect of 5-FU.

CLINICAL SIGNIFICANCE: Tests on tumor cells grown in vitro indicate that methotrexate inhibits the activity of FLD-URD, and by implication would also inhibit 5-FU. To date, there appears to be no clinical evidence to support these preliminary findings. Some recommended cancer chemotherapy regimens have included the combination of methotrexate and fluorouracil.

MANAGEMENT: Since the evidence to support this potential interaction is extremely preliminary, no course of action can be recommended at this time. However, one should be aware of the possibility of the interaction.

MERCAPTOPURINE (6-MP) INTERACTIONS

DRUGS   DISCUSSION

Allopurinol (Zyloprim)[5,10,19,20]

MECHANISM: Allopurinol is an effective inhibitor of the enzyme xanthine oxidase which is responsible for the metabolism of mercaptopurine to an inactive metabolite. Other mechanisms may be involved.

CLINICAL SIGNIFICANCE: Concomitant allopurinol-mercaptopurine administration appears to have the same result as giving a larger dose of mercaptopurine. Both antineoplastic activity and toxic effects are enhanced. At least one case has been reported in which the failure to decrease the dose of mercaptopurine during allopurinol therapy resulted in severe toxicity.[19] Some additional evidence has appeared which indicates that the pharmacokinetics of large intravenous doses of mercaptopurine are not affected by concomitant oral allopurinol administration.[5] The significance of this in patients receiving standard oral doses of mercaptopurine remains to be determined.

MANAGEMENT: When allopurinol and mercaptopurine are given concomitantly, the mercaptopurine dose may need to be reduced to as little as 25% of the usual dose.

METHOTREXATE INTERACTIONS

DRUGS   DISCUSSION

Ethanol (Alcohol, Ethyl)[6,7,8,13]

MECHANISM: It has been proposed that ethanol may enhance the possibility of methotrexate-induced hepatotoxicity.

DRUGS	DISCUSSION

CLINICAL SIGNIFICANCE: In one study of five cases of methotrexate-induced cirrhosis,[8] one patient ingested 28 to 85 g/week of ethanol and two ingested more than 85 g/week. This finding is consistent with the contention of others that ethanol may enhance the liver toxicity of methotrexate,[6,7] but certainly does not establish such an association. Also, a single case has been reported in which a patient on methotrexate developed respiratory failure and coma following a "cocktail."[13] A causal relationship was not established, however.

MANAGEMENT: Some workers feel strongly that ethanol should be avoided in patients receiving methotrexate,[6] and the manufacturer of methotrexate also recommends the avoidance of ethanol.[7] Even though the evidence for additive hepatotoxic effects is not conclusive, alcohol restriction is probably appropriate for most patients receiving methotrexate.

Para-aminobenzoic Acid (PABA)[7,11]

MECHANISM: PABA has been shown in vitro to displace methotrexate from plasma protein binding, thus increasing the free methotrexate concentrations.

CLINICAL SIGNIFICANCE: If this interaction occurs in humans, the increase of free methotrexate could result in severe toxicity since nearly toxic levels of methotrexate are used therapeutically. However, in the absence of clinical studies, it is impossible to determine if there is any danger in concomitant methotrexate and PABA administration.

MANAGEMENT: Until results of studies on man are available, it would be wise to give PABA with caution to patients receiving methotrexate or to avoid it, as the manufacturer recommends.[7] It should be noted that PABA is found in some proprietary analgesic mixtures.

Phenylbutazone (Butazolidin)[34]

MECHANISM: Not established. Although it has been proposed that phenylbutazone may displace methotrexate from plasma protein binding,[34] it also seems possible that phenylbutazone could reduce renal clearance of methotrexate. The ability of phenylbutazone and other nonsteroidal anti-inflammatory drugs to produce acute renal failure in occasional patients[44] might also result in accumulation of methotrexate.

CLINICAL SIGNIFICANCE: Two patients receiving methotrexate for psoriasis developed evidence of excessive methotrexate response during concomitant administration of phenylbutazone.[34] Both patients developed widespread cutaneous ulcerations, and one died following bone marrow depression and septicemia. Although the adverse responses seemed to be related to the concomitant use of phenylbutazone and methotrexate, the evidence is circumstantial.

METHOTREXATE INTERACTIONS (CONT.)

DRUGS	DISCUSSION

MANAGEMENT: Although only limited clinical evidence exists, the potential severity of the purported interaction indicates that phenylbutazone should be used only with caution in patients receiving methotrexate.

Probenecid (Benemid)[38,45,46]

MECHANISM: Probenecid appears to inhibit the renal excretion of methotrexate.

CLINICAL SIGNIFICANCE: Probenecid has been shown to considerably enhance serum methotrexate concentrations. Serum concentrations of methotrexate were considerably higher in four patients given probenecid (various doses) plus methotrexate (200 mg/m^2 bv IV bolus) than in four similar patients receiving methotrexate alone.[38] In a cross-over study of four patients, serum methotrexate levels were about 300% higher when probenecid (1.7 gm/m^2) was given with methotrexate as compared to methotrexate alone.[45] Although this interaction has not been studied in a large number of patients, the magnitude and predictability of the increases in serum methotrexate indicate that toxicity could occur if the interaction were not anticipated. Although probenecid inhibits the transfer of methotrexate from the cerebrospinal fluid in dogs,[46] this effect was not seen in a study of four patients.[45]

MANAGEMENT: Concomitant use of methotrexate and probenecid need not be avoided, but one should be alert for the necessity of reducing the dose of methotrexate in patients receiving both drugs.

Salicylates[7,11,12,21,22,31,35,38]

MECHANISM: Methotrexate undergoes renal tubular secretion that appears to be blocked by salicylates. Salicylates have also been shown to displace methotrexate from plasma protein binding, but the significance of this is not clear.

CLINICAL SIGNIFICANCE: Study in humans has shown a decreased clearance (about 35%) of methotrexate following salicylate administration as well as a decrease in plasma protein binding of about 30%.[12] Both of these factors would tend to increase the amount of active methotrexate and, therefore, toxicity. In another study[31] two patients receiving methotrexate and salicylate rapidly developed pancytopenia and died. A subsequent retrospective review of 176 patients who had received methotrexate infusions revealed that 66 patients also received salicylate in a dose greater than 600 mg/day. Of the seven patients who rapidly developed a severe pancytopenia, six were in the group who had received salicylates. Studies in mice also indicated that salicylates can enhance methotrexate toxicity.[31] One patient with psoriatic arthritis has been described who developed methotrexate hepatotoxicity while also taking moderate doses of aspirin for the arthritis.[21] Also, two elderly patients with psoriasis de-

METHOTREXATE INTERACTIONS (CONT.)

DRUGS	DISCUSSION

veloped signs of excessive methotrexate effect with concomitant aspirin therapy.[22] Another patient has been briefly described in whom aspirin ingestion was associated with a prolonged methotrexate half-life.[38] Taking all of the above evidence together, it appears that some patients on methotrexate may be adversely affected by concomitant salicylate therapy. Statements to the contrary[35] appear to arise from an inadequate review and/or analysis of the literature.

MANAGEMENT: On the basis of pharmacologic studies and initial clinical observations, it would be wise to administer salicylates to methotrexate-treated patients with caution or not at all. The manufacturer of methotrexate recommends that salicylates be avoided in patients receiving methotrexate.[7] Patients receiving methotrexate should be reminded of the many nonprescription mixtures that contain salicylates.

Vaccinations[16,17]

MECHANISM: Methotrexate may impair the immunologic response to smallpox vaccine resulting in generalized vaccinia. Other agents that may act as immunosuppressants (e.g., corticosteroids, other antineoplastic agents) could produce a similar effect.

CLINICAL SIGNIFICANCE: At least two cases of this interaction have been reported, with one patient receiving methotrexate,[16] and one receiving prednisone.[17] The reaction is potentially quite severe; death is possible. Since smallpox vaccine is no longer used, the primary importance of this interaction would be when other live vaccines such as measles, mumps, or rubella are used.

MANAGEMENT: Live vaccines should probably be avoided in patients receiving agents with immunosuppressive activity such as methotrexate.

PROCARBAZINE (MATULANE) INTERACTIONS

DRUGS	DISCUSSION

Central Nervous System Depressants[14,15]

MECHANISM: Procarbazine may augment the effects of central nervous system (CNS) depressants.

CLINICAL SIGNIFICANCE: The magnitude of enhanced CNS depression is not stated.

MANAGEMENT: CNS depressants should be administered cautiously in patients receiving procarbazine.

Ethanol (Ethyl Alcohol)[14,15]

MECHANISM: A disulfiram-like reaction reportedly may occur following ethanol ingestion in patients receiving procarbazine. Additive central nervous system depression may also occur.

PROCARBAZINE (MATULANE) INTERACTIONS (CONT.)

DRUGS	DISCUSSION

CLINICAL SIGNIFICANCE: These possible effects are listed by the manufacturer, but neither the incidence nor the magnitude of interaction is described.

MANAGEMENT: Patients should probably be warned of this possibility. From a medicolegal standpoint it should be noted that the manufacturer warns that ethanol "should not be used" in patients receiving procarbazine.

Sympathomimetics[28,32]

MECHANISM: Animal studies indicate that procarbazine inhibits monoamine oxidase.[28]

CLINICAL SIGNIFICANCE: If procarbazine inhibits monoamine oxidase in humans, one would expect potentially dangerous hypertensive episodes with administration of indirect acting sympathomimetics such as amphetamines, phenylpropanolamine, or ephedrine. However, clinical evidence to support such interactions is lacking. One patient receiving procarbazine developed a manic reaction following administration of lidocaine plus epinephrine for extraction of three teeth.[32] However, it seems unlikely that the epinephrine was responsible. More study is needed to determine if procarbazine is a monoamine oxidase inhibitor in humans.

MANAGEMENT: Until it is determined whether the interaction occurs in humans, sympathomimetics (especially indirect acting) should be used cautiously in patients receiving procarbazine.

TRIETHYLENETHIOPHOSPHORAMIDE (THIOTEPA) INTERACTIONS

DRUGS	DISCUSSION

Succinylcholine (Quelicin, Anectine)[4,9,18]

MECHANISM: Triethylenethiophosphoramide (TSPA) reportedly decreases pseudocholinesterase levels in the plasma, and succinylcholine is metabolized by pseudocholinesterase.

CLINICAL SIGNIFICANCE: It is not known whether pseudocholinesterase levels would be depressed sufficiently to prolong the effect of succinylcholine. In-vitro study seems to indicate that TSPA is not a very potent inhibitor of pseudocholinesterase.[18] No decrease in plasma pseudocholinesterase level was seen in one patient who received 255 mg instilled in the bladder.[4]

MANAGEMENT: Although present evidence indicates that any interaction may be slight, it may be wise to administer succinylcholine with caution to patients receiving TSPA.

References

1. Boston Collaborative Drug Surveillance Program: Allopurinol and cytotoxic drugs. Interaction in relation to bone marrow depression. JAMA 227:1036, 1974.
2. LYON GM: Allopurinol and cytotoxic agents (Letter). JAMA 228:1371, 1974.
3. KAPLAN SR, CALABRESI P: Immunosuppressive agents (first of two parts). N Engl J Med 289:952, 1973.
4. MONE JG, MATHIE WE: Qualitative and quantitative defects of pseudo-cholinesterase activity. Anaesthesia 22:55, 1967.
5. COFFEY JJ, et al: Effect of allopurinol on the pharmacokinetics of 6-mercaptopurine (NSC 755) in cancer patients. Cancer Res 32:1283, 1972.
6. PAI SH, et al: Severe liver damage caused by treatment of psoriasis with methotrexate. NY State J Med 73:2585, 1973.
7. Methotrexate. Product Information. Wayne, New Jersey, Lederle Laboratories, 1984.
8. TOBIAS H, AUERBACH R: Hepatotoxicity of long-term methotrexate therapy for psoriasis. Arch Intern Med 132:391, 1973.
9. SMITH RM Jr, et al: Succinylcholine-pantothenyl alcohol: a reappraisal. Anesth Analg Curr Res 48:205, 1969.
10. FREI E, LOO TL: Pharmacologic basis for the chemotherapy of leukemia. Pharmacol Physicians 1:1 (May) 1967.
11. DIXON RL, et al: Plasma protein binding of methotrexate and its displacement by various drugs. Fed Proc 24:454, 1965.
12. LIEGLER DG, et al: The effect of organic acids on renal clearance of methotrexate in man. Clin Pharmacol Ther 10:849, 1969.
13. GLASSNER J: Methotrexate and psoriasis (Letter). JAMA 210:1925, 1970.
14. Matulane. Product Information. Nutley, New Jersey, Roche Laboratories, 1984.
15. GOODMAN LS, GILMAN A (Eds): The Pharmacological Basis of Therapeutics. 4th Ed New York, Macmillan, 1970, pp. 1382–1383.
16. ALLISON J: Methotrexate and smallpox vaccination (Letter). Lancet 2:1250, 1968.
17. ROSENBAUM EH, et al: Vaccination of a patient receiving immunosuppressive therapy for lymphosarcoma. JAMA 198:737, 1966.
18. ZSIGMOND EK, ROBINS G: The effect of a series of anticancer drugs on plasma cholinesterase activity. Can Anaesth Soc J 19:75, 1972.
19. CALABRO JJ, CASTLEMAN B: Case records of the Massachusetts General Hospital (Case 4-1972). N Engl J Med 286:205, 1972.
20. BERNS A, et al: Hazard of combining allopurinol and thiopurine (Letter). N Engl J Med 286:730, 1972.
21. DUBIN HV, HARRELL ER: Liver disease associated with methotrexate treatment of psoriatic patients. Arch Dermatol 102:498, 1970.
22. BAKER H: Intermittent high dose oral methotrexate therapy in psoriasis. Br J Dermatol 82:65, 1970.
23. WOLFF H: Die Hemmung der Serumcholinesterase durch Cyclophosphamid (Endoxan). Klin Wochenschr 43:819, 1965.
24. WALKER IR, et al: Cyclophosphamide, cholinesterase and anaesthesia. Aust NZ J Med 2:247, 1972.
25. ANON: Clinicopathologic conference: hypertension and the lupus syndrome. Am J Med 49:519, 1970.

References (CONT.)

26. NIES AS, OATES JA: Clinicopathologic conference: hypertension and the lupus syndrome—revisited. Am J Med 51:812, 1971.
27. BAGLEY CM Jr, et al: Clinical pharmacology of cyclophosphamide. Cancer Res 33:226, 1973.
28. DEVITA VT, et al: Monoamine oxidase inhibition by a new carcinostatic agent, n-isopropyl-a-(2-methylhydrazine)-p-toluamide (MIH). Proc Soc Exp Biol Med 120:561, 1975.
29. RANDALL RF: Allopurinol (Letter). JAMA 229:638, 1974.
30. FABER OK, MOURIDSEN HT: Cyclophosphamide activation and corticosteroids (Letter). N Engl J Med 291:211, 1974.
31. MANDEL MA: The synergistic effect of salicylates on methotrexate toxicity. Plast Reconstr Surg 57:733, 1976.
32. MANN AM, HUTCHISON JL: Manic reaction associated with procarbazine hydrochloride therapy of Hodgkin's disease. Can Med Assoc J 97:1350, 1967.
33. MAUGH TH: Cancer chemotherapy: an unexpected drug interaction. Science 194:310, 1976.
34. ADAMS JD, HUNTER GA: Drug interactions in psoriasis. Aust J Dermatol 17:39, 1976.
35. TAYLOR JR, HALPRIN KM: Effect of sodium salicylate and indomethacin on methotrexate-serum albumin binding. Arch Dermatol 113:588, 1977.
36. LANE M, et al: Effect of food on fluorouracil (FU) absorption. ASCO abstracts (C-140), 1976, p. 271.
37. COHEN JL, et al: Clinical Pharmacology of oral and intravenous 5-fluorouracil (NSC 19893). Cancer Chemother Rep 58:723, 1974.
38. AHERNE GW, et al: Prolongation and enhancement of serum methotrexate concentrations by probenecid. Br Med J 1:1097, 1978.
39. KUHLMANN J, et al: Effects of cytotoxic drugs on plasma level and renal excretion of beta-acetyldigoxin. Clin Pharmacol Ther 30:518, 1981.
40. RIGGS, CE, et al: Doxorubicin pharmacokinetics: prochlorperazine and barbiturate effects. Clin Pharmacol Ther 31:263, 1982.
41. KOMUNE S, SNOW JB: Potentiating effects of cisplatin and ethacrynic acid in ototoxicity. Arch Otolaryngol 107:594, 1981.
42. STOLBACH L, et al: Evaluation of bone marrow toxic reaction in patients treated with allopurinol. JAMA 247:334, 1982.
43. KUHLMANN J, et al: Cytostatic drugs are without significant effect on digitoxin plasma level and renal excretion. Clin Pharmacol Ther 32:646, 1982.
44. GREENSTONE M, et al: Acute nephrotic syndrome with reversible renal failure after phenylbutazone. Br Med J 282:950, 1981.
45. HOWELL SB, et al: Effect of probenecid on cerebrospinal fluid methotrexate kinetics. Clin Pharmacol Ther 26:641, 1979.
46. RAMU A, et al: Probenecid inhibition of methotrexate excretion from cerebrospinal fluid in dogs. J Pharmacokinet Biopharm 6:389, 1978.
47. SELKER RG, et al: Bone-marrow depression with cimetidine plus carmustine. N Engl J Med 299:834, 1978.
48. VOLKIN RL, et al: Potentiation of carmustine-cranial irradiation-induced myelosuppression by cimetidine. Arch Intern Med 142:243, 1982.

References (CONT.)

49. FARBER BF, BRODY JP: Rapid development of aplastic anemia after intravenous chloramphenicol and cimetidine therapy. South Med J 74:1257, 1981.
50. SAZIE E, JAFFE JP: Severe granulocytopenia with cimetidine and phenytoin. Ann Intern Med 93:151, 1980.
51. AL-KAWAS FH, et al: Cimetidine and agranulocytosis. Ann Intern Med 90:992, 1979.

CHAPTER 8

Digitalis Drug Interactions

DIGITALIS INTERACTIONS

DRUGS	DISCUSSION

Amiloride (Midamor)[54]

MECHANISM: Amiloride appears to increase renal clearance and reduce nonrenal clearance of digoxin.

CLINICAL SIGNIFICANCE: Six healthy subjects were given a single dose of digoxin (15 mcg/kg body weight intravenously) with and without pretreatment with amiloride (10 mg/day for 8 days).[54] Amiloride administration was associated with an almost twofold increase in renal digoxin clearance, and the extrarenal clearance of digoxin was markedly reduced. The net effect of concurrent amiloride therapy was to decrease the total body digoxin clearance and to increase serum digoxin levels slightly. However, an evaluation of myocardial contractility indicated that amiloride suppresses the positive inotropic effect of digoxin. In these healthy subjects, the changes in digoxin pharmacokinetics caused by amiloride tended to offset each other, resulting in only a slight increase in serum digoxin levels. However, in a patient whose renal or extrarenal routes of elimination are severely compromised, the remaining route of elimination may assume greater importance. Thus, in a patient with impaired renal excretion of digoxin, amiloride might be expected to produce substantial increases in serum digoxin levels. Conversely, a patient with impaired extrarenal digoxin excretion might develop a *decreased* serum digoxin level due to an amiloride-induced increase in renal digoxin clearance. A reduction in the inotropic effect of digoxin by amiloride as observed in this study could be clinically important, but studies in patients receiving digoxin for congestive heart failure are needed to resolve this.

MANAGEMENT: In patients receiving both digoxin and amiloride, one should be alert for altered responses to digoxin.

Antacids, Oral[28,37,42-44,60]

MECHANISM: Some antacids appear to have the ability to impair the gastrointestinal absorption of digoxin.

CLINICAL SIGNIFICANCE: Studies of digoxin absorption in normal volunteers with and without concomitant antacid administration indicate that the following antacids can reduce digoxin bioavailability:

DRUGS	DISCUSSION

magnesium trisilicate, magnesium hydroxide, aluminum hydroxide.[43] The magnitude of the decreases in digoxin bioavailability (based on 6-day cumulative urinary excretion) would seem large enough to reduce the therapeutic response to digoxin in some patients. However, studies in patients receiving chronic digoxin therapy are needed to confirm the clinical importance of this interaction. A study in 12 subjects indicated that a magnesium-aluminum hydroxide antacid reduced the bioavailability of digoxin tablets but not digoxin capsules.[60] The absorption characteristics of lanatoside C may be affected by concomitant calcium carbonate administration,[42,44] but the *amount* of lanatoside C absorbed was not affected. The absorption of digoxin appeared to be inhibited by concomitant administration of magnesium peroxide in one patient.[37]

MANAGEMENT: One should be alert for reduced effect of digoxin in patients who are receiving concomitant antacid therapy. Spacing the doses in order to minimize mixing in the gastrointestinal tract may reduce the inhibitory effect of antacids on digoxin absorption. The use of digoxin capsules instead of tablets may minimize the interaction.

Barbiturates[14,19,61]

MECHANISM: Phenobarbital appears to enhance the metabolism of digitoxin to digoxin, presumably due to induction of hepatic microsomal enzymes.

CLINICAL SIGNIFICANCE: Decreased plasma digitoxin levels and a shortened digitoxin half-life have been demonstrated when phenobarbital is given to patients receiving digitoxin. The increased conversion of digitoxin to digoxin and other metabolites could decrease the therapeutic effect since digoxin has a much shorter half-life than digitoxin. However, in another study phenobarbital (100 mg/day) failed to affect serum digitoxin in healthy subjects.[61] Thus, more study is needed to determine the clinical consequences of this interaction.

MANAGEMENT: Pending the availability of further information, patients receiving both digitoxin and a barbiturate (or other enzyme inducer) should be watched for underdigitalization. The digitoxin dose should be increased if necessary. Digoxin would seem less likely to be affected by enzyme induction and may be preferable to digitoxin if this interaction becomes a problem.

Calcium Preparations[8,15,20]

MECHANISM: Calcium ion and digitalis have some similar effects on the myocardium. In fact, it is possible that the positive inotropic effect of digitalis is mediated via an effect on calcium.

CLINICAL SIGNIFICANCE: Parenteral calcium reportedly may precipitate cardiac arrhythmias in patients receiving digitalis glycosides. The death of two digitalized patients following administration of intravenous calcium preparations was apparently reported in 1936, but subsequent clinical descriptions of this interaction are lacking.

DIGITALIS INTERACTIONS (CONT.)

DRUGS	DISCUSSION

MANAGEMENT: On the basis of currently available evidence, parenteral calcium administration should generally be avoided in patients receiving digitalis glycosides. If it is given, the calcium should not be given rapidly or in large amounts in order to avoid high serum calcium levels.

Carbamazepine (Tegretol)[9]

MECHANISM: Not established.

CLINICAL SIGNIFICANCE: Bradycardia has been noted in patients receiving both carbamazepine and digitalis glycosides.[9] The possibility that this effect was due to the combined effects of both drugs was entertained, but a causal relationship was not established.

MANAGEMENT: No special precautions appear necessary until more is known about this possible interaction.

Cholestyramine (Questran)[10,21,22,39,49,50,61,62]

MECHANISM: Cholestyramine appears to bind digitoxin in the gut, thus interrupting the enterohepatic circulation of digitoxin and shortening its half-life.

CLINICAL SIGNIFICANCE: In a study of 15 subjects, seven received maintenance doses of cholestyramine following digitalization with digitoxin.[21] Serum levels of digitoxin and physiologic measurements of digitalis action both pointed to a reduced effect of digitoxin. In another study of six healthy subjects, cholestyramine (4 g eight times daily) reduced digoxin half-life from 142 to 84 hours.[62] Cholestyramine may also accelerate digitoxin elimination in cases of digitoxin overdose.[61] Determination of the magnitude and significance of this interaction in patients on chronic digitoxin therapy must await further study. Although single dose studies in normal volunteers indicate that cholestyramine inhibits the absorption of digoxin,[49] long-term studies have failed to demonstrate a consistent effect on serum digoxin.[39,50] In summary, there is evidence to indicate that the cholestyramine can impair absorption of digoxin and digitoxin, but the clinical impact in patients treated chronically has not been adequately assessed.

MANAGEMENT: Until more is known about this interaction, patients on digitalis glycosides (especially digitoxin) should be watched for underdigitalization if cholestyramine is also given. Giving the digitalis product 1½ to 2 hours before the cholestyramine may help lower the magnitude of the interaction.

Cimetidine (Tagamet)[74–78]

MECHANISM: Not established.

CLINICAL SIGNIFICANCE: In 11 hospitalized patients receiving digoxin for congestive heart failure, the addition of cimetidine (600 to

DRUGS	DISCUSSION

1200 mg/day) resulted in a 25% reduction in mean steady-state serum digoxin concentration.[74] However, no increase in the severity of congestive heart failure was noted. In another study, 11 healthy subjects were given single 1.25-mg doses of digoxin intravenously with and without pretreatment with cimetidine (1000 mg/day).[75] Cimetidine did not affect the pharmacokinetics of digoxin. Since gastric acid appears to be involved in the degradation of digoxin in the gut,[76,77] one might expect agents which reduce gastric acid to increase the gastrointestinal absorption of digoxin in patients with gastric hyperacidity. However, clinical evidence for such an effect appears to be lacking. A patient receiving digitoxin and quinidine developed digitoxin intoxication following initiation of cimetidine therapy.[78] The cimetidine probably increased the serum quinidine, which in turn would increase serum digitoxin concentration; however, the cimetidine may have also directly increased serum digitoxin levels by reducing its hepatic metabolism. In summary, there is some evidence from patients on chronic digoxin that cimetidine may reduce serum digoxin levels, but the magnitude of the effect appears to be insufficient to cause difficulties in most patients. Theoretically, cimetidine might be expected to inhibit the hepatic metabolism of digitoxin, but clinical evidence to support such an effect is scanty.

MANAGEMENT: Until this interaction is better described, one should be alert for evidence of altered response to digitalis glycosides if cimetidine therapy is initiated or discontinued.

Colestipol (Colestid)[22]

MECHANISM: Colestipol appears to bind digitalis glycosides in the gut, thus impairing their initial absorption and enterohepatic circulation.

CLINICAL SIGNIFICANCE: In four patients with digitoxin intoxication, colestipol appeared to reduce plasma digitoxin levels, presumably by interrupting enterohepatic circulation.[22] A similar effect was seen in one patient with digoxin intoxication, but one would expect digoxin to be less affected since it undergoes less enterohepatic circulation. Studies in patients receiving normal doses of digitalis glycosides are needed in order to evaluate the clinical importance of this interaction.

MANAGEMENT: Until this interaction is better described, one should be alert for evidence of underdigitalization if colestipol is given concomitantly with a digitalis glycoside (especially digitoxin). Giving the digitalis product 1½ to 2 hours before the colestipol may help lower the magnitude of the interaction.

Diazepam (Valium)[55]

MECHANISM: Not established.

CLINICAL SIGNIFICANCE: Not established. Preliminary results in a study of seven subjects indicated that diazepam increased digoxin half-life and reduced urinary digoxin excretion.[55] More data are needed to assess these findings.

DIGITALIS INTERACTIONS (CONT.)

MANAGEMENT: Until more is known, one should be alert for increased digoxin effect when diazepam is given concurrently.

Diuretics (Potassium-losing)[3,7,8,11,13,24–27,29,31,32,36,38,40,41]

MECHANISM: Diuretics such as furosemide (Lasix), ethacrynic acid (Edecrin), bumetanide (Bumex), chlorthalidone (Hygroton), metolazone (Zaroxolyn), and thiazides can produce potassium deficiencies with resultant predisposition to digitalis toxicity. The magnesium deficiency that can occur following diuretic therapy probably also contributes.

CLINICAL SIGNIFICANCE: This classic example of a drug interaction is well known but still occurs in patients receiving digitalis glycosides, especially since the introduction of the potent kaliuretics such as furosemide and ethacrynic acid. Jelliffe has presented data showing that, within a given range of serum digoxin concentrations, the incidence of digitalis toxicity increases as serum potassium levels decrease.[7] However, many patients on potassium-losing diuretics do not develop clinically important potassium depletion due to a variety of reasons such as low doses of diuretics and adequate potassium intake.

MANAGEMENT: The potassium and magnesium status of patients on concomitant diuretic-digitalis therapy should be closely monitored. Replacement potassium therapy should be undertaken if needed.

Edrophonium (Tensilon)[33]

MECHANISM: It is proposed that the additive vagomimetic effects of digitalis glycosides and edrophonium may cause excessive slowing of the heart rate.

CLINICAL SIGNIFICANCE: An 81-year-old woman on large doses of digoxin developed increasing atrioventricular block, bradycardia, and finally asystole when edrophonium (10 mg intravenously) was given.[33] It was proposed that the adverse cardiac response represented the combined effects of the digoxin and edrophonium.

MANAGEMENT: One should probably exercise greater caution when administering edrophonium injections to digitalized patients.

Food[45,46]

MECHANISM: None.

CLINICAL SIGNIFICANCE: Studies in healthy subjects demonstrated that ingestion of digoxin after food does not significantly change completeness of absorption but the peak serum concentration is lowered and the rate of absorption is delayed slightly.[45,46] In 21 patients receiving maintenance digoxin, a 4-week cross-over study revealed no difference in plasma concentrations whether the digoxin was given regularly after meals or in the fasting state.[46]

DRUGS	DISCUSSION

MANAGEMENT: No specific recommendations are necessary.

Glucose Infusions[15]

MECHANISM: Large infusions of carbohydrate may cause an intracellular shift of potassium with resultant decrease in serum potassium.

CLINICAL SIGNIFICANCE: Although clinical reports of interaction are lacking, it has been cautioned that a large intake of carbohydrate could worsen or precipitate impending digitalis toxicity.

MANAGEMENT: It would be prudent to avoid infusion of large amounts of carbohydrate to patients with digitalis toxicity, or to patients in whom digitalis toxicity is impending or suspected.

Heparin[12]

MECHANISM: Not established.

CLINICAL SIGNIFICANCE: Digitalis glycosides reportedly may antagonize the anticoagulant activity of heparin somewhat,[12] but no substantiating evidence was presented.

MANAGEMENT: No special precautions appear necessary.

Ibuprofen (Motrin)[56]

MECHANISM: Not established.

CLINICAL SIGNIFICANCE: In 12 patients stabilized on digoxin, addition of ibuprofen (1600 mg or more daily) resulted in approximately a 60% increase in serum digoxin after 1 week.[56] However, the increase was highly variable from patient to patient, and was not detectable after about a month of ibuprofen treatment. More study is needed to assess the incidence and magnitude of the interaction.

MANAGEMENT: Monitor for altered digoxin effect if ibuprofen is initiated or discontinued.

Kaolin-pectin **(Kaopectate and others)**[43,60,63]

MECHANISM: Kaolin-pectin appears to inhibit the gastrointestinal absorption of digoxin.

CLINICAL SIGNIFICANCE: Ten normal subjects were given digoxin (0.75 mg orally) with and without kaolin-pectin (60 ml orally).[43] Serum digoxin levels were considerably reduced in the presence of kaolin-pectin, as were the areas under the digoxin concentration curves and cumulative urinary digoxin excretion. In a subsequent study of seven healthy subjects on chronic digoxin, kaolin-pectin reduced digoxin bioavailability by 15% when the two drugs were given concurrently, but not when the digoxin was given 2 hours before the kaolin-pectin.[63] In another study of 12 healthy subjects kaolin-pectin

DIGITALIS INTERACTIONS (CONT.)

reduced the bioavailability of digoxin tablets but not digoxin capsules.[60] In summary, kaolin-pectin appears to produce a mild reduction in the bioavailability of digoxin tablets.

MANAGEMENT: Patients receiving digoxin should probably avoid more than occasional use of kaolin-pectin. When kaolin-pectin is used, it should probably not be given until 2 hours after digoxin tablets. The use of digoxin capsules may help minimize the interaction.

Metoclopramide (Reglan)[1,2,4,5,6]

MECHANISM: The gastrointestinal absorption of slowly dissolving brands of digoxin may be decreased by metoclopramide, which increases gastrointestinal motility.[4]

CLINICAL SIGNIFICANCE: In 11 patients on maintenance therapy with a slowly dissolving digoxin preparation, the addition of metoclopramide (30 mg/day for 10 days) resulted in a decreased serum digoxin level in all patients.[4] Although not tested directly, it seems likely that a more rapidly dissolving preparation (e.g., Lanoxin) would not be as much affected by drugs such as metoclopramide.

MANAGEMENT: In patients receiving chronic digoxin therapy, the addition of metoclopramide (or other drugs increasing gastrointestinal motility) should alert the practitioner to the possibility of decreased digoxin effect. The interaction can probably be minimized by the use of rapidly dissolving preparations such as Lanoxin tablets or digoxin capsules (e.g., Lanoxicaps).

Nifedipine (Procardia)[58,59,64]

MECHANISM: Not established.

CLINICAL SIGNIFICANCE: Nifedipine has been shown to substantially increase serum digoxin concentrations in one study, but other studies found no effect.[58,59,64] Although the reason for the conflicting results is not clear, one must assume that nifedipine may be capable of increasing serum digoxin levels in some patients until more data are available.

MANAGEMENT: Monitor for evidence of increased digoxin effect if nifedipine is given concurrently. Lower digoxin dose as needed.

Penicillamine (Cuprimine)[57]

MECHANISM: Not established.

CLINICAL SIGNIFICANCE: Patients stabilized on digoxin have developed reduced serum digoxin levels following penicillamine treatment.[57]

MANAGEMENT: One should be alert for evidence of altered digoxin effect if penicillamine is initiated or discontinued. Adjust digoxin dosage as necessary.

DIGITALIS INTERACTIONS (CONT.)

DRUGS	DISCUSSION

Phenylbutazone (Butazolidin)[23]

MECHANISM: Not established. Phenylbutazone appears to enhance the metabolism of digitoxin, probably by induction of hepatic microsomal enzymes.

CLINICAL SIGNIFICANCE: A preliminary study on digitoxin in one patient has shown decreased plasma digitoxin levels when phenylbutazone was administered. Study in more patients is needed to assess clinical significance of this effect. Also, the known ability of phenylbutazone to induce sodium retention should be considered carefully in the patient receiving digitalis glycosides.

MANAGEMENT: Patients receiving both digitoxin and phenylbutazone should be watched more closely for underdigitalization and phenylbutazone-induced sodium retention.

Propantheline (Pro-Banthine)[1,2,4–6,42]

MECHANISM: The gastrointestinal absorption of slowly dissolving brands of digoxin may be increased by propantheline, which decreases gastrointestinal motility.[4]

CLINICAL SIGNIFICANCE: In 13 patients on maintenance therapy with a slowly dissolving digoxin preparation, the addition of propantheline (15 mg/day for 10 days) resulted in an increased serum digoxin in nine of the patients.[4] Digoxin administered as a solution did not appear to be affected by propantheline, and subsequent study revealed that a more rapidly dissolving preparation (Lanoxin) was similarly unaffected by propantheline.[1] Since Lanoxin is by far the most widely used digoxin in the United States, most patients would probably not be significantly affected by this interaction. In another study[42] the total absorption of lanatoside C (given in solution) was not affected by pretreatment with an anticholinergic (oxyphencyclimine), although absorption was somewhat delayed.

MANAGEMENT: Patients receiving digoxin (other than rapidly dissolving brands such as Lanoxin) should be monitored for increased digoxin effect if anticholinergic drugs such as propantheline are added, and monitored for decreased digoxin effect when the anticholinergic is stopped.

Spironolactone (Aldactone)[30,34,65–73]

MECHANISM: Spironolactone may reduce the renal excretion of digoxin, produce false elevations in plasma digoxin by some methods, and possibly inhibit the positive inotropic effect of digitalis glycosides. Spironolactone also appears to enhance the metabolism of digitoxin.

CLINICAL SIGNIFICANCE: In nine patients on chronic digoxin therapy, spironolactone (100 mg/day for 10 days) increased the mean serum digoxin concentration from 0.8 mcg/L to 1.0 mcg/L.[65] The magnitude

DRUGS	DISCUSSION

of the increases was quite variable from patient to patient; in one patient, the digoxin concentration increased from 1.0 mcg/L to 3.5 mcg/L. Another study from the same laboratory in eight subjects also found a variable increase in serum digoxin after 5 days of spironolactone, 200 mg/day.[66] The assay used in these studies did not appear to be affected by spironolactone administration. However, several other studies have shown spironolactone to produce false increases in various serum digoxin assays.[67-72] It appears that digoxin assays using sheep antibody may be less likely to be affected by spironolactone than digoxin assays using rabbit antibody. However, spironolactone interference with digoxin assays cannot be ruled out unless the laboratory has performed serum digoxin assays on patients receiving chronic spironolactone in the absence of digoxin therapy. The half-life of digitoxin was reduced in several patients by the administration of spironolactone,[30] but the reduction was relatively small. Thus, most patients receiving digitoxin and spironolactone would probably not be adversely affected. In summary, there is substantial evidence that spironolactone may interfere with certain serum digoxin assays, and more limited evidence that spironolactone may produce a true increase in serum digoxin concentration.

MANAGEMENT: In patients receiving digoxin and spironolactone one should monitor the digoxin response by means other than serum digoxin concentrations, unless the digoxin assay used has been proven not to be affected by spironolactone therapy. Since there is some evidence that spironolactone may produce a *true* increase in serum digoxin levels, one should also be alert for evidence of enhanced digoxin effect in the presence of spironolactone therapy. To avoid the potential adverse interactions, one could use potassium supplements instead of spironolactone.

Succinylcholine (Anectine, Quelicin)[16-18,35]

MECHANISM: Not established. Succinylcholine appears to potentiate the cardiac effects of digitalis glycosides with respect to both conduction and increased ventricular irritability. It has been proposed but not proved that this is due to the effect on cholinergic receptors that release catecholamines. Also, depolarizing muscle relaxants may produce a sudden shift of potassium from inside the muscle cell to outside. If this occurred in the digitalized myocardium, arrhythmias could result. See also the description of the effect of succinylcholine on serum potassium.

CLINICAL SIGNIFICANCE: Cardiac arrhythmias have occurred following the administration of succinylcholine to fully digitalized patients. However, more study is needed to assess clinical significance.

MANAGEMENT: Pending availability of further information, succinylcholine should be used cautiously in digitalized patients. One manufacturer of succinylcholine states that it should not be used in digitalized patients unless absolutely necessary.

DIGITALIS INTERACTIONS (CONT.)

DRUGS	DISCUSSION

Sympathomimetics[15]

MECHANISM: Both sympathomimetics and digitalis glycosides may cause ectopic pacemaker activity. Thus, their concomitant use could increase the possibility of cardiac arrhythmias. Sympathomimetics with beta-receptor stimulant activity (e.g., epinephrine, isoproterenol) would be the most likely to produce this effect. Ephedrine has also been said to enhance the possibility of arrhythmias.[15]

CLINICAL SIGNIFICANCE: More clinical study of this interaction is needed, although theoretical considerations indicate that it may be clinically significant.

MANAGEMENT: Digitalized patients should be given sympathomimetics only with caution.

References

1. MANNINEN V, et al: Effect of propantheline and metoclopramide on absorption of digoxin (Letter). Lancet 1:1118, 1973.
2. MICHALOPOULOS CD, KOUTOULIDIS CV: Altered digoxin bioavailability (Letter). Lancet 1:167, 1974.
3. BELLER GA, et al: Correlation of serum magnesium levels and cardiac digitalis intoxication. Am J Cardiol 33:225, 1974.
4. MANNINEN V, et al: Altered absorption of digoxin in patients given propantheline and metoclopramide. Lancet 1:398, 1973.
5. THOMPSON WG: Altered absorption of digoxin in patients given propantheline and metoclopramide (Letter). Lancet 1:783, 1973.
6. MEDIN S, NYBERG L: Effect of propantheline and metoclopramide on absorption of digoxin (Letter). Lancet 1:1393, 1973.
7. JELLIFFE RW: Effect of serum potassium level upon risk of digitalis toxicity (Abstract). Ann Intern Med 78:821, 1973.
8. SCHICK D, SCHEUER J: Current concepts of therapy with digitalis glycosides. Part II. Am Heart J 87:391, 1974.
9. KILLIAN JM, FROMM GH: Carbamazepine in the treatment of neuralgia. Use and side effects. Arch Neurol 19:129, 1968.
10. THOMPSON WG: Effect of cholestyramine on absorption of 3H digoxin in rats. Am J Dig Dis 18:851, 1973.
11. GOOCH AS, et al: Influence of exercise on arrhythmias induced by digitalis-diuretic therapy in patients with atrial fibrillation. Am J Cardiol 33:230, 1974.
12. LEVINE WG: Heparin and oral anticoagulants, in, Goodman LS, Gilman A (Eds): The Pharmacological Basis of Therapeutics. 4th Ed., Macmillan, New York, 1970, pp. 1445–1463.
13. SELLER RH, et al: Digitalis toxicity and hypomagnesemia. Am Heart J 79:57, 1970.
14. JELLIFFE RW, BLANKENHORN DH: Effect of phenobarbital on digitoxin metabolism. Clin Res 14:160, 1966.
15. SHERROD TR: The cardiac glycosides. Hosp Practice 2:56, 1967.
16. DOWDY EG, et al: Effect of neuromuscular blocking agents on isolated digitalized mammalian hearts. Anesth Analg 44:608, 1965.

References (CONT.)

17. CURRAN FJ, et al: Report of a severe case of tetanus managed with large doses of intramuscular succinylcholine. Anesth Analg 47:218, 1968.
18. BIRCH AA Jr, et al: Changes in serum potassium response to succinylcholine following trauma. JAMA 210:490, 1969.
19. SOLOMON HM, ABRAMS WB: Interactions between digitoxin and other drugs in man. Am Heart J 83:277, 1972.
20. NOLA GT, et al: Assessment of the synergistic relationship between serum calcium and digitalis. Am Heart J 79:499, 1970.
21. CALDWELL JH, et al: Interruption of the enterohepatic circulation of digitoxin by cholestyramine. J Clin Invest 50:2638, 1971.
22. BAZZANO G, BAZZANO GS: Digitalis intoxication: treatment with a new steroid-binding resin. JAMA 220:828, 1972.
23. SOLOMON HM, et al: Interactions between digitoxin and other drugs in vitro and in vivo. Ann NY Acad Sci 179:362, 1971.
24. POOLE-WILSON PA, et al: Hypokalaemia, digitalis, and arrhythmias (Letter). Lancet 1:575, 1975.
25. SHAPIRO W, TAUBERT K: Hypokalaemia and digoxin-induced arrhythmias (Letter). Lancet 2:604, 1975.
26. BINNION PF: Hypokalaemia and digoxin-induced arrhythmias (Letter). Lancet 1:343, 1975.
27. CORBETT EC Jr: Hypokalaemia and digoxin-induced arrhythmias (Letter). Lancet 1:742, 1975.
28. LOO JC, et al: Effect of an antacid on absorption of digoxin in dogs (Letter). J Pharm Sci 64:1727, 1975.
29. SEMPLE P, et al: Furosemide and urinary digoxin clearance (Letter). N Engl J Med 293:612, 1975.
30. WIRTH KE, et al: Metabolism of digoxin in man and its modification by spironolactone. Eur J Clin Pharmacol 9:345, 1976.
31. MCALLISTER RG, et al: Effect of intravenous furosemide on the renal excretion of digoxin. J Clin Pharmacol 16:110, 1976.
32. STEINESS E, OLESEN KH: Cardiac arrhythmias induced by hypokalaemia and potassium loss during maintenance digoxin therapy. Br Heart J 38:167, 1976.
33. GOULD L, et al: Cardiac arrest during edrophonium administration. Am Heart J 81:437, 1971.
34. SOLYMOSS B, et al: Protection by spironolactone and oxandrolone against chronic digitoxin or indomethacin intoxication. Toxicol Appl Pharmacol 18:586, 1971.
35. PEREZ HR: Cardiac arrhythmia after succinylcholine. Anesth Analg 49:33, 1970.
36. STORSTEIN L: Renal excretion of digitoxin and its cardioactive metabolites. Clin Pharmacol Ther 16:14, 1974.
37. VANDERVIJGH WJF, et al: Reduced bioavailability of digoxin by magnesium perhydrol. Drug Intell Clin Pharm 10:680, 1976.
38. BROWN DD, et al: Effect of furosemide on the renal excretion of digoxin. Clin Pharmacol Ther 20:395, 1976.
39. HALL WH, et al: Effect of cholestyramine on digoxin absorption and excretion in man. Am J Cardiol 39:213, 1977.
40. BRATER DC, MORRELLI HF: Digoxin toxicity in patients with normokalemic potassium depletion. Clin Pharmacol Ther 22:21, 1977.

References (CONT.)

41. MALCOLM AD, et al: Digoxin kinetics during furosemide administration. Clin Pharmacol Ther 21:567, 1977.
42. ALDOUS S. THOMAS R: Absorption and metabolism of lanatoside C. Clin Pharmacol Ther 21:647, 1977.
43. BROWN DD, JUHL RP: Decreased bioavailability of digoxin due to antacids and kaolin-pectin. N Engl J Med 295:1034, 1976.
44. THOMAS R, ALDOUS S: The double peak in the plasma-drug curve after oral digoxin and lanatoside C. Lancet 2:1267, 1973.
45. GREENBLATT DJ, et al: Bioavailability of digoxin tablets and elixir in the fasting and postprandial states. Clin Pharmacol Ther 16:444, 1974.
46. WHITE RJ, et al: Plasma concentrations of digoxin after oral administration in the fasting and postprandial state. Br Med J 1:380, 1971.
47. KHALIL SAH: Bioavailability of digoxin in presence of antacids (Letter). J Pharm Sci 63:1641, 1974.
48. McELNAY JC, et al: Interaction of digoxin with antacid constituents (Letter). Br Med J 2:1554, 1978.
49. BROWN DD, et al: Decreased bioavailability of digoxin produced by dietary fiber and cholestyramine (Abstract). Am J Cardiol 39:297, 1977.
50. BAZZANO G, BAZZANO GS: Effect of digitalis-binding resins on cardiac glycoside plasma levels (Abstract). Clin Res 20:24, 1972.
51. WALDORFF S, et al: Spironolactone-induced changes in digoxin kinetics. Clin Pharmacol Ther 24:162, 1978.
52. LICHEY J, et al: The effect of oral spironolactone and intravenous carenoate-K on the digoxin radioimmunoassay. Int J Clin Pharmacol 15:557, 1977.
53. STEINESS E: Renal tubular secretion of digoxin. Circulation 50:103, 1974.
54. WALDORFF S, et al: Amiloride-induced changes in digoxin dynamics and kinetics: abolition of digoxin-induced inotropism with amiloride. Clin Pharmacol Ther 30:172, 1981.
55. CASTILLO-FERRANDO JR, et al: Digoxin levels and diazepam. Lancet 1:368, 1980.
56. QUATTROCCHI FP, et al: The effects of ibuprofen on serum digoxin concentrations. Drug Intell Clin Pharm 17:286, 1983.
57. MOEZZI B, et al: The effect of penicillamine on serum digoxin levels. Jap Heart J 19:366, 1978.
58. BELZ GG, et al: Digoxin plasma concentrations and nifedipine. Lancet 1:844, 1981.
59. PEDERSON KE, et al: Effect of nifedipine on digoxin kinetics in healthy subjects. Clin Pharmacol Ther 32:562, 1982.
60. ALLEN MD, et al: Effect of magnesium-aluminum hydroxide and kaolin-pectin on absorption of digoxin from tablets and capsules. J Clin Pharmacol 21:26, 1981.
61. PIERONI RE, FISHER JG: Use of cholestyramine resin in digitoxin toxicity. JAMA 245:1939, 1981.
62. CARRUTHERS SG, DUJOVNE CA: Cholestyramine and spironolactone and their combination in digitoxin elimination. Clin Pharmacol Ther 27:184, 1980.
63. ALBERT KS, et al: Influence of kaolin-pectin suspension on steady-state plasma digoxin levels. J Clin Pharmacol 21:449, 1981.

References (CONT.)

64. Zylber-Katz E, et al: Pharmacokinetic study of digoxin and nifedipine coadministration. Clin Pharmacol Ther 35:286, 1984.
65. Steiness E: Renal tubular secretion of digoxin. Circulation 50:103, 1974.
66. Waldorff S, et al: Spironolactone-induced changes in digoxin kinetics. Clin Pharmacol Ther 24:162, 1978.
67. Lichey J, et al: The influence of intravenous canrenoate on the determination of digoxin in serum by radio- and enzyme-immunoassay. Int J Clin Pharmacol Biopharm 17:61, 1979.
68. DiPiro JT, et al: Spironolactone interference with digoxin radioimmunoassay in cirrhotic patients. Am J Hosp Pharm 37:1518, 1980.
69. Silber B, et al: Spironolactone-associated digoxin radioimmunoassay interference. Clin Chem 25:48, 1979.
70. Huffman DH: The effect of spironolactone and canrenone on the digoxin radioimmunoassay. Res Commun Chem Pathol Pharmacol 9:787, 1974.
71. Muller H, et al: Cross reactivity of digitoxin and spironolactone in two radioimmunoassays for serum digoxin. Clin Chem 24:706, 1978.
72. Paladino JA, et al: Influence of spironolactone on serum digoxin concentration. JAMA 251:470, 1984.
73. Thomas RW, Maddox RR: The interaction of spironolactone and digoxin: A review and evaluation. Ther Drug Monit 3:117, 1981.
74. Fraley DS, et al: Effect of cimetidine on steady-state serum digoxin concentrations. Clin Pharm 2:163, 1983.
75. Ochs HR, et al: Cimetidine impairs clearance of creatinine but not of digoxin. Clin Pharmacol Ther 33:218, 1983.
76. Gault H, et al: Influence of gastric pH on digoxin biotransformation. I. Intragastric hydrolysis. Clin Pharmacol Ther 27:16, 1980.
77. McGilveray IJ, et al: Digoxin dosage in patients with gastric hyperacidity. Can Med Assoc J 121:704, 1979.
78. Polish LB, et al: Digitoxin-quinidine interaction: potentiation during administration of cimetidine. South Med J 74:634, 1981.

CHAPTER 9

Diuretic Drug Interactions

ACETAZOLAMIDE (DIAMOX) INTERACTIONS

DRUGS	DISCUSSION

Amphetamine[31,32]

MECHANISM: Acetazolamide tends to render the urine alkaline, resulting in an increased proportion of un-ionized amphetamine. Thus, renal tubular reabsorption of the amphetamine is increased, and more of the drug is eventually eliminated by hepatic metabolism.

CLINICAL SIGNIFICANCE: Well documented. Excretion of free amphetamine is extremely small in a highly alkaline urine, thus enhancing (or at least prolonging) the effect of the amphetamine. Individuals abusing amphetamines have made use of this property by ingesting sodium bicarbonate along with the amphetamine. Also, evidence from 11 patients with amphetamine psychosis indicates that with an alkaline urine, more amphetamine may be metabolized and these metabolites may contribute to the amphetamine psychosis.[32]

MANAGEMENT: It does not seem necessary to avoid concomitant use, but it should be realized that patients on acetazolamide may have enhanced effects from amphetamines.

Chlorthalidone (Hygroton)[29]

MECHANISM: Preliminary evidence indicates that acetazolamide may displace chlorthalidone from blood cells.

CLINICAL SIGNIFICANCE: Study in two normal subjects indicated that acetazolamide reduced the chlorthalidone content of blood cells and considerably reduced the plasma half-life of chlorthalidone.[29] The clinical effect of these pharmacokinetic changes has not been established.

MANAGEMENT: No special precautions appear necessary.

Ephedrine[61]

MECHANISM: Acetazolamide-induced alkalinization of the urine decreases the ionization of ephedrine, thus enhancing renal tubular reabsorption.

CLINICAL SIGNIFICANCE: Study in normal subjects given single doses of ephedrine have shown that urinary excretion of ephedrine is re-

DRUGS	DISCUSSION

duced when the urine is alkaline.[61] Short-term urinary alkalinization is unlikely to be clinically important, but ephedrine toxicity is possible if the urine remains alkaline for several days or longer.

MANAGEMENT: Monitor for evidence of ephedrine toxicity (e.g., nervousness, insomnia, excitability) if the urine remains alkaline for more than a day or two. Adjust ephedrine dose as needed.

Lithium Carbonate (Eskalith, Lithane, Lithonate)[4]

MECHANISM: Acetazolamide presumably impairs the proximal tubular reabsorption of lithium ions, thus increasing lithium excretion.

CLINICAL SIGNIFICANCE: Not established. It is possible that the increased lithium excretion could impair the therapeutic response to lithium carbonate but long-term studies are needed to confirm such an effect.

MANAGEMENT: No special precautions appear necessary.

Salicylates[34,62]

MECHANISM: It is proposed that carbonic anhydrase inhibitors such as acetazolamide, by reducing the blood pH, may produce a shift of salicylate from the plasma into the tissues.

CLINICAL SIGNIFICANCE: Animal studies indicate that acetazolamide may worsen salicylate intoxication by shifting salicylate into tissues. Also, patients receiving anti-arthritic doses of salicylates have developed evidence of central nervous system salicylate toxicity such as dizziness, lethargy, and disorientation during concurrent therapy with carbonic anhydrase inhibitors such as acetazolamide.[62]

MANAGEMENT: It has been recommended that acetazolamide be avoided in patients with salicylate intoxication.[34] In patients on large doses of salicylates, one should be alert for evidence of increased serum salicylate levels if carbonic anhydrase inhibitors are given concurrently. A reduction in salicylate dosage may be required.

BUMETANIDE INTERACTIONS

DRUGS	DISCUSSION

Indomethacin (Indocin)[56,58-60]

MECHANISM: Indomethacin inhibits prostaglandin synthesis, resulting in a tendency for the patient to retain sodium.

CLINICAL SIGNIFICANCE: Indomethacin reduces the natriuretic and diuretic response to bumetanide in both healthy subjects and patients with hypertension.[56,58-60] Prostaglandin inhibitors other than indomethacin (e.g., other nonsteroidal anti-inflammatory drugs) may have a similar effect on bumetanide, but few data are available.

BUMETANIDE INTERACTIONS (CONT.)

DRUGS	DISCUSSION

MANAGEMENT: Monitor for reduced diuretic and natriuretic response to bumetanide in the presence of indomethacin. Furosemide (Lasix) is also affected by indomethacin, and thus would not be a suitable non-interacting alternative. Aspirin may be less likely to interfere with bumetanide response, and may be worth trying in place of indomethacin if the interaction becomes troublesome.

Probenecid (Benemid)[55,56]

MECHANISM: Not established.

CLINICAL SIGNIFICANCE: Bumetanide diuresis may be slightly reduced in the presence of probenecid,[55] although this has not been a consistent finding.[56]

MANAGEMENT: No special precautions appear necessary, although one should be alert for the possibility of reduced bumetanide response.

CHLORTHALIDONE (HYGROTON) INTERACTIONS

DRUGS	DISCUSSION

Carbenoxolone[43]

MECHANISM: Chlorthalidone and carbenoxolone may have additive hypokalemic effects.

CLINICAL SIGNIFICANCE: A patient receiving carbenoxolone and chlorthalidone with no potassium supplementation developed a severe potassium deficiency with associated rhabdomyolysis and acute tubular necrosis.[43] It appears likely that the combination of carbenoxolone with any potassium wasting diuretic could produce a similar effect, especially in the absence of potassium supplementation.

MANAGEMENT: The potassium status of patients receiving carbenoxolone and a potassium wasting diuretic should be monitored closely. Potassium supplementation may be necessary.

Corticosteroids[3]

MECHANISM: Potassium-losing diuretics such as chlorthalidone may result in excessive potassium loss when given with corticosteroids.

CLINICAL SIGNIFICANCE: This interaction is based primarily on clinical observations rather than controlled trials, but there is little doubt that the combination can result in potassium depletion. This is especially true in patients with inadequate potassium intake.

MANAGEMENT: Special attention should be given to potassium balance when corticosteroids are given to patients receiving potassium-losing diuretics.

ETHACRYNIC ACID (EDECRIN) INTERACTIONS

DRUGS	DISCUSSION

Corticosteroids[3]

MECHANISM: Potent potassium-losing diuretics such as ethacrynic acid may result in excessive potassium loss when given with corticosteroids.

CLINICAL SIGNIFICANCE: This interaction is based primarily on clinical observations rather than controlled trials, but there is little doubt that the combination can result in severe potassium depletion. This is especially true in patients with inadequate potassium intake.

MANAGEMENT: Special attention should be given to the potassium balance when corticosteroids are given to patients receiving ethacrynic acid.

Lithium Carbonate (Eskalith, Lithane, Lithonate)[2,4]

MECHANISM: Lithium excretion decreases with sodium depletion, which in turn can be caused by sustained ethacrynic acid therapy.

CLINICAL SIGNIFICANCE: Acute experiments failed to demonstrate an effect of ethacrynic acid on lithium excretion.[4] However, one case of lithium intoxication has been reported which appeared to be due to furosemide (Lasix) plus dietary sodium restriction.[2] It seems reasonable that ethacrynic acid could have a similar effect.

MANAGEMENT: In patients receiving lithium carbonate, ethacrynic acid therapy should be undertaken cautiously, especially if dietary sodium is restricted. More frequent serum lithium determinations may be desirable.

FUROSEMIDE (LASIX) INTERACTIONS

DRUGS	DISCUSSION

Chloral Hydrate (Noctec)[41,44,45]

MECHANISM: Not established. Some plasma protein binding competition may be involved, but there is little supporting evidence.

CLINICAL SIGNIFICANCE: Six patients in a coronary care unit developed sweating, flushed skin, blood pressure variations, and uneasiness when furosemide (40 to 120 mg intravenously) was given in the presence of previous oral chloral hydrate.[44] In one patient, furosemide failed to produce the reaction when chloral hydrate was discontinued, but the reaction occurred again after chloral hydrate had been resumed. A subsequent retrospective study identified one probable and two possible cases of this interaction.[41] There is some evidence that hypoalbuminemia may increase the likelihood of symptoms from this interaction. It is not known whether oral furosemide could produce this reaction, but it is probably much less likely to do so than intravenous furosemide.

FUROSEMIDE (LASIX) INTERACTIONS (CONT.)

DRUGS	DISCUSSION

MANAGEMENT: Intravenous furosemide should be given with caution to any patient who has received chloral hydrate within the previous 24 hours.

Clofibrate (Atromid-S)[5,45]

MECHANISM: It is proposed that furosemide and clofibrate may compete for plasma albumin binding sites. Experimental evidence indicates that at plasma albumin concentrations below 2 g/100 ml the unbound fraction of furosemide increases considerably,[45] which lends support to a mechanism of protein binding competition in the patients described below.

CLINICAL SIGNIFICANCE: In several patients with nephrotic syndrome, hypoalbuminemia, and hyperlipoproteinemia, combined treatment with furosemide and clofibrate resulted in muscular symptoms (pain, stiffness, etc.) as well as a marked diuresis.[5] It seems likely that the competition for albumin binding between the two drugs and the hypoalbuminemia resulted in higher free levels of both drugs, thus causing the muscular syndrome and the pronounced diuresis. However, additional study will be required to establish conclusively that the interaction was responsible for the effects.

MANAGEMENT: Concomitant use of clofibrate and furosemide should be undertaken with some caution, especially if hypoalbuminemia is present.

Corticosteroids[3]

MECHANISM: Potent potassium-losing diuretics such as furosemide may result in excessive potassium loss when given with corticosteroids.

CLINICAL SIGNIFICANCE: This interaction is primarily based on clinical observations rather than controlled trials, but there is little doubt that the combination can result in severe potassium depletion. This is especially true in patients with inadequate potassium intake.

MANAGEMENT: Special attention should be given to the potassium balance when corticosteroids are given to patients receiving furosemide.

Indomethacin (Indocin)[52,53,72–81]

MECHANISM: It may be related to indomethacin-induced inhibition of prostaglandins.

CLINICAL SIGNIFICANCE: Indomethacin has been shown to inhibit the antihypertensive and diuretic effects of furosemide[74–76] in normal subjects and hypertensive patients.[74–76] In addition, patients with congestive heart failure maintained on furosemide have worsened after the addition of indomethacin therapy.[72,73] It seems likely that other nonsteroidal anti-inflammatory drugs would similarly inhibit

DRUGS	DISCUSSION

the response to furosemide, and there is some clinical evidence to support this view with drugs such as naproxen, ibuprofen, and large doses of salicylates.[77] There is also some clinical evidence indicating that sulindac may be less likely to interfere with the response to furosemide,[78-80] but the difference may only be relative.[81] In a study of eight patients with rheumatoid arthritis, furosemide (40 mg orally) was associated with lower plasma indomethacin levels following a single dose of indomethacin (50 mg orally).[52] However, since indomethacin plasma levels were measured for only 3 hours, one cannot conclude that the total effect of indomethacin would be decreased. In summary, indomethacin and most other nonsteroidal anti-inflammatory drugs appear to inhibit the diuretic and antihypertensive response to furosemide, and the interaction appears to be clinically important in at least some patients. The ability of furosemide to affect the response to indomethacin is not well established.

MANAGEMENT: One should be alert for evidence of reduced furosemide response in the presence of indomethacin or other nonsteroidal anti-inflammatory drugs (NSAIDs). If increasing the dose of furosemide does not achieve the desired response, one might consider trying a different NSAID (sulindac or salicylates may not affect furosemide to the same degree).

Lithium Carbonate (Eskalith, Lithane, Lithonate)[2,4,38,63]

MECHANISM: Lithium excretion decreases with sodium depletion, which in turn can be caused by sustained furosemide therapy.

CLINICAL SIGNIFICANCE: Although acute experiments failed to demonstrate an effect of furosemide on lithium excretion,[4] one case of lithium intoxication has been reported which appeared to be due to furosemide plus dietary sodium restriction.[2] Another case of purported furosemide-induced lithium intoxication has appeared,[38] but it does not seem clear that furosemide was responsible. In five normal subjects stabilized on lithium, furosemide (40 mg/day for 2 weeks) did not affect serum lithium levels, but a significant rise in serum lithium occurred during treatment with hydrochlorothiazide (50 mg/day for 2 weeks).[63] Larger doses of furosemide were not studied. Thus, there is relatively little evidence to indicate that furosemide affects serum lithium levels, but it is possible that the interaction occurs under certain circumstances.

MANAGEMENT: Although most patients are probably unaffected by this interaction, one should be alert for evidence of altered lithium levels if furosemide is initiated or discontinued.

Neuromuscular Blocking Agents[6,7,48,64]

MECHANISM: Not established.

CLINICAL SIGNIFICANCE: Three patients given tubocurarine during surgery developed enhanced neuromuscular blockade following ad-

FUROSEMIDE (LASIX) INTERACTIONS (CONT.)

DRUGS	DISCUSSION

ministration of furosemide.[48] Although mannitol was given concomitantly in most cases, it seems likely that the furosemide was primarily responsible. Animal studies indicate that low doses of furosemide enhance the neuromuscular blockade of tubocurarine and succinylcholine while high doses (1 to 4 mg/kg body weight) of furosemide antagonized the neuromuscular blockade.[64]

MANAGEMENT: One should be alert for altered dosage requirements for neuromuscular blocking agents in patients receiving furosemide.

Probenecid (Benemid)[46,47]

MECHANISM: Furosemide is apparently excreted primarily by active renal tubular secretion, which may be inhibited by concomitant probenecid therapy.

CLINICAL SIGNIFICANCE: Two studies have demonstrated an ability of probenecid to considerably reduce renal clearance of furosemide.[46,47] However, the ability of furosemide to increase urinary sodium excretion was minimally affected.

MANAGEMENT: No special precautions appear necessary.

SPIRONOLACTONE (ALDACTONE) INTERACTIONS

DRUGS	DISCUSSION

Ammonium Chloride[1,26]

MECHANISM: It is proposed that the inhibition of aldosterone by spironolactone may impair the ability of the kidney to secrete hydrogen ions, and in the presence of acidifying doses of ammonium chloride the combination may produce systemic acidosis.

CLINICAL SIGNIFICANCE: One patient treated with spironolactone, ammonium chloride, and potassium chloride developed acidosis,[1] and it was felt that the combination of spironolactone and ammonium chloride was at least partially responsible. The hyperkalemia caused by the spironolactone and potassium chloride may have contributed to the acidosis. A subsequent study in four normal volunteers showed that spironolactone pretreatment prevented the urinary acidification of ammonium chloride,[26] which is consistent with the ability of this combination to produce acidosis.

MANAGEMENT: The combination of spironolactone and acidifying doses of ammonium chloride should probably be given with some caution and with attention to the detection of acidosis.

Antipyrine[15,16]

MECHANISM: Spironolactone appears to stimulate the hepatic metabolism of antipyrine.

DRUGS	DISCUSSION

CLINICAL SIGNIFICANCE: In nine healthy subjects, the administration of spironolactone (100 mg/day for 14 days) resulted in a decreased antipyrine half-life in each case.[15] This raises the possibility that spironolactone might also stimulate the metabolism of other, more widely used drugs.

MANAGEMENT: The practitioner should consider the possibility that the clinical effect of antipyrine might be reduced somewhat by spironolactone, although no special precautions appear to be necessary.

Carbenoxolone[23]

MECHANISM: Not established.

CLINICAL SIGNIFICANCE: In one study of outpatients with chronic gastric ulcers treated with carbenoxolone, spironolactone appeared to inhibit both the side effects and ulcer healing of carbenoxolone.[23] Thiazide diuretics did not seem to affect the ulcer healing properties of carbenoxolone.

MANAGEMENT: Although clinical evidence is not extensive, it would probably be wise to avoid the use of spironolactone in patients receiving carbenoxolone.

Food[42]

MECHANISM: A possible explanation for enhanced bioavailability of spironolactone may be that food, by delaying gastric emptying, improves dissolution of the compound. Also, the solubility of spironolactone may be enhanced by cholic acids secreted in response to food.[42]

CLINICAL SIGNIFICANCE: Single dose studies in eight healthy men indicated that food enhanced the availability of spironolactone as evidenced by increased peak plasma concentrations and greater areas under the curve of canrenone, the major active metabolite of spironolactone.[42]

MANAGEMENT: It may be useful to dose spironolactone with food to enhance availability.[42]

Lithium Carbonate (Eskalith, Lithane, Lithonate)[33]

MECHANISM: Not established.

CLINICAL SIGNIFICANCE: In several patients with manic depressive illness, spironolactone (100 mg/daily) was associated with increasing serum lithium levels.[33] Studies in additional patients are needed to assess the clinical importance of these findings.

MANAGEMENT: Until this potential interaction is better described, one should be alert for evidence of altered serum lithium levels if spironolactone is given concomitantly.

DRUGS	DISCUSSION

Potassium Chloride[1,17-19,37]

MECHANISM: Spironolactone conserves potassium, and hyperkalemia may result if potassium supplements are also given.

CLINICAL SIGNIFICANCE: Severe or fatal hyperkalemia has been reported in patients receiving concomitant spironolactone and potassium chloride.[1,17-19] If the patient has significant renal disease, the combination of spironolactone and potassium chloride is especially likely to produce hyperkalemia. In one study patients with severe azotemia and on spironolactone plus potassium chloride, the incidence of hyperkalemia was 42%.[19] Another study has shown that the combined use of spironolactone and oral potassium chloride occurred in at least 104 patients during a 2-year period in one hospital.[37] A chart review of 25 of these patients revealed that 13 (52%) developed hyperkalemia.

MANAGEMENT: The combination of spironolactone and potassium chloride has been used successfully to treat severe potassium depletion. However, patients so treated must be monitored very closely to detect hyperkalemia. If azotemia is also present, the benefits of combined therapy would not seem likely to outweigh the risks in most patients.

Propoxyphene (Darvon)[39]

MECHANISM: Not established.

CLINICAL SIGNIFICANCE: A patient who had been receiving spironolactone for 4 years with no evidence of gynecomastia was given Darvon Compound (propoxyphene, aspirin, caffeine, phenacetin).[39] Two weeks later the patient complained of swollen, tender breasts and a pruritic rash, both of which resolved when spironolactone and the Darvon Compound were discontinued. Challenge with the Darvon Compound alone resulted in reappearance of the rash and the drug was discontinued. Readministration of the spironolactone alone did not produce breast changes but both gynecomastia and the rash reappeared when Darvon Compound was added to the spironolactone. Although the combination may have caused gynecomastia in this patient, few conclusions can be drawn until additional studies are done.

MANAGEMENT: No special precautions appear to be necessary at this time.

Salicylates[20-22,25,27,40]

MECHANISM: There is evidence that aspirin reduces the active renal tubular secretion of the active metabolite of spironolactone, canrenone.[27] This reduction in tubular secretion of canrenone is thought to reduce the pharmacologic activity of administered spironolactone.

CLINICAL SIGNIFICANCE: Aspirin has been shown to inhibit somewhat the natriuresis produced by spironolactone in humans[20,21,27] and animals.[22] However, the effect of spironolactone on urinary potas-

SPIRONOLACTONE (ALDACTONE) INTERACTIONS (CONT.)

DRUGS	DISCUSSION

sium excretion does not appear to be inhibited,[27] nor does the antihypertensive response to spironolactone appear to be affected.[40] The clinical importance of combined spironolactone and aspirin use is still not clear, but in most cases it is probably not large.

MANAGEMENT: It does not seem necessary to avoid aspirin use in patients receiving spironolactone. However, until the potential interaction is better defined, one should be alert for evidence of reduced spironolactone response if aspirin is taken concurrently.

Salt Substitutes[35,65]

MECHANISM: Salt substitutes contain large amounts of potassium and may result in hyperkalemia if taken by patients receiving potassium-retaining diuretics such as spironolactone.

CLINICAL SIGNIFICANCE: Two patients receiving spironolactone developed severe hyperkalemia with cardiac arrhythmias following excessive use of salt substitutes.[35] Another report described a 63-year-old man on furosemide and spironolactone who developed hyperkalemia during use of a salt substitute.[65]

MANAGEMENT: Patients receiving spironolactone should be warned against the use of salt substitutes unless recommended by their physician. If salt substitutes are used with spironolactone, intake of the salt substitute must be carefully controlled and the potassium status of the patient closely monitored.

THIAZIDE DIURETIC INTERACTIONS

DRUGS	DISCUSSION

Cholestyramine (Questran)[8,9,66]

MECHANISM: Cholestyramine is an anion-exchange resin that may bind acidic drugs such as thiazide diuretics in the gut.

CLINICAL SIGNIFICANCE: In six healthy subjects, 8 gm of cholestyramine reduced the total urinary excretion of a single 75 mg dose of hydrochlorothiazide by 85% and markedly reduced plasma hydrochlorothiazide concentrations.[66] Thus, cholestyramine would be expected to substantially reduce the therapeutic effect of hydrochlorothiazide, and probably also other thiazide diuretics.

MANAGEMENT: Administer thiazide diuretics at least 2 hours before the cholestyramine, and be alert for the need to increase the dose of the thiazide. Colestipol (Colestid) appears to inhibit hydrochlorothiazide absorption to a lesser extent than cholestyramine,[66] but one should still separate the doses to minimize the interaction.

THIAZIDE DIURETIC INTERACTIONS (CONT.)

DRUGS	DISCUSSION

Colestipol (Colestid)[10,66]

MECHANISM: Colestipol appears to inhibit the gastrointestinal absorption of chlorothiazide (Diuril).

CLINICAL SIGNIFICANCE: In ten patients with hyperlipoproteinemia, colestipol given at the same time as chlorothiazide or 1 hour after chlorothiazide resulted in considerable decreases in chlorothiazide absorption as measured by cumulative urinary excretion.[10] In six healthy subjects, 10 gm of colestipol reduced total urinary excretion of a single 75 mg dose of hydrochlorothiazide by 43% and also reduced plasma levels of the diuretic.[66] Thus, it seems likely that colestipol would inhibit the therapeutic response to thiazide diuretics.

MANAGEMENT: Administer the thiazide diuretic at least 2 hours before the colestipol; increase the thiazide dosage if needed.

Corticosteroids[3]

MECHANISM: Potassium-losing diuretics such as thiazides may result in excessive potassium loss when given with corticosteroids.

CLINICAL SIGNIFICANCE: This interaction is based primarily on clinical observations rather than on controlled trials, but there is little doubt that the combination can result in potassium depletion. This is especially true in patients with inadequate potassium intake.

MANAGEMENT: Special attention should be given to potassium balance when corticosteroids are given to patients receiving potassium-losing diuretics.

Cytotoxic agents[57]

MECHANISM: Not established. Thiazide diuretics theoretically could reduce renal methotrexate excretion.

CLINICAL SIGNIFICANCE: In 14 women with breast cancer receiving chemotherapy (cyclophosphamide, methotrexate, and 5-fluoracil) thiazide therapy appeared to enhance the myelosuppressive effect.[57] It is possible that if this interaction is real, it results from an effect of thiazides on one of the components (e.g., methotrexate) rather than cytotoxic agents in general.

MANAGEMENT: One should be alert for enhanced bone marrow suppression if thiazides are used concurrently with cytotoxic agents. Adjust cytotoxic drug dosage as needed.

Lithium Carbonate (Eskalith, Lithane, Lithonate)[2,4,24,28,30,33,36,50,51,63,67–70]

MECHANISM: It has been proposed that prolonged thiazide treatment causes a compensatory increase in proximal tubule reabsorption of sodium, resulting in increased lithium reabsorption as well.[24]

THIAZIDE DIURETIC INTERACTIONS (CONT.)

DRUGS	DISCUSSION

CLINICAL SIGNIFICANCE: Although bendroflumethiazide (Naturetin) did not affect urinary lithium excretion in short-term studies,[4] long-term thiazide therapy has been shown to decrease considerably renal lithium clearance.[24] The long-term thiazide therapy resulted in a 24% reduction in lithium clearance, which is of sufficient magnitude to result in elevated serum lithium levels and lithium toxicity. Indeed, serious lithium toxicity has resulted from thiazide diuretic therapy in several patients.[67,68,70] Since lithium and thiazide diuretics are both capable of increasing serum calcium levels, it is also possible that some patients on combined therapy may develop hypercalcemia.[69]

MANAGEMENT: Concomitant use of lithium carbonate and thiazide diuretics should be undertaken with caution. Serum lithium determinations should be performed and the lithium dose reduced as needed.

Skeletal Muscle Relaxants (Surgical)[11–13]

MECHANISM: Thiazides reportedly increase responsiveness to tubocurarine and gallamine, an effect that may be related to thiazide-induced potassium deficiency.

CLINICAL SIGNIFICANCE: Clinical reports describing this interaction appear to be lacking, although undocumented statements frequently occur indicating that the interaction is clinically significant.

MANAGEMENT: The possible increased response to nondepolarizing muscle relaxants plus the possible decreased arterial responsiveness to vasopressors dictates caution in performing surgery in patients receiving thiazides.

TRIAMTERENE (DYRENIUM) INTERACTIONS

DRUGS	DISCUSSION

Amantadine (Symmetrel)[71]

MECHANISM: Not established. There is some evidence that a triamterene-hydrochlorothiazide combination (Dyazide) may reduce the renal excretion of amantadine.

CLINICAL SIGNIFICANCE: A 61-year-old man developed evidence of amantadine toxicity (ataxia, agitation, hallucinations) 1 week after starting Dyazide therapy.[71] The symptoms resolved after stopping both drugs. When amantadine was restarted no symptoms occurred until Dyazide was added. Starting the Dyazide was also associated with a reduction in the renal excretion of amantadine, and an increase in serum amantadine concentration from 156 to 243 ng/ml. Although the Dyazide was probably responsible for the amantadine toxicity in this patient, it is not clear how often the interaction would occur in other patients receiving this combination. Also, it is not possible to determine, with available data, which of the components of the Diazide was responsible for the interaction.

DRUGS	DISCUSSION

MANAGEMENT: In patients receiving amantadine one should use triamterene or thiazide diuretics with caution. The amantidine dosage should be reduced as needed.

Indomethacin (Indocin)[54]

MECHANISM: It is proposed that indomethacin inhibits the prostaglandins that are normally secreted to protect against triamterene-induced nephrotoxicity.

CLINICAL SIGNIFICANCE: Four healthy subjects were given triamterene (200 mg/day for 3 days) with and without indomethacin (150 mg/day before and during triamterene).[54] Two of the subjects developed substantial reductions (62% and 72%) in creatinine clearance with concurrent administration of the drugs, but not with either drug alone. Triamterene was also associated with 60% and 69% reductions in urinary indomethacin excretion in these two subjects. Neither triamterene nor indomethacin appeared to affect the creatinine assay. The magnitude of the reductions in renal function in the two affected subjects following concurrent use of triamterene and indomethacin are sufficient to question the advisability of using the combination in practice. The authors indicate that nephrotoxicity was not seen when indomethacin was combined with furosemide (Lasix), hydrochlorothiazide, or spironolactone (Aldactone), and they suggest that these agents may be suitable alternatives in the patient receiving indomethacin. However, one should remember that indomethacin may inhibit the antihypertensive response to both furosemide and thiazides and may also reduce furosemide-induced natriuresis. Little is known regarding the effect of nonsteroidal anti-inflammatory drugs other than indomethacin on triamterene. Also, study in more people will be required to ascertain the incidence and magnitude of the nephrotoxic effect of combined use of indomethacin and triamterene.

MANAGEMENT: Until this interaction is better studied, one should carefully monitor renal function in patients on combined therapy with triamterene and nonsteroidal anti-inflammatory agents such as indomethacin. It is possible that spironolactone is less likely than triamterene to interact adversely with indomethacin, but this has not been established clinically.

Potassium Chloride[14]

MECHANISM: Triamterene conserves potassium, and hyperkalemia may result if potassium supplements are also given.

CLINICAL SIGNIFICANCE: Severe hyperkalemia has occasionally resulted from triamterene administration, and the addition of potassium supplements increases the likelihood of this adverse reaction. One case of pacemaker failure from hyperkalemia has been reported.[14] It resulted from the combined administration of potassium chloride and a preparation containing triamterene and hydro-

TRIAMTERENE (DYRENIUM) INTERACTIONS (CONT.)

DRUGS	DISCUSSION

chlorothiazide (Dyazide). Patients with azotemia would probably be more likely to manifest hyperkalemia from combined use of triamterene and potassium salts.

MANAGEMENT: It would be best to avoid the use of triamterene and potassium together. If combined use is felt to be necessary, potassium balance should be monitored very closely.

References

1. MASHFORD ML, ROBERTSON MB: Spironolactone and ammonium and potassium chloride (Letter). Br Med J 4:299, 1972.
2. HURTIG HI, DYSON WL: Lithium toxicity enhanced by diuresis (Letter). N Engl J Med 290:748, 1974.
3. THORN GW: Clinical considerations in the use of corticosteroids. N Engl J Med 274:775, 1966.
4. THOMSEN K, SCHOU M: Renal lithium excretion in man. Am J Physiol 215:823, 1968.
5. BRIDGMAN JF, et al: Complications during clofibrate treatment of nephrotic-syndrome hyperlipoproteinaemia. Lancet 2:506, 1972.
6. ANON: Lasix. Med Lett 9:6, 1967.
7. Lasix. Product Information. Somerville, New Jersey, Hoechst Pharmaceutical Co., 1984.
8. GALLO DG, et al: The interaction between cholestyramine and drugs. Proc Soc Exp Biol Med 120:60, 1965.
9. Questran. Product Information. Evansville, Indiana, Mead Johnson Laboratories, 1984.
10. KAUFFMAN RE, AZARNOFF DL: Effect of colestipol on gastrointestinal absorption of chlorothiazide in man. Clin Pharmacol Ther 14:886, 1973.
11. GODDARD JE, PHILLIPS OC: The influence of nonanesthetic drugs on the course of anesthesia. Penn Med J 68:48, 1965.
12. Esidrix. Product Information. Summit, New Jersey, CIBA Pharmaceutical Co., 1984.
13. SPHIRE RD: Gallamine: a second look. Anesth Analg 43:690, 1964.
14. O'REILLY MV, et al: Transvenous pacemaker failure induced by hyperkalemia. JAMA 228:336, 1974.
15. HUFFMAN DH, et al: The effect of spironolactone on antipyrine metabolism in man. Pharmacology 10:338, 1973.
16. TAYLOR SA, et al: Spironolactone—a weak enzyme inducer in man (Letter). J Pharm Pharmacol 24:578, 1972.
17. KALBIAN VV: Iatrogenic hyperkalemic paralysis with electrocardiographic changes. South Med J 67:342, 1974.
18. SHAPIRO S, et al: Fatal reactions among medical inpatients. JAMA 216:467, 1971.
19. GREENBLATT DJ, KOCH-WESER J: Adverse reactions to spironolactone: a report from The Boston Collaborative Drug Surveillance Program (Abstract). Clin Pharmacol Ther 14:136, 1973.

References (CONT.)

20. TWEEDDALE MG, OGILVIE RI: Antagonism of spironolactone-induced natriuresis by aspirin in man. N Engl J Med 289:198, 1973.
21. ELLIOT HC: Reduced adrenocortical steroid excretion rates in man following aspirin administration. Metabolism 11:1015, 1962.
22. HOFMANN LM, et al: Interactions of spironolactone and hydrochlorothiazide with aspirin in the rat and dog. J Pharmacol Exp Ther 180:1, 1972.
23. DOLL R, et al: Treatment of gastric ulcer with carbenoxolone: antagonistic effect of spironolactone. Gut 9:42, 1968.
24. PETERSEN V, et al: Effect of prolonged thiazide treatment on renal lithium clearance. Br Med J 2:143, 1974.
25. ALBERTI RL (Searle Laboratories): Personal Communication. July 21, 1975.
26. MANUEL MA, et al: An effect of spironolactone on urinary acidification in normal man. Arch Intern Med 134:472, 1974.
27. RAMSAY LE, et al: Influence of acetylsalicylic acid on the renal handling of a spironolactone metabolite in healthy subjects. Eur J Clin Pharmacol 10:43, 1976.
28. LEVY ST, et al: Lithium-induced diabetes insipidus: manic symptoms, brain and electrolyte correlates and chlorothiazide treatment. Am J Psychiatry 130:1014, 1973.
29. BEERMANN B, et al: Binding-site interaction of chlorthalidone and acetazolamide, two drugs transported by red blood cells. Clin Pharmacol Ther 17:424, 1975.
30. MACNEIL S, et al: Diuretics during lithium therapy (Letter). Lancet 1:1295, 1975.
31. ROWLAND M: Amphetamine blood and urine levels in man. J Pharm Sci 58:508, 1969.
32. ANGGARD E, et al: Amphetamine metabolism in amphetamine psychosis. Clin Pharmacol Ther 14:870, 1973.
33. BAER L, et al: Mechanisms of renal lithium handling and their relationship to mineralocorticoids: a dissociation between sodium and lithium ions. J Psychiatr Res 8:91, 1971.
34. HILL JB: Experimental salicylate poisoning: observations on effects of altering blood pH on tissue and plasma salicylate concentrations. Pediatrics 47:658, 1971.
35. YAP V, et al: Hyperkalemia with cardiac arrhythmia. JAMA 236:2775, 1976.
36. HIMMELHOCH JM, et al: Thiazide-lithium synergy in refractory mood swings. Am J Psychiatry 134:149, 1977.
37. SIMBORG DN: Medication prescribing on a university medical service— the incidence of drug combinations with potential adverse interactions. Johns Hopkins Med J 139:23, 1976.
38. OH TE: Frusemide and lithium toxicity. Anaesth Intensive Care 5(1):60, 1977.
39. LICATA AA, BARTTER FC: Spironolactone-induced gynecomastia related to allergic reaction to 'darvon compound' (Letter). Lancet 1:905, 1976.
40. HOLLIFIELD JW: Failure of aspirin to antagonize the antihypertensive effect of spironolactone in low-renin hypertension. South Med J 69:1034, 1976.
41. PEVONKA MP, et al: Interaction of chloral hydrate and furosemide. Drug Intell Clin Pharm 11:332, 1977.

References (CONT.)

42. MELANDER A, et al: Enhancement by food of canrenone bioavailability from spironolactone. Clin Pharmacol Ther 22:100, 1977.
43. DESCAMPS C: Rhabdomyolysis and acute tubular necrosis associated with carbenoxolone and diuretic treatment. Br Med J 1:272, 1977.
44. MALACH M, BERMAN N: Furosemide and chloral hydrate. Adverse drug interaction. JAMA 232:638, 1975.
45. PRANDOTA J, PRUITT AW: Furosemide binding to human albumin and plasma of nephrotic children. Clin Pharmacol Ther 17:159, 1975.
46. HONARI J, et al: Effects of probenecid on furosemide kinetics and natriuresis in man. Clin Pharmacol Ther 22:395, 1977.
47. HOMEIDA M, et al: Influence of probenecid and spironolactone on furosemide kinetics and dynamics in man. Clin Pharmacol Ther 22:402, 1977.
48. MILLER RD, et al: Enhancement of d-tubocurarine neuromuscular blockade by diuretics in man. Anesthesiology 45:442, 1976.
49. RICKER RR: Effect of hydrochlorothiazide on phosphorus during treatment with diphosphonate. Clin Pharmacol Ther 18:345, 1975.
50. HIMMELHOCH JM, et al: Adjustment of lithium dose during lithium-chlorothiazide therapy. Clin Pharmacol Ther 22:225, 1977.
51. CHAMBERS G, et al: Lithium used with a diuretic. Br Med J 3:805, 1977.
52. BROOKS PM, et al: The effect of frusemide on indomethacin plasma levels. Br J Clin Pharmacol 1:485, 1974.
53. Indocin®. Product Information, West Point, Pennsylvania, Merck Sharp & Dohme, 1984.
54. FAVRE L, et al: Reversible acute renal failure from combined triamterene and indomethacin: a study in healthy subjects. Ann Intern Med 96:317, 1982.
55. VELASQUEZ MT, et al: Effect of probenecid on the natriuresis and renin release induced by bumetanide in man. J Clin Pharmacol 21:657, 1981.
56. BRATER DC, et al: Interaction studies with bumetanide and furosemide. J Clin Pharmacol 21:647, 1981.
57. ORR LE: Potentiation of myelosuppression from cancer chemotherapy and thiazide diuretics. Drug Intell Clin Pharm 15:967, 1981.
58. BRATER DC, et al: Indomethacin and the response to butanemide. Clin Pharmacol Ther 27:421, 1980.
59. KAUFMAN J, et al: Bumetanide-induced diuresis and natriuresis: effect of prostaglandin synthetase inhibition. J Clin Pharmacol 21:663, 1981.
60. PEDRINELLI R, et al: Influence of indomethacin on the natriuretic and renin stimulating effect of bumetanide in essential hypertension. Clin Pharmacol Ther 28:722, 1980.
61. WILKINSON GR, BECKETT AH: Absorption, metabolism and excretion of the ephedrines in man. J Pharmacol Exp Ther 162:139, 1968.
62. ANDERSON CJ, et al: Toxicity of combined therapy with carbonic anhydrase inhibitors and aspirin. Am J Ophthalmol 86:516, 1978.
63. JEFFERSON JW, KALIN NH: Serum lithium levels and long-term diuretic use. JAMA 241:1134, 1979.
64. SCAPPATICCI KA, et al: Effects of furosemide on the neuromuscular junction. Anesthesiology 57:381, 1982.
65. MCCAUGHAN D: Hazards of non-prescription potassium supplements. Lancet 1:513, 1984.
66. HINNINGHAKE DB, et al: The effect of cholestyramine and colestipol on

the absorption of hydrochlorothiazide. Int J Clin Pharmacol Ther Toxicol 20:151, 1982.

67. SOLOMON K: Combined use of lithium and diuretics. South Med J 71:1098, 1978.

68. MEHTA BR, ROBINSON BHB: Lithium toxicity induced by triamterene-hydrochlorothiazide. Postgrad Med J 56:783, 1980.

69. SHEN F, SHERRARD DJ: Lithium-induced hyperparathyroidism: an alteration of the "set point." Ann Intern Med 96:63, 1982.

70. SOLOMON JG: Lithium toxicity precipitated by a diuretic. Psychosomatics 21:425, 1980.

71. WILSON TW, RAJPUT AH: Amantadine-Dyazide interaction. Can Med Assoc J 129:974, 1983.

72. ALLAN SG, et al: Interaction between diuretics and indomethacin. Br Med J 283:1611, 1981.

73. POE TE, et al: Interaction of indomethacin with furosemide. J Fam Pract 16:610, 1983.

74. BRATER DC: Analysis of the effect of indomethacin on the response to furosemide in man: effect of dose of furosemide. J Pharmacol Exp Ther 210:386, 1979.

75. SMITH DE, et al: Attenuation of furosemide's diuretic effect by indomethacin: pharmacokinetic evaluation. J Pharmacokinet Biopharm 7:265, 1979.

76. PATAK RV, et al: Antagonism of the effects of furosemide by indomethacin in normal and hypertensive man. Prostaglandins 10:649, 1975.

77. RAWLES JM: Antagonism between non-steroidal anti-inflammatory drugs and diuretics. Scott Med J 27:37, 1982.

78. CIABATTONI G, et al: Renal effects of anti-inflammatory drugs. Eur J Rheumatol Inflamm 3:210, 1980.

79. BUNNING RD, BARTH WF: Sulindac: a potentially renal-sparing nonsteroidal anti-inflammatory drug. JAMA 248:2864, 1982.

80. WONG DG, et al: Non-steroidal antiinflammatory drugs (NSAID) vs placebo in hypertension treated with diuretic and beta-blocker. Clin Pharmacol Ther 35:284, 1984.

81. ROBERTS DG, et al: Comparative effects of sulindac and indomethacin in humans. Clin Pharmacol Ther 35:269, 1984.

CHAPTER 10

Ethanol Interactions

ETHANOL (ALCOHOL) DRUG INTERACTIONS

DRUGS	DISCUSSION

Acetaminophen (Datril, Tylenol)[50,77-85]

MECHANISM: It is proposed that enzyme induction from prolonged intake of large amounts of alcohol results in enhanced formation of hepatotoxic metabolites of acetaminophen under conditions of acetaminophen overdose.

CLINICAL SIGNIFICANCE: Data from acetaminophen overdose in chronic alcoholics indicate that they are more susceptible to acetaminophen-induced hepatotoxicity.[77-80,82] These findings are consistent with the known ability of chronic alcoholism to result in enzyme induction and with the likelihood that enzyme induction results in accelerated formation of hepatotoxic acetaminophen metabolites. Whether alcoholism could predispose to hepatotoxicity in patients chronically receiving large therapeutic doses of acetaminophen is not established, but some of the reported cases have involved excessive therapeutic doses of acetaminophen rather than intentional overdoses.[77,78,82] In contrast to chronic alcohol abuse, acute alcohol intoxication tends to inhibit hepatic microsomal drug metabolism and thus might be expected to reduce the formation of toxic acetaminophen metabolites. Animal studies indicate that acute ethanol administration tends to protect against the hepatotoxicity of large doses of acetaminophen,[83,84] and ethanol intoxication may have contributed to a favorable outcome in a patient who took 60 gm of acetaminophen.[85] Finally, alcoholics may have lower bioavailability of acetaminophen, presumably due to increased first-pass metabolism.[81] This may partly explain the tendency of alcoholics to take large quantities of acetaminophen for therapeutic purposes.[77,78] In summary, substantial evidence indicates that chronic, excessive alcohol ingestion increases the toxicity of excessive therapeutic doses or overdoses of acetaminophen, while preliminary evidence indicates that acute alcohol intoxication protects against acetaminophen overdose toxicity.

MANAGEMENT: No special precautions appear necessary, but one should be aware that patients ingesting alcohol for prolonged periods may be more susceptible to hepatotoxicity from acetaminophen overdose.

ETHANOL (ALCOHOL) DRUG INTERACTIONS (CONT.)

DRUGS	DISCUSSION

Antidepressants, Tricyclic[2,9-12,38,57,58,86]

MECHANISM:
1. Combined central nervous system depression may account for the combined adverse effects on psychomotor performance.
2. One might expect prolonged intake of large amounts of alcohol to stimulate the metabolism of tricyclic antidepressants, but evidence to support such a mechanisms is lacking.
3. The anticholinergic effect of tricyclic antidepressants may delay gastric emptying, thus delaying the absorption of ethanol.[58]
4. Acute ethanol ingestion may inhibit the first-pass hepatic metabolism of tricyclic antidepressants.[86]

CLINICAL SIGNIFICANCE: During the initial part of therapy, amitriptyline and doxepin have been reported to add to the deleterious effect of alcohol on motor skill tests related to driving.[9,38,57] The evidence for doxepin is conflicting, however, with some indications that it is less likely to interact.[2] Nortriptyline and clomipramine are less sedative than amitriptyline, which may account for reports that they are less likely to enhance the adverse effects of ethanol on psychomotor skills.[38] Gastrointestinal complications of tricyclic antidepressants are reportedly more frequent if ethanol is consumed concomitantly.[11]

MANAGEMENT: Patients receiving tricyclic antidepressants should be informed that ethanol may produce a greater than expected impairment in psychomotor skills, especially during the first week of treatment. This warning is probably more important for the more sedative tricyclics such as amitriptyline and possibly doxepin.

Antipyrine[37,56,59]

MECHANISM: Chronic ethanol abuse can produce induction of hepatic microsomal enzymes resulting in enhanced antipyrine metabolism.

CLINICAL SIGNIFICANCE: Enhanced metabolism of antipyrene has been shown following intake of large amounts of ethanol (1 ml/kg/day for 21 days),[56] but not with more moderate ethanol intake.[37] Conversely, *acute* intoxication with ethanol would be expected to inhibit drug metabolism, including antipyrine. Also, in chronic alcoholics with significant liver damage, the ethanol-induced enzyme induction may be offset by diminished drug metabolizing capacity of the liver.[59] Since antipyrine is seldom used clinically, the primary significance of these findings relates to the concomitant use of ethanol and other drugs metabolized by hepatic microsomal enzymes.

MANAGEMENT: None required. See Clinical Significance.

Ascorbic Acid (Vitamin C)[60]

MECHANISM: It is proposed that the activity of alcohol dehydrogenase can be enhanced by increasing ascorbic acid saturation.

ETHANOL (ALCOHOL) DRUG INTERACTIONS (CONT.)

DRUGS	DISCUSSION

CLINICAL SIGNIFICANCE: In healthy volunteers, the clearance of ethanol was slightly enhanced by ascorbic acid administration (1 g/day for 2 weeks).[60]

MANAGEMENT: No precautions appear necessary.

Barbiturates[3–7,13,31,41,43,87]

MECHANISM:
1. Effect on ethanol: Phenobarbital appears to enhance the disappearance of ethanol from the blood, resulting in somewhat decreased blood ethanol concentrations.[3,13] The mechanism for this effect is not known. It may involve factors other than a direct increase in hepatic metabolism of ethanol.
2. Effect on barbiturates: Acute intoxication with ethanol appears to inhibit pentobarbital metabolism[7] while chronic ethanol ingestion appears to enhance the hepatic metabolism of pentobarbital.[5] It has also been proposed that ethanol may promote the penetration of barbiturates into tissues.[87]
3. Combined central nervous system depression.

CLINICAL SIGNIFICANCE: It is clear from the mechanisms just described (and probably others as yet undiscovered) that the interrelationships between ethanol and barbiturates are quite complex. Clinically the most important considerations are that they are both central nervous system depressants and that acute ethanol intoxication may impair barbiturate metabolism. Also, the enhanced drug metabolism with chronic ethanol intake[5] may partially explain the tolerance to barbiturates seen in chronic alcoholics.

MANAGEMENT: Although the precautions of combined ethanol-barbiturate use are well known, it bears repeating that the combination should be used cautiously with due attention to excessive central nervous system depression.

Benzodiazepines[1,40,42,48,49,52,61–72,88,89,99]

MECHANISM: Ethanol and benzodiazepines are likely to have additive central nervous system depressant activity. There is also evidence to indicate that ethanol may increase the absorption of diazepam[49,61] and reduce the hepatic metabolism of diazepam.[88,89] Finally, patients with alcoholic liver disease may eliminate benzodiazepines more slowly than those with normal liver function.[99]

CLINICAL SIGNIFICANCE: A number of studies have appeared demonstrating that benzodiazepines enhance the detrimental effects of ethanol on psychomotor skills and simulated driving.[1,48,52,61–66] Most of these studies have involved ethanol plus diazepam, although nitrazepam and bromazepam appear to have a similar effect when given with ethanol. Several studies have indicated that chlordiazepoxide may be less likely to enhance the adverse psychomotor effects of alcohol,[40,67–72] but it seems likely that this would occur with suffi-

ETHANOL (ALCOHOL) DRUG INTERACTIONS (CONT.)

DRUGS	DISCUSSION

cient doses of chlordiazepoxide. Ethanol also seems less likely to affect the hepatic metabolism of oxazepam than diazepam,[89] but additive central nervous system depression would be expected in either case. Many of the studies of the interaction between ethanol and benzodiazepines have differed with regard to degree of interaction. This is largely due to the many variables in the studies such as doses of drug and alcohol, type of test used, duration between drugs and testing, age of subjects, trial design, and chronic versus acute administration of drugs and/or ethanol. In summary, under the conditions that ethanol and benzodiazepines are normally used, one would expect some increase in the adverse psychomotor effects of alcohol. An exception to this would probably occur with the use of small doses of ethanol, benzodiazepine, or both agents.

MANAGEMENT: Patients receiving benzodiazepines should be warned against ingestion of moderate to large amounts of ethanol. Occasional ingestion of small amounts of ethanol probably causes little difficulty, unless alertness is required (as in driving) or the patient has a disease or condition that makes him sensitive to central nervous system depression.

Bromocriptine[74,75]

MECHANISM: Not established.

CLINICAL SIGNIFICANCE: Preliminary clinical evidence indicates that the combined use of ethanol and bromocriptine may increase the likelihood of gastrointestinal side effects or alcohol intolerance.[74,75]

MANAGEMENT: Current evidence indicates that it does not appear necessary to instruct patients on bromocriptine to abstain from ethanol. However, it would be prudent to warn them of the possibility so that they can discontinue ethanol if the reaction does occur.

Caffeine[35]

MECHANISM: Not established.

CLINICAL SIGNIFICANCE: In a study of 68 healthy subjects ethanol (0.75 g/kg body weight) and caffeine (300 mg/70 kg body weight) were given alone and in combination, followed by measurement of psychomotor skills.[35] Caffeine failed to reverse the detrimental effects of ethanol on performance with the exception of the reaction time tests. Thus, it does not appear that caffeine would be effective as an agent to "sober up" following excessive ethanol ingestion.

MANAGEMENT: One should be aware that coffee does not render the intoxicated person better able to drive a motor vehicle.

Chloral Hydrate (Noctec)[14-19]

MECHANISM: In-vitro studies[18] indicate that a metabolite of chloral hydrate (trichloroethanol) inhibits the metabolism of ethanol, while ethanol in turn appears to stimulate the formation of trichloroethanol and inhibit its conjugation with glucuronide.

CLINICAL SIGNIFICANCE: The concomitant administration of ethanol and chloral hydrate can result in elevations of both plasma trichloroethanol and blood ethanol.[18] Since all of these agents are central nervous system (CNS) depressants, the combination of chloral hydrate and ethanol has at least additive (and probably synergistic) CNS depressant activity. Performance of a complex motor task has been shown to be considerably more affected by chloral hydrate plus ethanol than by either agent taken alone.[19] Another type of reaction (flushing, tachycardia, headache) occasionally occurs when ethanol is ingested by a patient who has been receiving chloral hydrate.[15,19] This vasodilation reaction probably occurs to a lesser extent in many other patients who do not manifest the full symptomatic reaction.

MANAGEMENT: Patients should be made aware of the combined CNS depressant activity of ethanol and chloral hydrate. Patients with cardiovascular disease on chloral hydrate should be quite careful about ingesting ethanol since the tachycardia and hypotension of the vasodilation reaction could adversely affect their basic disease state.

Chloroform[47]

MECHANISM: It is proposed that prolonged intake of large amounts of ethanol may enhance the metabolism of chloroform to hepatotoxic metabolites.

CLINICAL SIGNIFICANCE: An alcoholic patient developed severe hepatotoxicity during prolonged ingestion of a chloroform-containing analgesic mixture. It was assumed that the hepatotoxicity resulted from combined toxicity of ethanol and chloroform, but there is no direct evidence to support this contention.

MANAGEMENT: Too little information is available.

Cimetidine (Tagamet)[94-98]

MECHANISM: Not established. Cimetidine probably inhibits hepatic ethanol metabolism and/or increases the gastrointestinal absorption of ethanol.

CLINICAL SIGNIFICANCE: Cimetidine has been shown to increase both peak plasma ethanol concentrations and the area under the plasma ethanol concentration time curve.[94,95] The magnitude of the increases in plasma ethanol have not been large, but they were sufficient to increase both objective and subjective ratings of ethanol intoxication. A 55-year-old man on 1200 mg/day of cimetidine developed an acute brain syndrome (disoriented, irritable, irrational) after drinking alcohol. He had regularly consumed alcohol prior to cimetidine therapy without developing such difficulties.[96] One must also consider the possibility of a pharmacodynamic interaction between cimetidine

DRUGS	DISCUSSION

and ethanol. The central nervous system toxicity that can follow cimetidine use in susceptible persons (e.g., the elderly, patients with renal disease or hepatic disease) may interact adversely with the central nervous system effects of ethanol. Further, acute ethanol intoxication is known to inhibit drug metabolism; thus, ethanol-induced inhibition of cimetidine metabolism could increase the serum cimetidine concentration which in turn would increase the likelihood of cimetidine-induced central nervous system toxicity. Ranitidine (Zantac) does not appear to affect the pharmacokinetics of ethanol,[95] and may be less likely than cimetidine to exhibit adverse central nervous system effects. Thus, one would expect ranitidine to be less likely than cimetidine to produce adverse psychiatric effects when combined with ethanol. On the positive side, cimetidine has been shown to attenuate the unpleasant cutaneous flushing and headaches that follow the use of certain alcoholic beverages in susceptible persons.[97,98] Assuming that this effect of cimetidine is due to H_2-receptor antagonism, one would expect ranititidine to have a similar effect.

MANAGEMENT: Patients receiving cimetidine do not need to abstain from ethanol, but they should be aware that the degree of ethanol intoxication may be greater than anticipated. In patients with moderate to heavy ethanol intake, ranitidine may be preferable since preliminary evidence indicates that it does not affect ethanol disposition.

Cromolyn (Intal)[51]

MECHANISM: None. See Clinical Significance.

CLINICAL SIGNIFICANCE: Results of psychomotor tests in subjects receiving cromolyn and ethanol failed to reveal evidence of a clinically significant interaction.[51]

MANAGEMENT: No special precautions appear necessary.

Disulfiram (Antabuse)[20,54,55]

MECHANISM: The pharmacologic and biochemical basis for the disulfiram-ethanol reaction has not been established.

CLINICAL SIGNIFICANCE: Among the signs and symptoms of the disulfiram-ethanol reaction are flushing, hypotension, nausea, tachycardia, vertigo, dyspnea, and blurred vision.[54,55] As little as 15 ml of ethanol reportedly can produce a mild reaction in some patients receiving disulfiram. Large amounts of ethanol may produce severe or even fatal reactions. Many oral liquid pharmaceutical preparations contain ethanol. Topically applied ethanol reportedly may also result in reactions, but the amount of ethanol required and the magnitude of the reaction requires further study.

MANAGEMENT: It would be prudent to advise patients receiving disulfiram to avoid all oral liquid pharmaceuticals unless they are known to be ethanol-free.

ETHANOL (ALCOHOL) DRUG INTERACTIONS (CONT.)

DRUGS	DISCUSSION

Glutethimide (Doriden)[3]

MECHANISM: One would expect additive central nervous system (CNS) depression with combined use of ethanol and glutethimide. Pharmacokinetic interaction has also been suggested (see Clinical Significance).

CLINICAL SIGNIFICANCE: The combined use of ethanol and glutethimide has been shown to *increase* blood ethanol concentration and *decrease* plasma glutethimide concentration.[3] Although these effects may prove to have clinical significance, it is probably more important to remember that both drugs are CNS depressants.

MANAGEMENT: Patients receiving glutethimide should be aware of the possible increased CNS depression with enthanol ingestion.

Meprobamate (Equanil, Miltown)[5-7,32-34]

MECHANISM: Acute intoxication with ethanol appears to inhibit meprobamate metabolism[7] while chronic ethanol ingestion appears to induce hepatic microsomal enzymes resulting in enhanced meprobamate metabolism.[5]

CLINICAL SIGNIFICANCE: Simultaneous use of ethanol and meprobamate may result in synergistic central nervous system (CNS) depression. The enhanced drug metabolism with chronic ethanol intake[5] may partially explain the tolerance to CNS depressants in chronic alcoholics.

MANAGEMENT: Patients should be made aware of the combined CNS depression of ethanol and meprobamate. Intake of large amounts of ethanol should be avoided.

Metoclopramide (Reglan)[76]

MECHANISM: Not established. Ethanol and metoclopramide may exhibit additive sedative effects.

CLINICAL SIGNIFICANCE: Study in seven healthy subjects indicated that metoclopramide (10 mg IV) may enhance the sedative effect of ethanol (70 mg/kg body weight).[76]

MANAGEMENT: Until more is known about this purported interaction, patients receiving metoclopramide should ingest ethanol with caution.

Milk[46]

MECHANISM: Milk probably delays gastric emptying, thus reducing the rate of absorption of ethanol.

CLINICAL SIGNIFICANCE: Ten subjects were given 25 ml of ethanol with either 720 ml of water or 720 ml of milk, and urinary excretion of ethanol was measured.[46] Both the urinary excretion data and subjec-

ETHANOL (ALCOHOL) DRUG INTERACTIONS (CONT.)

DRUGS	DISCUSSION

tive evaluation of behavior indicated that milk reduced the intoxicating effects of ethanol.

MANAGEMENT: Ingestion of milk prior to ethanol is probably effective in reducing the degree of intoxication. Other foods may have a similar effect.

Narcotic Analgesics[1,39]

MECHANISM: Not established.

CLINICAL SIGNIFICANCE: A study involving intravenous injection of meperidine in surgical patients and volunteers indicated that the volume of distribution of meperidine increased with increasing ethanol consumption.[39] It was proposed that this increase in volume of distribution might produce a decrease in the pharmacologic response to meperidine, but this remains speculative.

MANAGEMENT: No special precautions appear necessary.

Paraldehyde[45]

MECHANISM: Not established. Both ethanol and paraldehyde are metabolized to acetaldehyde. Since the disposition of both ethanol and acetaldehyde results in the conversion of NAD^+ to NADH, it is proposed that acidosis may result from changes in intermediary metabolism due to NAD^+ depletion.

CLINICAL SIGNIFICANCE: A patient developed metabolic acidosis following 3 months of combined ethanol and paraldehyde ingestion.[45] Paraldehyde intoxication has been associated with acidosis in previous reports, so the possible contributory role of ethanol in this case is difficult to assess.

MANAGEMENT: Obviously, excessive intake of either ethanol or paraldehyde should be avoided. Those with access to paraldehyde should be aware of the possibility that combined abuse may be more hazardous than either agent alone.

Phenothiazines[21,44,52,53,73]

MECHANISM: Ethanol and phenothiazines probably exhibit additive central nervous system depressant activity.

CLINICAL SIGNIFICANCE: Studies in normal subjects and patients indicate that chlorpromazine adds to the detrimental effects of ethanol on simulated driving[21] and various measures of coordination and judgment.[21,44] Subjective assessments of impairment and observation of behavior also indicate that chlorpromazine plus ethanol has a greater effect than ethanol alone. There is some evidence that thioridazine (Mellaril) may be less likely to add to the detrimental effects of ethanol on psychomotor skills.[21,52] It has also been proposed that ethanol may precipitate extrapyramidal reactions in patients receiving phenothiazines. Seven cases have been briefly described where akathisia or dystonia followed ingestion of moderate to large amounts of ethanol in the presence of phenothiazine therapy.[53] In summary, it appears likely that patients receiving antipsychotic doses of chlorpromazine would be more sensitive to the adverse effects of ethanol on psychomotor skills and behavior. Based on current evidence, thioridazine appears to be less likely to manifest this effect with ethanol, but the effects of other phenothiazines have not been well studied. More study is also needed to assess the ability of ethanol to induce extrapyramidal reactions in patients on phenothiazines.

MANAGEMENT: Patients receiving phenothiazines (especially large doses) should be aware that ethanol ingestion can result in impaired motor performance and driving ability. The possibility that ethanol might precipitate extrapyramidal reactions in certain susceptible patients receiving phenothiazines is another reason to limit ethanol intake.

Quinacrine (Atabrine)[8]

MECHANISM: Quinacrine reportedly inhibits aldehyde dehydrogenase to some extent, resulting in accumulation of acetaldehyde following ethanol ingestion.

CLINICAL SIGNIFICANCE: Not established. If acetaldehyde oxidation is inhibited sufficiently, an "Antabuse reaction" is possible.

MANAGEMENT: Too little clinical information is available to make a statement on management, but the possibility of interaction should be realized.

Salicylates[22-28,90-93]

MECHANISM: Ethanol appears to increase the gastrointestinal bleeding produced by salicylates. Both aspirin and ethanol individually damage the gastric mucosal barrier, and their combined use appears to result in additive or synergistic effects. Also, the ability of aspirin to prolong the bleeding time is enhanced by ethanol administration.

CLINICAL SIGNIFICANCE: Available evidence indicates that ethanol ingestion produces approximately a twofold increase in the minor gastric bleeding that regularly occurs with aspirin administration. It has not been established whether ethanol increases the likelihood of upper gastrointestinal hemorrhage due to aspirin, but indirect evidence indicates that it may. The clinical significance of the ethanol-induced increase in the bleeding time response to aspirin is not known, but the effect may be large enough in some patients to result in spontaneous bleeding.

MANAGEMENT: Concomitant use of ethanol and salicylates need not be avoided, but the possibility of enhanced gastrointestinal bleeding should be considered. When possible, one should avoid aspirin use

DRUGS	DISCUSSION

within 8 to 10 hours of heavy alcohol use. Some forms of salicylate appear to be less likely to produce gastric mucosal injury than standard aspirin tablets. Such products would include effervescent buffered products (e.g., Alka Seltzer), enteric-coated products (e.g., Ecotrin), choline salicylate (Arthropan), and salsalate (Disalcid). Theoretically, these preparations may be less likely to produce additive gastric mucosal damage than standard aspirin tablets. Also, salicylate-induced prolongation of the bleeding time can be avoided by using nonacetylated salicylates such as choline salicylate, sodium salicylate, or choline magnesium salicylate; ethanol-induced potentiation of salicylate bleeding time prolongation would thus not be a factor with these agents.

Tetrachloroethylene[29,30]

MECHANISM: A small amount of administered tetrachloroethylene is absorbed from the gastrointestinal tract, resulting in central nervous system (CNS) depression. This effect may be additive with that of alcohol.

CLINICAL SIGNIFICANCE: No case reports of interaction could be found, but, on the basis of theoretical considerations, concomitant administration probably does result in additive CNS depression.

MANAGEMENT: It is recommended that no ethanol be taken before or for 24 hours after tetrachloroethylene administration.

Tolazoline (Priscoline)[8]

MECHANISM: Tolazoline reportedly inhibits aldehyde dehydrogenase to some extent, resulting in accumulation of acetaldehyde following ethanol ingestion.

CLINICAL SIGNIFICANCE: Not established. If acetaldehyde oxidation is inhibited sufficiently, an "Antabuse reaction" is possible.

MANAGEMENT: Too little clinical information is available to make a statement on management, but the possibility of interaction should be realized.

Trichloroethylene[36]

MECHANISM: Not established.

CLINICAL SIGNIFICANCE: Industrial exposure to trichloroethylene has been associated with ethanol intolerance (e.g., flushing, lacrimation, blurred vision, and tachypnea).[36] It is possible that medical exposure could produce similar findings.

MANAGEMENT: Patients exposed to trichloroethylene should be warned of the potential adverse effects of ethanol ingestion.

References

1. LINNOILA M, HAKKINEN S: Effects of diazepam and codeine, alone and in combination with alcohol, on simulated driving. Clin Pharmacol Ther 15:368, 1974.
2. MILNER G, LANDAUER AA: The effects of doxepin, alone and together with alcohol, in relation to driving safety. Med J Aust 1:837, 1973.
3. MOULD GP, et al: Interaction of glutethimide and phenobarbitone with ethanol in man. J Pharm Pharmacol 24:894, 1972.
4. LIEBER CS: Hepatic and metabolic effects of alcohol (1966 to 1973). Gastroenterology 65:821, 1973.
5. MISRA PS, et al: Increase of ethanol, meprobamate and pentobarbital metabolism after chronic ethanol administration in man and in rats. Am J Med 41:346, 1971.
6. VALSRUB S: Alcohol-induced sensitivity and tolerance (Editorial). JAMA 219:508, 1972.
7. RUBIN E, et al: Inhibition of drug metabolism by acute ethanol intoxication: a hepatic microsomal mechanism. Am J Med 49:801, 1970.
8. AZARNOFF DL, HURWITZ A: Drug interactions. Pharmacol Physicians 4:1 (Feb.), 1970.
9. LANDAUER AA, et al: Alcohol and amitriptyline effects on skills related to driving behavior. Science 163:1467, 1969.
10. LOCKETT MF, MILNER G: Combining the antidepressant drugs. Br Med J 1:921, 1965.
11. MILNER G: Gastrointestinal side effects and psychotropic drugs. Med J Aust 2:153, 1969.
12. LAURIE W: Alcohol as a cause of sudden unexpected death. Med J Aust 1:1224, 1971.
13. MEZEY E, ROBLES EA: Effects of phenobarbital administration on rates of ethanol clearance and on ethanol-oxidizing enzymes in man. Gastroenterology 66:248, 1974.
14. KAPLAN HL, et al: Chloral hydrate and alcohol metabolism in human subjects. J Forensic Sci 12:295, 1967.
15. CHAPMAN AH: Reaction to alcohol and chloral hydrate (Questions and Answers). JAMA 167:273, 1958.
16. FREEMAN J, SCHULMAN MP: Reactions of chloral hydrate and ethanol with alcohol dehydrogenase from human liver (Abstract). Fed Proc 29:275ABS, 1970.
17. GESSNER PK, CABANA BE: A study of the interaction of the hypnotic effects and of the toxic effects of chloral hydrate and ethanol. J Pharmacol Exp Ther 174:247, 1970.
18. SELLERS EM, et al: Interaction of chloral hydrate and ethanol in man. I. Metabolism. Clin Pharmacol Ther 13:37, 1972.
19. SELLERS EM, et al: Interaction of chloral hydrate and ethanol in man. II. Hemodynamics and performance. Clin Pharmacol Ther 13:50, 1972.
20. FERNANDEZ D: Another esophageal rupture after alcohol and disulfiram (Letter). N Engl J Med 286:610, 1972.
21. MILNER G, LANDAUER AA: Alcohol, thioridazine and chlorpromazine effects on skills related to driving behaviour. Br J Psychiatry 118:351, 1971.
22. GOULSTON K, COOKE AR: Alcohol, aspirin and gastrointestinal bleeding. Br Med J 4:664, 1968.

References (CONT.)

23. BOUCHIER IND, WILLIAMS HS: Determination of faecal blood-loss after combined alcohol and sodium-acetylsalicylate intake. Lancet 1:178, 1969.
24. MOULD G: Faecal blood-loss after sodium acetylsalicylate taken with alcohol (Letter). Lancet 1:1268, 1969.
25. WOOD PHN: Faecal blood-loss after sodium acetylsalicylate taken with alcohol (Letter). Lancet 1:677, 1969.
26. DOBBING J: Faecal blood-loss after sodium acetylsalicylate taken with alcohol (Letter). Lancet 1:527, 1969.
27. BABB RR, WILBUR RS: Aspirin and gastrointestinal bleeding. An opinion. Calif Med 110:440, 1969.
28. LEONARDS JR, LEVY G: Reduction or prevention of aspirin-induced occult gastrointestinal blood loss in man. Clin Pharmacol Ther 10:571, 1969.
29. ROLLO IM: Drugs used in the therapy of helminthiasis. In Goodman LS, Gilman A (Eds): The Pharmacological Basis of Therapeutics. 4th Ed. New York, Macmillan, 1970, pp. 1067–1094.
30. ANON: Thiabendazole (mintezol)—a new anthelmintic. Med Lett 9:99, 1967.
31. JOHNSTONE RE, et al: Respiratory interaction of alcohol (Letter). JAMA 233:770, 1975.
32. ASHFORD JR, COBBY JM: Drug Interactions. The effects of alcohol and meprobamate applied singly and jointly in human subjects. III. J Stud Alcohol Supplement 7:140, 1975.
33. COBBY JM, ASHFORD JR: Drug Interactions. The effects of alcohol and meprobamate applied singly and jointly in human subjects. IV. J Stud Alcohol Supplement 7:162, 1975.
34. ASHFORD JR, CARPENTER JA: Drug Interactions. The effects of alcohol and meprobamate applied singly and jointly in human subjects. V. J Stud Alcohol Supplement 7:177, 1975.
35. FRANKS HM, et al: The effect of caffeine on human performance, alone and in combination with ethanol. Psychopharmacology 45:177, 1975.
36. PARDYS S, BROTHMAN M: Trichlorethylene and alcohol: a straight flush (Letter). JAMA 229:521, 1974.
37. VESTAL RE, et al: Antipyrine metabolism in man: influence of age, alcohol, caffeine, and smoking. Clin Pharmacol Ther 18:425, 1975.
38. SEPPALA T, et al: Effect of tricyclic antidepressants and alcohol on psychomotor skills related to driving. Clin Pharmacol Ther 17:515, 1975.
39. MATHER LE, et al: Meperidine kinetics in man. Intravenous injection in surgical patients and volunteers. Clin Pharmacol Ther 17:21, 1975.
40. REGGIANI G, et al: Some aspects of the experimental and clinical toxicology of chlordiazepoxide. Toxicity and side-effects of psychotropic drugs. Amsterdam, Excerpta Medica Foundation, 1968, pp. 79–97.
41. MEZEY E: Effect of phenobarbital administration on ethanol oxidizing enzymes and on rates of ethanol degradation. Biochem Pharmacol 20:508, 1971.
42. ROSINGA WM: Interaction of drugs and alcohol in relation to traffic safety. In Meyer L, and Peck HM (Eds): Drug Induced Disease. Vol. 3. Amsterdam, Excerpta Medica Foundation, 1968, pp. 295–306.
43. MILNER G: Interaction between barbiturates, alcohol and some psychotropic drugs. Med J Aust 1:1204, 1970.

References (CONT.)

44. ZIRKLE GA, et al: Effects of chlorpromazine and alcohol on coordination and judgment. JAMA 168:1496, 1959.

45. HADDEN JW, METZNER RJ: Pseudoketosis and hyperacetaldehydemia in paraldehyde acidosis. Am J Med 47:642, 1969.

46. MILLER DS, et al: Effect of ingestion of milk on concentrations of blood alcohol. Nature 212:1051, 1966.

47. STATHERS GM: The synergistic effect of ethanol and chlorodyne in producing hepatotoxicity. Med J Aust 2:1134, 1970.

48. SARRIO I, et al: Interaction of drugs with alcohol on human psychomotor skills related to driving: effect of sleep deprivation or two weeks' treatment with hypnotics. J Clin Pharmacol 15:52, 1975.

49. HAYES SL, et al: Ethanol and oral diazepam absorption. N Engl J Med 296:186, 1977.

50. EMBY DJ, FRASER BN: Hepatotoxicity of paracetamol enhanced by ingestion of alcohol: report of two cases. S Afr Med J 51:208, 1977.

51. CRAWFORD WA, et al: The effect of disodium cromoglycate on human performance, alone and in combination with ethanol. Med J Aust 1:997, 1976.

52. SAARIO I: Psychomotor skills during subacute treatment with thioridazine and bromazepam, and their combined effects with alcohol. Ann Clin Res 8:117, 1976.

53. LUTZ EG: Neuroleptic-induced akathisia and dystonia triggered by alcohol. JAMA 236:2422, 1976.

54. EIENBAAS RM: Drug Therapy Reviews: management of the disulfiram-alcohol reaction. Am J Hosp Pharm 34:827, 1977.

55. KITSON TM: The disulfiram-ethanol reaction: a review. J Stud Alcohol 38:96, 1977.

56. VESELL ES, et al: Genetic and environmental factors affecting ethanol metabolism in man. Clin Pharmacol Ther 12:192, 1971.

57. SEPPALA T: Psychomotor skills during acute and two-week treatment with mianserin (ORG GB 94) and amitriptyline, and their combined effects with alcohol. Ann Clin Res 9:66, 1977.

58. HALL RC, et al: The effect of desmethylimipramine on the absorption of alcohol and paracetamol. Postgrad Med J 52:139, 1976.

59. SOTANIEMI EA, et al: Histological changes in the liver and indices of drug metabolism in alcoholics. Eur J Clin Pharmacol 11:295, 1977.

60. KRASNER N, et al: Ascorbic-acid saturation and ethanol metabolism. Lancet 2:693, 1974.

61. MACLEOD SM, et al: Diazepam actions and plasma concentrations following ethanol ingestion. Eur J Clin Pharmacol 11:345, 1977.

62. LINNOILA M: Effects of diazepam, chlordiazepoxide, thioridazine, haloperidole, flupenthixole and alcohol on psychomotor skills related to driving. Ann Med Exp Biol Fenn 51:125, 1973.

63. LINNOILA M: Drug interaction on psychomotor skills related to driving: hypnotics and alcohol. Ann Med Exp Biol Fen 51:118, 1973.

64. LINNOILA M, MATTILA MJ: Drug interaction on psychomotor skills related to driving: diazepam and alcohol. Eur J Clin Pharmacol 5:186, 1973.

65. MORLAND J, et al: Combined effects of diazepam and ethanol on mental and psychomotor functions. Acta Pharmacol Toxicol 34:5, 1974.

66. LINNOILA M, et al: Effect of treatment with diazepam or lithium and alcohol on psychomotor skills related to driving. Eur J Clin Pharmacol 7:337, 1974.

315

References (CONT.)

67. HUGHES FW, et al: Comparative effect in human subjects of chlordiazepoxide, diazepam, and placebo on mental and physical performance. Clin Pharmacol Ther 6:139, 1965.
68. HOFFER A: Lack of potentiation by chlordiazepoxide (Librium) of depression or excitation due to alcohol. Can Med Assoc J 87:920, 1962.
69. BETTS TA, et al: Effect of four commonly-used tranquilizers on lowspeed driving performance tests. Br Med J 4:580, 1972.
70. DUNDEE JW, et al: Alcohol and the benzodiazepines. The interaction between intravenous ethanol and chlordiazepoxide and diazepam. Q J Stud Alcohol 32:960, 1971.
71. GOLDBERG L: Behavioral and physiological effects of alcohol on man. Psychom Med 28:570, 1966.
72. MILLER AI, et al: Effects of combined chlordiazepoxide and alcohol in man. Quart J Stud Alcohol 24:9, 1963.
73. SUTHERLAND VC, et al: Cerebral metabolism in problem drinkers under the influence of alcohol and chlorpromazine hydrochloride. J Appl Physiol 15:189, 1960.
74. WASS JA, et al: Long-term treatment of acromegaly with bromocriptine. Br Med J 1:875, 1977.
75. AYRES J, MAISEY MN: Alcohol increases bromocriptine's side effects. N Engl J Med 302:806, 1980.
76. BATEMAN DN, et al: Pharmacokinetic and concentration-effect studies with intravenous metoclopramide. Br J Clin Pharmacol 6:401, 1978.
77. BARKER JD Jr, et al: Chronic excessive acetaminophen use and liver damage. Ann Intern Med 87:299, 1977.
78. McCLAIN CJ, et al: Potentiation of acetaminophen hepatoxicity by alcohol. JAMA 244:251, 1980.
79. JOHNSON MW, et al: Alcoholism, nonprescription drugs and hepatoxicity. The risk from unknown acetaminophen ingestion. Am J Gastroenterol 76:530, 1981.
80. McJUNKIN B, et al: Fatal massive hepatic necrosis following acetaminophen overdose. JAMA 236:1874, 1976.
81. DIETZ AJ Jr, et al: Acetaminophen kinetics in the alcoholic. Clin Pharmacol Ther 31:218, 1982.
82. LICHT J, et al: Apparent potentiation of acetaminophen hepatotoxicity by alcohol. Ann Intern Med 92:511, 1980.
83. SATO C, et al: Prevention of acetaminophen-induced hepatotoxicity by acute ethanol administration in the rat: comparison with carbon tetrachloride-induced hepatotoxicity. J Pharmacol Exp Ther 218:805, 1981.
84. SATO C, LIEBER CS: Mechanism of the preventive effect of ethanol on acetaminophen-induced hepatotoxicity. J Pharmacol Exp Ther 218:811, 1981.
85. LYONS L, et al: Treatment of acetaminophen overdosage with N-acetylcysteine. N Engl J Med 296:174, 1977.
86. DORIAN P, et al: Amitriptyline and ethanol: pharmacokinetic and pharmacodynamic interaction. Eur J Clin Pharmacol 25:325, 1983.
87. STEAD AH, MOFFAT AC: Quantification of the interaction between barbiturates and alcohol and interpretation of fatal blood concentrations. Hum Toxicol 2:5, 1983.
88. SELLERS EM, et al: Intravenous diazepam and oral ethanol interaction. Clin Pharmacol Ther 28:638, 1980.

References (CONT.)

89. SELLERS EM, et al: Different effects on benzodiazepine disposition by disulfiram and ethanol. Arzneimmittelforsch 30:882, 1980.
90. DESCHEPPER PJ, et al: Gastrointestinal blood loss after diflunisal and after aspirin: effect of ethanol. Clin Pharmacol Ther 23:669, 1978.
91. CARANASOS GJ, et al: Drug-induced illness leading to hospitalization. JAMA 228:713, 1974.
92. DEYKIN D, et al: Ethanol potentiation of aspirin-induced prolongation of the bleeding time. N Engl J Med 306:852, 1982.
93. NEEDHAM CD, et al: Aspirin and alcohol in gastrointestinal haemorrhage. Gut 12:819, 1971.
94. FEELY J, WOOD AJJ: Effects of cimetidine on the elimination and actions of ethanol. JAMA 247:2819, 1982.
95. SEITZ HK, et al: Increased blood ethanol levels following cimetidine but not ranitidine. Lancet 1:760, 1983.
96. HARKNESS LL, GILLER EL Jr: Cimetidine psychotoxicity without significant medical illness: case report. J Clin Psychiatry 44:75, 1983.
97. TAN OT, et al: Blocking of alcohol-induced flush with a combination of H_1 and H_2 histamine antagonists. Lancet 2:365, 1979.
98. GLASER D, DE TARNOWSKY GO Jr: Cimetidine and red-wine headaches. Ann Intern Med 98:413, 1983.
99. JUHL RP, et al: Alprazolam pharmacokinetics in alcoholic liver disease. J Clin Pharmacol 24:113, 1984.

CHAPTER 11

Hormone Interactions

ANABOLIC STEROID INTERACTIONS

DRUGS	DISCUSSION

Corticosteroids[50,51]

MECHANISM: Not established.

CLINICAL SIGNIFICANCE: Methandrostenolone (Dianabol) has been reported to enhance the therapeutic and toxic response to corticosteroid therapy in patients with rheumatoid arthritis.[50,51] Reports involving anabolic steroids other than methandrostenolone appear to be lacking.

MANAGEMENT: One should be alert for evidence of enhanced corticosteroid response if methandrostenolone is given.

Oxyphenbutazone (Tandearil)[11-13]

MECHANISM: Not established. Oxyphenbutazone plasma levels may be increased by methandrostenolone (Dianabol), perhaps by an effect on the volume of distribution and/or inhibition of metabolism. Phenylbutazone does not appear to be affected by methandrostenolone, which may be due to competition between phenylbutazone and its major metabolite (oxyphenbutazone) for plasma protein binding.

CLINICAL SIGNIFICANCE: Considerable increases in plasma oxyphenbutazone levels have been reported in several patients who also received methandrostenolone. However, clinical reports of toxicity from this interaction are lacking. Although phenylbutazone does not appear to interact with methandrostenolone, not enough information is available to make a definite statement.

MANAGEMENT: Until more is known concerning the toxic potential of this interaction, caution should be observed in concomitant administration of oxyphenbutazone and methandrostenolone.

CORTICOSTEROID INTERACTIONS

DRUGS	DISCUSSION

Antacids[63-66]

MECHANISM: Antacids possibly reduce the gastrointestinal absorption of corticosteroids.

CORTICOSTEROID INTERACTIONS (CONT.)

DRUGS	DISCUSSION

CLINICAL SIGNIFICANCE: Although some clinical studies have shown that antacids may reduce the absorption of corticosteroids such as prednisone and dexamethasone,[63,64] other studies have found no interaction.[65,66] Even if the interaction does occur, a patient stabilized on both a corticosteroid and an antacid is not likely to be adversely affected since the corticosteroid dose would probably be titrated to the appropriate level.

MANAGEMENT: Monitor for the need to alter corticosteroid dose if antacids are started, stopped, or if antacid dosage schedule is changed relative to corticosteroid doses.

Barbiturates[32–34,38,39,41,43,44,67]

MECHANISM: Phenobarbital appears to enhance the metabolism of corticosteroids, probably due to phenobarbital-induced induction of hepatic microsomal enzymes. It has also been suggested that hypoxemia can cause enzyme induction.[34] Thus, it is possible that in asthmatic patients, barbiturates could initiate a vicious circle by decreasing corticosteroid effect resulting in worsening of asthma, hypoxemia and thus increasing enzyme induction.

CLINICAL SIGNIFICANCE: Three prednisone-dependent asthmatics were shown to develop worsening of asthma following initiation of phenobarbital administration.[32] This reversed when the phenobarbital was withdrawn. Results of subsequent pharmacokinetic studies in several patients using phenobarbital and dexamethasone were consistent with the view that phenobarbital enhances corticosteroid metabolism by enzyme induction. In another study, renal transplant patients receiving phenobarbital and/or phenytoin eliminated prednisolone more rapidly than 12 control patients not receiving these drugs.[67] Another report described a decrease in renal allograft survival in patients receiving phenobarbital, presumably due to phenobarbital-induced increases in prednisone disposition with resultant reduced immunosuppression.[38] Phenobarbital has also been shown to reduce the half-life of methylprednisolone.[39] Thus, substantial evidence is accumulating to indicate that barbiturates can reduce the effects of corticosteroids.

MANAGEMENT: If does not seem necessary to avoid concomitant use of corticosteroids and barbiturates, but one should be alert for reduced corticosteroid response if barbiturates or other enzyme inducers are given concomitantly. It may be necessary to increase the corticosteroid dose.

Cholestyramine (Questran)[62]

MECHANISM: Cholestyramine may inhibit the gastrointestinal absorption of hydrocortisone.

CLINICAL SIGNIFICANCE: Ten healthy subjects were given hydrocortisone (50 mg orally) with and without concurrent cholestyramine (4 to

CORTICOSTEROID INTERACTIONS (CONT.)

DRUGS	DISCUSSION

8 g orally).[62] The 4-g dose of cholestyramine reduced the area under the hydrocortisone plasma concentration time curve by 35% over 200 minutes; the effect was greater with the 8-g dose of cholestyramine. Thus, it appears that cholestyramine reduces the extent of hydrocortisone absorption, but multiple dose studies will be required to determine the clinical importance of these findings.

MANAGEMENT: Separate doses of oral hydrocortisone from cholestyramine so as to avoid mixing in the gastrointestinal tract. Be alert for evidence of reduced hydrocortisone response and increase dose as needed.

Cromolyn (Intal)[48]

MECHANISM: None.

CLINICAL SIGNIFICANCE: Cromolyn therapy produced a slight decrease in the clearance of dexamethasone in four asthmatic patients,[48] but the magnitude of the change seems insufficient to produce any clinical effect.

MANAGEMENT: No special precautions appear necessary.

Ephedrine[46]

MECHANISM: Not established.

CLINICAL SIGNIFICANCE: Nine patients with asthma were given dexamethasone before and after ephedrine (100 mg/day for 3 weeks).[46] Ephedrine therapy was associated with a 36% decrease in dexamethasone half-life and a 42% increase in the metabolic clearance rate for dexamethasone. The effect of ephedrine on the disposition of other corticosteroids is not known. In the same study, theophylline did not appear to affect dexamethasone disposition in seven patients.

MANAGEMENT: One should be alert for diminished responses to dexamethasone (and possibly other corticosteroids) if ephedrine is given concomitantly. Some have suggested that theophylline may be preferable to ephedrine as a bronchodilator in steroid-dependent asthmatics.

Estrogen[1,16,45,68]

MECHANISM: Not established. It is possible that the estrogen-induced increase in serum cortisol-binding globulin retards the normally rapid metabolism of hydrocortisone.

CLINICAL SIGNIFICANCE: Estrogen administration has been shown to enhance the anti-inflammatory effect of hydrocortisone in patients with chronic inflammatory skin diseases.[16] When estrogen was added, a three- to twentyfold reduction in the dose of corticosteroid was possible. There is also some evidence that women taking oral contraceptives may have a lower metabolic clearance rate for prednisolone than subjects not receiving oral contraceptives.[45] In another study[1] estrogen administration consistently enhanced the glucosuric effect of hydrocortisone administered to nine diabetic subjects. However, the glucosuric effect of prednisone, prednisolone, dexamethasone, and methylprednisolone were not consistently affected by estrogen. Finally, the pharmacokinetics of prednisolone (40 mg intravenously) were compared in eight women receiving oral contraceptives, five healthy women not on oral contraceptives, and eight healthy men.[68] The plasma clearance of total prednisolone in women on oral contraceptives was about 50% less than that seen in the other two groups, and the area under the plasma concentration time curve for free prednisolone was about twice that of the other two groups. Thus, there is substantial evidence that estrogens and oral contraceptives can enhance the effect of corticosteroids.

MANAGEMENT: In patients receiving both corticosteroids and an estrogen one should be alert for evidence of excessive corticosteroid effects. It may be necessary to reduce the dose of the corticosteroid.

Food[49]

MECHANISM: None.

CLINICAL SIGNIFICANCE: A cross-over study of two commercial prednisone tablets in four healthy volunteers indicated food did not affect absorption of prednisone as indicated by a comparison of the fasted versus the nonfasted mean plasma prednisolone concentrations.[49]

MANAGEMENT: None necessary.

Indomethacin (Indocin)[28,42]

MECHANISM: The combined effects of indomethacin and corticosteroids may result in increased incidence and/or severity of gastrointestinal ulceration. Indomethacin apparently does not displace cortisol from protein binding[42] as was previously suggested.

CLINICAL SIGNIFICANCE: In one study, the use of prednisone in conjunction with indomethacin appeared to increase the tendency for gastric ulceration in six patients.[28]

MANAGEMENT: It has been suggested that it might be advisable to avoid concomitant use of indomethacin and corticosteroids.[34] However, since many patients will undoubtedly receive this combination, a more realistic precaution would be to watch more closely for gastrointestinal ulceration in such patients.

Phenylbutazone (Butazolidin)[52]

MECHANISM: Not established.

CLINICAL SIGNIFICANCE: In three healthy subjects receiving phenylbutazone an intravenous injection of hydrocortisone was associated

DRUGS	DISCUSSION

with an increase in the urinary excretion of oxidized metabolites of phenylbutazone.[52] However, the clinical significance of these findings remains to be established. One should also consider the possibility that combined use of phenylbutazone and corticosteroids may increase the likelihood of gastrointestinal ulceration as compared to that seen with either drug alone.

MANAGEMENT: No special precautions appear to be necessary, but one should consider the possibility that the likelihood of gastrointestinal ulceration may be increased.

Salicylates[18–20,36,37,69]

MECHANISM: Not established. It has been proposed that corticosteroids may decrease blood salicylate concentrations by increasing glomerular filtration rate (GFR) and decreasing tubular reabsorption of water. Although corticosteroids have been associated with increased GFR[36,37] it remains to be shown that this is responsible for the change in salicylate excretion. Indeed, there is evidence to indicate that corticosteroids may enhance the metabolism of salicylates.[69] Aspirin has been shown to decrease corticosteroid conjugation but the clinical significance of this effect is not known.

CLINICAL SIGNIFICANCE: Decreasing corticosteroid dosage in patients who are also on large doses of salicylates may result in an increasing serum salicylate level with the possibility of salicylate intoxication. One report described four cases that may represent examples of this corticosteroid-salicylate interaction.[18] In another study, corticosteroids appeared to lower serum salicylate levels to below the desired therapeutic range in several patients.[69] Also, gastrointestinal ulceration may be more likely in patients receiving salicylates and corticosteroids than in patients receiving either drug alone.

MANAGEMENT: Corticosteroids and salicylates are frequently administered together and their concomitant use is not contraindicated. However, salicylate dosage requirements may be higher in the presence of corticosteroids, and patients should be watched for salicylate intoxication if the corticosteroid dosage is reduced. The possibility that concomitant therapy may increase the incidence or severity of gastrointestinal ulceration should be kept in mind.

Vitamin A[20,27]

MECHANISM: Not established. Topical vitamin A can reverse the impairment of wound healing seen in patients receiving corticosteroids, perhaps by restoring the normal inflammatory reaction in the wound. The possibility has been suggested that systemic vitamin A could inhibit the anti-inflammatory effect of systemic corticosteroids.

CLINICAL SIGNIFICANCE: It appears fairly well established that topical vitamin A has a beneficial effect on wound healing in patients on corticosteroid therapy. Vitamin A does not appear to enhance wound

CORTICOSTEROID INTERACTIONS (CONT.)

DRUGS	DISCUSSION

healing in patients not receiving corticosteroids. The ability of systemic vitamin A to reactivate inflammation that has been controlled by corticosteroids is a matter of speculation, although one possible example of this interaction has been observed. Animal studies indicate that systemic vitamin A does not prevent corticosteroid-induced increased sensitivity to infection.[27]

MANAGEMENT: Until more information is available systemic vitamin A should be administered with some caution to patients receiving corticosteroids.

ESTROGEN/ORAL CONTRACEPTIVE INTERACTIONS

DRUGS	DISCUSSION

Aminocaproic Acid (Amicar)[23,26]

MECHANISM: Theoretically, an inhibitor of fibrinolysis (aminocaproic acid) with agents that can increase clotting factors (oral contraceptives) could lead to a hypercoagulable state.

CLINICAL SIGNIFICANCE: This interaction is based on theoretical considerations; clinical reports of interaction are lacking.

MANAGEMENT: Pending availability of further information, some caution should be observed in concomitant administration of aminocaproic acid and oral contraceptives.

Antidepressants, Tricyclic[4-7,71]

MECHANISM: It has been proposed that estrogens may effect the metabolism of tricyclic antidepressants[6] but direct evidence for such a mechanism is lacking.

CLINICAL SIGNIFICANCE: Not established. Women on low-dose oral contraceptives have an imipramine bioavailability of 44%, versus 27% in women not on oral contraceptives.[71] Evidence has been presented that ethinyl estradiol (50 μg daily) may impair the response to imipramine (150 mg daily) and increase side effects, while lower doses of estrogen (25 μg daily) had a favorable effect.[4] A subsequent case was briefly described[7] which reportedly represented an example of this interaction. However, Beaumont[5] has failed to find an adverse interaction between oral contraceptives and clomipramine (Anafranil). This may have been due to the lower dose of estrogens in oral contraceptives compared with the previous studies. Obviously, more evidence needs to be presented in order to evaluate the clinical significance.

MANAGEMENT: Although clinical evidence for an interaction is preliminary, one should watch for alteration of tricyclic antidepressant effect if estrogens are also given.

DRUGS	DISCUSSION

Antipyrine[8,21,22,53]

MECHANISM: It is proposed that estrogens and oral contraceptives impair antipyrine metabolism.

CLINICAL SIGNIFICANCE: Several clinical studies have shown that estrogens and oral contraceptives decrease the metabolism of antipyrine. It seems likely that the interaction does occur.

MANAGEMENT: Since antipyrine is seldom used in the United States, the main significance of these findings is that oral contraceptives may have the potential for inhibiting the metabolism of other drugs.

Barbiturates[3,25,40,54]

MECHANISM: Phenobarbital has been shown to increase the metabolism of estrogens in animals, and it is probable that a similar effect occurs in humans.

CLINICAL SIGNIFICANCE: Isolated cases have appeared of epileptic patients receiving combinations of anticonvulsants (including barbiturates) who have become pregnant while taking oral contraceptives. It is likely that low-dose oral contraceptives that have smaller amounts of steroids would be most likely to be rendered less effective by adequate doses of a potent microsomal enzyme inducer.

MANAGEMENT: If it is important that pregnancy be avoided in a patient receiving barbiturates it would probably be wise to use alternative methods of contraception in addition to or instead of oral contraceptives. If barbiturates and oral contraceptives are used concomitantly, spotting or breakthrough bleeding may be an indication that significant enzyme induction is occurring.

Benzodiazepines[55–57,70]

MECHANISM: Oral contraceptives appear to inhibit the metabolism of some benzodiazepines and enhance the metabolism of other benzodiazepines.

CLINICAL SIGNIFICANCE: The mean half-life of chlordiazepoxide (Librium) was 24.3 hours in seven women receiving oral contraceptives (50 to 100 mcg estrogen), compared to a mean of 14.8 hours in 11 women not receiving oral contraceptives. Although the difference was not statistically significant, it seems likely that oral contraceptives do inhibit chlordiazepoxide metabolism. The disposition of diazepam (Valium) (10 mg IV) was compared in eight women receiving low dose (50 mcg estrogen) oral contraceptives and eight women not receiving oral contraceptives. The women receiving oral contraceptives had a longer mean diazepam half-life (69 hours versus 47 hours) and lower total metabolic clearance (0.27 ml/min/kg body weight versus 0.45 ml/min/kg body weight) than those not receiving oral contraceptives. The magnitude of these changes seems large enough to increase the clinical response to diazepam. The disposition of lorazepam

ESTROGEN/ORAL CONTRACEPTIVE
INTERACTIONS (CONT.)

DRUGS	DISCUSSION

(Ativan) (2 mg IV) was compared in eight women receiving oral contraceptives and nine comparable women not on oral contraceptives. Unlike the results seen with chlordiazepoxide and diazepam, oral contraceptives appeared to *enhance* the metabolism of lorazepam. The lorazepam half-life was shorter (4.8 hours versus 13.4 hours) and lorazepam clearance was higher (302 ml/min versus 78 ml/min) in the presence of oral contraceptives. The magnitude of these changes would appear to be sufficient to reduce the clinical response to lorazepam. However, more details are needed to assess the clinical importance of this preliminary report. The disposition of oxazepam (Serax) (45 mg orally) was compared in eight women receiving oral contraceptives and nine comparable women not receiving oral contraceptives. As with lorazepam, the metabolism of oxazepam appeared to be enhanced by concurrent use of oral contraceptives. The oxazepam half-life was shorter (6.8 hours versus 12.4 hours) and the clearance was higher (191 ml/min versus 81 ml/min) in those taking oral contraceptives. The report was preliminary, but the results indicate that oxazepam response may be reduced. In another preliminary report, low-dose oral contraceptives enhanced temazepam elimination.[70] Although the effect of oral contraceptives on other benzodiazepines is not established, one would theoretically expect an increased effect from benzodiazepines which undergo oxidative metabolism in the liver: e.g., alprazolam (Xanax), halazepam (Paxipam), prazepam (Centrax), clorazepate (Tranxene), and flurazepam (Dalmane). Conversely, one might expect a reduced effect from benzodiazepines which undergo glucuronide conjugation.

MANAGEMENT: In patients on oral contraceptives, one should be alert for evidence of enhanced effect of chlordiazepoxide, diazepam, and most other benzodiazepines except those which undergo glucuronide conjugation (e.g., lorazepam, oxazepam, and temazepam).

Caffeine[58]

MECHANISM: Not established. Oral contraceptives may reduce caffeine metabolism.

CLINICAL SIGNIFICANCE: The pharmacokinetics of caffeine (250 mg orally) was compared in nine women on oral contraceptives and nine women not on oral contraceptives. The half-life of caffeine was longer (10.7 hours versus 6.2 hours) and the total plasma clearance lower in women taking oral contraceptives than in women not on oral contraceptives. Thus, caffeine may be expected to have a somewhat greater effect in women receiving oral contraceptives.

MANAGEMENT: No special precautions appear to be necessary.

Clofibrate (Atromid-S)[9]

MECHANISM: Not established.

CLINICAL SIGNIFICANCE: One case report has appeared describing a patient with type IV hyperlipoproteinemia controlled on clofibrate therapy who developed a return of elevated serum cholesterol and triglyceride after taking an oral contraceptive.[9] The incidence of this effect and the effect of oral contraceptives on other types of hyperlipidemias are not known.

MANAGEMENT: Although little clinical evidence is available, patients with hyperlipidemias (treated or not) should be monitored for worsening of clinical and laboratory parameters if oral contraceptives are started.

Meperidine (Demerol)[29,30,35]

MECHANISM: Not established. See Clinical Significance.

CLINICAL SIGNIFICANCE: Preliminary information from urinary excretion data indicated that subjects on oral contraceptives excreted more unchanged meperidine while controls tended to excrete more of the demethylated metabolite.[29] However, subsequent study failed to confirm these findings.[35]

MANAGEMENT: No special precautions appear to be necessary.

Mineral Oil[24]

MECHANISM: Theoretically, mineral oil could impair absorption of estrogens and oral contraceptives.

CLINICAL SIGNIFICANCE: Not established. Some patients with prostatic carcinoma receiving oral estrogens have had exacerbations when mineral oil was taken. Whether the mineral oil was responsible or whether oral contraceptives could be affected remains to be established.

MANAGEMENT: No special precautions appear to be necessary, but all patients should be discouraged from excessive intake of mineral oil.

Phenothiazines[10]

MECHANISM: Not established. It has been proposed that estrogens might decrease the elimination rate of phenothiazines.

CLINICAL SIGNIFICANCE: Following the observation of a dystonic reaction to prochlorperazine (Compazine) in a patient with morning sickness (and presumably high estrogen levels), the effect of conjugated estrogens (Premarin) on butaperazine blood levels was measured in four postmenopausal schizophrenic patients.[10] The plasma levels of butaperazine were increased following estrogen treatment, as was the area under the plasma level-time curve. However, these are preliminary results and further study is needed to assess the clinical significance.

MANAGEMENT: No special precautions appear necessary at this time.

Smoking[59–61]

MECHANISM: Not established.

ESTROGEN/ORAL CONTRACEPTIVE
INTERACTIONS (CONT.)

DRUGS	DISCUSSION

CLINICAL SIGNIFICANCE: Considerable epidemiologic evidence indicates that smoking increases the risk of cardiovascular adverse effects associated with oral contraceptive use (e.g., stroke, myocardial infarction, thromboembolism).[59,60] The risk increases in persons older than 35 years and in patients smoking more than 15 cigarettes per day. Smoking does not appear to alter the metabolism of the progestogens or estrogens found in oral contraceptives.[61]

MANAGEMENT: Women on oral contraceptives should be encouraged not to smoke; if they continue to smoke, they should use an alternative form of contraceptive.

Thyroid Hormones[14,15]

MECHANISM: Estrogens tend to increase serum thyroxine-binding globulin. Thus, in a patient with a nonfunctioning thyroid gland who is receiving thyroid replacement therapy, free thyroxine may be decreased when estrogens are started, thus increasing thyroid requirements. However, if the patient's thyroid gland has sufficient function, the decreased free thyroxine will result in a compensatory increase in thyroxine output by the thyroid.

CLINICAL SIGNIFICANCE: This interaction is based largely on theoretical considerations rather than clinical observations. Thus, the clinical significance remains to be established.

MANAGEMENT: Physicians should be alert to the possibility that patients without a functioning thyroid gland who are on thyroid replacement therapy may need to increase their thyroid dose if estrogens or oral contraceptives are given.

THYROID HORMONE INTERACTIONS

DRUGS	DISCUSSION

Cholestyramine (Questran)[31]

MECHANISM: Cholestyramine binds both thyroxine and triiodothyronine in the intestine, thus impairing absorption of these thyroid hormones. In-vitro studies indicate that the binding is not easily reversed.

CLINICAL SIGNIFICANCE: Decreased thyroid hormone absorption due to cholestyramine was suspected in one patient and later documented in patients and volunteers using radioactive thyroxine. In-vitro studies showed triiodothyronine to be similarly bound by cholestyramine.

MANAGEMENT: This study shows that 4 to 5 hours should elapse between administration of cholestyramine and thyroid hormones.

Ketamine (Ketaject, Ketalar)[17]

MECHANISM: Not established.

THYROID HORMONE INTERACTIONS (CONT.)

DRUGS	DISCUSSION

CLINICAL SIGNIFICANCE: In two patients receiving thyroid replacement therapy, the administration of ketamine was followed by marked hypertension and tachycardia.[17] Although less severe increases in blood pressure and heart rate may occur following ketamine alone, it was felt that the thyroid replacement therapy was involved in these cases. More study is needed to assess clinical significance.

MANAGEMENT: Until more is known about this possible interaction, ketamine should probably be administered with caution to patients on thyroid replacement therapy. If a reaction does occur, on the basis of the response of the two patients just described,[17] propranolol may be useful.

References

1. NELSON DH, et al: Potentiation of the biologic effect of administered cortisol by estrogen treatment. J Clin Endocrinol Metab 23:261, 1963.
2. CARTER D, et al: Effect of oral contraceptives on drug and vitamin D_3 metabolism (Abstract). Clin Pharmacol Ther 15:202,1974.
3. JANZ D, SCHMIDT D: Anti-epileptic drugs and failure of oral contraceptives (Letter). Lancet 1:1113, 1974.
4. PRANGE AJ Jr, et al: Estrogen may well affect response to antidepressant (Medical News). JAMA 219:143, 1972.
5. BEAUMONT G: Drug interactions with clomipramine (Anafranil). J Int Med Res 1:480, 1973.
6. SOMANI SM, KHURANA RC: Mechanism of estrogen-imipramine interaction (Letter). JAMA 223:560, 1973.
7. KHURANA RC: Estrogen-imipramine interaction (Letter). JAMA 222:702, 1972.
8. SOTANIEMI EA, et al: Drug metabolism and androgen control therapy in prostatic cancer. Clin Pharmacol Ther 14:413, 1973.
9. ROBERTSON-RINTOUL J: Raised serum-lipids and oral contraceptives (Letter). Lancet 2:1320, 1972.
10. EL-YOUSEF MK, MANIER DH: Estrogen effects on phenothiazine derivative blood levels (Letter). JAMA 228:827, 1974.
11. HVIDBERG EF, et al: Studies of the interaction of phenylbutazone, oxyphenbutazone and methandrostenolone in man. Proc Soc Exp Biol Med 129:438, 1968.
12. WEINER M, et al: Drug interactions: The effect of combined administration on the half-life of coumarin and pyrazolone drugs in man. Fed Proc 24:153, 1965.
13. WEINER M, et al: Effect of steroids on disposition of oxyphenbutazone in man. Proc Soc Exp Biol Med 124:1170, 1967.
14. MARGULIS RR, LEACH RG: Effect of oral contraceptives on thyroid function (Questions and Answers). JAMA 206:2326, 1968.
15. WIENER JD: Thyroid hormones and protein-bound iodine (Letter). JAMA 207:1717, 1969.
16. SPANGLER AS, et al: Enhancement of the anti-inflammatory action of hydrocortisone by estrogen. J Clin Endocrinol 29:650, 1969.

References (CONT.)

17. Kaplan JA, Cooperman LH: Alarming reactions to ketamine in patients taking thyroid medication—treatment with propranolol. Anesthesiology 35:229, 1971.
18. Klinenberg JR, Miller F: Effect of corticosteroids on blood salicylate concentration. JAMA 194:601, 1965.
19. Elliott HC: Reduced adrenocortical steroid excretion rates in man following aspirin administration. Metabolism 11:1015, 1962.
20. Hunt TK, et al: Effect of vitamin A on reversing the inhibitory effect of cortisone on healing of open wounds in animals and man. Ann Surg 170:633, 1969.
21. O'Malley K, et al: Increased antipyrine half-life in women taking oral contraceptives. Scott Med J 15:454, 1970.
22. O'Malley K, et al: Impairment of human drug metabolism by oral contraceptive steroids. Clin Pharmacol Ther 13:552, 1972.
23. Elgee NJ: Medical aspects of oral contraceptives. Ann Intern Med 72:409, 1970.
24. Swyer GIM: Liquid paraffin and oral contraception (Notes and Queries). Practitioner 202:592, 1969.
25. Conney AH: Pharmacological implications of microsomal enzyme induction. Pharmacol Rev 19:317, 1967.
26. Anon: Aminocaproic acid in haemophilia and in menorrhagia. Drug Ther Bull 5:63, 1967.
27. Stephens FO, et al: Effect of cortisone and vitamin A on wound infection. Am J Surg 121:569, 1971.
28. Emmanuel JH, Montgomery RD: Gastric ulcer and the antiarthritic drugs. Postgrad Med J 47:227, 1971.
29. Crawford JS, Rudofsky S: Some alterations in the pattern of drug metabolism associated with pregnancy, oral contraceptives, and the newly-born. Br J Anaesth 38:446, 1966.
30. Crawford JS, Hooi HWY: Binding of bromsulphthalein by serum albumin from pregnant women, neonates and subjects on oral contraceptives. Br J Anaesth 40:723, 1968.
31. Northcutt RC, et al: The influence of cholestyramine on thyroxin absorption. JAMA 208:1857, 1969.
32. Brooks SM, et al: Adverse effects of phenobarbital on corticosteroid metabolism in patients with bronchial asthma. N Engl J Med 286:1125, 1972.
33. Falliers CJ: Corticosteroids and phenobarbital in asthma (Letter). N Engl J Med 287:201, 1972.
34. Sotaniemi E, et al: Increased clearance of tolbutamide from the blood of asthmatic patients. Ann Allerg 29:139, 1971.
35. Stambaugh JE Jr, Wainer IW: Drug interactions I: meperidine and combination oral contraceptives. J Clin Pharmacol 15:46, 1975.
36. George CRP: Nonspecific enhancement of glomerular filtration by corticosteroids (Letter). Lancet 2:728, 1974.
37. Polak A, Lavender S: Nonspecific enhancement of glomerular filtration by corticosteroids (Letter). Lancet 2:841, 1974.
38. Wassner SJ, et al: The adverse effect of anticonvulsant therapy on renal allograft survival. J Pediatr 88:134, 1976.
39. Stjernholm MR, Katz FH: Effects of diphenylhydantoin, phenobarbital and diazepam on the metabolism of methylprednisolone and its sodium succinate. J Clin Endocrinol Metab 41:887, 1975.

References (CONT.)

40. ROBERTON YR, JOHNSON ES: Interactions between oral contraceptives and other drugs: a review. Curr Med Res Opin 3:647, 1976.
41. BERMAN ML, GREEN OC: Acute stimulation of cortisol metabolism by pentobarbital in man. Anesthesiology 34:365, 1971.
42. HVIDBERG E, et al: Influence of indomethacin on the distribution of cortisol in man. Eur J Clin Pharmacol 3:102, 1971.
43. SOUTHERN AL, et al: Effect of N-phenylbarbital (phetharbital) on the metabolism of testosterone and cortisol in man. J Clin Endocrinol Metab 29:251, 1969.
44. BROOKS PM, et al: Effects of enzyme induction on metabolism of prednisolone. Clinical and laboratory study. Ann Rheum Dis 35:339, 1976.
45. KOZOWER M, et al: Decreased clearance of prednisolone, a factor in the development of corticosteroid side effects. J Clin Endocrinol Metab 38:407, 1974.
46. BROOKS SM, et al: The effects of ephedrine and theophylline on dexamethasone metabolism in bronchial asthma. J Clin Pharmacol 17:308, 1977.
47. TOPPOZADA M, et al: Uterine response to prostaglandin E_2 under oral contraceptives. Contraception 13:749, 1976.
48. BROOKS SM, et al: The effects of disodium cromoglycate on dexamethasone metabolism. Am Rev Respir Dis 114:1191, 1976.
49. TEMBO AV, et al: Effect of food on the bioavailability of prednisone. J Clin Pharmacol 16:620, 1976.
50. CLARK GM, MILLS D: Corticosteroid therapy of rheumatoid arthritis supplemented with methandrostenolone. Arthritis Rheum 5:156, 1962.
51. MILLS D, CLARK GM: The effect of methandrostenolone on excretion of compound F (Abstract). Arthritis Rheum 4:426, 1961.
52. AARBAKKE J, et al: Increased oxidation of phenylbutazone during hydrocortisone infusion in man. Br J Clin Pharmacol 4:621, 1977.
53. CARTER DE, et al: Effect of oral contraceptives on plasma clearance. Clin Pharmacol Ther 18:700, 1975.
54. HEMPEL E, KLINGER W: Drug stimulated biotransformation of hormonal steroid contraceptives: clinical implications. Drugs 12:442, 1976.
55. ROBERTS RK, et al: Disposition of chlordiazepoxide: sex differences and effects of oral contraceptives. Clin Pharmacol Ther 25:826, 1979.
56. ABERNETHY DR, et al: Impairment of diazepam metabolism by low-dose estrogen-containing oral contraceptive steroids. N Engl J Med 306:791, 1982.
57. PATWARDHAN R, et al: Induction of glucuronidation by oral contraceptive steroids (ocs). Clin Res 29:861A, 1981.
58. PATWARDHAN RV, et al: Impaired elimination of caffeine by oral contraceptive steroids. J Lab Clin Med 95:603, 1980.
59. FREDRICKSEN H, RAVENHOLT RT: Thromboembolism, oral contraceptives and cigarettes. Public Health Rep 85:197, 1970.
60. Ovulen®. Product Information. Chicago, Searle Laboratories, 1984.
61. CRAWFORD FE, et al: Oral contraceptive steroid plasma concentrations in smokers and nonsmokers. Br Med J 282:1829, 1981.
62. JOHANSSON C, et al: Interaction by cholestyramine on the uptake of hydrocortisone in the gastrointestinal tract. Acta Med Scand 204:509, 1978.
63. NAGGAR VF, et al: Effect of concomitant administration of magnesium

References (CONT.)

trisilicate on GI absorption of dexamethasone in humans. J Pharm Sci 67:1029, 1978.

64. URBINE M, et al: Decreased bioavailability of prednisone due to antacids in patients with chronic active liver disease and in healthy volunteers. Gastroenterology 80:661, 1981.

65. LEE DAH, et al: The effect of concurrent administration of antacids on prednisolone absorption. Br J Clin Pharmacol 8:92, 1979.

66. TANNER AR, et al: Concurrent administration of antacids and prednisolone: Effect on serum levels of prednisolone. Br J Clin Pharmacol 7:397, 1979.

67. GAMBERTOGLIO J, et al: Enhancement of prednisolone elimination by anticonvulsants in renal transplant recipients. Clin Pharmacol Ther 31:228, 1982.

68. BOEKENOOGEN SJ, et al: Prednisolone disposition and protein binding in oral contraceptive users. J Clin Endocrinol Metab 56:702, 1983.

69. GRAHAM GG, et al: Patterns of plasma concentrations and urinary excretion of salicylate in rheumatoid arthritis. Clin Pharmacol Ther 22:410, 1977.

70. STOEHR GP, et al: The effect of low-dose estrogen-containing oral contraceptives on the pharmacokinetics of triazolam, alprazolam, temazepam, and lorazepam (Abstract). Drug Intell Clin Pharm 18:495, 1984.

71. ABERNETHY DR, et al: Imipramine disposition in users of oral contraceptive steroids. Clin Pharmacol Ther 6:792, 1984.

CHAPTER 12

Monoamine Oxidase Inhibitor Interactions

MONOAMINE OXIDASE INHIBITOR INTERACTIONS

DRUGS	DISCUSSION

Amphetamines[4,12-14,17-19]

MECHANISM: Monoamine oxidase inhibitors (MAOI) tend to increase the amount of norepinephrine present in storage sites of the adrenergic neuron. The subsequent administration of agents that result in catecholamine release (e.g., amphetamines) results in liberation of a larger amount of norepinephrine to react with the receptor. It is probable that MAOI with intrinsic amphetamine-like activity (e.g., phenelzine, tranylcypromine) are more dangerous in combination with amphetamines. Pargyline and nialamide do not have amphetamine-like pharmacologic actions. Furazolidone (Furoxone), also an MAOI, has been shown to increase pressor sensitivity to amphetamine.[17,18]

CLINICAL SIGNIFICANCE: Fatalities and near-fatalities have occurred in patients receiving amphetamines and an MAOI concomitantly. Tranylcypromine appears to be the most dangerous MAOI in this regard. One patient developed a fever of 109.4°F following administration of tranylcypromine plus dextroamphetamine.[12] Another patient on phenelzine developed headache, hypertension, and a fatal cerebral hemorrhage following ingestion of 20 mg of dextroamphetamine.[19] Cardiac arrhythmias, flushing, vomiting, and seizures have also been reported.

MANAGEMENT: Amphetamines should not be given to patients receiving MAOI. Phentolamine (Regitine) appears to be the logical therapy for severe hypertension from this interaction since it would block the excessive alpha stimulation of the released norepinephrine.[14]

Anticholinergic Agents[15]

MECHANISM: Not established. The activity of anticholinergic drugs is reported to be potentiated by MAOI.

CLINICAL SIGNIFICANCE: MAOI reportedly may potentiate antiparkinson anticholinergic agents, but clinical documentation is lacking.

MANAGEMENT: Too little is known to make a statement on management.

MONOAMINE OXIDASE INHIBITOR INTERACTIONS (CONT.)

DRUGS	DISCUSSION

Antidepressants, Tricyclic[5-7,15,43-46,50-52,56,57,78-82]

MECHANISM: The mechanism has not been established. See Clinical Significance.

CLINICAL SIGNIFICANCE: Severe reactions have been reported with the concomitant administration of an MAOI and a tricyclic antidepressant, usually when the tricyclic is added to established MAOI therapy. The symptoms that have been observed include excitation, hyperpyrexia, and convulsions; fatalities have occurred. In most of the reports of severe reactions, excessive doses of one or more drugs were used, the tricyclic antidepressant was given parenterally, or other psychotropic drugs were also being given. However, Beaumont[7] briefly reports three patients who were thought to have died as a result of an interaction between clomipramine (Anafranil) and MAOI, two of whom were receiving "therapeutic" doses of both drugs. Still, there is convincing evidence[5,51,52,56,57,79-82] that MAOI and some tricyclic antidepressants can be given safely together in most patients if the following precautions are used:
1. avoid large doses
2. give the drugs orally
3. avoid clomipramine and imipramine
4. monitor the patient closely

Thus, it appears that reactions can occur following combined use of MAOI and tricyclics, but the incidence and severity of reactions appear lower than suspected earlier. Also, tricyclic antidepressants could theoretically reduce the danger of indirectly acting sympathomimetics or tyramine in patients receiving MAOI, since tricyclic antidepressants may inhibit the uptake of the sympathomimetic by the adrenergic neuron.

MANAGEMENT: It is clear that concomitant use can no longer be considered contraindicated. However, when combined use is contemplated, any possible benefit of the combination should be weighed against the known hazards of these agents. Further, one should remember that a potentially lethal combination (in overdose) will be at the disposal of suicide-prone patients.

Barbiturates[8,15]

MECHANISM: Not established. It is possible that MAOI inhibit the metabolism of barbiturates.

CLINICAL SIGNIFICANCE: A patient receiving tranylcypromine (30 mg/day for 3 weeks) became semicomatose for 36 hours following the administration of amylobarbital (250 mg intramuscularly).[8] Subsequent animal studies indicated that tranylcypromine may prolong amylobarbital hypnosis. However, little is known concerning the effect of normal oral doses of barbiturates in patients receiving MAOI.

MANAGEMENT: Barbiturates should be given with some caution to patients receiving MAOI.

MONOAMINE OXIDASE INHIBITOR INTERACTIONS (CONT.)

DRUGS	DISCUSSION

Benzodiazepines[59,75]

MECHANISM: Not established.

CLINICAL SIGNIFICANCE: A patient receiving phenelzine (Nardil) and chlordiazepoxide (Librium) developed massive edema, and it was proposed that the drug combination may have been responsible.[59] Another patient was subsequently reported who developed edema while receiving isocarboxazid (Marplan) and chlordiazepoxide.[75] Although the drug combinations may have contributed to the edema, such an association is still very tentative.

MANAGEMENT: No special precautions appear necessary.

Carbamazepine (Tegretol)[48]

MECHANISM: Because of the structural similarity between carbamazepine and the tricyclic antidepressants, the possibility exists that carbamazepine may also be dangerous in patients receiving MAOI.

CLINICAL SIGNIFICANCE: No clinical reports of interaction have appeared; only theoretical considerations are involved.

MANAGEMENT: Pending availability of further information, it would be prudent to avoid concomitant use of carbamazepine and an MAOI. Since the manufacturer lists concomitant administration of these drugs under contraindications, medicolegal considerations must be taken into account.

Cyclamates[20]

MECHANISM: Cyclamate is converted in part to cyclohexylamine in the intestine. Cyclohexylamine is a pressor amine and theoretically could result in an adverse drug interaction in patients receiving MAOI.

CLINICAL SIGNIFICANCE: This interaction is postulated from theoretical considerations rather than clinical reports of interactions. Also, due to the restrictions on cyclamates in the United States, concomitant use with MAOI would seldom occur.

MANAGEMENT: Pending the availability of further information, patients receiving MAOI should probably be advised to limit cyclamate consumption.

Dextromethorphan[49]

MECHANISM: Not established.

CLINICAL SIGNIFICANCE: A single case has been reported in which a patient receiving phenelzine developed nausea, coma, hypotension, and hyperpyrexia following ingestion of 2 ounces of a cough syrup containing dextromethorphan. Death may have been due to the combination of hyperpyrexia and cerebral hypoxia. Drug interaction was

DRUGS	DISCUSSION

suspected but not proved to be the precipitating factor in this reaction.

MANAGEMENT: Until more information is available, patients on MAOI should be instructed to avoid preparations containing dextromethorphan.

Doxapram (Dopram)[21,22]

MECHANISM: Not established.

CLINICAL SIGNIFICANCE: The adverse cardiovascular effects of doxapram (e.g., hypertension, arrhythmias) are reportedly potentiated by MAOI.

MANAGEMENT: Pending the availability of further information, caution should be used in giving MAOI and doxapram concomitantly.

Ephedrine[14,15,23,24,86]

MECHANISM: MAOI tend to increase the amount of norepinephrine present in storage sites of the adrenergic neuron. The subsequent administration of agents that result in catecholamine release (e.g., ephedrine) results in liberation of a larger amount of norepinephrine to react with the receptor.

CLINICAL SIGNIFICANCE: Severe hypertensive reactions may occur with concomitant administration. At least one death has been attributed to this interaction. The combination of ephedrine and MAOI was used intentionally to increase blood pressure in four patients with postural hypotension, but resulted in excessive supine hypertension.[86]

MANAGEMENT: Ephedrine should be avoided in patients receiving MAOI due to the difficulty of selecting a dose that will be therapeutic but not toxic. Phentolamine (Regitine) appears to be the logical therapy for severe hypertension from this interaction since it would block the excessive alpha stimulation of the released norepinephrine.[14]

Epinephrine (Adrenaline)[1,2,14,15]

MECHANISM: The termination of the pharmacologic response to epinephrine is not primarily dependent on monoamine oxidase. Thus, exogenous epinephrine should not be appreciably affected by administration of MAOI. The small enhancement of epinephrine that may be seen is possibly due to a "denervation supersensitivity" induced by the MAOI.

CLINICAL SIGNIFICANCE: In one study in four healthy subjects (two receiving phenelzine and two receiving tranylcypromine), the administration of epinephrine did not significantly affect heart rate or blood pressure.[1] Thus, although extensive study of this interaction has not been conducted in man, available evidence indicates that epinephrine is not significantly potentiated by MAO inhibition.

MONOAMINE OXIDASE INHIBITOR INTERACTIONS (CONT.)

DRUGS	DISCUSSION

MANAGEMENT: No sympathomimetic can be given with impunity to patients receiving MAOI. However, epinephrine is not likely to produce severe reactions if it is administered with care.

Ethanol (Alcohol, Ethyl)[15,23,47]

MECHANISM: There is no known mechanism for any interaction between ethanol itself and MAOI. However, some alcoholic beverages (e.g., Chianti wine) may contain considerable amounts of tyramine. In the presence of MAO inhibition, the normally rapid metabolism of tyramine in the intestine and liver is impaired, resulting in a markedly enhanced pressor response to tyramine.

CLINICAL SIGNIFICANCE: Although the effect of ethanol may be enhanced somewhat in the presence of MAO inhibition, too little information is available to assess the clinical significance. However, the danger of tyramine-containing alcoholic beverages is definite. Fatal hypertensive crises may result.

MANAGEMENT: Since the patient is not likely to be able to assess the tyramine content of a given drink (especially drinks with many ingredients), it would be wise to advise patients receiving MAOI to avoid alcoholic beverages.

Food[60-74,83-86]

MECHANISM: Tyramine in foods is normally metabolized by monoamine oxidase in the gut wall and liver before reaching the systemic circulation. In the presence of MAOI, excessive amounts of tyramine may reach the systemic circulation, resulting in an excessive pressor response. The excessive pressor response can occur following a single dose of an MAOI.[84]

CLINICAL SIGNIFICANCE: Blackwell[60] described 11 tranylcypromine-treated patients who experienced hypertensive crises following ingestion of cheddar cheese (raw or cooked) and in one case "marmite" (a yeast extract that reportedly contains 1.5 mg of tyramine per gram). The food products were eaten within one-half to 2-hours of the attack, and in some instances as little as 22 g of cheese was ingested. Chicken liver ingestion was associated with severe hypertensive crises in six patients receiving tranylcypromine.[61] The tyramine content of the chicken livers was analyzed by two different methods, with the amount ranging from 94 mcg/g to 113 mcg/g. However, other chicken livers obtained by the authors did not contain significant amounts of tyramine, indicating that tyramine may be formed during storage of the liver. Nuessle[63] reported that a similar type of hypertensive crisis occurred when a patient had eaten pickled herring while on tranylcypromine. The tyramine content of pickled herring was reported to be 3.03 mg/g. In seven hospitalized patients marked potentiation of the pressor effects of tyramine hydrochloride occurred in patients receiving MAOI.[66] As little as 6 mg of tyramine given orally produced

DRUGS	DISCUSSION

hypertension. In another report a patient on phenelzine experienced a hypertensive crisis an hour after ingesting the beverage, "Bovril."[69] Ingestion of whole broad beans (Vicia faba) has been associated with hypertensive crisis in several patients[70,71] presumably due to the dopa content of the beans.

MANAGEMENT: Patients receiving MAOI should be instructed to avoid foods that may have a high tyramine content. Estimates of the tyramine content of foods and beverages have been published.[66,72,83] Foods to be avoided include cheeses (especially aged), wines (especially red), caviar, herring (dried or pickled), canned figs, fermented or spoiled meat (including salami, pepperoni, summer sausage), fava beans, yeast extracts, avocados (especially if overripe), and yogurt.

Norepinephrine (Levarterenol, Levophed)[1,2,14,15,23]

MECHANISM: Catechol-0-methyltransferase (COMT) appears to be much more important in the metabolism of exogenous levarterenol than is monoamine oxidase. Thus, administered levarterenol should not be appreciably affected by MAO inhibition. The small enhancement of levarterenol that may be seen is possibly due to a "denervation supersensitivity" induced by the MAOI.

CLINICAL SIGNIFICANCE: In one study in four healthy subjects (two receiving phenelzine and two receiving tranylcypromine), the administration of levarterenol did not significantly affect heart rate or blood pressure.[1] Only patients with decreased blood pressure from the MAOI have manifested a somewhat increased response to levarterenol.

MANAGEMENT: No sympathomimetic can be given with impunity to patients receiving an MAOI. However, levarterenol is not likely to produce severe reactions if it is administered with care.

Levodopa (L-DOPA)[9,25–27,39–41,55,58,76]

MECHANISM: Levodopa is the precursor of dopamine, which in turn is converted into norepinephrine. A major pathway of degradation of dopamine involves monoamine oxidase; thus, MAOI will decrease dopamine degradation while levodopa increases dopamine formation. Norepinephrine formation is also likely to be increased by levodopa. It is likely that the adverse cardiovascular effects seen with concomitant levodopa and MAOI administration are due to increased storage and release of dopamine, norepinephrine, or both.

CLINICAL SIGNIFICANCE: Hypertension, flushing of the face, pounding of the heart, and lightheadedness have been reported with concomitant administration of nialamide and levodopa to normal volunteers.[25] One patient receiving phenelzine manifested hypertension when given 50 mg of levodopa but not when given 25 mg of levodopa.[39] Preliminary evidence also indicates that the addition of MAOI to patients on levodopa may result in worsening of akinesia and tremor.[40] A favorable use of the interaction has been reported in two patients with idiopathic orthostatic hypotension given levodopa and tranylcypromine.[9,76] However, one patient developed palpitations, a diastolic pressure of 150 mm Hg, and two small retinal hemorrhages.[9] Also, it appears that carbidopa may inhibit the hypertensive reaction to levodopa in patients receiving MAOI.[55] Another report describes favorable effects in parkinsonism with a combination of levodopa, a decarboxylase inhibitor (benserazide), and an MAOI (L-Deprenil).[58]

MANAGEMENT: The concomitant use of levodopa and MAOI should generally be avoided. If they are given concomitantly and hypertension ensues, the results of one case indicate that phentolamine (Regitine) may reverse the hypertension.[39] The use of a decarboxylase inhibitor (e.g., carbidopa) with levodopa apparently prevents the hypertensive reactions, so it would be desirable to use such agents with levodopa if use of an MAOI is anticipated.

Meperidine (Demerol)[3,10,11,13–15,32,33]

MECHANISM: The mechanism is not established, although some have been proposed.[3,10]

CLINICAL SIGNIFICANCE: When meperidine is given to a patient receiving an MAOI, severe reactions, generally immediate, with excitation, sweating, rigidity and hypertension, may occur. However, some patients develop hypotension and coma, which are apparently due to potentiation of the pharmacologic effects of meperidine. Although several deaths that were apparently due to this interaction have been reported, most patients probably do not react adversely to the combination.[3] Other narcotics (e.g., morphine) are not likely to cause such severe reactions. Thus, although they cannot be used with impunity, they are much preferable to meperidine.

MANAGEMENT: Meperidine should probably be avoided in patients receiving MAOI. Morphine and other narcotics may be given cautiously, and, preferably, in reduced dose.

Metaraminol (Aramine)[15,77]

MECHANISM: Metaraminol is an indirect acting sympathomimetic producing its pressor effect by releasing norepinephrine, which reacts with the adrenergic receptor. Since MAOI tend to increase the amount of norepinephrine present in storage sites of the adrenergic neuron, patients receiving MAOI would be expected to manifest an enhanced response to metaraminol.

CLINICAL SIGNIFICANCE: A hypertensive patient who had a hypotensive episode while receiving pargyline (Eutonyl) was given metaraminol (4 mg intramuscularly). Within 10 minutes his systolic blood pressure was 300 mm Hg; he lost consciousness and developed an irregular cardiac rhythm.[77]

MANAGEMENT: Metaraminol should be avoided in patients receiving MAOI. Levarterenol (Levophed) is likely to be a safer pressor agent to use.

Methotrimeprazine (Levoprome)[15,38]

MECHANISM: Not established.

CLINICAL SIGNIFICANCE: A fatal reaction has occurred in a patient receiving pargyline and methotrimeprazine, but drug interaction was not unequivocally established as the cause.

MANAGEMENT: Although the interaction is not well documented, the possibility of a fatal reaction contraindicates concomitant use.

Methylphenidate (Ritalin)[15,31]

Methylphenidate has amphetamine-like pharmacologic activity. The general discussion for the amphetamines (see p. 332) would apply to methylphenidate, but reactions may be less severe.

Phenothiazines[15,29]

MECHANISM: Not established. It is possible that MAOI inhibit the metabolism of phenothiazines.

CLINICAL SIGNIFICANCE: Increased side effects of the phenothiazines (e.g., extrapyramidal reactions) reportedly may occur with concomitant use of MAOI and phenothiazines. However, several studies have appeared in which this combination was used to treat various psychiatric disorders. In at least one of these (tranylcypromine plus trifluoperazine), side effects of both agents were reportedly *decreased* by using them in combination.[29] It has also been proposed that trifluoperazine protects against tyramine-induced hypertensive crises in patients receiving tranylcypromine. If this is true, it may be due to the alpha-adrenergic blocking effect of the phenothiazine. In summary, it appears that some combinations of MAOI and phenothiazines are beneficial. It should be kept in mind, however, that this does not rule out the possibility that other combinations may prove to increase side effects.

MANAGEMENT: No special precautions appear necessary, but physicians should be alert for side effects in patients when untried combinations of a phenothiazine and MAOI are used.

Phenylephrine (Neo-Synephrine)[1,2,15,23,30,86]

MECHANISM: Phenylephrine appears to act primarily by direct action on adrenergic receptors, with relatively little indirect activity. However, phenylephrine is metabolized by MAO in the intestine and liver. Thus, normal oral doses of phenylephrine in the presence of MAO inhibition would be expected to be markedly enhanced. Parenteral

DRUGS	DISCUSSION

doses of phenylephrine would not be expected to be affected appreciably since much smaller doses are used (because of decreased exposure to intestinal and hepatic monoamine oxidase).

CLINICAL SIGNIFICANCE: In one clinical study of this interaction, MAO inhibition markedly enhanced the hypertensive response to oral phenylephrine.[23] On three occasions, it was necessary to use phentolamine to abate the severe hypertension. As expected from the preceding discussion of mechanisms, parenteral (in this case intravenous) administration of phenylephrine resulted in only a moderate potentiation of the pressor response. In a subsequent study in four healthy subjects, pretreatment with MAOI resulted in a two- to two-and-one-half-fold increase in the pressor response to phenylephrine.[1] In another study of four patients with hypotension, phenylephrine produced a pronounced pressor response when combined with an MAOI.[86] Thus, the evidence is convincing that a significant interaction exists.

MANAGEMENT: Oral phenylephrine should be avoided in patients receiving MAOI. It should be noted that phenylephrine is found in many nonprescription cold remedies. Parenteral phenylephrine should be used with great care in patients on MAOI. The effect of phenylephrine-containing nose sprays has not been studied, but they should probably be avoided until information on their safety is available.

Phenylpropanolamine (Propadrine)[34–37,53]

MECHANISM: Phenylpropanolamine resembles ephedrine in pharmacologic actions. Thus, the MAOI-induced increases in norepinephrine storage in the adrenergic neuron results in liberation of larger amounts of norepinephrine to react with the receptor site when phenylpropanolamine is given.

CLINICAL SIGNIFICANCE: Several case reports have appeared in the literature describing this interaction. Headache, vomiting, and elevated blood pressure have been the major findings. One patient receiving 45 mg/day of phenelzine (Nardil) developed a cardiac arrhythmia following a single dose of a phenylpropanolamine-containing decongestant (Sinutab).[53] Severe reactions (e.g., marked hypertension) appear more likely with standard dosage forms of phenylpropanolamine while the sustained-release preparations are more likely to produce headache, vomiting, etc.

MANAGEMENT: Phenylpropanolamine should not be given to patients receiving MAOI.

Pseudoephedrine (Sudafed)[78]

MECHANISM: MAOI tend to increase the amount of norepinephrine in storage sites of the adrenergic neuron. Subsequent displacement of these increased stores of norepinephrine by indirect acting sympathomimetics (e.g., pseudoephedrine) can result in an exaggerated response.

DRUGS	DISCUSSION

CLINICAL SIGNIFICANCE: A fatal reaction has purportedly occurred following ingestion of a single dose of pseudoephedrine in a patient receiving a monoamine oxidase inhibitor,[78] but no details were given. Although there is little clinical evidence of interaction, the one fatal case in addition to theoretical considerations would indicate that the interaction is real.

MANAGEMENT: Patients receiving MAOI should be instructed to avoid ingestion of pseudoephedrine.

Succinylcholine (Anectine, Quelicin)[42]

MECHANISM: A preliminary report indicates that phenelzine (an MAOI) may decrease plasma pseudocholinesterase to the subnormal range. Thus, succinylcholine may have an enhanced effect since it is metabolized by pseudocholinesterase.

CLINICAL SIGNIFICANCE: One case report has appeared in which a patient on phenelzine developed prolonged apnea following administration of succinylcholine. This patient and three others receiving phenelzine were shown to have decreased pseudocholinesterase levels. However, based on information from this preliminary study, other MAOI do not appear to affect pseudocholinesterase.

MANAGEMENT: Pending availability of further information, succinylcholine should be administered with caution to patients receiving phenelzine (Nardil).

References

1. BOAKES AJ, et al: Interactions between sympathomimetic amines and antidepressant agents in man. Br Med J 1:311, 1973.
2. BOAKES AJ: Sympathomimetic amines and antidepressant agents (Letter). Br Med J 2:114, 1973.
3. EVANS-PROSSER CDG: The use of pethidine and morphine in the presence of monoamine oxidase inhibitors. Br J Anaesthesiol 40:279, 1968.
4. ZECK P: The dangers of some antidepressant drugs (Letter). Med J Aust 2:607, 1961.
5. KLINE NS: Experimental use of monoamine oxidase inhibitors with tricyclic antidepressants (Questions and Answers). JAMA 227:807, 1974.
6. MITCHELL JR, et al: Guanethidine and related agents. III. Antagonism by drugs which inhibit the norepinephrine pump in man. J Clin Invest 49:1596, 1970.
7. BEAUMONT G: Drug interactions with clomipramine (Anafranil). J Int Med Res 1:480, 1973.
8. DOMINO EF, et al: Barbiturate intoxication in a patient treated with a MAO inhibitor. Am J Psychiatry 118:941, 1962.
9. SHARPE J, et al: Idiopathic orthostatic hypotension treated with levo-

References (CONT.)

dopa and MAO inhibitor: a preliminary report. Can Med Assoc J 107:296, 1972.

10. JOUNELA AJ, KIVIMAKI T: Possible sensitivity to meperidine in phenylketonuria (Letter). N Engl J Med 288:1411, 1973.

11. GESSNER PK, SOBLE AG: Studies on the role of brain 5-hydroxytryptamine in the interaction between tranylcypromine and meperidine (Abstract). Fed Proc 29:685abs, 1970.

12. KRISKO I, et al: Severe hyperpyrexia due to tranylcypromineramphetamine toxicity. Ann Intern Med 70:559, 1969.

13. BROWNLEE G, WILLIAMS GW: Potentiation of amphetamine and pethidine by monoaminoxidase inhibitors. Lancet 1:669, 1963.

14. GOLDBERG LI: Monoamine oxidase inhibitors. Adverse reactions and possible mechanisms. JAMA 190:456, 1964.

15. SJOQVIST F: Psychotropic drugs (2). Interaction between monoamine oxidase (MAO) inhibitors and other substances. Proc R Soc Med 58:967, 1965.

16. LEVY J, MICHEL-BER E: Difficulties and complications caused in man by monoamine oxidase (MAO) inhibitors, with special reference to their specific and secondary pharmacological effects. In Toxicity and Side-effects of Psychotropic Drugs. Amsterdam, Excerpta Medica Foundation, 1968, pp. 223–245.

17. PETTINGER WA, et al: Inhibition of monoamine oxidase in man by furazolidone. Clin Pharmacol Ther 9:442, 1968.

18. PETTINGER WA, OATES JA: Supersensitivity to tyramine during monoamine oxidase inhibition in man. Mechanism at the level of the adrenergic neuron. Clin Pharmacol Ther 9:341, 1968.

19. LLOYD JTA, WALKER DRH: Death after combined dexamphetamine and phenelzine (Letter). Br Med J 2:168, 1965.

20. ANON: The safety of cyclamate—an artificial sweetner. Med Lett 17:85, 1969.

21. ANON: Doxapram (Dopram)—an analeptic. Med Lett 11:7, 1969.

22. FRANZ DN: Central nervous system stimulants. In GOODMAN LS, GILMAN A (Eds): The Pharmacological Basis of Therapeutics. 4th Ed. New York, Macmillan, 1970, p. 355.

23. ELLIS J, et al: Modification by monoamine oxidase inhibitors of the effect of some sympathomimetics on blood pressure. Br Med J 2:75, 1967.

24. MARK LC, et al: Hypotension following use of monoamine oxidase inhibitor. NY J Med 67:570, 1967.

25. FRIEND DG, et al: The action of L-dihydroxyphenylalanine in patients receiving nialamide. Clin Pharmacol Ther 6:362, 1965.

26. COTZIAS GC, et al: L-dopa in Parkinson's syndrome. N Engl J Med 281:272, 1969.

27. COTZIAS GC: Metabolic modification of some neurologic disorders. JAMA 210:1255, 1969.

28. KLAWANS HL Jr: The pharmacology of parkinsonism. a review. Dis Nerv Syst 29:805, 1968.

29. HEDBERG DL, et al: Tranylcypromine-trifluoperazine combination in the treatment of schizophrenia. Am J Psychiatry 127:1141, 1971.

References (CONT.)

30. LADER MH, et al: Interactions between sympathomimetic amines and a new monoamine oxidase inhibitor. Psychopharmacologia 18:118, 1970.
31. Ritalin. Product Information, CIBA Pharmaceutical Co., 1984.
32. VIGRAN IM: Dangerous potentiation of meperidine hydrochloride by pargyline hydrochloride. JAMA 187:953, 1964.
33. ANON: Analgesics and monoamine-oxidase inhibitors. Br Med J 4:284, 1967.
34. CUTHBERT MF, et al: Cough and cold remedies: potential danger to patients on monoamine oxidase inhibitors. Br Med J 1:404, 1969.
35. TONKS CM, LLOYD AT: Hazards with monoamine-oxidase inhibitors (Letter). Br Med J 1:589, 1965.
36. MASON AMS, BUCKLE RM: "Cold" cures and monoamine-oxidase inhibitors (Letter). Br Med J 1:845, 1969.
37. HUMBERSTONE PM: Hypertension from cold remedies (Letter). Br Med J 1:846, 1969.
38. BARSA JA, SAUNDERS, JC: A comparative study of tranylcypromine and pargyline. Psychopharmacologia 6:295, 1964.
39. HUNTER KR, et al: Monoamine oxidase inhibitors and L-DOPA. Br Med J 3:388, 1970.
40. KOTT E, et al: Excretion of dopa metabolites (Letter). N Engl J Med 284:395, 1971.
41. GOLDBERG LI, WHITSETT TL: Cardiovascular effects of levodopa. Clin Pharmacol Ther 12:376, 1971.
42. BODLEY PO, et al: Low serum-pseudocholinesterase levels complicating treatment with phenelzine. Br Med J 3:510, 1969.
43. LOCKETT MF, MILNER G: Combining the antidepressant drugs. Br Med J 1:921, 1965.
44. BRACHFELD J, et al: Imipramine-tranylcypromine incompatibility, near fatal toxic reaction. JAMA 186:1172, 1963.
45. JARECKI HG: Combined amitriptyline and phenelzine poisoning. Am J Psychiatry 120:189, 1963.
46. SARGENT W: Combining the antidepressant drugs (Letter). Br Med J 1:251, 1965.
47. MACLEOD I: Fatal reaction to phenelzine. Br Med J 1:1554, 1965.
48. Tegretol. Product Information, Geigy Pharmaceuticals, 1984.
49. RIVERS N, HORNER B: Possible lethal reaction between nardil and dextromethorphan (Letter). Can Med Assoc J 103:85, 1970.
50. SIMMONS AV, et al: Case of self-poisoning with multiple antidepressant drugs. Lancet 1:214, 1970.
51. WINSTON F: Combined antidepressant therapy. Br J Psychiatry 118:301, 1971.
52. SCHUCKIT U, et al: Tricyclic antidepressants and monoamine oxidase inhibitors. Combination therapy in the treatment of depression. Arch Gen Psychiatry 24:509, 1971.
53. TERRY R, et al: Sintab (Letter). Med J Aust 2:763, 1975.
54. ANON: Foods potentially harmful to patients taking MAO inhibitors. Med Lett 18:32 (March 26) 1976.
55. TEYCHENNE PF, et al: Interactions of levodopa with inhibitors of monoamine oxidase and L-aromatic amino acid decarboxylase. Clin Pharmacol Ther 18:273, 1975.

References (CONT.)

56. Spiker DG, Pugh DD: Combining tricyclic and monoamine oxidase inhibitor antidepressants. Arch Gen Psychiatry 33:828, 1976.
57. Ananth J, Luchins D: A review of combined tricyclic and MAOI therapy. Compr Psychiatry 18(3):221, 1977.
58. Birkmayer W, et al: Implications of combined treatment with 'madopar' and L-deprenil in parkinson's disease. Lancet 1:439, 1977.
59. Goonewardene A, Toghill PJ: Gross oedema occurring during treatment for depression. Br Med J 2:879, 1977.
60. Blackwell B: Hypertensive crises due to monoamine-oxidase inhibitors. Lancet 2:849, 1963.
61. Hedberg DL, et al: Six cases of hypertensive crises in patients on tranylcypromine after eating chicken livers. Am J Psychiatry 122:933, 1966.
62. Davies EB: Tranylcypromine and cheese (Letter). Lancet 2:691, 1963.
63. Nuessle WF, et al: Pickled herring and tranylcypromine reaction (Letter). JAMA 192:726, 1965.
64. Asatoor AM, et al: Tranylcypromine and cheese (Letter). Lancet 2:733, 1963.
65. Blackwell B, et al: Effects of yeast extract after monoamine oxidase inhibition. Lancet 1:940, 1965.
66. Horwitz D, et al: Monoamine oxidase inhibitors, tyramine, and cheese. JAMA 188:1108, 1964.
67. Tedeschi DH, Fellows EJ: Monoamine oxidase inhibitors: augmentation of pressor effects of peroral tyramine. Science 144:1225, 1964.
68. Cuthill JM, et al: Death associated with tranylcypromine and cheese. Lancet 1:1076, 1964.
69. Harper M: Toxic effects of monoamine-oxidase inhibitors (Letter). Lancet 2:312, 1964.
70. Blomley DJ: Monoamine-oxidase inhibitors (Letter). Lancet 2:1181, 1964.
71. Hodge JV, et al: Monoamine-oxidase inhibitors, broad beans, and hypertension (Letter). Lancet 1:1108, 1964.
72. Sen NP: Analysis and significance of tyramine in foods. J Food Sci 34:22, 1969.
73. Marley E, et al: Interactions of monoamine-oxidase inhibitors, amines, foodstuffs. Adv Pharmacol Chemother 8:185, 1970.
74. Selvey N: Pressor action of tyramine-containing foods (Questions and Answers). JAMA 238:976, 1977.
75. Pathak SK: Gross oedema during treatment for depression (Letter). Br Med J 2:1220, 1977.
76. Corder CN, et al: Postural hypotension: adrenergic responsivity and levodopa therapy. Neurology 27:921, 1977.
77. Horler AR, Wynne NA: Hypertensive crisis due to pargyline and metaraminol. Br Med J 3:460, 1965.
78. Wright SP: Hazards with monoamine-oxide inhibitors: a persistent problem (Letter). Lancet 1:284, 1978.
79. White K: Tricyclic overdose in a patient given combined tricyclic-MAOI treatment. Am J Psychiatry 135:1411, 1978.
80. Young JPR, et al: Controlled trial of trimipramine, monoamine oxidase inhibitors, and combined treatment in depressed outpatients. Br Med J 2:1315, 1979.

References (CONT.)

81. WHITE K, et al: Combined monoamine oxidase inhibitor-tricyclic antidepressant treatment: a pilot study. Am J Psychiatry 137:1422, 1980.
82. WHITE K: Combined tricyclic and monoamine-oxidase inhibitor antidepressant treatment. West J Med 138:406, 1983.
83. Monoamine oxidase inhibitors for depression. Med Lett 22:58, 1980.
84. PEET M, et al: The interaction of tyramine with a single dose of tranylcypromine in healthy volunteers. Br J Clin Pharmacol 11:212, 1981.
85. ELSWORTH JD, et al: Deprenyl administration in man: a selective monoamine oxidase B inhibitor without the "cheese effect." Psychopharmacology 57:33, 1978.
86. DAVIES B, et al: Pressor amines and monoamine-oxidase inhibitors for treatment of postural hypotension in autonomic failure. Limitations and hazards. Lancet 1:172, 1978.

CHAPTER 13

Phenothiazine Interactions

PHENOTHIAZINES

DRUGS	DISCUSSION

Amphetamines[1,2,3,43]

MECHANISM: Not established. Phenothiazines reportedly inhibit the "amine pump" mechanism responsible for the uptake of various amines, including amphetamines, into the adrenergic neuron.[1] If a similar process occurs in the central nervous system, the central effects of amphetamines could be antagonized.

CLINICAL SIGNIFICANCE: Amphetamines have been shown to adversely affect schizophrenic symptoms in patients receiving chlorpromazine.[43] Also, it has been observed that obese schizophrenic patients taking phenothiazines and other psychotherapeutic agents do not respond to dextroamphetamine therapy for weight reduction.[3] Also, the expected alterations in sleep patterns were not seen. It is possible that tricyclic antidepressants could have a similar effect in reducing the anorectic action of amphetamines. On the positive side, chlorpromazine has been used successfully in the treatment of amphetamine overdose. In summary, amphetamines may inhibit the antipsychotic effect of phenothiazines, and phenothiazines may inhibit the anorectic effect of amphetamines.

MANAGEMENT: Due to the mutually inhibitory effects of amphetamines and phenothiazines, it would be best to avoid concurrent use.

Antacids, Oral[4,5,10,44]

MECHANISM: Antacids may inhibit the absorption of orally administered phenothiazines.

CLINICAL SIGNIFICANCE: In one study of ten patients receiving large doses of chlorpromazine, the concomitant administration of an antacid (Aludrox) resulted in 10% to 45% decreases in urinary chlorpromazine excretion.[10] Information from another study indicates that an antacid containing magnesium trisilicate and aluminum hydroxide may result in decreased blood levels of chlorpromazine given as an oral suspension.[4] Thus, a decreased therapeutic response to chlorpromazine seems possible, and one possible case of this has been reported.[4] In one preliminary report antacids did not affect the absorption of chlorpromazine,[44] but until more studies are done one should assume that antacids are capable of reducing the gastrointestinal absorption of chlorpromazine (and possibly other phenothiazines).

PHENOTHIAZINES (CONT.)

DRUGS	DISCUSSION

MANAGEMENT: On the basis of these studies, it would seem wise to space the administration of oral phenothiazines and antacids so that mixing in the gastrointestinal tract will be minimized.

Anticholinergics[9,27,29-32,45-50]

MECHANISM: Several potential mechanisms exist for interactions of phenothiazines and anticholinergic agents: (1) inhibition of the antipsychotic effect of the phenothiazine; (2) additive anticholinergic effects; and (3) possible inhibition of the gastrointestinal absorption of phenothiazines by anticholinergics.

CLINICAL SIGNIFICANCE: There is some evidence that anticholinergic agents may inhibit the therapeutic response to phenothiazines, possibly through a direct inhibitory effect on the therapeutic effect of the phenothiazine.[50] However, there is also evidence that anticholinergics may reduce the gastrointestinal absorption of chlorpromazine. For example, trihexyphenidyl has been shown to reduce plasma chlorpromazine levels in schizophrenic patients,[9] and orphenadrine has been shown to reduce plasma levels and pharmacologic response of chlorpromazine.[31] The additive anticholinergic effects of phenothiazines and anticholinergics may also result in paralytic ileus[48,49] or heat stroke,[45-47] either one of which may be fatal. However, it is not known whether the risk of ileus or heat stroke is higher in patients taking phenothiazines plus anticholinergics as compared to the risk in patients taking either drug alone.

MANAGEMENT: These data further support the contention that anticholinergics should not be used routinely in patients receiving phenothiazines. If the combination is used, one should be alert for evidence of reduced phenothiazine effects, and for symptoms which may signal the onset of adynamic ileus (e.g., constipation, abdominal pain and distention). Patients on phenothiazines and anticholinergics should also take precautions to avoid heat stroke.

Antidepressants, Tricyclic[6,21,22,33,51,52]

MECHANISM: It is proposed that phenothiazines may inhibit the metabolism of tricyclic antidepressants.[6,21] Evidence has also been presented indicating that tricyclic antidepressants may inhibit phenothiazine metabolism.[22,52]

CLINICAL SIGNIFICANCE: Pharmacologic studies in schizophrenics have shown increased plasma levels and decreased urinary excretion of tricyclic antidepressants when phenothiazines were given concomitantly.[6] In one study of four patients, extremely high tricyclic antidepressant levels were found during concurrent therapy with imipramine and fluphenazine decanoate,[51] although there was a curious absence of adverse effects from these elevated levels. In another study of eight patients, butaperazine plasma levels were higher when desipramine (Norpramin) was given concomitantly.[22] The effect was

DRUGS	DISCUSSION

seen in the six patients who received 150 mg/day of desipramine or more, but not in the two patients who received less than 150 mg/day. In seven schizophrenic patients receiving chlorpromazine (300 mg daily), the addition of nortriptyline (150 mg daily) increased plasma chlorpromazine levels, reduced blood pressure, and markedly reduced the therapeutic response to chlorpromazine as measured by the In-patient Multidimensional Psychiatric Scale (IMPS).[52] In light of this growing evidence of pharmacokinetic and pharmacodynamic interactions between phenothiazines and tricyclic antidepressants, one might question the rationale of combination products containing both agents (e.g., Etrafon, Triavil). Clearly, more study is needed to ascertain that any purported benefit of combined use outweighs the risk.

MANAGEMENT: In patients receiving combined therapy with phenothiazines and tricyclic antidepressants, one should be alert for evidence of increased toxicity and reduced therapeutic response.

Attapulgite[7]

MECHANISM: Attapulgite appears to inhibit the gastrointestinal absorption of promazine.[7]

CLINICAL SIGNIFICANCE: Repeated studies in a single subject demonstrated that an antidiarrheal mixture of attapulgite and pectin could impair the absorption of promazine as measured by urinary promazine excretion.[7] The effect of such antidiarrheal preparations on the absorption of other phenothiazines is not known.

MANAGEMENT: Although evidence is preliminary, it would be wise to separate doses of phenothiazines from preparations containing attapulgite to minimize mixing in the gastrointestinal tract. Examples of products containing attapulgite include Rheaban, Diar-Aid, Polymagma, and Diarkote.

Barbiturates[10,20,31,57]

MECHANISM: Barbiturates presumably increase the metabolism of chlorpromazine by induction of hepatic microsomal enzymes. The fact that urinary excretion of the conjugated fraction of chlorpromazine is increased following phenobarbital supports this view.

CLINICAL SIGNIFICANCE: Phenobarbital has been shown to increase the urinary excretion of chlorpromazine,[10] and also reduce plasma chlorpromazine levels.[20,31] In a crossover study involving 12 patients on chlorpromazine (300 mg/day), phenobarbital (150 mg/day) was associated with considerable reductions in plasma chlorpromazine levels.[31] The therapeutic significance of these findings has not been determined, but it appears reasonable to assume that the antipsychotic effect of chlorpromazine may be somewhat reduced. There is also some evidence that thioridazine may reduce serum phenobarbital levels.[57]

PHENOTHIAZINES (CONT.)

MANAGEMENT: It does not seem necessary to avoid concomitant use of phenothiazines and barbiturates, but one should be alert for evidence of reduced effect of either drug if the combination is used.

Chlorphentermine (Pre-Sate)[37]

MECHANISM: Not established.

CLINICAL SIGNIFICANCE: A cross-over study in 30 obese psychiatric patients indicated that neither chlorphentermine nor phenmetrazine results in weight loss in the presence of chlorpromazine therapy.[37] This indicates, but does not prove, that phenothiazines inhibit the anorexic effect of chlorphentermine (see also Phenmetrazine, p. 351, and Amphetamines, p. 346).

MANAGEMENT: It may be desirable to use weight reduction methods other than anorexic drugs in patients receiving phenothiazines. Anorexic drugs are generally felt to be of limited value in any patient, so limiting their use in these patients should pose few problems.

Cimetidine (Tagamet)[40]

MECHANISM: Not established. It is possible that cimetidine impairs the gastrointestinal absorption of chlorpromazine (Thorazine).

CLINICAL SIGNIFICANCE: In eight patients on chlorpromazine (75 to 450 mg daily), administration of cimetidine 1.0 gm/day for 7 days decreased steady state chlorpromazine levels by a mean of 35%.[40] Although the magnitude of the reduction may be expected to reduce chlorpromazine response in some patients, this was not assessed in the study.

MANAGEMENT: Until more is known about this potential interaction one should be alert for evidence of reduced chlorpromazine response in the presence of cimetidine therapy.

Hydroxyzine (Atarax, Vistaril)[18]

MECHANISM: Not established.

CLINICAL SIGNIFICANCE: One double blind trial in 19 psychotic patients gave preliminary evidence that hydroxyzine might impair the therapeutic response to phenothiazines.[18] However, determination of the clinical significance must await further study.

MANAGEMENT: No special precautions appear necessary until more is known about this possible interaction.

Levodopa (L-Dopa)[1,11,12,14,19,23,35]

MECHANISM: Not established. A well-documented side effect of phenothiazines is the production of extrapyramidal symptoms. It has been

PHENOTHIAZINES (CONT.)

proposed that phenothiazines may block dopamine receptors in the central nervous system.

CLINICAL SIGNIFICANCE: The therapeutic response of patients with parkinsonism to levodopa reportedly may be inhibited by phenothiazines. Buterophenones (e.g., Haloperidol) may have a similar effect. It has also been reported that chlorpromazine (200 mg/day for 3 days) can inhibit the ability of levodopa to stimulate growth hormone secretion.[23]

MANAGEMENT: On the basis of current evidence, it would appear wise to avoid administration of phenothiazines to patients receiving levodopa.

Lithium Carbonate (Lithane, Lithonate)[15,24,26,28,34,39,53–55]

MECHANISM: Not established.

CLINICAL SIGNIFICANCE: Several pharmacokinetic interactions between phenothiazines and lithium have been described: lithium-induced reductions in plasma chlorpromazine levels; phenothiazine-induced increases in the red cell (and perhaps brain) uptake of lithium; and chlorpromazine-induced increases in renal lithium excretion. The clinical outcome of these mechanisms would be difficult to predict, but one should be alert for altered response to either drug with combined use. In addition to the pharmacokinetic interactions, clinical reports indicate that, in acute manic patients, concurrent therapy with lithium and phenothiazines (especially thioridazine) may predispose to neurotoxicity (e.g., delirium, seizures, encephalopathy) or an increase in the likelihood of extrapyramidal symptoms. The combined use of haloperidol and lithium has been implicated in the production of severe neurotoxic symptoms (hyperpyrexia, confusion, and irreversible brain damage) in a small number of patients, but a definite cause and effect relationship between the drug combination and the neurotoxicity has not been established.

MANAGEMENT: It would be preferable to avoid the concurrent use of lithium and neuroleptics (especially thioridazine or haloperidol) in patients with acute manic symptoms. Chronic therapy with these combinations appears less likely to result in an adverse interaction. Although the clinical importance of the pharmacokinetic interactions of phenothiazines and lithium are not well established, one should be alert for evidence of reduced phenothiazine response in the presence of lithium therapy.

Narcotic Analgesics[36,42]

MECHANISM: Not established.

CLINICAL SIGNIFICANCE: The combination of phenothiazines and narcotic analgesics is known to result in enhanced respiratory depression and hypotension. Ten healthy subjects were given a single dose of

PHENOTHIAZINES (CONT.)

intramuscular meperidine (26 mg/m^2) with and without concurrent intramuscular chlorpromazine (30 mg/m^2).[42] Chlorpromazine did not alter the pharmacokinetics of meperidine, but did increase the urinary excretion of normeperidine. The meperidine-chlorpromazine combination was also associated with considerably more lethargy and a greater hypotensive response than the meperidine-placebo combination. Two of the subjects on meperidine and chlorpromazine developed severe orthostatic hypotension. Although these toxic effects were associated with evidence of increased normeperidine formation, the role of normeperidine in production of these effects is not clear. For example, one cannot rule out the possibility that the adverse effects resulted from the combined pharmacologic effect of chlorpromazine and meperidine itself.

MANAGEMENT: One should be alert for evidence of excessive central nervous system depression, hypotension, and respiratory depression if meperidine and chlorpromazine are used concurrently.

Orphenadrine (Norflex)[8,13,31]

MECHANISM: Not established.

CLINICAL SIGNIFICANCE: A single case has been reported in which a patient receiving both orphenadrine and chlorpromazine developed severe symptomatic hypoglycemia. Subsequent studies in this patient indicated that combined therapy with these agents may result in an enhanced hypoglycemic response to a tolbutamide test (1.0 g intravenously). Also, the anticholinergic effect of orphenadrine may reduce phenothiazine plasma levels (see Anticholinergics, p. 347). It is interesting that there was no mention of adverse effects due to drug interaction concerning six patients who were receiving orphenadrine and fluphenazine.[8]

MANAGEMENT: In patients on concomitant use of phenothiazines and orphenadrine, one should be alert for evidence of excessive anticholinergic effects (especially ileus), reduced phenothiazine plasma levels or hypoglycemia.

Phenmetrazine (Preludin)[37,38]

MECHANISM: Not established.

CLINICAL SIGNIFICANCE: A double-blind controlled study in psychiatric patients indicated that chlorpromazine reduced the ability of phenmetrazine to produce a weight loss.[38] Another study in 30 obese psychiatric patients yielded similar results.[37] Thus, it does appear that chlorpromazine (and possibly other phenothiazines) can reduce the efficacy of phenmetrazine, such as it is.

MANAGEMENT: It is probably desirable to use weight reduction methods other than anorexic drugs in patients receiving phenothiazines. Anorexic drugs are probably of limited value in most patients, so limiting their use in these patients should pose few problems.

PHENOTHIAZINES (CONT.)

DRUGS	DISCUSSION

Phenylpropanolamine[25,56]

MECHANISM: Not established.

CLINICAL SIGNIFICANCE: A 27-year-old woman on chronic thioridazine (100 mg daily) was found dead 2 hours after taking one decongestant capsule containing 50 mg of phenylpropanolamine and 4 mg of chlorpheniramine. However, thioridazine alone has been associated with sudden death, and a cause and effect relationship between the purported drug interaction and the death was not established.

MANAGEMENT: Although there is very little evidence to support the existence of this interaction, the severity of the reaction dictates caution in the concurrent use of thioridazine (and possibly other phenothiazines) and sympathomimetics such as phenylpropanolamine.

Smoking[40,41]

MECHANISM: Smoking may enhance the hepatic metabolism of phenothiazines.

CLINICAL SIGNIFICANCE: In an epidemiologic study of the frequency of drowsiness attributed to oral chlorpromazine (Thorazine), only 3% of heavy smokers (> 20 cigarettes/day) developed drowsiness, while the frequency in light smokers (20 cigarettes/day or less) and nonsmokers was 11% and 16%, respectively. In another study, the frequency of hypotension in patients on chlorpromazine was 0% in heavy smokers, 8% in light smokers, and 10% in nonsmokers. It seems unlikely that smoking would decrease chlorpromazine side effects selectively, without affecting the therapeutic response to chlorpromazine. However, the effects of smoking on the therapeutic response to phenothiazines have not been systematically studied.

MANAGEMENT: One should be alert for evidence of increased phenothiazine dosage requirements in smokers.

Succinylcholine (Anectine, Quelicin)[16,17]

MECHANISM: Not established. There has been some evidence to indicate that phenothiazines lower serum and erythrocyte cholinesterase levels, resulting in an enhanced neuromuscular blockade of succinylcholine.

CLINICAL SIGNIFICANCE: Not established. A single case[16] has been reported in which promazine (25 mg intravenously) given to a patient who had received 550 mg of succinylcholine during surgery was followed by prolonged apnea. This neuromuscular blockade appeared to respond to edrophonium. Also, Sphire[17] has stated that chlorpromazine may enhance the response to muscle relaxants, but substantiating information was not given.

352

PHENOTHIAZINES (CONT.)

DRUGS	DISCUSSION

MANAGEMENT: Pending availability of further information, promazine and presumably other phenothiazines should be administered with caution to patients who have received succinylcholine.

References

1. KLAWANS HL Jr: The pharmacology of parkinsonism. A review. Dis Nerv Syst 29:805, 1968.
2. ESPELIN DE, DONE AK: Amphetamine poisoning: effectiveness of chlorpromazine. N Engl J Med 278:1361, 1968.
3. MODELL W, HUSSAR AE: Failure of dextroamphetamine sulfate to influence eating and sleeping patterns in obese schizophrenic patients. Clinical and pharmacological significance. JAMA 193:275, 1965.
4. FANN WE: Chlorpromazine: effects of antacids on its gastrointestinal absorption. J Clin Pharmacol 13:388, 1973.
5. FANN WE, et al: The effects of antacids on the blood levels of chlorpromazine (Abstract). Clin Pharmacol Ther 14:135, 1973.
6. GRAM LF, OVERO KF: Drug interaction: inhibitory effect of neuroleptics on metabolism of tricyclic antidepressants in man. Br Med J 1:463, 1972.
7. SORBY DL, LIU G: Effects of adsorbents on drug absorption. II. Effect of an antidiarrhea mixture on promazine absorption. J Pharm Sci 55:504, 1966.
8. FLEMING P, et al: Levodopa in drug-induced extrapyramidal disorders (Letter). Lancet 2:1186, 1970.
9. RIVERA-CALIMLIM L, et al: Effects of mode of management on plasma chlorpromazine in psychiatric patients. Clin Pharmacol Ther 14:978, 1973.
10. FORREST FM, et al: Modification of chlorpromazine metabolism by some other drugs frequently administered to psychiatric patients. Biol Psychiatry 2:53, 1970.
11. COTZIAS GC, et al: L-DOPA in Parkinson's syndrome (Letter). N Engl J Med 281:272, 1969.
12. JENKINS RB, GROH RH: Psychic effects in patients treated with levodopa (Letter). JAMA 212:2265, 1970.
13. BUCKLE RM, GUILLEBAUD J: Hypoglycaemic coma occurring during treatment with chlorpromazine and orphenadrine. Br Med J 4:599, 1967.
14. YARYURA-TOBIAS JA, et al: Action of L-DOPA in drug-induced extrapyramidalism. Dis Nerv Syst 31:60, 1970.
15. ZALL H, et al: Lithium carbonate: a clinical study. Am J Psychiatry 125:549, 1968.
16. REGAN AG, ALDRETE JA: Prolonged apnea after administration of promazine hydrochloride following succinylcholine infusion. Anesth Analg 46:315, 1967.
17. SPHIRE RD: Gallamine: a second look. Anesth Analg 43:690, 1964.
18. ROSS EK, PRIEST RG: The effect of hydroxyzine on phenothiazine therapy. Dis Nerv Syst 31:412, 1970.

References (CONT.)

19. YAHR MD, DUVOISIN RC: Drug therapy of Parkinsonism. N Engl J Med 287:20, 1972.
20. CURRY SH, et al: Factors affecting chlorpromazine plasma levels in psychiatric patients. Arch Gen Psychiatry 22:209, 1970.
21. GRAM LF, et al: Influence of neuroleptics and benzodiazepines on metabolism of tricyclic antidepressants in man. Am J Psychiatry 131:863, 1974.
22. EL-YOUSEF MK, MANIER DH: Tricyclic antidepressants and phenothiazines (Letter). JAMA 229:1419, 1974.
23. MIMS RB, et al: Inhibition of L-dopa-induced growth hormone stimulation by pyridoxine and chlorpromazine. J Clin Endocrinol Metab 40:256, 1975.
24. CRAMMER JL, et al: Blood levels and management of lithium treatment. Br Med J 3:650, 1974.
25. ALEXANDER CS: Epinephrine not contraindicated in cardiac arrest attributed to phenothiazine (Questions and Answers). JAMA 236:405, 1976.
26. KERZNER B, RIVER-CALIMLIM L: Lithium and chlorpromazine (CPZ) interaction. Clin Pharmacol Ther 19:109, 1976.
27. RIVERA-CALIMLIM, et al: Clinical response and plasma levels: effect of dose, dosage schedules and drug interactions on plasma chlorpromazine levels. Am J Psychiatry 133:6, 1976.
28. SLETTEN I, et al: The effect of chlorpromazine on lithium excretion in psychiatric subjects. Curr Ther Res 8:441, 1966.
29. GERSHON S, et al: Interaction between some anticholinergic agents and phenothiazines. Clin Pharmacol Ther 6:749, 1965.
30. AIPERT M, et al: Anticholinergic exacerbation of phenothiazine-induced extrapyramidal syndrome. Am J Psychiatry 133:1073, 1976.
31. LOGA S, et al: Interactions of orphenadrine and phenobarbitone with chlorpromazine: plasma concentrations and effects in man. Br J Clin Pharmacol 2:197, 1975.
32. RIVERA-CALIMLIM L: Chlorpromazine-trihexyphenidyl interaction. Drug Therapy 6:196, 1976.
33. OVERO KF, et al: Interaction of perphenazine with the kinetics of nortriptyline. Acta Pharmacol Toxicol 40:97, 1977.
34. STRAYHORN JM, NASH JL: Severe neurotoxicity despite "therapeutic" serum lithium levels. Dis Nerv Syst 38:107, 1977.
35. CAMPBELL JB: Long-term treatment of Parkinson's disease with levodopa. Neurology 20:18, 1970.
36. SWETT C, et al: Hypotension due to chlorpromazine. Arch Gen Psychiatry 34:661, 1977.
37. SLETTEN IW, et al: Weight reduction with chlorphentermine and phenmetrazine in obese psychiatric patients during chlorpromazine therapy. Curr Ther Res 9:570, 1967.
38. REID AA: Pharmacological antagonism between chlorpromazine and phenmetrazine in mental hospital patients. Med J Aust 1:187, 1964.
39. RIVERA-CALIMLIM L, et al: Effect of lithium on plasma chlorpromazine levels. Clin Pharmacol Ther 23:451, 1978.
40. HOWES CA, et al: Reduced steady-state plasma concentrations of chlorpromazine and indomethacin in patients receiving cimetidine. Eur J Clin Pharmacol 24:99, 1983.

References (CONT.)

41. SWETT C Jr: Drowsiness due to chlorpromazine in relation to cigarette smoking. Arch Gen Psychiatry 31:211, 1974.
42. STAMBAUGH JE, WAINER IW: Drug interaction: meperidine and chloropromazine, a toxic combination. J Clin Pharmacol 21:140, 1981.
43. CASEY JF, et al: Combined drug therapy of chronic schizophrenics. Am J Psychiatry 117:997, 1961.
44. PINELL OC, et al: Drug-drug interaction of chlorpromazine and antacid. Clin Pharmacol Ther 23:125, 1978.
45. MANN SC, BOGER WP: Psychotropic drugs, summer heat and humidity, and hyperpyrexia: a danger restated. Am J Psychiatry 135:1097, 1978.
46. WESTLAKE RJ, RASTEGAR A: Hyperpyrexia from drug combinations. JAMA 225:1250, 1973.
47. ZELMAN S, GUILLAN R: Heat stroke in phenothiazine-treated patients: a report of three fatalities. Am J Psychiatry 126:1787, 1970.
48. GIORDANO J, et al: Fatal paralytic ileus complicating phenothiazine therapy. South Med J 68:351, 1975.
49. WARNES J, et al: Adynamic ileus during psychoactive medication: a report of three fatal and five severe cases. Can Med Ass J 96:1112, 1967.
50. SINGH MM, SMITH JM: Reversal of some therapeutic effects of an antipsychotic agent by an antiparkinsonian drug. J Nerv Ment Dis 157:50, 1973.
51. SIRIS SG, et al: Plasma imipramine concentrations in patients receiving concomitant fluphenazine decanoate. Am J Psychiatry 139:104, 1982.
52. LOGA S, et al: Interaction of chlorpromazine and nortriptyline in patients with schizophrenia. Clin Pharmacokinet 6:454, 1981.
53. GHADIRIAN AM, LEHMANN HE: Neurological side effects of lithium: organic brain syndrome, seizures, extrapyramidal side effects, and EEG changes. Compr Psychiatry 21:327, 1981.
54. SPRING S, FRANKEL, M: New data on lithium and haloperidol incompatibility. Am J Psychiatry 138:818, 1981.
55. KAMLANA SH, et al: Lithium: some drug interactions. Practitioner 224:1291, 1980.
56. CHOUINARD G, et al: Death attributed to ventricular arrhythmia induced by thioridazine in combination with a single Contac-C capsule. Can Med Ass J 119:729, 1978.
57. GAY PE, MADSEN JA: Interaction between phenobarbital and thioridazine. Neurology 33:1631, 1983.

CHAPTER 14

Salicylate Drug Interactions

SALICYLATE INTERACTIONS

DRUGS	DISCUSSION

Acetaminophen (Datril, Tylenol)[43,44]

MECHANISM: Not established.

CLINICAL SIGNIFICANCE: A study of 21 subjects who were given various combinations of aspirin and acetaminophen demonstrated that acetaminophen increased blood levels of unhydrolyzed aspirin but not total salicylate.[43] It was proposed that the increase in unhydrolyzed aspirin would increase the therapeutic effect; however, it has also been suggested that combinations of aspirin with either acetaminophen or phenacetin may increase the likelihood of analgesic nephropathy.[44]

MANAGEMENT: No special precautions appear necessary. However, in the absence of a proven advantage of combined therapy over either agent alone, it may be better to use one agent or the other.

Ammonium Chloride[1,2,36,37]

MECHANISM: Sufficient doses of ammonium chloride can acidify the urine, thus increasing the renal tubular reabsorption of salicylate and possibly increasing plasma salicylate concentrations.

CLINICAL SIGNIFICANCE: In patients receiving large doses of salicylate, urinary acidification with ammonium chloride may increase serum salicylate somewhat. However, if the urine is acidic before the ammonium chloride therapy (as it usually is), the changes are likely to be small. Considerable increases in serum salicylate seem likely only if the ammonium chloride is given to a patient receiving large doses of salicylate who has an initial urine pH of above 6.5.[36,37]

MANAGEMENT: Although this interaction is likely to occur only rarely, one should be alert for evidence of increased serum salicylate levels when drugs that acidify the urine are given to patients on large doses of salicylates (e.g., over 3 g daily).

Antacids, Oral[7,25,27,36,37]

MECHANISM: The ability of antacids to alkalinize the urine results in reduced renal tubular reabsorption of salicylate, which may result in

SALICYLATE INTERACTIONS (CONT.)

reduced serum salicylate levels. It has also been proposed that antacids might cause premature disruption of the coating of enteric-coated aspirin or perhaps increase gastric emptying resulting in earlier release of the aspirin in the intestine.[7]

CLINICAL SIGNIFICANCE: Study in three children with rheumatic fever receiving large doses of salicylate indicated that concurrent administration of an antacid (magnesium and aluminum hydroxide) was associated with reduced serum salicylate levels.[25] Subsequent study in nine normal subjects given large doses of choline salicylate showed that magnesium and aluminum hydroxide was associated with reduced steady state salicylate levels.[37] Another study in six healthy subjects showed that magnesium and aluminum hydroxide (Maalox) resulted in earlier peak urinary excretion rate of aspirin administered in enteric coated form (Ecotrin).[7] This may indicate earlier or more rapid release of aspirin, the clinical significance of which is not yet established.

MANAGEMENT: In patients receiving larger doses of salicylates, one should be alert for alteration in serum salicylate levels if antacids are started or stopped.

Ascorbic Acid (Vitamin C)[1,2,36–38]

MECHANISM: It was previously thought that ascorbic acid could render the urine acidic, thus increasing the renal tubular reabsorption of salicylate and increasing plasma salicylate concentrations. However, more recent studies have failed to confirm that ascorbic acid acidifies the urine.[36,37]

CLINICAL SIGNIFICANCE: One study in nine normal subjects receiving choline salicylate (daily dose equivalent to 3.75 g of aspirin) showed that ascorbic acid (3 g/day) did not affect serum salicylate levels.[37] This is consistent with the findings that ascorbic acid (4 to 6 g/day) did not consistently reduce urine pH.[38] Also, salicylate levels are not likely to be increased by urinary acidification if the patient has an acidic urine prior to administration of the acidifier.

MANAGEMENT: No special precautions appear necessary.

Cimetidine (Tagamet)[54–56]

MECHANISM: Not established.

CLINICAL SIGNIFICANCE: Cimetidine has been shown to slightly increase serum salicylate concentrations and bioavailability following administration of enteric-coated aspirin.[54,55] However, the magnitude of the increases do not appear to be sufficient to produce adverse effects. In another study of six subjects, cimetidine appeared to increase the absorption rate of aspirin three of the subjects, but there was no significant change in the group as a whole.[56] The type of aspirin used was not stated. In summary, there is little evidence that cimetidine

DRUGS	DISCUSSION

has a clinically important effect on aspirin absorption, although an effect of cimetidine on aspirin metabolism cannot yet be ruled out.

MANAGEMENT: No special precautions appear to be necessary at this point, but one should be alert for evidence of altered serum salicylate levels in the presence of cimetidine therapy.

Fenoprofen (Nalfon)[3,31]

MECHANISM: Not established.

CLINICAL SIGNIFICANCE: In healthy subjects ingesting fenoprofen and aspirin the area under the fenoprofen plasma curve was reduced by single doses of aspirin and more so by multiple aspirin doses.[3] There was also evidence that the half-life of fenoprofen was decreased by multiple doses (but not single doses) of aspirin. However, the clinical significance of these findings remains to be determined.

MANAGEMENT: Until the clinical importance of this interaction is established, special precautions would not seem necessary.

Food[33-35]

MECHANISM: The delayed rate of absorption of aspirin may be a result of reduced rate of gastric emptying and adsorption of aspirin by food particles.[33]

CLINICAL SIGNIFICANCE: In a study of eight volunteer subjects, food has been shown to affect absorption of effervescent aspirin as indicated by delayed and reduced plasma salicylate levels in the first hour following administration.[33] In another study of five different commercial aspirin preparations in 25 subjects, serum salicylate levels were about twice as high in fasting versus nonfasting conditions at 10 and 20 minutes following administration of the aspirin.[34] Spiers and Malone found similar food-induced decreases in serum salicylate when calcium aspirin (1.5 g) was given to nonfasting and fasting subjects.[35] This may be of clinical significance if rapid analgesia is desired.

MANAGEMENT: For rapid analgesia, one should not take aspirin on a full stomach.

Gold[28]

MECHANISM: Not established.

CLINICAL SIGNIFICANCE: In one study aspirin (3.9 g/day) was given with and without gold to patients with rheumatoid arthritis.[28] Serum aspartate aminotransferase levels were higher in the patients also receiving gold, leading the authors to conclude that gold therapy may predispose to aspirin hepatotoxicity. More study is needed.

MANAGEMENT: No special precautions appear necessary.

SALICYLATE INTERACTIONS (CONT.)

Heparin[8,9,23,32,39,46,47]

MECHANISM: Aspirin has been shown to inhibit platelet function, thus impairing one of the hemostatic mechanisms that the heparin-treated patient depends on to prevent bleeding.

CLINICAL SIGNIFICANCE: Deykin has advised that aspirin be "scrupulously avoided" in patients receiving heparin.[9] Others[8] have noted the possible dangers of combined use of heparin and aspirin, especially if thrombocytopenia is present. In an epidemiologic study of 2,656 patients receiving heparin therapy, major bleeding was 2.4-fold more common in patients who received aspirin than in those who received no aspirin.[46] Also, serious bleeding was noted in 8 of 12 patients given aspirin in addition to heparin to prevent deep vein thrombosis following hip surgery.[39] In summary, both theoretical considerations and clinical data indicate an increased risk of bleeding if aspirin is added to heparin therapy. The risk versus benefit of the use of aspirin to prevent thrombosis in conjunction with heparin is not clearly established at this time.

MANAGEMENT: Aspirin should be used only with caution in patients receiving heparin and only if substantial therapeutic benefit is expected from the aspirin. Acetaminophen (Tylenol) is often an adequate substitute for aspirin for mild analgesia and antipyresis. If a salicylate is required in a patient receiving heparin and the platelet effects of aspirin are not desired, a nonacetylated salicylate could be used to avoid inhibition of platelet function. Such salicylates would include choline salicylate (Arthropan), salsalate (Disalcid), magnesium salicylate, and sodium salicylate.

Ibuprofen (Advil, Motrin, Nuprin, Rufen)[45]

MECHANISM: Not established.

CLINICAL SIGNIFICANCE: Aspirin appears to substantially reduce serum ibuprofen concentrations, but does not appear to inhibit the therapeutic response to ibuprofen.[45]

MANAGEMENT: No special precautions appear necessary.

Indomethacin (Indocin)[3,10–13,20–22,29,30,48–52]

MECHANISM: Although the mechanism is not established, it seems likely that aspirin has some inhibitory effect on the gastrointestinal absorption of indomethacin.

CLINICAL SIGNIFICANCE: Using 14C-indomethacin, aspirin was found to decrease serum and urine levels of indomethacin, and increase fecal excretion.[13] In another study of ten healthy subjects, 1200 mg of aspirin three times daily resulted in a 20% reduction in plasma levels of indomethacin after a single dose, but the reduction was not as large when the indomethacin was given in multiple doses.[48] Subsequent study of this interaction seemed to discount the existence of interac-

DRUGS	DISCUSSION

tion,[12] but the timing of the doses and the blood sampling were such that an interaction could have escaped their detection. When the indomethacin is given rectally and the aspirin is given orally, no interaction could be detected.[10] Finally, Rubin and associates[3] found oral aspirin to decrease peak indomethacin plasma concentrations, although the area under the plasma concentration-time curve was not significantly affected. In summary, oral aspirin does appear to have some inhibitory effect on the gastrointestinal absorption of indomethacin. Although one clinical study indicated that 1500 mg daily of aspirin inhibited the anti-inflammatory response to indomethacin,[49] subsequent double-blind clinical studies indicated that aspirin had no effect[50] or actually increased[51] the anti-inflammatory response to indomethacin in patients with rheumatic diseases. Thus, the bulk of the evidence indicates that aspirin is unlikely to adversely affect the anti-inflammatory effects of indomethacin in patients with rheumatic disease. Also, preliminary evidence indicates that sodium salicylate may reduce indomethacin-induced gastrointestinal blood loss.[52]

MANAGEMENT: No special precautions appear to be necessary at this time.

Intrauterine Contraceptive Devices (IUDs)[40-42]

MECHANISM: Not established. The contraceptive efficacy of IUDs may be related to an inflammatory reaction, which would be inhibited by salicylates.

CLINICAL SIGNIFICANCE: Isolated cases of unwanted pregnancy during IUD use have occurred in women taking aspirin[40] or other anti-inflammatory drugs such as corticosteroids.[40-42] However, it has not been established that the anti-inflammatory drugs were responsible for the contraceptive failure.

MANAGEMENT: Until more information is available, women using IUDs should consider using another form of contraception during short-term therapy with salicylates or other anti-inflammatory drugs. If the anti-inflammatory drug is used chronically, one should consider the possibility that the IUD failure rate may be somewhat increased when selecting a contraceptive method.

Naproxen (Naprosyn, Naxen)[14,53]

MECHANISM: It is proposed that aspirin may compete with naproxen for plasma protein binding, thereby increasing the renal clearance of naproxen.[14]

CLINICAL SIGNIFICANCE: In healthy subjects, aspirin has been shown to produce a small decrease in plasma naproxen levels.[14] However, the magnitude of the change indicates that the interaction is not likely to have much effect on the therapeutic response to naproxen. A double-blind study in 36 patients with rheumatoid arthritis indicated that naproxen plus aspirin was more effective than aspirin alone.[53]

SALICYLATE INTERACTIONS (CONT.)

However, since the combination of naproxen and aspirin was not compared with naproxen alone, it is not possible to conclude that aspirin does not affect the response to naproxen.

MANAGEMENT: On the basis of current evidence, no special precautions appear to be necessary.

Para-aminobenzoic Acid (PABA)[15]

MECHANISM: PABA appears to block the formation of salicyluric acid from salicylic acid, resulting in increased salicylate blood levels.

CLINICAL SIGNIFICANCE: PABA has been combined with salicylates in a number of proprietary analgesic mixtures. Excessive salicylate levels probably do not often occur as a result of this interaction.

MANAGEMENT: No action is needed, but one should be aware that PABA may increase serum salicylate levels.

Phenylbutazone (Butazolidin)[4,6,26]

MECHANISM: Phenylbutazone inhibits the uricosuria that usually follows large doses of salicylates. It is also possible that salicylates compete with phenylbutazone for plasma protein binding.

CLINICAL SIGNIFICANCE: In four non-gouty patients, uricosuria resulted from administration of 5 g/day of aspirin. When 200, 400, and 600 mg per day administration of phenylbutazone had been added during the next 3 days, serum urate rose from an average of 4 mg per 100 ml to 6 mg per 100 ml.[6] A similar effect was seen when phenylbutazone was given first. A patient with a history of gout may be more likely to be adversely affected by this interaction.

MANAGEMENT: It is not necessary to avoid concomitant administration of salicylates and phenylbutazone, but the physician should be aware of the possibility of interaction.

Probenecid (Benemid)[4,5,16–18,24]

MECHANISM: Salicylates inhibit the uricosuric activity of probenecid as well as other uricosuric agents. Preliminary evidence indicates that salicylates and probenecid may share a common binding site on the plasma albumin molecule.

CLINICAL SIGNIFICANCE: Well documented. Probenecid uricosuria may be considerably inhibited by large doses of salicylates. Doses of salicylate that do not produce serum salicylate levels above 5 mg/100 ml do not appear to significantly affect probenecid uricosuria. Thus, occasional analgesic doses of salicylate may be insufficient to interact with probenecid. Also, probenecid appears to inhibit the uricosuria that usually follows large doses of salicylates.

MANAGEMENT: More than occasional small doses of salicylates should be avoided in patients receiving probenecid.

SALICYLATE INTERACTIONS (CONT.)

DRUGS	DISCUSSION

Sulfinpyrazone (Anturane)[5,6,19]

MECHANISM: Salicylates inhibit the uricosuric effect of sulfinpyrazone.

CLINICAL SIGNIFICANCE: Sulfinpyrazone uricosuria may be considerably inhibited by large doses of salicylates. Sulfinpyrazone also appears to inhibit the uricosuria that usually follows large doses of salicylates.

MANAGEMENT: More than occasional small doses of salicylates should be avoided in patients receiving sulfinpyrazone.

Sulindac (Clinoril)[49,57]

MECHANISM: Not established.

CLINICAL SIGNIFICANCE: Although aspirin reportedly reduces the plasma levels of the active sulfide metabolite of sulindac,[57] available evidence indicates that aspirin does not appreciably affect the antiinflammatory response to sulindac.[49,57] However, a possible increase in the incidence of adverse gastrointestinal effects with the combination compared to sulindac alone has prompted the manufacturer of sulindac to recommend against combining it with aspirin.[57]

MANAGEMENT: Until clinical evidence of a positive effect of the combination is available, it would be prudent to avoid concurrent use of sulindac and aspirin.

References

1. LEVY G, TSUCHIYA T: Salicylate accumulation kinetics in man. N Engl J Med 287:430, 1972.
2. LEVY G, LEONARDS JR: Urine pH and salicylate therapy (Letter). JAMA 217:81, 1971.
3. RUBIN A, et al: Interactions of aspirin with nonsteroidal antiinflammatory drugs in man. Arthritis Rheum 16:635, 1973.
4. BLUESTONE R, et al: Effect of drugs on urate binding to plasma proteins. Br Med J 4:590, 1969.
5. SMITH MJH, SMITH PK: The Salicylates. A Critical Bibliographic Review. New York, Interscience Publishers, 1966, pp. 86–90.
6. OYER JH, et al: Suppression of salicylate-induced uricosuria by phenylbutazone. Am J Med Sci 251:1, 1966.
7. FELDMAN S, CARLSTEDT BC: Effect of antacid on absorption of enteric-coated aspirin (Letter). JAMA 227:660, 1974.
8. NICLASSON P-M, et al: Thrombocytopenia and bleeding—complications in severe cases of meningococcal infection treated with heparin, dextran 70 and chlorpromazine. Scand J Infect Dis 4:183, 1972.
9. DEYKIN D: The use of heparin. N Engl J Med 280:937, 1969.
10. LINDQUIST B, et al: Effect of concurrent administration of aspirin and

References (CONT.)

indomethacin on serum concentrations. Clin Pharmacol Ther 15:247, 1974.

11. YESAIR DW, et al: Comparative effects of salicylic acid, phenylbutazone, probenecid and other anions on the metabolism, distribution and excretion of indomethacin by rates. Biochem Pharmacol 19:1591, 1970.

12. CHAMPION GD, et al: The effect of aspirin on serum indomethacin. Clin Pharmacol Ther 13:239, 1972.

13. JEREMY R, TOWSON J: Interaction between aspirin and indomethacin in the treatment of rheumatoid arthritis. Med J Aust 2:127, 1970.

14. SEGRE EJ, et al: Naproxen-aspirin interactions in man. Clin Pharmacol Ther 15:374, 1974.

15. SMITH MJH, SMITH PK: Op. cit., pp. 34–43.

16. ROBINSON WD: Current status of the treatment of gout. JAMA 164:1670, 1957.

17. PASCALE LR, et al: Therapeutic value of probenecid (Benemid) in gout. JAMA 149:1188, 1952.

18. PASCALE LR, et al: Inhibition of the uricosuric action of Benemid by salicylate. J Lab Clin Med 45:771, 1955.

19. YU TF, et al: Mutual suppression of the uricosuric effects of sulfinpyrazone and salicylate: a study in interactions between drugs. J Clin Invest 42:1330, 1963.

20. BROOKS PM, et al: Indomethacin-aspirin interaction: a clinical appraisal. Br Med J 3:69, 1975.

21. KALDESTAD E, et al: Interaction of indomethacin and acetylsalicylic acid as shown by the serum concentrations of indomethacin and salicylate. Eur J Clin Pharmacol 9:199, 1975.

22. LEI BW, et al: The influence of aspirin on the absorption and disposition of indomethacin. Clin Pharmacol Ther 19:110, 1976.

23. RUBENSTEIN JJ: Aspirin, heparin and hemorrhage (Letter). N Engl J Med 294:1122, 1976.

24. BOGER WP, et al: Probenecid and salicylates: the question of interaction in terms of penicillin excretion. J Lab Clin Med 45:478, 1955.

25. LEVY G, et al: Decreased serum salicylate concentrations in children with rheumatic fever treated with antacid. N Engl J Med 293:323, 1975.

26. CHIGNELL CF, STARKWEATHER DK: Optical studies of drug-protein complexes V. The interaction of phenylbutazone, flufenamic acid, and dicoumarol with acetylsalicylic acid-treated human serum albumin. Mol Pharmacol 7:229, 1971.

27. STRICKLAND-HODGE B, et al: The effects of antacids on enteric coated salicylate preparations. Rheumatol Rehab 15:148, 1976.

28. DAVIS JD, et al: Fenoprofen, aspirin, and gold induction in rheumatoid arthritis. Clin Pharmacol Ther 21:52, 1977.

29. KENDALL MJ, et al: Xylose test: effect of aspirin and indomethacin. Br Med J 1:553, 1971.

30. BARRACLOUGH DRE, et al: Salicylate therapy and drug interaction in rheumatoid arthritis. Aust NZ J Med 5:518, 1975.

31. GRUBER CM: Clinical pharmacology of fenoprofen: a review. J Rheumatol (Supplement)2:8, 1976.

32. SCHONDORF TH, HEY D: Combined administration of low dose heparin

References (CONT.)

and aspirin as prophylaxis of deep vein thrombosis after hip joint surgery. Haemostasis 5:250, 1976.

33. VOLANS GN: Effects of food on the absorption of effervescent aspirin. Br J Clin Pharmac 1:137, 1974.
34. WOOD JH: Effect of food on aspirin absorption (Letter). Lancet 2:212, 1967.
35. SPIERS ASD, MALONE HF: Effect of food on aspirin absorption (Letter). Lancet 1:440, 1967.
36. KLINENBERG JR, MILLER F: Effect of corticosteroids on blood salicylate concentration. JAMA 194:601, 1965.
37. HANSTEN PD, HAYTON WL: Effect of antacids and ascorbic acid on serum salicylate concentration. J Clin Pharmacol 24:326, 1980.
38. MCLEOD DC, NAHATA MC: Inefficacy of ascorbic acid as a urinary acidifier (Letter). N Engl J Med 296:1413, 1977.
39. YETT HS, et al: The hazards of aspirin plus heparin (Letter). N Engl J Med 298:1092, 1978.
40. BUHLER M, PAPIERNIK E: Successive pregnancies in women fitted with intrauterine devices who take antiinflammatory drugs. Lancet 1:483, 1983.
41. INKELES DM, HANSEN RI: Unexpected pregnancy in a woman using an intrauterine device and receiving steroid therapy. Ann Ophthalmol 14:975, 1982.
42. ZERNER J, et al: Failure of an intrauterine device concurrent with administration of corticosteroids. Fertil Steril 27:1467, 1976.
43. COTTY VF, et al: Augmentation of human blood acetylsalicylate concentrations by the simultaneous administration of acetaminophen with aspirin. Toxicol Appl Pharmacol 41:7, 1977.
44. WILSON DR, GAULT MH: Declining incidence of analgesic nephropathy in Canada. Can Med Ass J 127:500, 1982.
45. GRENNAN DM, et al: The aspirin-ibuprofen interaction in rheumatoid arthritis. Br J Clin Pharmacol 8:497, 1979.
46. WALKER AM, JICK H: Predictors of bleeding during heparin therapy. JAMA 244:1209, 1980.
47. HEIDEN D, et al: Heparin bleeding, platelet dysfunction, and aspirin. JAMA 246:330, 1981.
48. KWAN KC, et al: Effects of concomitant aspirin administration on the pharmacokinetics of indomethacin in man. J Pharmacokinet Biopharm 6:451, 1978.
49. PAWLOTSKY Y, et al: Comparative interaction of aspirin with indomethacin and sulindac in chronic rheumatic diseases. Eur J Rheumatol Inflamm 1:18, 1978.
50. TORGYAN S, et al: A comparative study with indomethacin and combined indomethacin-sodium salicylate in rheumatoid arthritis. Int J Clin Pharmacol Biopharm 17:439, 1979.
51. ALVAN, G, EKSTRAND R: Clinical effects of indomethacin and additive clinical effect of indomethacin during salicylate maintenance therapy. Scand J Rheumatol [Suppl] 39:29, 1981.
52. TORGYAN S, et al: Reduction of indomethacin-induced gastrointestinal blood loss by sodium salicylate in man. Int J Clin Pharmacol 16:610, 1978.

References (CONT.)

53. WILLKENS RF, SEGRE EJ: Combination therapy with naproxen and aspirin in rheumatoid arthritis. Arthritis Rheum 19:677, 1976.
54. PATON TW, et al: Effect of cimetidine on bioavailability of enteric-coated aspirin tablets. Clin Pharm 2:165, 1983.
55. WILLOUGHBY JS, et al: The effect of cimetidine on enteric-coated ASA disposition. Clin Pharmacol Ther 33:268, 1983.
56. KHOURY W, et al: The effect of cimetidine on aspirin absorption. Gastroenterology 76:1169, 1979.
57. Clinoril. Product Information. West Point, Pennsylvania, Merck, Sharp & Dohme, 1984.

CHAPTER 15

Tricyclic Antidepressant Interactions

TRICYCLIC ANTIDEPRESSANT INTERACTIONS

DRUGS	DISCUSSION

Acetazolamide (Diamox)[12,13,36,40]

MECHANISM: Acetazolamide tends to render the urine alkaline, resulting in an increased proportion of un-ionized drug. Thus, renal tubular reabsorption of the tricyclic antidepressant is increased.

CLINICAL SIGNIFICANCE: In the patient with normal hepatic metabolism of tricyclic antidepressants, fluctuations in urinary pH would probably have little clinical effect since relatively small amounts of tricyclic antidepressants are excreted unchanged in the urine.

MANAGEMENT: No special precautions appear to be necessary.

Ammonium Chloride[12,13,36,40]

MECHANISM: Ammonium chloride tends to acidify the urine, resulting in an increased proportion of ionized drug. Thus, tubular reabsorption of the tricyclic antidepressant is decreased.

CLINICAL SIGNIFICANCE: In the patient with normal hepatic metabolism of tricyclic antidepressants, fluctuations in urinary pH would probably have little clinical effect since relatively small amounts of tricyclic antidepressants are excreted unchanged in the urine.

MANAGEMENT: No special precautions appear to be necessary.

Amphetamines[6,38]

MECHANISM: Not established. However, in view of the effect of norepinephrine in patients receiving tricyclic antidepressants (see p. 372), it seems likely that amphetamines would have an enhanced effect in patients on tricyclics due to the release of norepinephrine.

CLINICAL SIGNIFICANCE: Amphetamine abuse in patients receiving tricyclic antidepressants reportedly may be fatal,[38] but case reports of such an effect appear to be lacking.

MANAGEMENT: Even though clinical evidence is scanty, theoretical considerations would dictate caution in the administration of amphetamines to patients receiving tricyclic antidepressants.

TRICYCLIC ANTIDEPRESSANT INTERACTIONS (CONT.)

DRUGS	DISCUSSION

Anticholinergics[7-9,41,60]

MECHANISM: Tricyclic antidepressants may display additive anticholinergic effects with anticholinergic drugs such as antihistamines, phenothiazines, antiparkinson drugs, glutethimide (Doriden), and meperidine (Demerol).

CLINICAL SIGNIFICANCE: Combined use of tricyclic antidepressants and other anticholinergics is not uncommon, at least in the elderly.[60] The adverse effects of excessive cholinergic blockade are usually minor (e.g., dry mouth, constipation, etc.). However, the possibility of precipitating adynamic ileus, urinary retention, or acute glaucoma should be considered, especially in older patients. Additive anticholinergic effects would be more likely with antidepressants possessing greater anticholinergic activity such as amitriptyline, nortriptyline, imipramine, trimipramine, doxepin, and maprotiline. Antidepressants with less anticholinergic effect would include trazodone, protriptyline, desipramine, and especially amoxapine.

MANAGEMENT: Serious complications are not likely to occur if the practitioner is alert to the possibility of excessive anticholinergic activity. If additive anticholinergic effects become troublesome, use an antidepressant with low anticholinergic activity (see Clinical Significance). Also, an alternative drug can usually be found for the agent that is adding to the anticholinergic effect of the tricyclic antidepressant. A method has been described by which drug-induced dry mouth may be treated with a pilocarpine syrup.[9] Also, pyridoxine reportedly may prevent some of the anticholinergic side effects of tricyclic antidepressants.[41]

Barbiturates[4,10,16,25,27,28,33-35,39,45]

A. With Therapeutic Doses of Tricyclic Antidepressant:

MECHANISM: Barbiturates appear to stimulate the metabolism of tricyclic antidepressants and may decrease their blood levels.

CLINICAL SIGNIFICANCE: Several reports have described individual patients who manifested considerable decreases in serum levels of tricyclic antidepressants in the presence of a barbiturate. Subsequent study in patients receiving protriptyline confirmed that tricyclic antidepressant serum levels may be lower in the presence of barbiturate therapy.[45]

MANAGEMENT: Patients on tricyclic antidepressants probably respond better in the absence of barbiturates, and it has been recommended that barbiturates be avoided in such patients.[10] Benzodiazepines do not appear to affect tricyclic antidepressant serum levels (see p. 368).

B. With Toxic Doses of Tricyclic Antidepressant:

MECHANISM: Barbiturates may potentiate the adverse effects of toxic doses of tricyclic antidepressants (e.g., respiratory depression). It is possible that they are both competing for the same hydroxylating enzymes.

DRUGS	DISCUSSION

CLINICAL SIGNIFICANCE: This effect has been reported in only a few patients, but probably represents a real interaction.

MANAGEMENT: Barbiturates should probably not be used in patients with tricyclic antidepressant toxicity. Diazepam (Valium) is felt by some to be the agent of choice to treat the convulsions of tricyclic antidepressant toxicity,[27] while others have used paraldehyde.[28]

Benzodiazepines[4,14,15,22,26,32,43,45,65]

MECHANISM: Not established.

CLINICAL SIGNIFICANCE: Additive sedation or enhanced atropine-like effects reportedly may occur with concomitant use of chlordiazepoxide and a tricyclic antidepressant. Several case reports have appeared describing this interaction.[14,15,65] However, the drugs have been used together in clinical trials without mention of serious complications. Thus, it would appear that if the interaction does occur, it is in a very small proportion of patients and is not especially severe. Kline[32] states that it is safe to combine chlordiazepoxide with tricyclic antidepressants. Most studies indicate that plasma levels of tricyclic antidepressants are not affected by administration of benzodiazepines such as diazepam, chlordiazepoxide, or nitrazepam.[43,45]

MANAGEMENT: No special precautions appear to be necessary.

Cimetidine (Tagamet)[54-59]

MECHANISM: Cimetidine probably impairs the hepatic metabolism of tricyclic antidepressants.

CLINICAL SIGNIFICANCE: A woman who was receiving 1200 mg/day of cimetidine unexpectedly developed severe anticholinergic symptoms (e.g., severe dry mouth, urinary retention, blurred vision) when 100–125 mg/day of imipramine therapy was started.[54] Similar symptoms were seen when the imipramine was replaced by 125 mg/day of desipramine. The disposition of imipramine was then studied with and without cimetidine in this patient; the half-life and steady-state serum concentrations of imipramine were approximately doubled in the presence of cimetidine. Another report describes a man who was receiving both cimetidine and nortriptyline. When the cimetidine was discontinued, the steady-state serum concentration of nortriptyline decreased from 104 mg/L to 75 mg/L.[55] For this patient, the steady-state serum concentration of nortriptyline was, on average, 42% higher while he was taking cimetidine. In another case a patient receiving 1200 mg/day of cimetidine and 300 mg/day of imipramine developed a 58% decrease in the steady-state serum concentration of imipramine 7–10 days after cimetidine was stopped; the serum concentration of imipramine then increased by about threefold 5 to 7 days after cimetidine was resumed.[56] A preliminary report described six healthy subjects who were given imipramine with and without cimetidine.[57] Cimetidine increased the half-life of imipramine by 43% and reduced imipramine clearance by 41%. Furthermore, the bioavailability of imipramine was 40% when given alone and 75% when given in combination with cimetidine. In another study, six healthy men were given single 100-mg oral doses of imipramine or nortriptyline with and without pretreatment with cimetidine, 300 mg four times daily for 2 days.[58] Imipramine clearance decreased and bioavailability increased in the presence of cimetidine. Nortriptyline pharmacokinetics were only minimally affected by cimetidine pretreatment in this single dose study, but plasma levels of the major metabolite of nortriptyline (10-hydroxynortriptyline) were substantially increased. In another report, a 65-year-old man developed breast cancer while receiving cimetidine and doxepin.[59] The authors suggest that the malignant change may have resulted from the combined effects of the two drugs, since each drug individually has been associated with breast hyperplasia. In summary, the evidence indicates that cimetidine inhibits the elimination of imipramine, desipramine, and nortriptyline. Little clinical information is available on the effect of cimetidine on related antidepressants such as amitriptyline, amoxapine, protriptyline, doxepin, trimipramine, maprotiline, or trazodone. However, theoretical considerations would indicate that their elimination might also be reduced by cimetidine therapy.

MANAGEMENT: In patients stabilized on tricyclic antidepressants who are then given cimetidine, one should be alert for evidence of tricyclic antidepressant toxicity (e.g., severe dry mouth, blurred vision, urinary retention, tachycardia, constipation, and postural hypotension). If cimetidine is discontinued or its dose substantially reduced in a patient stabilized on both a tricyclic antidepressant and cimetidine, the patient should be monitored for an inadequate response to the tricyclic antidepressant. In patients who are already receiving cimetidine and are about to begin a course of therapy with a tricyclic antidepressant, one should consider using conservative antidepressant doses until the patient's response to therapy can be evaluated. Ranitidine (Zantac) is probably less likely than cimetidine to interact with tricyclic antidepressants, but clinical studies are lacking.

Disulfiram (Antabuse)[20,21,29,30,61]

MECHANISM: Unknown.

CLINICAL SIGNIFICANCE: Two patients on disulfiram therapy developed acute organic brain syndrome following addition of amitriptyline therapy.[61] Symptoms included confusion, disorientation, hallucinations, and memory loss, but a cause and effect relationship between drug interaction and the symptoms was not established. Also, amitriptyline is said to enhance the alcohol reaction in patients taking disulfiram. However, controlled studies are needed to confirm this finding.

MANAGEMENT: Although evidence to support the existence of a drug interaction is scanty, one should be alert for evidence of organic brain syndrome in patients on combined therapy.

TRICYCLIC ANTIDEPRESSANT INTERACTIONS (CONT.)

DRUGS	DISCUSSION

Epinephrine (Adrenalin)[2,3,44]

MECHANISM: Not established.

CLINICAL SIGNIFICANCE: Intravenous infusions of epinephrine to healthy subjects receiving imipramine have resulted in a two- to four-fold increase in the pressor response to epinephrine.[2] In addition, several instances of cardiac dysrhythmias were observed. In another study in six healthy subjects, protriptyline (60 mg/day for 4 days) pretreatment considerably enhanced the pressor response to epinephrine infusions.[44] It is not known what effect tricyclic antidepressant pretreatment would have on the response to epinephrine administered by other methods and/or in smaller doses.

MANAGEMENT: Patients receiving tricyclic antidepressants should be given intravenous epinephrine only with great caution and beginning with small doses. Some caution should also be exercised if the epinephrine is administered by other routes.

Ethchlorvynol (Placidyl)[31]

MECHANISM: Unknown.

CLINICAL SIGNIFICANCE: Concomitant administration of ethchlorvynol and amitriptyline reportedly may result in transient delirium. However, the clinical significance cannot be determined with the amount of information presented.

MANAGEMENT: Pending accumulation of further information, concomitant administration of ethchlorvynol and tricyclic antidepressants should be undertaken with some caution.

Haloperidol (Haldol)[1,43]

MECHANISM: It is proposed that haloperidol inhibits the metabolism of tricyclic antidepressants.

CLINICAL SIGNIFICANCE: In two schizophrenic patients, haloperidol (12 to 20 mg/day) resulted in a decrease in total urinary radioactivity after oral administration of ^{14}C-imipramine.[1] In another study,[43] the metabolism of nortriptyline appeared to be inhibited in a patient receiving haloperidol (16 mg/day). The clinical significance of this finding has not been established, and the result may be favorable in some cases.

MANAGEMENT: No special precautions appear to be necessary.

Isoproterenol (Isuprel)[2,46]

MECHANISM: Not established.

CLINICAL SIGNIFICANCE: A patient on concurrent therapy with amitriptyline and isoproterenol died following complications of a cardiac arrhythmia.[46] Although the death was thought to result from the com-

DRUGS	DISCUSSION

bined effects of the two drugs, the patient was apparently using excessive quantities of isoproterenol prior to the arrhythmia. Thus, it is difficult to ascertain whether the death resulted from the isoproterenol alone or the isoproterenol-amitriptyline combination. Further, a study of the effects of isoproterenol with and without tricyclic antidepressant pretreatment indicated minimal interaction, although one of the four patients developed tachycardia while on the combination.[46]

MANAGEMENT: No special precautions appear to be necessary, but one should consider the possibility that tricyclic antidepressants may increase the likelihood of arrhythmias following isoproterenol in certain predisposed patients.

Levodopa (Dopar, Larodopa)[42,47,48]

MECHANISM: It is proposed that tricyclic antidepressants slow gastric emptying, thus enhancing the degradation of levodopa to inactive products within the gut.

CLINICAL SIGNIFICANCE: The absorption of a single dose of levodopa was studied before and after imipramine (100 mg/day for 3 days).[47] The results indicated that the bioavailability of intact levodopa was impaired in the presence of imipramine, although definite conclusions could not be reached. An inhibitory effect of tricyclic antidepressants on levodopa absorption would be consistent with the effect of other anticholinergics on levodopa absorption, but the clinical importance of this purported interaction is not established.

MANAGEMENT: It would not seem necessary to avoid the concomitant use of levodopa and tricyclic antidepressants. However, one should be alert for altered levodopa effect if tricyclics are started or stopped.

Lithium Carbonate[49]

MECHANISM: Possible additive lowering of the seizure threshold.

CLINICAL SIGNIFICANCE: A patient on 300 mg/day of amitriptyline (Elavil) developed grand mal seizures after addition of 900 mg/day of lithium (plasma lithium level, 0.8 to 0.9 mEq/L).[49] The seizures recurred following rechallenge. However, if the seizures resulted from the combined effects of the two drugs, they must occur very rarely. Lithium and tricyclic antidepressants are frequently used together with no ill effects.

MANAGEMENT: No special precautions appear necessary, but one should consider the possibility of interaction if seizures occur in a patient on the combination.

Meperidine (Demerol)[18]

MECHANISM: Tricyclic antidepressants reportedly enhance meperidine-induced respiratory depression. This effect is probably similar in

DRUGS	DISCUSSION

nature to that seen with concomitant meperidine and phenothiazine administration.

CLINICAL SIGNIFICANCE: More study is needed to determine the magnitude of this effect.

MANAGEMENT: Pending further information, caution should be observed with concomitant administration of meperidine and tricyclic antidepressants in patients with lung disease or in patients in whom respiratory depression may be especially dangerous.

Methylphenidate (Ritalin)[11,19,23,24,63]

MECHANISM: Methylphenidate appears to inhibit the metabolism of tricyclic antidepressants and may increase their blood levels appreciably.

CLINICAL SIGNIFICANCE: Clinical examples of tricyclic antidepressant toxicity in patients also receiving methylphenidate have not appeared in the literature, but they may occur. In some reports, the methylphenidate-induced increases in tricyclic antidepressant blood levels have resulted in improved antidepressant response. Some patients apparently do not manifest elevated tricyclic antidepressant levels following methylphenidate administration.[19,63]

MANAGEMENT: This interaction may result in enhanced antidepressant effect. However, patients receiving both methylphenidate and a tricyclic antidepressant should be watched for signs of excessive tricyclic antidepressant effects.

Norepinephrine (Levarterenol, Levophed)[2,3,5,44,62]

MECHANISM: Not established.

CLINICAL SIGNIFICANCE: Intravenous infusions of norepinephrine to healthy subjects receiving imipramine have resulted in a four- to eightfold increase in the pressor response to norepinephrine.[2] Similarly, Mitchell and associates[5] found a several-fold increase in the pressor response to norepinephrine in patients receiving desipramine, amitriptyline, or protriptyline. In another study in six healthy subjects, protriptyline (60 mg/day for 4 days) pretreatment produced a marked increase in the pressor response to infusions of norepinephrine.[44] Thus, this interaction appears to be well documented with a variety of tricyclic antidepressants.

MANAGEMENT: Patients receiving tricyclic antidepressants should be given intravenous norepinephrine only with great caution and beginning with small doses.

Phenylbutazone (Butazolidin)[37]

MECHANISM: Desipramine appears to inhibit the gastrointestinal absorption of phenylbutazone.

CLINICAL SIGNIFICANCE: Preliminary study in four subjects indicates that peak plasma phenylbutazone levels can be considerably delayed by the prior administration of desipramine. However, total phenylbutazone absorption (based on urinary excretion of oxyphenbutazone) did not appear to be affected. Thus, under the conditions of multiple dosing of phenylbutazone, this interaction may not produce clinically detectable impairment of phenylbutazone effect. More study is needed.

MANAGEMENT: Until more is known about this interaction, patients might be watched for decreased phenylbutazone effect if desipramine (or other tricyclic antidepressants) is given.

Phenylephrine (Neo-Synephrine)[2,3,62]

MECHANISM: Not established.

CLINICAL SIGNIFICANCE: Intravenous infusions of phenylephrine to healthy subjects receiving imipramine have resulted in a two- to threefold increase in the pressor response to phenylephrine.[2] The effect of tricyclic antidepressant pretreatment on the response to *oral* phenylephrine is not known.

MANAGEMENT: Patients receiving tricyclic antidepressants should be given parenteral phenylephrine only with caution, and one should also be alert for enhanced responses to oral phenylephrine.

Propoxyphene (Darvon, Darvocet-N)[50]

MECHANISM: Propoxyphene appears to inhibit the metabolism of doxepin (Adapin, Sinequan).

CLINICAL SIGNIFICANCE: In one case report an 89-year-old man on chronic doxepin in a dose of 150 mg/day developed a doubling of his plasma doxepin level following propoxyphene therapy (65 mg every 6 hours).[50] The increased plasma doxepin was associated with lethargy, which reversed after propoxyphene therapy was discontinued. Ten healthy subjects were then given antipyrine (1.2 g IV) with and without propoxyphene (65 mg every 4 hours for eight doses, starting 8 hours before the antipyrine). Propoxyphene prolonged the antipyrine half-life from 12.2 to 15.2 hours and reduced the total antipyrine clearance from 0.63 to 0.53 ml/minute/kg body weight. These results are consistent with previous studies indicating that propoxyphene can impair the hepatic metabolism of carbamazepine (Tegretol) and possibly other drugs. It should be noted that the studies showing inhibition of drug metabolism due to propoxyphene have involved propoxyphene doses of 65 mg three to six times daily. The effect of lower and/or sporadic doses of propoxyphene on drug metabolism is not clear, but such doses would probably be less likely to interact. It is not known whether tricyclic antidepressants other than doxepin would be affected by propoxyphene, but it certainly seems possible.

DRUGS	DISCUSSION

MANAGEMENT: One should be alert for evidence of enhanced doxepin (or other tricyclic) effect if propoxyphene is given concurrently.

Smoking[51-53,64]

MECHANISM: Smoking may enhance the hepatic metabolism of tricyclic antidepressants.

CLINICAL SIGNIFICANCE: Although no difference in the steady state plasma levels of nortriptyline between smokers and nonsmokers was observed in one study,[51] two subsequent studies involving large numbers of patients demonstrated lower plasma levels of amitriptyline, desipramine, imipramine, and nortriptyline in smokers than in nonsmokers.[52,53] Preliminary results from another study indicated that smokers have a higher percentage of free plasma nortriptyline than nonsmokers.[64] Thus, it is possible that the plasma free antidepressant concentration is not significantly affected, even though the total plasma level may be reduced. Although a precise relationship between tricyclic antidepressant plasma levels and therapeutic effect is not established, the magnitude of the decreases in plasma drug concentrations associated with smoking appears large enough to interfere with efficacy in some patients.

MANAGEMENT: No special precautions appear to be necessary, but one should be aware that smoking may alter the response to tricyclic antidepressants.

References

1. GRAM LF, OVERO KF: Drug interaction: inhibitory effect of neuroleptics on metabolism of tricyclic antidepressants in man. Br Med J 1:463, 1972.
2. BOAKES AJ, et al: Interactions between sympathomimetic amines and antidepressant agents in man. Br Med J 1:311, 1973.
3. BOAKES AJ: Sympathomimetic amines and antidepressant agents (Letter). Br Med J 2:114, 1973.
4. SILVERMAN G, BRAITHWAITE R: Interaction of benzodiazepines with tricyclic antidepressants (Letter). Br Med J 4:111, 1972.
5. MITCHELL JR, et al: Guanethidine and related agents. III. Antagonism by drugs which inhibit the norepinephrine pump in man. J Clin Invest 49:1596, 1970.
6. BEAUMONT G: Drug interactions with clomipramine (Anafranil). J Int Med Res 1:480, 1973.
7. KESSELL A, et al: Side effects with a new hypnotic: drug potentiation. Med J Aust 2:1194, 1967.
8. MILNER G: Gastro-intestinal side effects and psychotropic drugs. Med J Aust 2:153, 1969.
9. AYD FJ Jr (Ed): Rx tip: relieving drug-induced oral and pharyngeal dryness. Int Drug Ther Newslett 2:24, 1967.

References (CONT.)

10. Burrows GD, Davies B: Antidepressants and barbiturates (Letter). Br Med J 4:113, 1971.
11. Wharton RN, et al: A potential clinical use for the interaction of methylphenidate with tricyclic antidepressants. Am J Psychiatry 127:1619, 1971.
12. Weiner IM, Mudge GH: Renal tubular mechanisms for excretion of organic acids and bases. Am J Med 36:743, 1964.
13. Milne MD: Influence of acid-base balance on efficacy and toxicity of drugs. Proc R Soc Med 58:961, 1965.
14. Abdou FA: Elavil-Librium combination. Am J Psychiatry 120:1204, 1964.
15. Kane FJ Jr, Taylor TW: A toxic reaction to combined Elavil-Librium therapy. Am J Psychiatry 119:1179, 1963.
16. Borden EC, Rostand SG: Recovery from massive amitriptyline overdosage (Letter). Lancet 1:1256, 1968.
17. Porter AMW: Body height and imipramine side effects. Br Med J 2:406, 1968.
18. Goodman LS, Gilman A (Eds): The Pharmacological Basis of Therapeutics. 4th Ed. New York, Macmillan, 1970, pp. 255–260.
19. Zeidenberg P, et al: Clinical and metabolic studies with imipramine in man. Am J Psychiatry 127:1321, 1971.
20. Pullar-Strecker H: Drug interactions in alcoholism treatment (Letter). Lancet 1:735, 1969.
21. MacCallum WAG: Drug interactions in alcoholism treatment (Letter). Lancet 1:313, 1969.
22. Anon: General practitioner clinical trials. Chlordiazepoxide with amitriptyline in neurotic depression. Practitioner 202:437, 1969.
23. Garrettson LK, et al: Methylphenidate interactions with both anticonvulsants and ethyl biscoumacetate. JAMA 207:2053, 1969.
24. Anon: Methylphenidate (Ritalin). Med Lett Drugs Ther 11:47, 1969.
25. Alexanderson B, et al: Steady state plasma levels of nortriptyline in twins: influence of genetic factors and drug therapy. Br Med J 4:764, 1969.
26. Haider I: A comparative trial of Ro 4-6270 and amitriptyline in depressive illness. Br J Psychiatry 113:993, 1967.
27. Crocker J, Morton B: Tricyclic (antidepressant) drug toxicity. Clin Toxicol 2:397, 1969.
28. Noble J, Matthew H: Acute poisoning by tricyclic antidepressants: clinical features and management of 100 patients. Clin Toxicol 2:403, 1969.
29. Burnett GB, Reading HW: Drug interactions in alcoholism treatment (Letter). Lancet 1:415, 1969.
30. Glatt MM: Drug interactions in alcoholism treatment (Letter). Lancet 1:627, 1969.
31. Hussar DA: Tabular compilation of drug interactions. Am J Pharm 141:107, 1969.
32. Kline NS: Psychochemotherapeutic drug combinations (Questions and Answers). JAMA 210:1928, 1969.
33. Sjoqvist F, et al: Plasma level of monomethylated tricyclic antidepressants and side-effects in man. In Toxicity and Side-effects of Psychotropic Drugs. Amsterdam, Excerpta Medica Foundation, 1968, pp. 246–257.

References (CONT.)

34. HAMMER W, et al: A comparative study of the metabolism of desmethylimipramine, nortriptyline, and oxyphenbutazone in man. Clin Pharmacol Ther 10:44, 1969.
35. ANON: Metabolism of drugs. Br Med J 1:767, 1970.
36. SJOQVIST F: The pH-dependent excretion of monomethylated tricyclic antidepressants in dogs and man. Clin Pharmacol Ther 10:826, 1969.
37. CONSOLO S, et al: Delayed absorption of phenylbutazone caused by desmethylimipramine in humans. Eur J Pharmacol 10:239, 1970.
38. RAISFELD IH: Cardiovascular complications of antidepressant therapy. Am Heart J 83:129, 1972.
39. ROYDS RB, KNIGHT AH: Tricyclic antidepressant poisoning. Practitioner 204:282, 1970.
40. GRAM LF, et al: Imipramine metabolism: pH dependent distribution and urinary excretion. Clin Pharmacol Ther 12:239, 1971.
41. ARNOLD SE, et al: Tricyclic antidepressants and peripheral anticholinergic activity. Psychopharmacology 74:325, 1981.
42. JEFFERSON JW: A review of the cardiovascular effects and toxicity of tricyclic antidepressants. Psychosom Med 37:160, 1975.
43. GRAM LF, et al: Influence of neuroleptics and benzodiazepines on metabolism of tricyclic antidepressants in man. Am J Psychiatry 131:863, 1974.
44. SVEDMYR N: The influence of a tricyclic antidepressive agent (protriptyline) on some of the circulatory effects of noradrenaline and adrenaline in man. Life Sci 7:77, 1968.
45. MOODY JP, et al: Pharmacokinetic aspects of protriptyline plasma levels. Eur J Clin Pharmacol 11:51, 1977.
46. KADAR D: Amitriptyline and isoproterenol: fatal drug combination (Letter). Can Med Assoc J 112:556, 1975.
47. MORGAN JP, et al: Imipramine-mediated interference with levodopa absorption from the gastrointestinal tract in man. Neurology 25:1029, 1975.
48. RAMPTON DS: Hypertensive crisis in a patient given sinemet, metoclopramide, and amitriptyline. Br Med J 3:607, 1977.
49. SOLOMON JG: Seizures during lithium-amitriptyline therapy. Postgrad Med 66:145, 1979.
50. ABERNETHY DR, et al: Impairment of hepatic drug oxidation by propoxyphene. Ann Intern Med 97:223, 1982.
51. NORMAN TR, et al: Cigarette smoking and plasma nortriptyline levels. Clin Pharmacol Ther 21:453, 1977.
52. LINNOILA M, et al: Effect of alcohol consumption and cigarette smoking on antidepressant levels of depressed patients. Am J Psychiatry 138:841, 1981.
53. PEREL JM, et al: Pharmacodynamics of imipramine and clinical outcome in depressed patients. In Gottschalk L, Merlis S (Eds): Pharmacokinetics of Psychoactive Drugs. New York, Spectrum, 1975.
54. MILLER DD, MACKLIN M: Cimetidine-imipramine interaction: a case report. Am J Psychiatry 140:351, 1983.
55. MILLER DD, et al: Cimetidine's effect on steady-state serum nortriptyline concentrations. Drug Intell Clin Pharm 17:904, 1983.
56. SHAPIRO PA: Cimetidine-imipramine interaction: case report and comments. Am J Psychiatry 141:152, 1984.

References (CONT.)

57. ABERNETHY DR, et al: Imipramine-cimetidine interaction: impairment of clearance and enhanced bioavailability. Clin Pharmacol Ther 33:237, 1983.

58. HENAUER SA, HOLLISTER LE: Cimetidine interaction with imipramine and nortriptyline. Clin Pharmacol Ther 35:183, 1984.

59. SMEDLEY HM: Malignant breast change in man given two drugs associated with breast hyperplasia. Lancet 2:638, 1981.

60. BLAZER DG, et al: The risk of anticholinergic toxicity in the elderly: a study of prescribing practices in two populations. J Gerontology 38:31, 1983.

61. MAANY I, et al: Possible toxic interaction between disulfiram and amitriptyline. Arch Gen Psychiatry 39:743, 1982.

62. GHOSE K: Sympathomimetic amines and tricyclic antidepressant drugs. Neuropharmacology 19:1251, 1980.

63. DRIMMER EJ, et al: Desipramine and methylphenidate combination treatment for depression: case report. Am J Psychiatry 140:241, 1983.

64. PERRY PJ, et al: The effects of smoking on nortriptyline plasma levels in depressed patients (Abstract). Drug Intell Clin Pharm 17:449, 1983.

65. BERESFORD TP, et al: Adverse reactions to a benzodiazepine-tricyclic antidepressant compound. J Clin Psychopharmacol 1:392, 1981.

CHAPTER 16

Miscellaneous Interactions

ACETAMINOPHEN (TYLENOL) INTERACTIONS

DRUGS	DISCUSSION

Anticholinergics[196,197]

MECHANISM: Anticholinergics slow gastric emptying, thus reducing the rate of acetaminophen absorption from the intestine.

CLINICAL SIGNIFICANCE: Acetaminophen (1.5 gm orally) was given to six patients with and without pretreatment with propantheline (Pro-Banthine), 30 mg intravenously.[196,197] The rate of absorption of acetaminophen was considerably slower in the presence of propantheline, but the extent of acetaminophen absorption did not appear to be affected. Oral administration of propantheline is likely to have a similar effect. One might expect other agents with anticholinergic activity such as tricyclic antidepressants, antihistamines, and phenothiazines also to delay acetaminophen absorption. Since acetaminophen is often used for acute relief of pain or fever, one would expect anticholinergics to delay the onset of the therapeutic response to acetaminophen. However, this has not been studied clinically.

MANAGEMENT: One should be aware that the onset of acetaminophen effect may be delayed in patients receiving anticholinergics so that excessive repeated doses of acetaminophen are not given.

Barbiturates[204–209]

MECHANISM: Barbiturates appear to enhance the metabolism of acetaminophen.

CLINICAL SIGNIFICANCE: The fate of acetaminophen (1.0 gm orally and intravenously) was compared in six healthy subjects and six epileptic patients receiving chronic anticonvulsant therapy (e.g., barbiturates, carbamazepine, primidone).[204] The epileptic patients had lower oral acetaminophen bioavailability and a shorter serum acetaminophen half-life following its intravenous administration. Although clinical evidence is lacking, one might expect that patients taking enzyme-inducing drugs would experience a reduced therapeutic response to acetaminophen. With acetaminophen overdoses, however, one would expect long-term phenobarbital therapy to increase the conjugation of acetaminophen to its nontoxic glucuronide metabolite, as well as its oxidative biotransformation to the hepatotoxic metabolite. The overall effect of these two opposing mechanisms is not predictable, but available evidence indicates that phenobarbital pretreatment tends to increase the hepatotoxicity of toxic acetaminophen doses. Phenobarbital has been shown to increase the hepatotoxicity and nephrotoxicity of acetaminophen overdose in rats,[205,206] but evidence from humans is limited to isolated case reports.[207,208] In summary, patients who chronically receive barbiturates may experience a somewhat reduced effect from therapeutic doses of acetaminophen and perhaps increased toxicity from acetaminophen overdose.

MANAGEMENT: Until more is known about this interaction, large doses of acetaminophen should be administered with caution to patients on barbiturate therapy.

Charcoal[202]

MECHANISM: Activated charcoal reduces the gastrointestinal absorption of acetaminophen.

CLINICAL SIGNIFICANCE: Activated charcoal in large oral doses (5 to 10 g) considerably reduces the gastrointestinal absorption of acetaminophen. However, the effect of smaller doses of activated charcoal (as found in antidiarrheals and antiflatulants) on acetaminophen absorption is not established.

MANAGEMENT: One should separate therapeutic doses of acetaminophen from doses of activated charcoal to avoid possible inhibition of acetaminophen absorption.

Cholestyramine (Questran)[203]

MECHANISM: Cholestyramine inhibits the gastrointestinal absorption of acetaminophen.

CLINICAL SIGNIFICANCE: In four healthy subjects, concurrent administration of cholestyramine (12 g orally) markedly reduced plasma levels of acetaminophen (2.0 g orally).[203] It seems likely that colestipol (Colestid) would similarly reduce plasma acetaminophen levels.

MANAGEMENT: Give acetaminophen 1 hour or more before cholestyramine or colestipol to minimize the inhibition of acetaminophen absorption.

Diazepam (Valium)[212]

MECHANISM: Not established.

CLINICAL SIGNIFICANCE: A preliminary study in four subjects indicated that acetaminophen (3.0 g/day for 5 days) somewhat reduced the 96-hour urinary excretion of diazepam and its metabolites following a single 10-mg dose of diazepam.[212] The effect was greater in the two female subjects, but additional study is needed to confirm these results and to define the magnitude of the interaction.

MANAGEMENT: No special precautions appear necessary at this point.

DRUGS	DISCUSSION

Food[164-166]

MECHANISM: The delay in absorption may be due to the delayed entry of the drug into the intestine, or it may be due to a delay in tablet disintegration and dissolution.[164,165] Pectin found in the high carbohydrate test meal may retard absorption by adsorption as well as retard absorption through increased viscosity, and slow distribution throughout gastric fluids.[166]

CLINICAL SIGNIFICANCE: Reports of the administration of 1.0 g of acetaminophen with food in four adult male volunteers demonstrated a considerable reduction in the rate of absorption of the drug with little change in the total amount of acetaminophen absorbed. The meal consisted of 200 ml orange juice, 30 g cornflakes, and Pop Tarts.[164,165] In another study[166] high carbohydrate test meals (crackers, jelly, and dates) significantly delayed absorption of acetaminophen as measured by urinary excretion. It was noted that high protein, high lipid, or balanced meals appeared to have little inhibitory effect on the rate of absorption.

MANAGEMENT: For rapid analgesia acetaminophen should not be taken with meals, especially meals high in carbohydrates.

Metoclopramide[6,7]

MECHANISM: It is proposed that metoclopramide increases the absorption rate of acetaminophen by stimulating gastric emptying.[6]

CLINICAL SIGNIFICANCE: Although the absorption rate of acetaminophen has been shown to be increased by metoclopramide in healthy subjects,[6,7] the *amount* of acetaminophen absorbed did not seem to be affected. Thus, the onset of analgesia may be somewhat sooner, but it is unlikely that most patients would be significantly affected by this interaction.

MANAGEMENT: No special precautions appear to be necessary.

Propantheline (Pro-Banthine)[6,7]

MECHANISM: It is proposed that propantheline decreases the absorption rate of acetaminophen by delaying gastric emptying.[6]

CLINICAL SIGNIFICANCE: Although the absorption rate of acetaminophen has been shown to be decreased by propantheline in studies done in six patients,[6,7] the *amount* of acetaminophen absorbed did not seem to be affected. The six patients received 30 mg of propantheline intravenously; the effect of standard oral doses of propantheline on acetaminophen absorption remains to be established.

MANAGEMENT: No special precautions appear to be necessary, but one should be aware that the onset of acetaminophen effect may be slightly delayed in patients receiving anticholinergics.

ALLOPURINOL (ZYLOPRIM) INTERACTIONS

DRUGS	DISCUSSION

Iron Preparations[13,30]

MECHANISM: Early animal studies reportedly indicated that allopurinol may increase hepatic iron concentration.

CLINICAL SIGNIFICANCE: There does not appear to be any clinical evidence of an increase in hepatic iron stores, and some animal studies have failed to demonstrate such an effect.

MANAGEMENT: No special precautions appear to be necessary.

Probenecid (Benemid)[8,14,170]

MECHANISM:
1. Allopurinol (or one of its metabolites) appears to inhibit the metabolism of probenecid.[14,170]
2. Probenecid appears to enhance the renal elimination of the active metabolite of allopurinol (alloxanthine).[8]

CLINICAL SIGNIFICANCE: The clinical significance of these mechanisms has not been established, and combined therapy with these two drugs has been used to advantage. However, it is possible that an occasional patient might manifest toxicity or lack of response due to the increased plasma probenecid levels and decreased plasma alloxanthine levels. In one study, two of five subjects developed a 50% increase in probenecid half-life with allopurinol administration, while in the other three subjects there was little change.[170]

MANAGEMENT: No special precautions appear to be necessary.

AMMONIUM CHLORIDE INTERACTIONS

DRUGS	DISCUSSION

Ephedrine[235]

MECHANISM: With acidification of the urine by ammonium chloride, ephedrine will be more ionized, thus reducing its renal tubular reabsorption and increasing its urinary excretion.

CLINICAL SIGNIFICANCE: In normal subjects given single doses of ephedrine, acidification of the urine with ammonium chloride resulted in considerably increased urinary excretion rates of ephedrine as compared to excretion with alkaline urine.[235]

MANAGEMENT: No special precautions appear necessary, but one should be aware that changes in urine pH may somewhat alter ephedrine serum levels.

Narcotic Analgesics[108,133]

MECHANISM: Methadone is a weak base that is more ionized (and thus more easily excreted) when the urine is made acidic (e.g., by ammonium chloride administration).

AMMONIUM CHLORIDE INTERACTIONS (CONT.)

DRUGS	DISCUSSION

CLINICAL SIGNIFICANCE: Studies of urinary excretion of methadone in a number of patients on methadone maintenance indicate that renal methadone clearance is considerably higher if the urine is acidic.[108,133] The magnitude of the increase appears sufficient to affect the response to methadone.

MANAGEMENT: If patients on methadone maintenance receive doses of ammonium chloride large enough to acidify the urine (e.g., several grams daily) one should be alert for reduced methadone effect.

Phenylpropanolamine (Propadrine)[235]

MECHANISM: With acidification of the urine by ammonium chloride, phenylpropanolamine will be more ionized, thus reducing its renal tubular reabsorption and increasing its urinary excretion.

CLINICAL SIGNIFICANCE: In normal subjects given single doses of phenylpropanolamine, acidification of the urine with ammonium chloride resulted in considerably increased urinary excretion rates of phenylpropanolamine as compared to excretion with alkaline urine.[235]

MANAGEMENT: No special precautions appear necessary, but one should be aware that changes in urine pH may somewhat alter phenylpropanolamine serum levels.

Pseudoephedrine (Sudafed)[140]

MECHANISM: With acidification of the urine by ammonium chloride, pseudoephedrine will be more ionized, thus reducing its renal tubular reabsorption and increasing its urinary excretion.

CLINICAL SIGNIFICANCE: Studies in three volunteers given a single dose of pseudoephedrine (180 mg) showed that acidification of the urine with ammonium chloride reduced the half-life of pseudo-ephedrine.[140] Although the reduction in plasma levels of pseudo-ephedrine were sufficient to inhibit the clinical response, this has not been reported.

MANAGEMENT: No special precautions appear necessary, but one should be aware that changes in urine pH may alter plasma pseudo-ephedrine levels.

AMPHETAMINE INTERACTIONS

DRUGS	DISCUSSION

Haloperidol (Haldol)[31-33,91]

MECHANISM: Haloperidol has many of the pharmacologic properties of the phenothiazines, and reportedly antagonizes the stimulant effects of amphetamines. Haloperidol apparently inhibits the "amine

DRUGS	DISCUSSION

pump" mechanism responsible for the uptake of various amines, including amphetamines, into the adrenergic neuron. If a similar process occurs in the central nervous system, the central effects of amphetamines could be antagonized.

CLINICAL SIGNIFICANCE: An uncontrolled study in eight patients indicated that haloperidol inhibited amphetamine-induced symptoms, and may be of value in treatment of amphetamine abuse.[94] The effect of haloperidol on the therapeutic response to amphetamines (e.g., obesity) is not clear.

MANAGEMENT: Pending availability of further information, amphetamines might be expected to be somewhat less active in patients receiving haloperidol.

Lithium Carbonate (Lithane, Lithonate)[90,98,112]

MECHANISM: Not established.

CLINICAL SIGNIFICANCE: Flemenbaum[90] has reported two cases of apparent lithium-carbonate-induced inhibition of amphetamine "highs." He also described a patient who had previously achieved weight reduction from amphetamines, but failed to do so when lithium was also being given. Although these findings suggest the possibility of interaction, confirmation is needed.

MANAGEMENT: Although evidence for interaction is scanty, the possibility should be kept in mind.

Norepinephrine (Levarterenol, Levophed)[139]

MECHANISM: Not established.

CLINICAL SIGNIFICANCE: In six patients with a history of amphetamine abuse, administration of amphetamine considerably enhanced the pressor response to intravenous norepinephrine.[139] This was shown with both intravenous administration of amphetamine and following large oral doses of amphetamine for several days. The effect of chronic amphetamine use in normal "therapeutic" doses on the pressor response to norepinephrine was not studied.

MANAGEMENT: In patients ingesting large amounts of amphetamines one should be alert for an enhanced pressor response to intravenous norepinephrine. Until more information is available some caution should also be observed in patients receiving "normal" doses of amphetamines.

Sodium Bicarbonate[9,34,35]

MECHANISM: Sufficient doses of sodium bicarbonate can render the urine alkaline, resulting in an increased proportion of un-ionized amphetamine. Thus, renal tubular reabsorption of the amphetamine is increased, and more of the drug is eventually eliminated by hepatic metabolism.

AMPHETAMINE INTERACTIONS (CONT.)

DRUGS	DISCUSSION

CLINICAL SIGNIFICANCE: Well documented. Excretion of free amphetamine is extremely small in a highly alkaline urine, thus enhancing (or at least prolonging) the effect of the amphetamine. Individuals abusing amphetamines have made use of this property by ingesting sodium bicarbonate along with the amphetamine.

MANAGEMENT: It should be realized that patients on urinary alkalinizers may have enhanced effects from amphetamines.

ANTACID, ORAL INTERACTIONS

DRUGS	DISCUSSION

Benzodiazepines[99]

MECHANISM: Magnesium-aluminum hydroxide appears to reduce the *rate* of chlordiazepoxide (Librium) absorption, but not the total amount absorbed.

CLINICAL SIGNIFICANCE: In ten normal subjects the absorption of chlordiazepoxide (25 mg orally) was measured with and without concomitant administration of magnesium-aluminum hydroxide (Maalox).[99] Chlordiazepoxide absorption was delayed by the antacid but the completeness of absorption was not reduced. Data from some studies indicate that antacids may reduce the rate and extent of the gastrointestinal absorption of clorazepate, but this has not been a consistent finding.

MANAGEMENT: No special precautions appear necessary.

Cimetidine (Tagamet)[189-191]

MECHANISM: Antacids appear to inhibit the gastrointestinal absorption of cimetidine and ranitidine.

CLINICAL SIGNIFICANCE: Concurrent administration of antacids may reduce the extent of cimetidine absorption, thus lowering serum cimetidine levels.[189,191] However, the extent to which the therapeutic response to cimetidine would be affected has not been established.

MANAGEMENT: Separate doses of cimetidine and antacids. The interaction is minimal if the cimetidine is given with a meal and the antacid one hour or more after the meal.

Diflunisal (Dolobid)[232-234]

MECHANISM: Antacids reduce the extent of gastrointestinal absorption of diflunisal.

CLINICAL SIGNIFICANCE: Single-dose studies in fasting healthy subjects have shown that aluminum hydroxide reduces diflunisal bioavailability by about 25% to 40%,[232,233] and magnesium-aluminum hydroxide reduced diflunisal bioavailability by about 15% to 20%.[234]

ANTACID, ORAL INTERACTIONS (CONT.)

DRUGS	DISCUSSION

Repeated doses of magnesium-aluminum hydroxide lowered diflunisal bioavailability by about 30%.[234] Magnesium hydroxide slightly *increased* diflunisal bioavailability,[232] but neither aluminum hydroxide nor magnesium-aluminum hydroxide affected diflunisal bioavailability in the fed state. In summary, aluminum-containing antacids tend to reduce diflunisal bioavailability under fasting conditions.

MANAGEMENT: If antacids and diflunisal are used together, administration of diflunisal with meals may minimize the interaction.

Indomethacin (Indocin)[119,131,185]

MECHANISM: Some antacids appear to inhibit the gastrointestinal absorption of indomethacin.

CLINICAL SIGNIFICANCE: Studies in normal volunteers have indicated that aluminum and magnesium-containing antacids decrease the gastrointestinal absorption of indomethacin.[119,131,185] However, the magnitude of the decreases in plasma indomethacin was not large and the clinical impact of this interaction remains to be established.

MANAGEMENT: It would not appear necessary to avoid the concomitant use of indomethacin and antacids. However, one should be alert for evidence of reduced indomethacin effect in patients so treated.

Iron Preparations[49,51,169]

MECHANISM: Not established. It is possible that the magnesium trisilicate forms poorly soluble substances with the oral iron, thus decreasing iron absorption.[51] Antacids containing carbonate reportedly may have a similar effect.[49]

CLINICAL SIGNIFICANCE: It has been reported clinically that patients with iron deficiency anemia do not respond to oral iron therapy as expected if agents such as magnesium trisilicate are given concomitantly. A subsequent study of nine patients also indicated that magnesium trisilicate impairs the absorption of simultaneously administered ferrous sulfate. However, the evidence presented was not conclusive enough to establish unequivocally that an interaction occurred. In-vitro studies are consistent with the above clinical evidence, indicating reduced iron availability in the presence of certain antacids.[169]

MANAGEMENT: The administration of magnesium trisilicate and oral iron preparations should be spaced as far apart as possible. Pending availability of further information, the same precaution should be observed with other antacids.

Levodopa (L-DOPA)[4,15–18,92,144]

MECHANISM: Levodopa appears to be metabolized in the stomach. Thus, antacids that speed gastric emptying may decrease the amount of levodopa degradation before absorption in the small intestine.

ANTACID, ORAL INTERACTIONS (CONT.)

DRUGS	DISCUSSION

CLINICAL SIGNIFICANCE: In patients with slow gastric emptying, excessive breakdown of levodopa may occur in the stomach. Antacids may enhance gastric emptying in some of these patients, thus increasing the amount of levodopa absorbed. However, evidence to date does not indicate that patients on levodopa with normal gastric emptying would be significantly affected by antacid administration.

MANAGEMENT: No special precautions appear to be necessary in most cases. However, practitioners should remember that antacids might increase levodopa absorption in an occasional patient.

Lithium carbonate (Eskalith, Lithane, Lithonate)[172]

MECHANISM: None.

CLINICAL SIGNIFICANCE: A study in six healthy subjects indicated that an aluminum-magnesium hydroxide antacid did not affect lithium absorption.[172]

MANAGEMENT: No special precautions appear necessary.

Naproxen (Naprosyn)[107]

MECHANISM: Some antacids may delay the absorption of naproxen.

CLINICAL SIGNIFICANCE: A study in 14 healthy subjects indicated that magnesium oxide and aluminum hydroxide may delay naproxen absorption.[107] However, plasma naproxen levels were not measured long enough to determine whether the completeness of naproxen absorption was affected. Sodium bicarbonate appeared to *increase* the absorption rate of naproxen, while magnesium-aluminum hydroxide (Maalox) seemed to have minimal effects. The clinical significance of these findings cannot be determined until studies are done which indicate whether the bioavailability of naproxen is affected.

MANAGEMENT: No special precautions appear to be necessary at this point.

Penicillamine (Cuprimine)[241]

MECHANISM: Antacids may reduce the gastrointestinal absorption of penicillamine.

CLINICAL SIGNIFICANCE: Six healthy subjects were given penicillamine (500 mg orally) with and without 30 ml of an antacid containing magnesium-aluminum hydroxides and simethicone (Maalox Plus).[241] The antacid reduced urinary recovery of penicillamine, indicating that penicillamine bioavailability was reduced.

MANAGEMENT: Until more is known about this interaction it would be prudent to give antacids 2 hours after penicillamine.

ANTACID, ORAL INTERACTIONS (CONT.)

DRUGS	DISCUSSION

Sodium Polystyrene Sulfonate Resin (Kayexalate)[77,85,93]

MECHANISM: It has been proposed that sodium polystyrene sulfonate resin (SPSR) binds the magnesium or calcium found in "nonsystemic" antacids. This prevents the normally occurring combination of magnesium or calcium with bicarbonate ions in the small intestine. Thus, the neutralization of bicarbonate ions by the magnesium or calcium that normally balances the neutralization of gastric acid by the antacid is impaired, resulting in systemic alkalosis.

CLINICAL SIGNIFICANCE: A study of 11 patients has demonstrated considerable elevation of plasma bicarbonate following the concomitant use of SPSR with magnesium-containing (Maalox) and calcium-containing (calcium carbonate) antacids.[77] The increases in blood and urine pH seen could alter the disposition of a number of drugs that are weak acids and bases. In a subsequent study, this interaction was used to advantage in the treatment of a patient with metabolic acidosis.[85] Also a patient receiving magnesium hydroxide (milk of magnesia) and SPSR developed severe alkalosis, presumably as a result of this interaction.[93]

MANAGEMENT: Concomitant use of SPSR with magnesium- or calcium-containing antacids should be undertaken with caution, especially in patients in whom systemic alkalinization may be dangerous. Rectal use of SPSR may avoid the interaction.

ANTICHOLINERGIC INTERACTIONS

DRUGS	DISCUSSION

Haloperidol (Haldol)[10]

MECHANISM: Not established.

CLINICAL SIGNIFICANCE: One study in ten schizophrenic patients indicated that the addition of benztropine (Cogentin) to haloperidol therapy resulted in an increase in "social avoidance behavior."[10] Some of the other therapeutic effects of haloperidol (e.g., cognitive and perceptual) did not appear to be adversely affected. Trihexyphenidyl (Artane) apparently had a similar inhibitory effect on the therapeutic response to haloperidol in schizophrenic patients.

MANAGEMENT: If this interaction proves to be real, it is yet another argument against the routine use of anticholinergic drugs in patients receiving antipsychotic drugs such as phenothiazines and haloperidol.

Levodopa (Dopar, Larodopa, L-DOPA)[4,106]

MECHANISM: Sufficient doses of anticholinergics may delay gastric emptying, thus increasing the degradation of levodopa in the stomach and decreasing the amount of levodopa delivered to the small intestine for absorption.

DRUGS	DISCUSSION

CLINICAL SIGNIFICANCE: Trihexyphenidyl has been shown to reduce the bioavailability of levodopa in a few patients.[106] Also, a single patient was described who required large doses of levodopa (7 g/day) while taking homatropine concomitantly.[4] When the homatropine was stopped, levodopa toxicity appeared, and the patient was subsequently stabilized on 4 g/day of levodopa. However, anticholinergic agents that gain access to the central nervous system are used to relieve the symptoms of parkinsonism, and this favorable effect would tend to offset the reduction in levodopa bioavailability.

MANAGEMENT: Patients should be watched for decreased levodopa effect when anticholinergics are used in doses that may be sufficient to decrease gastrointestinal motility. When anticholinergic therapy is stopped in a patient treated with levodopa, the practitioner should increase his vigilance toward detecting levodopa toxicity.

Methotrimeprazine (Levoprome)[29]

MECHANISM: Not established.

CLINICAL SIGNIFICANCE: Extrapyramidal symptoms have been reported in six patients premedicated with scopolamine and methotrimeprazine. Other anticholinergics presumably would have a similar effect.

MANAGEMENT: Anticholinergics should be administered with caution to patients receiving methotrimeprazine.

Potassium salts[163,187,188]

MECHANISM: Anticholinergic-induced slowing of gastrointestinal motility may increase the contact time of solid potassium chloride dosage forms with the gastrointestinal mucosa.

CLINICAL SIGNIFICANCE: Forty-eight healthy subjects received potassium chloride (2.4 gm tid for 7 days) as a wax-matrix (Slow-K) or microencapsulated (Micro-K) product with and without concurrent treatment with 2.0 mg tid of glycopyrrolate (Robinul).[187] The anticholinergic agent (glycopyrrolate) was associated with a considerable increase in upper gastrointestinal lesions detected by endoscopy following use of the wax-matrix preparation. The microencapsulated product was associated with less mucosal injury overall and did not appear to be affected by concurrent glycopyrrolate therapy. However, the manufacturer of a wax-matrix potassium chloride product has presented preliminary data that purportedly refute the findings of less mucosal damage with the microencapsulated product.[188] Further, it has been proposed that glycopyrrolate itself may produce gastric mucosal damage.[163] More study is needed on this interaction.

MANAGEMENT: Until the conflicting data are resolved, it would be prudent to avoid wax-matrix potassium chloride (and possibly other solid dosage forms of potassium chloride) in patients with slowed gas-

ANTICHOLINERGIC INTERACTIONS (CONT.)

DRUGS	DISCUSSION

trointestinal motility due to anticholinergic agents, other drugs, or disease.

ANTIPYRINE INTERACTIONS

DRUGS	DISCUSSION

Barbiturates[2,114,127]

MECHANISM: Barbiturates appear to enhance the metabolism of antipyrine due to induction of hepatic microsomal enzymes.

CLINICAL SIGNIFICANCE: In a study of 19 healthy subjects, amobarbital has been shown to decrease antipyrine half-life by 35%.[2] Another study of this interaction in fraternal and identical twins[127] indicated that genetic influences may be important in the degree to which phenobarbital enhances the metabolism of antipyrine. Thus, the therapeutic effect of antipyrine might be expected to be decreased by concomitant barbiturate administration. However, systemic antipyrine is seldom used in therapy.

MANAGEMENT: No special precautions appear to be necessary.

Food[105,151]

MECHANISM: Not established.

CLINICAL SIGNIFICANCE: Vestal[105] in his study of 307 healthy subjects of different age groups reported that coffee or tea intake can shorten the plasma half-life of antipyrine as indicated by a higher metabolic clearance rate of the drug in subjects with a high intake of these beverages. Studies in normal volunteers indicate that low carbohydrate-high protein diets decrease the plasma half-life of antipyrine when compared to the half-life obtained with the volunteers' usual home diet. Supplementing standard diets with protein decreased the plasma half-life, whereas supplementing standard diets with carbohydrate increased the plasma half-life of antipyrine.[151] Since antipyrine is seldom used in therapy, these findings are primarily of interest as they might relate to other drugs.

MANAGEMENT: None appears to be necessary.

BARBITURATE INTERACTIONS

DRUGS	DISCUSSION

Central Nervous System (CNS) Depressants[171]

MECHANISM: Additive effects may be seen with concomitant use of barbiturates and other depressants.

CLINICAL SIGNIFICANCE: Barbiturates are likely to add to the CNS depression of a variety of agents such as ethanol, sedative-hypnotics,

BARBITURATE INTERACTIONS (CONT.)

DRUGS	DISCUSSION

narcotic analgesics, and antihistamines. See also Barbiturates Plus Ethanol, p. 305, and Barbiturates Plus Phenothiazines, p. 348.

MANAGEMENT: Physicians should be alert for additive CNS depressant effects, especially in patients who may be especially susceptible (e.g., those with severe chronic lung disease).

Cimetidine (Tagamet)[229]

MECHANISM: Not established. Phenobarbital may enhance cimetidine elimination.

CLINICAL SIGNIFICANCE: Study in healthy subjects indicates that phenobarbital (100 mg/day for 3 weeks) reduces plasma cimetidine concentration and enhances total cimetidine clearance.[229] However, the magnitude of the changes was small and not likely to be sufficient to reduce the clinical response to cimetidine.

MANAGEMENT: No special precautions appear necessary.

Dexpanthenol (Ilopan)[36,37]

MECHANISM: Not established.

CLINICAL SIGNIFICANCE: Although adverse reactions had reportedly occurred following concurrent use of dexpanthenol and barbiturates, there is little evidence to support the existence of the interaction.

MANAGEMENT: No special precautions appear necessary.

Disulfiram (Antabuse)[109]

MECHANISM: None known.

CLINICAL SIGNIFICANCE: Although disulfiram is known to increase phenytoin plasma levels, in at least one patient serum phenobarbital was not altered by disulfiram administration.[109]

MANAGEMENT: No special precautions appear to be necessary.

Methoxyflurane (Penthrane)[104,173]

MECHANISM: It has been proposed that induction of hepatic microsomal enzymes by barbiturates may stimulate the metabolism of methoxyflurane to nephrotoxic metabolites.

CLINICAL SIGNIFICANCE: In a study of the effects of methoxyflurane on renal function in 13 patients, one patient had been receiving an enzyme inducer (secobarbital, 100 mg/day).[104] The secobarbital-treated patient developed nonoliguric renal insufficiency along with serum inorganic fluoride levels considerably higher than the mean of the other twelve patients. The proposal that the barbiturate may have predisposed this patient to methoxyflurane nephrotoxicity is consistent with previous studies in animals. Another patient has been described who may also have represented an example of this interaction.[173]

MANAGEMENT: It has been proposed that methoxyflurane be avoided in patients who are receiving enzyme inducers such as barbiturates. It should be remembered that enzyme induction dissipates slowly following discontinuation of the inducing agent, usually returning to normal within 2 to 3 weeks.

Narcotic Analgesics[113,128,138,159]

MECHANISM: It has been proposed that barbiturates enhance the metabolism of meperidine to the toxic metabolite, normeperidine.[128] Also, barbiturates and narcotic analgesics may exhibit additive or synergistic central nervous system depression.[138]

CLINICAL SIGNIFICANCE: A patient who had been receiving phenobarbital developed prolonged sedation when given meperidine.[128] Previous meperidine administration prior to phenobarbital therapy had not resulted in excessive central nervous system (CNS) depression. Subsequent study in patients and a normal volunteer indicated that phenobarbital enhances the demethylation of meperidine to normeperidine. It is not yet clear whether the enhanced CNS depression was due to increased normeperidine levels, or simply due to the combined depressant effects of the phenobarbital and meperidine.

MANAGEMENT: It may be necessary to reduce the dosage of one or both drugs when significant amounts of barbiturates and narcotic analgesics are used concomitantly. Additional caution may be necessary when using the combination of phenobarbital and meperidine.

Phenmetrazine (Preludin)[227]

MECHANISM: Not established.

CLINICAL SIGNIFICANCE: Amobarbital (90 mg/day) appeared to inhibit the weight-reducing ability of phenmetrazine in 50 patients.[227] The effect of barbiturates on the response to other anorexiants is not established, but may be similar.

MANAGEMENT: In view of the limited usefulness of anorexiants in the treatment of obesity it should not be difficult to avoid concurrent use with barbiturates.

Phenylbutazone (Butazolidin)[116,174]

MECHANISM: Barbiturates appear to stimulate the metabolism of phenylbutazone through induction of hepatic microsomal enzymes.

CLINICAL SIGNIFICANCE: Studies in a large number of healthy subjects[116] and patients with sickle cell anemia[174] indicate that phenobarbital reduces the half-life of phenylbutazone. This effect seemed to be most marked in patients who had longer phenylbutazone half-

BARBITURATE INTERACTIONS (CONT.)

lives prior to the phenobarbital.[116] The effect of the reduced half-life on the therapeutic response to phenylbutazone has not been established.

MANAGEMENT: It does not seem necessary to avoid concomitant use of barbiturates and phenylbutazone, but one should be alert for evidence of reduced phenylbutazone effect if the combination is used.

Probenecid (Benemid)[228]

MECHANISM: Not established.

CLINICAL SIGNIFICANCE: Probenecid prolonged thiopental anesthesia in a study of 86 patients.[228]

MANAGEMENT: One should anticipate the possibility that the duration of thiopental anesthesia may be longer than expected in patients receiving probenecid.

Propoxyphene (Darvon, Darvocet-N)[242]

MECHANISM: Propoxyphene appears to inhibit the hepatic metabolism of phenobarbital.

CLINICAL SIGNIFICANCE: In four epileptic patients on chronic phenobarbital, propoxyphene (65 mg three times a day) increased mean phenobarbital levels by 20% after 1 week.[242]

MANAGEMENT: Monitor for evidence of enhanced phenobarbital effect if propoxyphene is given concurrently. Lower phenobarbital dose as needed.

Pyridoxine (Vitamin B_6)[97]

MECHANISM: Not established. It is proposed that pyridoxine administration might enhance the activity of pyridoxal-phosphate dependent enzymes,[97] thus enhancing phenobarbital metabolism.

CLINICAL SIGNIFICANCE: Reductions in serum phenobarbital levels were noted in several epileptic patients when given pyridoxine (200 mg/day for 4 weeks).[97] Studies in additional patients are required to determine whether pyridoxine does have the ability to reduce serum phenobarbital levels.

MANAGEMENT: No special precautions appear necessary at this point.

Theophylline[160,184,186]

MECHANISM: Phenobarbital may enhance the metabolism of theophylline by induction of hepatic microsomal enzymes.

CLINICAL SIGNIFICANCE: A study in 12 healthy men indicated that phenobarbital (1.5 mg/kg body weight for 2 weeks) did *not* affect the disposition of theophylline (4.5 mg/kg body weight intravenously).[184]

BARBITURATE INTERACTIONS (CONT.)

DRUGS	DISCUSSION

Subsequent study in six healthy subjects indicated that phenobarbital somewhat enhanced the serum clearance of theophylline.[186] It may be that the duration of phenobarbital administration in the first study (2 weeks) was insufficient to produce maximal enzyme induction. In another report, secobarbital appears to have increased the clearance of theophylline in an infant.[160] It seems unlikely that this interaction would be clinically important with acute theophylline therapy. However, patients receiving chronic theophylline therapy might develop impaired control of their asthma.

MANAGEMENT: In patients receiving chronic theophylline therapy the initiation or discontinuation of phenobarbital (and possibly other barbiturates) should alert one to the possibility of altered theophylline effect. The logic of dosage forms containing both theophylline and a barbiturate has also been questioned.

BENZODIAZEPINE INTERACTIONS

DRUGS	DISCUSSION

Cimetidine (Tagamet)[111,278-290]

MECHANISM: Cimetidine appears to inhibit the hepatic metabolism of some benzodiazepines.

CLINICAL SIGNIFICANCE: Cimetidine reduces the plasma clearance of diazepam, chlordiazepoxide, desmethyldiazepam, and probably also alprazolam and triazolam.[278-283,287,289] Since clorazepate, halazepam, and prazepam are metabolized to active desmethyldiazepam, they would also interact with cimetidine. Clondazepam and flurazepam undergo oxidative metabolism in the liver, and their elimination is probably also reduced by cimetidine. Although some studies have found an increased sedative effect of diazepam in the presence of cimetidine,[278] others have found minimal effects of cimetidine on the response to diazepam.[111,283,285] The pharmacokinetics of benzodiazepines that undergo glucuronide conjugation such as lorazepam, oxazepam, and temazepam do not appear to be affected by cimetidine therapy.[289,290] In summary, plasma levels of several benzodiazepines and/or their active metabolites may be increased by cimetidine, but the degree to which the pharmacologic response to the benzodiazepines is increased is not well established.

MANAGEMENT: One should be alert for evidence of altered benzodiazepine response if cimetidine is initiated or discontinued. Ranitidine appears to be less likely to interact with benzodiazepines than cimetidine.

Disulfiram (Antabuse)[230,231]

MECHANISM: Disulfiram inhibits the hepatic metabolism of some benzodiazepines.

393

BENZODIAZEPINE INTERACTIONS (CONT.)

DRUGS	DISCUSSION

CLINICAL SIGNIFICANCE: Disulfiram (500 mg/day for about 2 weeks) has been shown to reduce the clearance and prolong the half-life of both chlordiazepoxide (Librium) and diazepam (Valium).[230] The magnitude of these changes appears to be sufficient to enhance the pharmacologic response to the benzodiazepines, but this was not assessed. Other benzodiazepines that undergo oxidative metabolism such as alprazolam (Xanax), clonazepam (Clonopin), clorazepate (Tranxene), flurazepam (Dalmane), halazepam (Paxipam), prazepam (Centrax), and triazolam (Halcion) are probably also affected by disulfiram treatment, but studies are not available. Oxazepam (Serax) and lorazepam (Ativan) are converted to inactive glucuronides, a process which does not appear to be affected by disulfiram.[230,231] Temazepam (Restoril) also undergoes glucuronide conjugation and would not be expected to be affected by disulfiram.

MANAGEMENT: One should be alert for evidence of enhanced benzodiazepine response in patients receiving disulfiram. Some patients may require a reduction in benzodiazepine dosage.

Food[147–149]

MECHANISM: It has been proposed that the increase in serum diazepam following food is related to secretion of the drug in gastric fluid with subsequent reabsorption and/or enterohepatic circulation of the drug.[147,148] Food intake has been shown not to alter the binding of diazepam to plasma proteins.[149]

CLINICAL SIGNIFICANCE: Studies in healthy volunteers receiving *intravenous* diazepam have demonstrated that serum concentrations of diazepam increased following food intake.[147,148] Determinations of the effect of food on the late impairment of psychomotor skills have demonstrated that food intake at 3 hours after injection of diazepam causes an increase in cumulative reaction times and an increase in the number of mistakes in tests involving reactive skills and co-ordinative skills. Peak increases in serum concentrations were shown to occur 2 hours after subjects had eaten with as much as 50% increase in serum diazepam when compared with the fasted state.[148]

MANAGEMENT: Although the possibility exists that food intake can enhance the effect of diazepam, no special precautions appear necessary at this time.

Levodopa (Dopar, Larodopa, L-DOPA)[1,5,244]

MECHANISM: Not established.

CLINICAL SIGNIFICANCE: Hunter and colleagues[5] briefly describe one levodopa-treated patient who manifested deterioration of his parkinsonism when diazepam was started. A similar deterioration has apparently been observed in three other levodopa-treated patients who were given diazepam.[1] Another patient well controlled on levodopa, benztropine, and diphenhydramine developed an acute exacerbation

BENZODIAZEPINE INTERACTIONS (CONT.)

of the disease following the administration of chlordiazepoxide, with return of control 5 days after the chlordiazepoxide was stopped.[244] Thus, several case reports indicate that benzodiazepines are capable of inhibiting the antiparkinson effects of levodopa, but little is known regarding the incidence of the interaction or the factors which make it more likely to occur.

MANAGEMENT: One should be alert for evidence of reduced antiparkinson effect of levodopa in the presence of benzodiazepine therapy. If the interaction occurs, the benzodiazepine should probably be discontinued.

Lithium Carbonate (Eskalith, Lithane, Lithonate)[132]

MECHANISM: Not established.

CLINICAL SIGNIFICANCE: A patient repeatedly became hypothermic while taking lithium and diazepam but did not manifest hypothermia when taking either drug alone.[132] It seems quite likely that the drug combination was responsible for the reaction in this patient, but it is not known whether it is an idiosyncratic reaction or one that may be expected in a significant number of other patients so treated.

MANAGEMENT: Although clinical evidence of interaction is quite scanty, one should be alert for evidence of hypothermia in patients receiving both diazepam and lithium.

Methaqualone Plus Diphenhydramine (Mandrax)[43]

MECHANISM: Not established.

CLINICAL SIGNIFICANCE: Not established. A single case has been reported in which a patient recovering from an overdose of a combination product of methaqualone and diphenhydramine developed apnea following diazepam (10 mg intravenously) administration.

MANAGEMENT: Diazepam (and other benzodiazepines) should be given with caution to patients with pre-existing respiratory depression.

Naproxen (Naprosyn)[136]

MECHANISM: None known.

CLINICAL SIGNIFICANCE: A double blind cross-over study in 24 healthy subjects indicated that diazepam and naproxen do not interact as measured by various psychological tests.[136] However, the results of this single dose study do not necessarily apply to the clinical situation of chronic use of one or both drugs.

MANAGEMENT: No special precautions appear necessary.

BENZODIAZEPINE INTERACTIONS (CONT.)

DRUGS	DISCUSSION

Neuromuscular Blocking Agents[42,83,84,110]

MECHANISM: Not established. Study in normal volunteers given diazepam indicates that the drug may directly inhibit the contractile mechanism of skeletal muscle.[110]

CLINICAL SIGNIFICANCE: Preliminary clinical study indicated that diazepam increased the duration of action of gallamine, and decreased the duration of succinylcholine activity.[42] However, subsequent work[83,84] has not substantiated these findings, and it appears likely that diazepam itself does not significantly affect the response to neuromuscular blocking agents. An *inhibition* of neuromuscular blockage has been reported when the injectable form of diazepam was given intraarterially, an effect presumably due to one or more of the preservatives, solvents, etc. that are found in this preparation. The effect of intravenous or intramuscular doses of diazepam on the response to neuromuscular blockers under clinical conditions remains to be determined.

MANAGEMENT: On the basis of current evidence, special precautions do not appear necessary with concomitant use of these drugs. However, physicians should be alert for any unusual effects.

Smoking[213–217]

MECHANISM: Smoking may enhance the hepatic metabolism of some benzodiazepines.

CLINICAL SIGNIFICANCE: An epidemiologic study of the incidence of drowsiness due to chlordiazepoxide (Librium) and diazepam (Valium) showed that drowsiness was less likely to occur in smokers.[213] This effect was directly proportional to the number of cigarettes smoked per day. However, the results of studies of the effects of smoking on benzodiazepine pharmacokinetics have not been consistent. Early reports indicate that the pharmacokinetics of diazepam and chlordiazepoxide are unaffected by smoking,[214,215] whereas later studies show an increased clearance of diazepam and lorazepam in smokers.[216,217] Diazepam clearance is less likely to be increased in elderly smokers.[216]

MANAGEMENT: One should be aware that larger doses of benzodiazepines may be required in smokers to achieve sedative effects equivalent to those obtained in nonsmokers.

CALCIUM INTERACTIONS

DRUGS	DISCUSSION

Calcium channel blockers[198–201]

MECHANISM: Increasing the extracellular calcium concentration may antagonize the pharmacologic response to calcium channel blockers.

CALCIUM INTERACTIONS (CONT.)

DRUGS	DISCUSSION

CLINICAL SIGNIFICANCE: A patient with atrial fibrillation controlled with verapamil developed a return of the arrhythmia following administration of calcium adipinate (1.2 g/day) and calciferol (3000 IU/day).[198] Calcium infusions have also been used with success to treat overdoses of verapamil.[199–201] Thus, the evidence indicates that administration of calcium may reduce the response to verapamil and probably other calcium-channel blockers. However, the amount of calcium required and the magnitude of the reduction in effect cannot be determined from available data.

MANAGEMENT: In patients receiving calcium-channel blockers, one should be alert for evidence of reduced response if calcium products are given concurrently.

CHOLESTYRAMINE (QUESTRAN) INTERACTIONS

DRUGS	DISCUSSION

Iron Preparations[82]

MECHANISM: Cholestyramine may bind iron in the gastrointestinal tract, thus preventing its absorption.

CLINICAL SIGNIFICANCE: Not established. A single case report and animal studies indicate that cholestyramine may impair the absorption of dietary iron. The significance of these findings to concomitant therapy with oral iron and cholestyramine remains to be established.

MANAGEMENT: Very little is known about the possibility of this interaction. However, until more is known, it might be prudent to space doses of cholestyramine and oral iron so that mixing in the gastrointestinal tract is minimized.

Loperamide (Imodium)[237]

MECHANISM: Cholestyramine possibly binds with loperamide, thus reducing the gastrointestinal absorption of loperamide.

CLINICAL SIGNIFICANCE: In one patient with an ileostomy, cholestyramine appeared to inhibit the ability of loperamide to reduce fluid loss from the ileostomy.[237] However, more study is needed to assess the clinical importance of this interaction.

MANAGEMENT: Until more is known about this purported interaction, loperamide should be administered 2 or more hours before cholestyramine.

Phenylbutazone (Butazolidin)[38,39]

MECHANISM: Cholestyramine is an anion-exchange resin that may bind acidic drugs such as phenylbutazone in the gut.

397

CHOLESTYRAMINE (QUESTRAN) INTERACTIONS (CONT.)

DRUGS	DISCUSSION

CLINICAL SIGNIFICANCE: Not established. Preliminary animal studies indicate that the absorption of phenylbutazone may be delayed, but not necessarily decreased, by the concomitant oral administration of cholestyramine. Under conditions of repetitive dosing in humans, cholestyramine may or may not have an effect on the therapeutic response to phenylbutazone.

MANAGEMENT: Pending availability of further information, it would be prudent to administer phenylbutazone at least 1 hour before the cholestyramine.

CIMETIDINE (TAGAMET) INTERACTIONS

DRUGS	DISCUSSION

Food[161]

MECHANISM: Not established.

CLINICAL SIGNIFICANCE: Cimetidine is absorbed more slowly when taken with meals. A study involving 6 healthy male volunteers given a dose of 300 mg of cimetidine demonstrated that food delayed the therapeutic blood concentrations of the drug and had little effect on the time the concentration of drug was maintained above the therapeutic level. The delayed absorption of cimetidine by food appears to be beneficial by maintaining effective blood concentrations during the period between meals.

MANAGEMENT: Based on these findings it would appear to be advantageous to take cimetidine with meals.

Narcotic Analgesics[302-308]

MECHANISM: Not established. The hepatic metabolism of certain narcotic analgesics may be inhibited by cimetidine. Also, the effects of histamine released in response to narcotic analgesics may be partially inhibited by cimetidine. Finally, additive effects might be seen in the central nervous system.

CLINICAL SIGNIFICANCE: Isolated cases have appeared that may have represented cimetidine-induced increases in the respiratory depression and sedation that may follow administration of narcotic analgesics.[302,303] Also, in-vitro studies indicate that cimetidine may inhibit the hepatic microsomal metabolism of meperidine and fentanyl.[304,305] However, morphine disposition was not affected by cimetidine pretreatment in seven healthy men,[306] probably because morphine undergoes glucuronidation, a metabolic process not affected by cimetidine. Cimetidine may inhibit some of the cardiovascular effects of histamine, which is released in response to administration of narcotic analgesics.[307,308] In summary, cimetidine does not appear to inhibit the hepatic metabolism of narcotic analgesics such as morphine which undergo glucuronide conjugation, but limited

DRUGS	DISCUSSION

as morphine which undergo glucuronide conjugation, but limited data indicate that the metabolism of other narcotics might be inhibited by cimetidine. Pharmacologic interactions between cimetidine and narcotic analgesics are also possible, but not well studied.

MANAGEMENT: Until these interactions are better described, one should be alert for evidence of enhanced respiratory and central nervous system depression in the presence of combined therapy with cimetidine and narcotic analgesics.

Nifedipine (Procardia)[310]

MECHANISM: Cimetidine may inhibit the hepatic metabolism of nifedipine.

CLINICAL SIGNIFICANCE: In a preliminary study of seven healthy volunteers, 7 days of concurrent treatment with cimetidine (100 mg/day) and nifedipine (40 mg/day) considerably increased the peak plasma levels and area under the plasma concentration-time curve of nifedipine.[310] In seven hypertensive patients, cimetidine appeared to increase the antihypertensive response to nifedipine. The significance of this interaction cannot be determined from the preliminary data available, but a clinically important increase in nifedipine effect seems possible.

MANAGEMENT: Until more information is available, one should be alert for evidence of altered nifedipine response if cimetidine therapy is initiated or discontinued.

Theophylline[161,263-277]

MECHANISM: Cimetidine inhibits the hepatic metabolism of theophylline.

CLINICAL SIGNIFICANCE: Pharmacokinetic studies have consistently shown that cimetidine reduces theophylline plasma clearance, increases theophylline half-life, and increases plasma theophylline levels.[263-268] Moreover, several case reports have appeared describing elevated plasma theophylline levels and/or theophylline toxicity during cimetidine therapy.[269-277] One fatality has been described, an elderly man in whom cimetidine-induced theophylline toxicity may have played a role.[277] Since cimetidine begins to reduce theophylline elimination as soon as therapeutic serum levels of cimetidine are achieved, a new steady state serum theophylline level will usually be observed by the second day of cimetidine therapy. However, it may take longer in some patients (e.g., patients whose theophylline half-life is relatively long to begin with and/or those patients who develop a marked increase in theophylline half-life due to cimetidine).

MANAGEMENT: One may need to adjust the dose of theophylline when cimetidine is initiated or discontinued, or if the cimetidine dose is changed. In a patient already receiving cimetidine, initial doses of theophylline should be conservative until the dosage requirement is

CIMETIDINE (TAGAMET) INTERACTIONS (CONT.)

DRUGS	DISCUSSION

determined. Serum theophylline determinations would be useful in following this interaction. Ranitidine (Zantac) does not appear to affect theophylline disposition and thus would be preferrable to cimetidine in patients receiving theophylline.

Verapamil (Calan, Isoptin)[309]

MECHANISM: Cimetidine may reduce the hepatic metabolism of verapamil.

CLINICAL SIGNIFICANCE: In a preliminary study in nine healthy subjects, pretreatment with cimetidine (1200 mg/day for 5 days) reduced the clearance of verapamil (given as 10 mg intravenously) and increased verapamil half-life from 3.4 hours to 5.1 hours.[309] The significance of this interaction cannot be determined from the preliminary data available, but a clinically important increase in verapamil effect seems possible.

MANAGEMENT: Until more information is available, one should be alert for evidence of altered verapamil response if cimetidine therapy is initiated or discontinued.

CYCLOSPORINE (SANDIMMUNE) INTERACTIONS

DRUGS	DISCUSSION

Corticosteroids[296-297]

MECHANISM: Not established.

CLINICAL SIGNIFICANCE: Preliminary evidence indicates that cyclosporine reduces the plasma clearance of prednisolone in renal transplant patients, and may thus increase prednisolone effects.[296] In another preliminary study, plasma cyclosporine levels were increased in the presence of methylprednisolone.[297]

MANAGEMENT: One should be alert for evidence of increased response to both cyclosporine and corticosteroids if the two drugs are used concurrently.

Ketoconazole (Nirzoral)[298,299,300]

MECHANISM: Not established. Ketoconazole may inhibit cyclosporin metabolism.

CLINICAL SIGNIFICANCE: Blood cyclosporine concentrations increased following initiation of ketoconazole therapy in one patient, and returned to baseline values after discontinuation of ketoconazole.[298] These findings were supported by animal studies.[299]

MANAGEMENT: One should be alert for evidence of excessive cyclosporine effect (e.g., nephrotoxicity) in the presence of ketokonazole therapy. Reduce the cyclosporine dosage as needed.

CYCLOSPORINE (SANDIMMUNE) INTERACTIONS (CONT.)

DRUGS	DISCUSSION

Melphalan (Alkeran)[300]

MECHANISM: Not established.

CLINICAL SIGNIFICANCE: Renal failure occurred in 13 of 17 patients who received cyclosporine and high-dose melphalan therapy; the authors felt the reactions resulted from a drug interaction between cyclosporine and melphalan.[300]

MANAGEMENT: Monitor renal function carefully in patients receiving concurrent therapy with cyclosporine and melphalan.

Sulfamethoxazole/Trimethoprim (Bactrim, Septra)[301]

MECHANISM: Not established.

CLINICAL SIGNIFICANCE: Preliminary epidemiologic evidence indicates that cyclosporine and sulfamethoxazole/trimethoprim may exhibit synergistic nephrotoxic effects.[301] More study is needed.

MANAGEMENT: One should be alert for evidence of nephrotoxicity with combined use of cyclosporine and sulfamethoxazole/trimethoprim.

DAPSONE (AVLOSULFAN) INTERACTIONS

DRUGS	DISCUSSION

Probenecid (Benemid)[76]

MECHANISM: Probenecid appears to inhibit the renal excretion of dapsone.

MECHANISM: One preliminary study has shown dapsone serum levels to be raised when probenecid is also given. Dapsone serum levels were increased about 50% over control levels after 4 hours and 25% after 8 hours.

MANAGEMENT: One should be alert for evidence of elevated dapsone serum levels, and the possible necessity of a reduction in dapsone dose.

DISULFIRAM (ANTABUSE) INTERACTIONS

DRUGS	DISCUSSION

Paraldehyde[40,41]

MECHANISM: Paraldehyde is thought to be depolymerized to acetaldehyde by the liver. Thus, disulfiram would theoretically impair the disposition of acetaldehyde by inhibition of acetaldehyde dehydrogenase.

CLINICAL SIGNIFICANCE: Although clinical reports of this interaction are lacking, animal studies and theoretical considerations indicate that the interaction may be clinically significant.

DISULFIRAM (ANTABUSE) INTERACTIONS (CONT.)

DRUGS	DISCUSSION

MANAGEMENT: Pending the availability of further information, the concomitant administration of paraldehyde and disulfiram should be undertaken with great care or, preferably, avoided completely.

DOPAMINE (INTROPIN) INTERACTIONS

DRUGS	DISCUSSION

Ergot Alkaloids[175]

MECHANISM: The combined use of these two vasoconstrictors may result in excessive peripheral vasoconstriction.

CLINICAL SIGNIFICANCE: A patient has been described who developed gangrene of both hands and feet following administration of ergonovine (ergometrine) and dopamine infusions.[175] It was felt that the gangrene was a result of the combined effect of the drugs, although either drug alone can cause gangrene in sufficient dosage.

MANAGEMENT: It has been proposed that dopamine and ergot alkaloids such as ergonovine should not be used concomitantly.[175]

DYPHYLLINE (LUFYLLIN) INTERACTIONS

DRUGS	DISCUSSION

Probenecid (Benemid)[192,193]

MECHANISM: Probenecid appears to inhibit the renal excretion of dyphylline.

CLINICAL SIGNIFICANCE: In twelve healthy subjects pretreatment with probenecid (1.0 g orally) approximately doubled the half-life of dyphylline and reduced dyphylline clearance by almost 50%.[192] If this interaction is sustained during multiple dosing, an excessive serum level of dyphylline could result.

MANAGEMENT: One should be alert for evidence of altered dyphylline effect if probenecid is started or stopped. Theophylline does not appear to interact with probenecid,[193] and may thus be a suitable alternative to dyphylline if one wishes to avoid this interaction.

ECHOTHIOPHATE IODIDE (PHOSPHOLINE IODIDE) INTERACTIONS

DRUGS	DISCUSSION

Procaine[48]

MECHANISM: Prolonged ophthalmic use of echothiophate results in reduced pseudocholinesterase activity, which could result in reduced hydrolysis of procaine.

ECHOTHIOPHATE IODIDE (PHOSPHOLINE IODIDE) INTERACTIONS (CONT.)

DRUGS	DISCUSSION

CLINICAL SIGNIFICANCE: Not established. Patients with inherited atypical plasma cholinesterase have developed severe reactions (e.g., unconsciousness, cardiovascular collapse) following the local injection of procaine. It seems reasonable to assume that echothiophate-induced depression of pseudocholinesterase activity could predispose the patient to reactions following procaine. It is possible that some "anaphylactic" reactions to local anesthetics may actually be due to drug-induced or hereditary reduction of pseudocholinesterase activity.

MANAGEMENT: Although little clinical information is available concerning this interaction, patients using echothiophate should be given procaine injections with caution. It may be wise to use a local anesthetic other than procaine in such patients.

Succinylcholine (Anectine)[19,44–47,130,183]

MECHANISM: Prolonged ophthalmic use of echothiophate iodide results in reduced activity of pseudocholinesterase, the enzyme responsible for the metabolism of succinylcholine. Preliminary study indicates that pralidoxime may reverse the lowered pseudocholinesterase levels without affecting the control of the glaucoma by echothiophate.

CLINICAL SIGNIFICANCE: Prolonged apnea and death are possible with the administration of succinylcholine to patients with echothiophate-induced depression of pseudocholinesterase. This would be more likely in patients on long-term echothiophate therapy, and may be most significant with short procedures (e.g., electroshock therapy).

MANAGEMENT: Patients receiving echothiophate iodide should be given succinylcholine only with caution. It may be wise to measure pseudocholinesterase activity prior to succinylcholine administration; a simple test for pseudocholinesterase has been described.[47] In patients on echothiophate, it would be preferable to use an agent other than succinylcholine if possible.

EPHEDRINE INTERACTIONS

DRUGS	DISCUSSION

Sodium bicarbonate[235]

MECHANISM: Sodium bicarbonate-induced alkalinization of the urine decreases the ionization of ephedrine, thus enhancing renal tubular reabsorption.

CLINICAL SIGNIFICANCE: Study in normal subjects given single doses of ephedrine has shown that urinary excretion of ephedrine is reduced when the urine is alkaline.[235] Short-term urinary alkalinization is unlikely to be clinically important, but ephedrine toxicity is possible if the urine remains alkaline for several days or longer.

EPHEDRINE INTERACTIONS (CONT.)

DRUGS	DISCUSSION

MANAGEMENT: Monitor for evidence of ephedrine toxicity (e.g., nervousness, insomnia, excitability) if the urine remains alkaline for more than a day or two. Adjust ephedrine dose as needed.

Theophylline[20,102,103,123]

MECHANISM: Not established.

CLINICAL SIGNIFICANCE: Study in asthmatic children has shown that the addition of ephedrine to theophylline therapy considerably increased the incidence of adverse reactions such as insomnia, nervousness, and gastrointestinal complaints.[102] Although ephedrine appeared to increase side effects, it did not increase the efficacy of treatment. A subsequent study in 16 asthmatic children found that ephedrine enhanced the bronchodilating effects of theophylline but did not enhance toxicity.[123] The latter study used lower doses of ephedrine, which may account for the conflicting results. More study is needed to assess the clinical importance of this interaction.

MANAGEMENT: One should be alert for evidence of increased adverse reactions (e.g., insomnia, nervousness, gastrointestinal symptoms) when ephedrine is added to theophylline therapy. Avoiding fixed dose combinations of ephedrine and theophylline would facilitate achieving the optimal dose of each drug.

GLUTETHIMIDE (DORIDEN) INTERACTIONS

DRUGS	DISCUSSION

Smoking[218]

MECHANISM: Not established.

CLINICAL SIGNIFICANCE: A study in seven normal subjects indicated that glutethimide had a greater detrimental effect on a tracking psychomotor test in smokers than in nonsmokers. The results of pharmacokinetic studies in these subjects were consistent with an increase in glutethimide absorption in the smokers, but the number of subjects is too small to arrive at definite conclusions.

MANAGEMENT: No special precautions appear necessary.

HALOPERIDOL (HALDOL) INTERACTIONS

DRUGS	DISCUSSION

Lithium Carbonate (Eskalith, Lithane, Lithonate)[101,120–122,180,245–256]

MECHANISM: Not established. It has been proposed that haloperidol and lithium could have a combined inhibitory effect on striatal adenylate cyclase.[120]

HALOPERIDOL (HALDOL) INTERACTIONS (CONT.)

DRUGS	DISCUSSION

CLINICAL SIGNIFICANCE: Four patients with mania developed encephalopathy (e.g., lethargy, fever, confusion, extrapyramidal symptoms) following the combined use of lithium carbonate and high doses of haloperidol.[101] Two of the patients developed permanent brain damage and the other two patients developed persistent dyskinesias. A similar case of severe rigidity, fever, mutism, and an irreversible dyskinesia was associated with the combined use of lithium and haloperidol.[245] Extrapyramidal symptoms were also noted in ten other patients who received combined therapy with haloperidol (maximum dose, 30 mg/day) and lithium (serum lithium always below 1.2 mmol/L).[246] Another report described seven patients who developed an unexpected degree of extrapyramidal symptoms while receiving lithium and haloperidol.[121] Others[247] observed a patient who developed a severe acute brain syndrome while receiving lithium-haloperidol therapy and cite another report of three patients on such therapy who developed dyskinesias and other neurologic toxicity. Several other cases have been reported as examples of lithium-haloperidol interaction.[254–256] Thomas and colleagues analyzed the Wechsler adult intelligence scale in seven patients receiving lithium plus haloperidol and compared the results to patients receiving lithium plus chlorpromazine.[248] The results indicated possible brain damage in the lithium-haloperidol group, but, this report was only preliminary, and more detailed study of this phenomenon is needed.[249,250] Most of the above cases were relatively isolated events that occurred within a much larger group of lithium-haloperidol treated patients who did not manifest such effects. Further, several epidemiologic studies have failed to detect evidence supporting an adverse lithium-haloperidol interaction.[122,180,251,252] However, negative epidemiologic evidence does not disprove the occurrence of this interaction in specific predisposed persons and one must assume that under certain conditions the combination may be detrimental to the patient. Factors that probably increase the likelihood of an adverse drug interaction are large doses of one or both drugs; the presence of acute mania; failure to discontinue drugs when adverse effects occur; pre-existing brain damage; a history of extrapyramidal symptoms with neuroleptic therapy alone; the concurrent use of anticholinergic antiparkinson drugs; and the presence of other physiologic disturbances such as infection, fever, or dehydration.

MANAGEMENT: It has been recommended that neuroleptics such as haloperidol be used alone for initial control of acute mania symptoms and that lithium be added as the neuroleptic dosage is reduced.[246,253] If haloperidol and lithium are used concomitantly, careful attention should be given to the dose of both agents as well as to early detection of neurotoxicity, particularly in the presence of predisposing factors described above.

HEPARIN INTERACTIONS

DRUGS	DISCUSSION

Intramuscular Injections[21,78]

MECHANISM: Intramuscular injections of drugs to patients receiving heparin may result in hematomas and bleeding into adjacent areas.

CLINICAL SIGNIFICANCE: In one study of elderly women receiving IV heparin, intramuscular administration of other drugs into the buttocks appeared to be at least partly responsible for the observed bleeding into the hip and groin.[78]

MANAGEMENT: If possible, intramuscular administration of drugs should be avoided during the period in which intravenous heparin exerts its effect, especially in elderly women.

Smoking[219]

MECHANISM: Not established.

CLINICAL SIGNIFICANCE: In a study of factors affecting heparin pharmacokinetics in 20 patients with thromboembolic disease, it was found that smokers had shorter heparin half-lives (0.62 hours versus 0.97 hours) and more rapid heparin elimination rates than nonsmokers. Thus, smoking may be one of the factors affecting dosage requirements for heparin. However, more study is needed to determine the incidence and magnitude of this purported interaction.

MANAGEMENT: No special precautions appear necessary at this point.

INDOMETHACIN (INDOCIN) INTERACTIONS

DRUGS	DISCUSSION

Food[119,167,168]

MECHANISM: Not established.

CLINICAL SIGNIFICANCE: Studies in healthy adult volunteers have shown that mean peak serum concentrations of indomethacin are delayed and decreased by food when compared with levels achieved under fasting conditions.[119,167] However, the significance of these findings to patients on long-term indomethacin therapy is not clear. The psychological and/or real advantage of taking the drug with meals to reduce gastrointestinal symptoms probably outweighs the disadvantage of possible delays or decreases in absorption.

MANAGEMENT: No specific recommendations appear necessary.

Lithium carbonate[239,240]

MECHANISM: Indomethacin reduces renal lithium excretion, probably due to indomethacin-induced prostaglandin inhibition.

CLINICAL SIGNIFICANCE: Indomethacin (150 mg/day) has been shown to reduce renal lithium clearance and increase plasma lithium

DRUGS	DISCUSSION

levels.[239,240] The magnitude of the increases appears sufficient to cause lithium toxicity in some patients.

MANAGEMENT: Monitor plasma lithium concentrations carefully if indomethacin (or another nonsteroidal anti-inflammatory drug) is initiated or discontinued.

Phenylpropanolamine[236]

MECHANISM: Not established. Indomethacin-induced inhibition of prostaglandins may make patients more susceptible to hypertensive stimuli such as sympathomimetics.

CLINICAL SIGNIFICANCE: A single 25-mg dose of indomethacin resulted in hypertension and headache in a patient on chronic phenylpropanolamine.[236] A re-challenge was positive, indicating that the interaction was probably responsible for the hypertensive episodes in this patient. However, it is not known how often the interaction would occur in other persons.

MANAGEMENT: Until more information is available, blood pressure should be monitored in patients receiving concurrent therapy with sympathomimetics (such as phenylpropanolamine) and prostaglandin inhibitors (such as indomethacin). If blood pressure is increased one or both drugs should be discontinued if possible.

Probenecid (Benemid)[50,89,257]

MECHANISM: Indomethacin appears to undergo renal tubular secretion that may be blocked by probenecid.

CLINICAL SIGNIFICANCE: One study in six subjects demonstrated that indomethacin blood levels may be considerably increased by concomitant probenecid administration.[50] The half-life of indomethacin alone was 10.1 hours, and it increased to 17.6 hours when probenecid was also given. Preliminary information from another study gave similar results.[89] However, there is evidence that the increased plasma indomethacin levels may be associated with an increased therapeutic response without a corresponding increase in side effects.[257] Thus, the interaction may be favorable in at least some patients.

MANAGEMENT: No special precautions appear to be necessary.

Vaccinations[22]

MECHANISM: It is proposed that the anti-inflammatory effect of indomethacin may alter the response to smallpox vaccination.

CLINICAL SIGNIFICANCE: A single case has been reported in which a 60-year-old man receiving indomethacin developed a severe reaction to a smallpox vaccination.[22] However a cause and effect relationship has not been established. Since smallpox vaccine is no longer used,

INDOMETHACIN (INDOCIN) INTERACTIONS (CONT.)

DRUGS	DISCUSSION

the only implications of these findings would be for other live vaccines such as measles, mumps, and rubella.

MANAGEMENT: Although clinical evidence is very scanty, practitioners should be aware that indomethacin therapy may predispose patients to reactions from live vaccines.

IRON PREPARATION INTERACTIONS

DRUGS	DISCUSSION

Pancreatic Extracts[80]

MECHANISM: Pancreatic extracts apparently contain a substance that inhibits iron absorption.

CLINICAL SIGNIFICANCE: Not established. A very preliminary study indicates that the serum iron response to oral iron is decreased by concomitant administration of various pancreatic extracts and purified pancreatic enzymes.

MANAGEMENT: No special precautions appear necessary, but the possibility of interaction should be realized.

Penicillamine (Cuprimine)[126,258]

MECHANISM: Oral iron preparations appear to inhibit the absorption of penicillamine.

CLINICAL SIGNIFICANCE: In a study using increased urinary copper excretion as a measure of penicillamine effect, five healthy subjects were given iron alone, penicillamine alone, and iron plus penicillamine.[126] The results indicated that iron reduced the pharmacologic effect of penicillamine on urinary copper excretion, presumably by reducing oral absorption of penicillamine. In another study in six healthy men, ferrous sulfate (300 mg orally) reduced plasma penicillamine levels to 35% of control values.[258]

MANAGEMENT: Patients receiving penicillamine (e.g., for rheumatoid arthritis) should space doses of oral iron so as to minimize mixing in the gastrointestinal tract. One should also be alert for evidence of reduced penicillamine response, and adjust penicillamine dose as needed.

Vitamin E[52]

MECHANISM: Not established.

CLINICAL SIGNIFICANCE: A preliminary study indicates that vitamin E may impair the hematologic response to iron therapy in children with iron deficiency anemia. More study is needed to confirm this finding.

IRON PREPARATION INTERACTIONS (CONT.)

DRUGS	DISCUSSION

MANAGEMENT: Pending availability of further information, patients with iron deficiency anemia who are receiving iron therapy should be observed for this effect if vitamin E is given concomitantly.

KAOLIN INTERACTIONS

DRUGS	DISCUSSION

Pseudoephedrine (Sudafed)[3]

MECHANISM: Kaolin probably has the ability to absorb pseudoephedrine, thus inhibiting its gastrointestinal absorption.

CLINICAL SIGNIFICANCE: A study in six healthy subjects has shown that pseudoephedrine absorption (as measured by cumulative urinary excretion) can be slightly decreased by concomitant administration of a kaolin suspension.[3] The magnitude of the effect does not seem sufficient to have much effect on the therapeutic response to pseudoephedrine.

MANAGEMENT: No special precautions appear to be necessary.

LEVODOPA (L-DOPA) INTERACTIONS

DRUGS	DISCUSSION

Food[100,145,146]

MECHANISM: Delayed absorption of levodopa following protein intake may be attributable to competition for intestinal absorption as well as change in pH or gastric emptying time.[145] The competition for absorption may occur following hydrolysis of protein since levodopa is absorbed and transported by the same mechanisms that transport other large, neutral amino acids.[145,146]

CLINICAL SIGNIFICANCE: Morgan[145] reported that peak plasma concentrations of levodopa were less in a patient following a small protein meal (milk and crackers) than in other patients taking the drug in the fasting state. A delay in absorption and urinary excretion was observed in the fed patient. Gillespie[146] reported that in eight patients with parkinsonism high intakes of protein (2 g/kg body weight/day) tended to cancel the therapeutic effects of levodopa whereas low protein intakes (0.5 g/kg body weight/day) tended to potentiate and stabilize the therapeutic effects of the drug. These data suggest that there may be loss of clinical improvement in patients receiving levodopa who ingest large amounts of protein daily.

MANAGEMENT: Although it has been suggested that greater absorption and therapeutic effect might be achieved if levodopa were administered away from meals,[145] most standard texts recommend that the drug be taken with meals to slow absorption and thus reduce the central emetic effect. Patients on levodopa should probably avoid

LEVODOPA (L-DOPA) INTERACTIONS (CONT.)

DRUGS	DISCUSSION

high protein diets as well as diets with widely fluctuating protein intake.

Methionine[176]

MECHANISM: Not established.

CLINICAL SIGNIFICANCE: Fourteen parkinsonian patients receiving levodopa were placed on a restricted L-methionine diet for 8 days and then given either placebo (seven patients) or methionine (seven patients) in a dose of 4.5 g/day.[176] Patients receiving placebo demonstrated little change, with some subjective improvement in three patients. However, five of the seven patients on methionine developed a worsening of their parkinsonism. Thus, based on this initial study, it appears that L-methionine may inhibit the clinical response to levodopa in parkinsonism. Doses of methionine similar to the dose used in this study have been used to acidify the urine.

MANAGEMENT: Large doses of methionine should probably be avoided in parkinsonian patients receiving levodopa.

Papaverine[177-179]

MECHANISM: Not established. It has been suggested that papaverine might block dopamine receptors.

CLINICAL SIGNIFICANCE: Several parkinsonian patients maintained on levodopa have developed worsening of their parkinsonism following papaverine administration.[177,179] The therapeutic response to levodopa returned 5 to 10 days after the papaverine was stopped.

MANAGEMENT: Papaverine should probably be avoided in patients with parkinsonism, especially if they are receiving levodopa. In most cases it should not be difficult to find a therapeutic alternative to papaverine.

Phenylbutazone (Butazolidin)[1]

MECHANISM: Not established.

CLINICAL SIGNIFICANCE: A single patient has been described in whom phenylbutazone appeared to antagonize the therapeutic response to levodopa.[1]

MANAGEMENT: Clinical evidence is too scanty to make a statement on management, but practitioners should be alert for this potential interaction.

Phenylephrine (Neo-Synephrine)[54]

MECHANISM: Not established. It has been proposed that levodopa or its metabolites may competitively inhibit agents that act on alpha-adrenergic receptors (e.g., phenylephrine).

LEVODOPA (L-DOPA) INTERACTIONS (CONT.)

DRUGS	DISCUSSION

CLINICAL SIGNIFICANCE: Levodopa administration has been shown to reduce the mydriasis following topical phenylephrine. It is not known whether other responses to phenylephrine would be inhibited.

MANAGEMENT: Too little information is available concerning clinical significance to make a statement on management.

Pyridoxine (Vitamin B$_6$)[11,23–25,55,56,86–88,94,134,135,142]

MECHANISM: Pyridoxine appears to enhance the metabolism of levodopa, thus decreasing the amount available to the site of action in the brain.

CLINICAL SIGNIFICANCE: It has been observed by many workers that pyridoxine reverses the levodopa-induced improvement in Parkinson's syndrome. Doses as small as 10 to 25 mg of pyridoxine may be sufficient to produce this effect. This antagonism apparently does not occur if the patient is also receiving a peripheral decarboxylase inhibitor such as carbidopa.[11,25,87,88]

MANAGEMENT: Pyridoxine and vitamin preparations containing pyridoxine should be avoided in patients receiving levodopa, unless a peripheral decarboxylase inhibitor (e.g., carbidopa) is also being given.

LITHIUM CARBONATE INTERACTIONS

DRUGS	DISCUSSION

Levarterenol (Levophed, Norepinephrine)[129]

MECHANISM: Not established.

CLINICAL SIGNIFICANCE: Eight patients with manic depressive illness were given levarterenol (norepinephrine) before and after 7 to 10 days of lithium carbonate treatment.[129] Lithium decreased the pressor response to levarterenol by 22%. This effect would not seem likely to cause clinical difficulties.

MANAGEMENT: No special precautions appear to be necessary.

Mazindol (Sanorex)[195]

MECHANISM: Not established. Mazindol-induced anorexia with decreased fluid and sodium intake might reduce renal lithium excretion.

CLINICAL SIGNIFICANCE: A patient on chronic lithium therapy developed ataxia and lethargy progressing to stupor with muscle fasciculations following addition of 2 mg/day of mazindol.[195] Serum lithium was 3.2 mEq/L; previous lithium levels were below 1.3 mEq/L. The temporal relationship of the reaction indicates that mazindol may have been involved, but definitive conclusions cannot be drawn from a single case.

411

LITHIUM CARBONATE INTERACTIONS (CONT.)

DRUGS	DISCUSSION

MANAGEMENT: If patients on lithium therapy are given anorexic agents such as mazindol, one should ensure that intake of fluid and sodium is not severely compromised.

Neuromuscular Blocking Agents[137,181,182,259]

MECHANISM: Not established.

CLINICAL SIGNIFICANCE: A patient on chronic lithium carbonate therapy developed prolonged apnea (4 hours) following the use of succinylcholine during surgery.[182] Lithium has also been reported to enhance the neuromuscular blocking activity of pancuronium.[181] Studies in dogs indicate that lithium can prolong the neuromuscular blockade of succinylcholine, decamethonium, and pancuronium.[137] However, some have questioned the clinical importance of this interaction.[259]

MANAGEMENT: In patients receiving chronic lithium carbonate therapy, one should be aware that the action of neuromuscular blocking agents may be prolonged.

Piroxicam (Feldene)[194]

MECHANISM: Not established. Piroxicam-induced prostaglandin inhibition may inhibit renal lithium excretion.

CLINICAL SIGNIFICANCE: A 56-year-old woman stabilized on lithium for 10 years developed elevated serum lithium levels and symptoms of lithium toxicity after starting piroxicam therapy.[194] The same patient was subsequently studied under controlled conditions while on lithium 750 mg/day and starting therapy with 20 mg/day of piroxicam. The serum lithium increased to 1.5 mmol/L (therapeutic range, 0.8 to 1.4 mmol/L) after starting piroxicam, and fell to 1.0 mmol/L a few weeks after discontinuation of piroxicam. It seems likely that piroxicam was responsible for the changes in serum lithium levels in this patient given the temporal relationship and the known effect of other prostaglandin inhibitors on lithium disposition. However, additional study will be required to determine if this interaction would predictably occur in patients receiving the two drugs.

MANAGEMENT: One should be alert for evidence of altered lithium effect if piroxicam is initiated or discontinued. Serum lithium determinations would be useful in monitoring this interaction.

Potassium Iodide[26,95,141,143]

MECHANISM: It is proposed that lithium carbonate and iodide preparations may have synergistic hypothyroid activity.

CLINICAL SIGNIFICANCE: Several patients have been described in whom potassium iodide appeared to act synergistically with lithium carbonate in producing hypothyroidism.[26,95,141,143]

LITHIUM CARBONATE INTERACTIONS (CONT.)

DRUGS	DISCUSSION

MANAGEMENT: It has been suggested that lithium carbonate and potassium iodide should not be used together. If concomitant use is employed, the practitioner certainly should be alert for signs of hypothyroidism.

Sodium Bicarbonate[28]

MECHANISM: Sodium bicarbonate appears to increase the renal excretion of lithium. This may be partly due to the sodium content of the sodium bicarbonate (see section on Sodium Chloride below).

CLINICAL SIGNIFICANCE: Not established. It is possible that the increased lithium excretion could impair the therapeutic response to lithium carbonate.

MANAGEMENT: Patients on combined therapy should be monitored for decreased lithium effect. Lithium blood levels may be helpful in this regard.

Sodium Chloride[12,57,81,96,115]

MECHANISM: The excretion of lithium appears to be proportional to the intake of sodium chloride.

CLINICAL SIGNIFICANCE: Patients on salt-restricted diets who receive lithium carbonate are prone to the development of lithium toxicity. Increasing sodium intake has been associated with reduced therapeutic response to lithium as well as a decrease in side effects.[115] Large doses of sodium chloride increase lithium excretion and have been recommended by some for the treatment of lithium intoxication.

MANAGEMENT: Extremely large or small sodium chloride intake should be avoided in patients receiving lithium carbonate. Patients on severe salt-restricted diets should probably not be given lithium carbonate.

Theophylline[28,260]

MECHANISM: Aminophylline appears to increase the renal excretion of lithium in single dose studies.

CLINICAL SIGNIFICANCE: Not established. Single dose studies in normal subjects indicate that aminophylline may enhance the renal excretion of lithium.[28] Also, theophylline therapy was associated with decreased serum lithium levels and a worsening of manic symptoms in one patient.[260] More study is needed to determine the incidence and magnitude of this interaction.

MANAGEMENT: One should be alert for evidence of reduced lithium response in the presence of theophylline therapy.

LITHIUM CARBONATE INTERACTIONS (CONT.)

DRUGS	DISCUSSION

Urea (Ureaphil)[28]

MECHANISM: Urea appears to increase the renal excretion of lithium in single dose studies.

CLINICAL SIGNIFICANCE: Single dose studies in normal subjects indicate that urea may enhance the renal excretion of lithium.[28] However, the clinical significance of this finding is not clear.

MANAGEMENT: Although clinical documentation is scanty, one should be alert for evidence of reduced lithium response in the presence of urea therapy.

METAPROTERENOL (ALUPENT) INTERACTIONS

DRUGS	DISCUSSION

Food[150]

MECHANISM: None known.

CLINICAL SIGNIFICANCE: Presence of food in the stomach has been shown to have very little effect on the bronchodilating activity of metaproterenol as judged by spirometric tests in a study of eight asthmatic adolescents given the drug in either the fasting or nonfasting state.[150]

MANAGEMENT: None required.

METHOCARBAMOL (ROBAXIN) INTERACTIONS

DRUGS	DISCUSSION

Pyridostigmine Bromide (Mestinon)[58]

MECHANISM: Not established.

CLINICAL SIGNIFICANCE: A single case has been reported in which methocarbamol may have impaired the therapeutic effect of pyridostigmine bromide in a patient with myasthenia gravis.

MANAGEMENT: Pending availability of further information, methocarbamol should be used with caution in myasthenic patients receiving pyridostigmine bromide.

METHOTRIMEPRAZINE (LEVOPROME) INTERACTIONS

DRUGS	DISCUSSION

Central Nervous System (CNS) Depressants[29]

MECHANISM: Methotrimeprazine is a CNS depressant and may potentiate the effect of other CNS depressants.

METHOTRIMEPRAZINE (LEVOPROME) INTERACTIONS (CONT.)

DRUGS	DISCUSSION

CLINICAL SIGNIFICANCE: The CNS depressant effects of thiopental, morphine, and anesthetic gases have been shown clinically to be enhanced by the concomitant use of methotrimeprazine. It is likely that other drugs that depress the CNS would be similarly affected.

MANAGEMENT: CNS depressants should be used with caution in conjunction with methotrimeprazine. The possibility that dosage of the CNS depressant may require reduction should be kept in mind.

Skeletal Muscle Relaxants (Surgical)[29]

MECHANISM: Not established.

CLINICAL SIGNIFICANCE: Methotrimeprazine has reportedly been shown clinically to prolong curare-induced muscle relaxation. The possibility of undesirable side effects from concomitant use of succinylcholine and methotrimeprazine has also been mentioned.

MANAGEMENT: Pending availability of further information, skeletal muscle relaxants should be used with added caution in patients receiving methotrimeprazine.

MINERAL OIL INTERACTIONS

DRUGS	DISCUSSION

Vitamin A[27]

MECHANISM: It has been proposed that mineral oil may impair the gastrointestinal absorption of vitamin A.

CLINICAL SIGNIFICANCE: Although many feel that vitamin A absorption is affected by mineral oil, a review of the literature by Cohen[27] failed to reveal evidence for such an effect.

MANAGEMENT: Although evidence for an interaction appears to be lacking, it may be wise to separate doses of vitamin A and mineral oil in order to minimize mixing in the gastrointestinal tract.

NAPROXEN (ANAPROX, NAPROSYN) INTERACTIONS

DRUGS	DISCUSSION

Probenecid (Benemid)[238]

MECHANISM: Probenecid may inhibit both the renal excretion and hepatic metabolism of naproxen.

CLINICAL SIGNIFICANCE: Six healthy subjects received naproxen (500 mg orally) with and without probenecid pretreatment.[238] Probenecid increased plasma naproxen levels by 50%. The degree to which this would increase naproxen toxicity and/or efficacy is not established.

NAPROXEN (ANAPROX, NAPROXYN) INTERACTIONS (CONT.)

DRUGS	DISCUSSION

MANAGEMENT: One should be aware that naproxen dosage requirements may be lower in patients receiving probenecid concurrently.

NARCOTIC ANALGESIC INTERACTIONS

DRUGS	DISCUSSION

Dexpanthenol (Ilopan)[64-67]

MECHANISM: Not established.

CLINICAL SIGNIFICANCE: The manufacturer of Ilopan indicates that its use with "antibiotics, narcotics and barbiturates" may result in "allergic reactions."[66] However, the observation that hundreds of patients were receiving these drugs and pantothenyl alcohol with no apparent ill effects[64] led to an inquiry to the manufacturer for information on the nature of the interaction. The response indicated that there is little evidence to support the existence of drug interaction.[67]

MANAGEMENT: Although the clinical significance of this interaction is questionable, physicians should realize that the product information contains the warning.

Neuromuscular Blocking Agents[72,73]

MECHANISM: The central respiratory depressant effect of narcotics adds to the neuromuscular blockade of muscle relaxants.

CLINICAL SIGNIFICANCE: Clinical impressions have indicated that atelectasis and increased degree of respiratory depression may occur with concomitant use of narcotic analgesics and neuromuscular blocking agents. This has been supported by pharmacologic studies in man.[72]

MANAGEMENT: Narcotic analgesics should be used with care in patients receiving skeletal muscle relaxants.

NEUROMUSCULAR BLOCKING AGENTS

DRUGS	DISCUSSION

Dexpanthenol (Ilopan)[65,66]

MECHANISM: See Clinical Significance.

CLINICAL SIGNIFICANCE: Dexpanthenol apparently prolonged the effects of succinylcholine in one patient.[66] However, a subsequent study of this purported interaction using six patients failed to detect any unusual respiratory embarrassment or muscle-twitch depression.[65]

MANAGEMENT: No special precautions appear to be necessary.

416

NEUROMUSCULAR BLOCKING AGENTS (CONT.)

Magnesium Salts[68-70,118]

MECHANISM: The magnesium ion possesses neuromuscular blocking activity itself, presumably by decreasing acetylcholine release from motor nerve terminals. This theoretically would result in at least additive, and perhaps potentiating effects with muscle relaxants such as succinylcholine, tubocurarine, and decamethonium.

CLINICAL SIGNIFICANCE: At least two case reports have appeared in which excessive neuromuscular blockade occurred in patients receiving magnesium sulfate and a neuromuscular blocking agent. A partially controlled study of patients who had cesarean section indicated that considerably less succinylcholine was required in those patients who were treated with magnesium sulfate. This effect was not seen in the small number of patients who received tubocurarine instead of succinylcholine. There is also clinical evidence that administration of magnesium sulfate may attenuate succinylcholine-induced hyperkalemia and muscle fasciculations.[118] More study is needed.

MANAGEMENT: Caution should be exercised in giving magnesium sulfate and other neuromuscular blocking agents concomitantly. Intravenous administration of calcium may partially ameliorate the excessive neuromuscular blockade that may occur.

Procaine[71]

MECHANISM: Not established. It has been proposed that procaine may displace succinylcholine from plasma protein binding. Also, procaine and succinylcholine are both metabolized by plasma pseudocholinesterase; large doses of procaine might competitively inhibit the metabolism of succinylcholine.

CLINICAL SIGNIFICANCE: Intravenous procaine has been shown to enhance the neuromuscular blocking action of succinylcholine. However, the doses of procaine required to produce a clinically significant effect were larger than those normally used in anesthetic practice.

MANAGEMENT: Some caution should be observed in the administration of large doses of procaine to patients receiving succinylcholine.

Thiamine[75]

MECHANISM: Not established.

CLINICAL SIGNIFICANCE: Sphire[75] states that thiamine may enhance the response to muscle relaxants, but substantiating information is not given.

MANAGEMENT: No special precautions appear necessary.

Trasylol[74,117]

MECHANISM: Not established.

NEUROMUSCULAR BLOCKING AGENTS (CONT.)

DRUGS	DISCUSSION

CLINICAL SIGNIFICANCE: Three cases have been reported in which apnea followed the use of trasylol in patients who had recently received muscle relaxants (e.g., succinylcholine, tubocurarine).[74] However, these findings were not supported in subsequent animal studies.[117]

MANAGEMENT: Until this purported interaction is better described, the concomitant use of trasylol and neuromuscular blocking agents should be undertaken with caution.

ORPHENADRINE (NORFLEX) INTERACTIONS

DRUGS	DISCUSSION

Propoxyphene (Darvon)[53,59–64]

MECHANISM: Not established. If the interaction exists, it may be due to an undefined combined effect on the central nervous system. Another possibility is the production of hypoglycemia. Hypoglycemic activity has been attributed to both propoxyphene[63] and orphenadrine.[53] It is interesting to note that the possible symptoms of this interaction are mental confusion, anxiety, and tremors, all of which may occur during a hypoglycemic episode. Another possibility is that propoxyphene impairs the hepatic metabolism of orphenadrine.

CLINICAL SIGNIFICANCE: Not established. Although the manufacturers of the drugs warn about this interaction,[59,60] communications with physicians from both companies indicate that evidence for an interaction is not impressive.[61,62] The warning is apparently based on a few reports of reactions to the manufacturer following the use of both drugs.[62] The author has observed two possible cases of this interaction, but in both cases other drugs were also being taken. There is little doubt that many patients have received these two drugs concomitantly with no apparent adverse effects, and it may be that if the interaction occurs it is only in an occasional predisposed patient.

MANAGEMENT: Although there is relatively little clinical information to support the existence of interaction, physicians should be aware of the possibility of an interaction.

PENTAZOCINE (TALWIN) INTERACTIONS

DRUGS	DISCUSSION

Smoking[220,221]

MECHANISM: Smoking may enhance the hepatic metabolism of pentazocine.

CLINICAL SIGNIFICANCE: Smokers required larger doses of pentazocine than nonsmokers when pentazocine was used as a supplement for nitrous oxide anasthesia in 41 patients.[220] Another study in 70 healthy

PENTAZOCINE (TALWIN) INTERACTIONS (CONT.)

DRUGS	DISCUSSION

subjects showed that smokers metabolized 40% more pentazocine than nonsmokers as measured by cumulative urinary pentazocine excretion.[221] These results are consistent with a smoking-induced increase in the hepatic metabolism of pentazocine.

MANAGEMENT: A larger dose of pentazocine may be required by smokers than nonsmokers to obtain an equivalent analgesic response.

PHENACETIN INTERACTIONS

DRUGS	DISCUSSION

Food[152]

MECHANISM: It appears that charcoal-broiled beef stimulates the metabolism of phenacetin.[152]

CLINICAL SIGNIFICANCE: In a study of nine normal volunteers it has been shown that a diet that contains charcoal-broiled beef lowered plasma phenacetin levels but had little effect on plasma levels of phenacetin's major metabolite.[152] These results indicate that charcoal-broiled beef decreases the bioavailability of phenacetin by enhancing metabolism in the gastrointestinal tract and/or by enhancing metabolism in the first pass through the liver.

MANAGEMENT: None required.

PROBENECID (BENEMID) INTERACTIONS

DRUGS	DISCUSSION

Sulfinpyrazone (Anturane)[79]

MECHANISM: Probenecid markedly inhibits the renal tubular secretion of sulfinpyrazone and its major metabolite.

CLINICAL SIGNIFICANCE: Not established. In this study, no additive uricosuric activity was noted. The possibility of increased toxicity needs further study.

MANAGEMENT: No special precautions appear necessary at this point.

PROPOXYPHENE (DARVON) INTERACTIONS

DRUGS	DISCUSSION

Food[162]

MECHANISM: The delay in absorption has been attributed to slower gastric emptying and/or the physical barrier produced by the food mass.[162]

CLINICAL SIGNIFICANCE: The effect of meal composition on the absorption of propoxyphene has been studied in six healthy volunteers.[162]

PROPOXYPHENE (DARVON) INTERACTIONS (CONT.)

DRUGS	DISCUSSION

On an empty stomach, peak plasma levels occurred at about 2 hours, while both high carbohydrate and high fat meals delayed peak times to about 3 hours and high protein to about 4 hours. Although the absorption rate of the drug was decreased by food, high carbohydrate and high protein meals slightly increased the overall bioavailability of propoxyphene.

MANAGEMENT: If rapid analgesia is required, it would be preferable to take propoxyphene on an empty stomach.

Smoking[261,262]

MECHANISM: Smoking may enhance the hepatic metabolism of propoxyphene.

CLINICAL SIGNIFICANCE: In an epidemiologic study of the efficacy of propoxyphene, the drug was rated ineffective in 20% of heavy smokers (> 20 cigarettes/day), 15% of light smokers (20 cigarettes/day or less), and 10% of nonsmokers.[262] These results are consistent with a smoking-induced reduction in propoxyphene effect, but confirmation is needed.

MANAGEMENT: One should be alert for evidence of inadequate propoxyphene analgesia in smokers (especially heavy smokers); selection of an alternative analgesic may be appropriate in such patients.

PROPYLTHIOURACIL INTERACTIONS

DRUGS	DISCUSSION

Food[125]

MECHANISM: Not established.

CLINICAL SIGNIFICANCE: A study involving eight healthy volunteers demonstrated that the degree of propylthiouracil absorption is subject to considerable interindividual variation in either the fasted or nonfasted state. In some individuals food appeared to enhance absorption of propylthiouracil while in others food appeared to decrease absorption.[125]

MANAGEMENT: The marked patient variation precludes making a general recommendation concerning the method of administration of propylthiouracil with respect to meals. However, food should be considered a potential cause of altered propylthiouracil response.

PSEUDOEPHEDRINE (SUDAFED) INTERACTIONS

DRUGS	DISCUSSION

Sodium Bicarbonate[140]

MECHANISM: Alkalinization of the urine with sodium bicarbonate results in less ionization of pseudoephedrine, thus increasing its renal tubular reabsorption and reducing its urinary excretion.

PSEUDOEPHEDRINE (SUDAFED) INTERACTIONS (CONT.)

DRUGS	DISCUSSION

CLINICAL SIGNIFICANCE: Studies in three normal subjects given a single dose of pseudoephedrine (180 mg) showed that alkalinization of the urine with sodium bicarbonate approximately doubled the half-life of pseudoephedrine.[140]

MANAGEMENT: No special precautions appear necessary, but one should be aware that alkalinization of the urine may prolong the effect of pseudoephedrine.

RANITIDINE (ZANTAC) INTERACTIONS

DRUGS	DISCUSSION

Theophylline[291-295]

MECHANISM: None.

CLINICAL SIGNIFICANCE: Although ranitidine was thought to have increased plasma theophylline levels in one case,[291] subsequent analysis of the case shed doubt on ranitidine as a cause.[292] Further, three clinical studies in healthy subjects failed to find an effect of ranitidine on theophylline disposition.[293-295]

MANAGEMENT: No special precautions appear necessary.

THEOPHYLLINE INTERACTIONS

DRUGS	DISCUSSION

Carbamazepine (Tegratol)[243]

MECHANISM: Carbamazepine probably stimulates the hepatic metabolism of theophylline.

CLINICAL SIGNIFICANCE: In a 11-year-old girl maintained on theophylline, the administration of carbamazepine was associated with subtherapeutic theophylline levels and worsening of asthma symptoms.[243] Also, the theophylline half-life was about 3 hours while she was receiving carbamazepine, and about 6 hours when she was not receiving carbamazepine. These findings are consistent with the known ability of carbamazepine to produce enzyme induction, and the known susceptibility of theophylline to enzyme induction. However, further studies will be needed to determine the incidence and magnitude of this interaction.

MANAGEMENT: One should be alert for evidence of altered theophylline serum levels if carbamazepine is initiated or discontinued.

Food[124,151,158]

MECHANISM: Not established. It is proposed that high protein diets enhance the hepatic biotransformation of theophylline, while high carbohydrate diets reduce theophylline biotransformation.[151]

DRUGS	DISCUSSION

CLINICAL SIGNIFICANCE: Studies in normal volunteers indicate that low carbohydrate-high protein diets decrease the plasma half-life of theophylline about 35% to 40% when compared to the half-life obtained on the volunteers' usual home diet.[124,151] Supplementing standard diets with protein decreased the plasma half-life, whereas supplementing standard diets with carbohydrate increased the plasma half-life.[151] In another study involving six healthy male volunteers it was noted that absorption of theophylline from a solid dosage form was faster after a high protein meal than after a high fat or high carbohydrate meal.[158] However, the difference in serum theophylline levels was significant only during the first 2 hours after dosing, and total absorption of theophylline was only minimally affected.

MANAGEMENT: Patients receiving theophylline should be warned against making major changes in their protein or carbohydrate intake without informing their physician.

Smoking[222-226]

MECHANISM: Smoking stimulates the hepatic metabolism of theophylline.

CLINICAL SIGNIFICANCE: Numerous studies have shown that the elimination of theophylline is considerably more rapid in smokers than in nonsmokers.[222,223] Smoking shortens theophylline half-life, increases total body theophylline clearance, and reduces theophylline serum levels. Adverse reactions to theophylline tend to occur less frequently in smokers than in nonsmokers,[224] which is consistent with smoking-induced reductions in serum theophylline. The smoking-induced increase in theophylline elimination tends to dissipate somewhat when patients stop smoking, but this occurs slowly over a period of months.[225,226]

MANAGEMENT: Smokers require larger maintenance doses of theophylline than nonsmokers in order to achieve adequate serum theophylline levels.

Vidarabine (Vira-A)[210,211]

MECHANISM: Not established. It has been proposed that vidarabine inhibits the metabolism of theophylline.

CLINICAL SIGNIFICANCE: A woman with a history of congestive heart failure and chronic obstructive pulmonary disease developed increased serum theophylline concentrations 4 days after beginning therapy with vidarabine (Vira-A) for diffuse cutaneous herpes zoster.[210] The half-life of theophylline appeared to be prolonged in the presence of vidarabine. The authors ruled out several other obvious causes of altered theophylline disposition, but the patient was acutely ill and received theophylline in varying doses, routes, and formulations during her hospital stay. Also, in view of reports of possible inhibition of theophylline metabolism by various viral infections,[211] one

THEOPHYLLINE INTERACTIONS (CONT.)

DRUGS	DISCUSSION

wonders if the diffuse herpes zoster infection may have affected theophylline metabolism in this case. More study is needed to determine whether this purported interaction is real.

MANAGEMENT: Until more data are available, one should be alert for evidence of altered theophylline serum levels if vidarabine is used concurrently.

ZINC INTERACTIONS

DRUGS	DISCUSSION

Food[153-157]

MECHANISM: In-vitro experiments indicate zinc is precipitated by phosphate and phytate at pH values approximating the pH values of the intestinal lumen.[153] The high phosphorous and calcium content of dairy products and the high phytate content of brown bread may contribute to inhibition of zinc absorption.[153]

CLINICAL SIGNIFICANCE: A study which involved healthy volunteers demonstrated zinc absorption was reduced as much as 50% when taken with coffee.[153] In this same study it was shown that brown bread and dairy products, specifically milk and cheese, decreased zinc absorption. This may be of clinical significance since milk is many times prescribed with zinc to reduce gastrointestinal irritation.[153] In a group of healthy young volunteers the absorption of zinc when administered with a meal or even 45 minutes after a meal was markedly reduced when compared with the fasted state.[155]

MANAGEMENT: If zinc is to be administered with food to give better patient tolerance, consideration should be given to avoid foods high in calcium, phosphorous, and/or phytate content.

VERAPAMIL INTERACTIONS

DRUGS	DISCUSSION

Digitalis glycosides[318-323]

MECHANISM: Verapamil appears to inhibit the renal excretion of digoxin, but other mechanisms may also be involved (e.g., reduced, nonrenal digoxin elimination). Verapamil and digitalis glycosides may also have additive pharmacodynamic effects such as inhibition of atrioventricular conduction.

CLINICAL SIGNIFICANCE: Numerous studies have shown that verapamil increases serum digoxin concentration by an average of about 70%.[318-322] The increase has been shown in both patients and healthy subjects, and with both chronic and single doses of the drugs. The interaction appears to be dose-related; verapamil doses of 240 mg/day produce larger increases in serum digoxin than doses of 160 mg/

VERAPAMIL INTERACTIONS (CONT.)

DRUGS	DISCUSSION

day.[322] In one patient on chronic digoxin, the administration of verapamil (5 mg by slow intravenous injection) resulted in asystole.[323] It was proposed that the asystole was a result of the combined effects of verapamil and digoxin on atrioventricular conduction.

MANAGEMENT: One should be alert for evidence of increased serum digoxin concentration in the presence of verapamil therapy. Also, one should monitor for additive pharmacodynamic effects (e.g., slowed atrioventricular conduction), especially if the verapamil is given intravenously.

References

1. WODAK J, et al: Review of 12 months' treatment with L-DOPA in Parkinson's disease, with remarks on unusual side effects. Med J Aust 2:1277, 1972.
2. STEVENSON JH, et al: Changes in human drug metabolism after long-term exposure to hypnotics. Br Med J 4:322, 1972.
3. LUCAROTTI RL, et al: Enhanced pseudoephedrine absorption by concurrent administration of aluminum hydroxide gel in humans. J Pharm Sci 61:903, 1972.
4. FERMAGLICH J, O'DOHERTY DS: Effect of gastric motility on levodopa. Dis Nerv Syst 33:624, 1972.
5. HUNTER KR, et al: Use of levodopa with other drugs. Lancet 2:1283, 1970.
6. NIMMO J, et al: Pharmacological modification of gastric emptying: effects of propantheline and metoclopramide on Paracetamol absorption. Br Med J 1:587, 1973.
7. NIMMO J: The influence of metoclopramide on drug absorption. Postgrad Med J (July Supplement) 49:25, 1973.
8. ELION GB, et al: Renal clearance of oxipurinol, the chief metabolite of allopurinol. Am J Med 45:69, 1968.
9. ANGGARD E, et al: Amphetamine metabolism in amphetamine psychosis. Clin Pharmacol Ther 14:870, 1973.
10. SINGH MM, SMITH JM: Reversal of some therapeutic effects of an antipsychotic agent by an antiparkinsonism drug. J Nerv Ment Dis 157:50, 1973.
11. FAHN S: "On-off" phenomenon with levodopa therapy in parkinsonism. Neurology 24:431, 1974.
12. HURTIG HI, DYSON WL: Lithium toxicity enhanced by diuresis (Letter). N Engl J Med 290:748, 1974.
13. GRACE ND, et al: Effect of allopurinol on iron mobilization. Gastroenterology 59:103, 1970.
14. TJANDRAMAGA TB, CUCINELL SA: Interaction of probenecid and allopurinol in gouty subjects (Abstract). Fed Proc 30:392, 1971.
15. RIVERA-CALIMLIM L, et al: L-DOPA absorption and metabolism by the human stomach (Abstract 379). Pharmacologist 12:269, 1970.
16. DUJOVNE CA, et al: The stomach as an important factor in the metabolism and effectiveness of L-DOPA in parkinsonian patients (Abstract). Gastroenterology 58:1039, 1970.

References (CONT.)

17. RIVERA-CALIMLIM L, et al: L-DOPA absorption and metabolism by the human stomach (Abstract). J Clin Invest 49:79a, 1970.
18. RIVERA-CALIMLIM L, et al: L-DOPA treatment failure: explanation and correction. Br Med J 4:93, 1970.
19. MONE JG, MATHIE WE: Qualitative and quantitative defects of pseudocholinesterase activity. Anaesthesia 22:55, 1967.
20. WEINBERGER M, BRONSKY E: Interaction of ephedrine and theophylline (Abstract). Clin Pharmacol Ther 15:223, 1974.
21. GENTON E: Guidelines for heparin therapy. Ann Intern Med 80:77, 1974.
22. MADDOCKS AC: Indomethacin and vaccination (Letter). Lancet 2:210, 1973.
23. BIANCHINE JR, et al: Levodopa and pyridoxine co-administration: differential metabolic effect in parkinsonian and normal subjects (Abstract). Ann Intern Med 78:830, 1973.
24. CARTER AB: Pyridoxine and parkinsonism (Letter). Br Med J 4:236, 1973.
25. MARS H: Levodopa, carbidopa, and pyridoxine in parkinson disease. Metabolic interactions. Arch Neurol 30:444, 1974.
26. SHOPSIN B, et al: Iodine and lithium-induced hypothyroidism. Documentation of synergism. Am J Med 55:695, 1973.
27. COHEN H: Mineral oil, vitamin A, and carotene. Genesis and correction of a common misconception. J Med Soc NJ 67:111, 1970.
28. THOMSEN K, SCHOU M: Renal lithium excretion in man. Am J Physiol 215:823, 1968.
29. Levoprome®. Product information. Wayne, New Jersey, Lederle Laboratories, 1966.
30. Zyloprim®. Product Information. Research Triangle Park, North Carolina, Burroughs Wellcome & Co., 1978.
31. ANON: Haloperidol. Med Let 9:70, 1967.
32. GOODMAN LS, GILMAN A (Eds): The Pharmacological Basis of Therapeutics. 5th Ed. New York, Macmillan, 1975, pp. 166–167.
33. KLAWANS HL, Jr: The pharmacology of parkinsonism. A review. Dis Nerv Syst 29:805, 1968.
34. ROWLAND M: Amphetamine blood and urine levels in man. J Pharm Sci 58:508, 1969.
35. MILNE MD: Influence of acid-base balance on efficacy and toxicity of drugs. Proc R Soc Med 58:961, 1965.
36. Ilopan®. Product Information. Adria Laboratories, Dublin, Ohio, 1984.
37. WORTON AG: Personal communication, 1968.
38. GALLO DG, et al: The interaction between cholestyramine and drugs. Proc Soc Exp Biol Med 120:60, 1965.
39. Questran®. Product Information. Evansville, Indiana, Mead Johnson Laboratories, 1973.
40. GOODMAN LS, GILMAN A (Eds): The Pharmacological Basis of Therapeutics. 5th Ed. New York, Macmillan, 1975, pp. 131–132.
41. HADDEN JW, METZNER RJ: Pseudoketosis and hyperacetaldehydemia in paraldehyde acidosis. Am J Med 47:642, 1969.
42. FELDMAN SA, CRAWLEY BE: Interaction of diazepam with the muscle-relaxant drugs. Br Med J 2:336, 1970.
43. DOUGHTY A: Unexpected danger of diazepam (Letter). Br Med J 2:239, 1970.

References (CONT.)

44. Cavallaro RJ, et al: Effect of ecothiophate therapy on metabolism of succinylcholine in man. Anesth Analg 47:570, 1968.
45. Kinyon GE: Anticholinesterase eye drops—need for caution (Letter). N Engl J Med 280:53, 1969.
46. Lipson ML, et al: Oral administration of pralidoxime chloride in echothiophate iodide therapy. Arch Ophthal 82:830, 1969.
47. Cohen PJ, et al: A simple test for abnormal pseudocholinesterase. Anesthesiology 32:281, 1970.
48. Zsigmond EK, Eilderton TE: Abnormal reaction to procaine and succinylcholine in a patient with inherited atypical plasma cholinesterase. Case report. Can Anaesth Soc J 15:498, 1968.
49. Azarnoff DL, Hurwitz A: Drug interactions. Pharmacol Physicians 4:1 (Feb.), 1970.
50. Skeith MD, et al: The renal excretion of indomethacin and its inhibition by probenecid. Clin Pharmacol Ther 9:89, 1968.
51. Hall GJL, Davis AE: Inhibition of iron absorption by magnesium trisilicate. Med J Aust 2:95, 1969.
52. Melhorn DK, Gross S: Relationships between iron-dextran and vitamin E in an iron deficiency anemia in children. J Lab Clin Med 74:789, 1969.
53. Buckle RM, Guillebaud J: Hypoglycaemic coma occurring during treatment with chlorpromazine and orphenadrine. Br Med J 4:599, 1967.
54. Godwin-Austen RB, et al: Mydriatic responses to sympathomimetic amines in patients treated with L-DOPA. Lancet 2:1043, 1969.
55. Duvoisin RC, et al: Pyridoxine reversal of L-DOPA effects in parkinsonism. Trans Am Neurol Assoc 94:81, 1969.
56. Cotzias GC: Metabolic modification of some neurologic disorders. JAMA 210:1255, 1969.
57. Platman SR, Fieve RR: Lithium retention and excretion. The effect of sodium and fluid intake. Arch Gen Psychiatry 20:285, 1969.
58. Podrizki A: Methocarbamol and myasthenia gravis. JAMA 205:938, 1968.
59. Norflex®. Product Information. Northridge, California, Riker Laboratories, 1984.
60. Darvon®. Product Information. Indianapolis, Indiana, Eli Lilly and Co., 1978.
61. Maxwell SB: Personal communication, March 31, 1970.
62. Silverglade A: Personal communication. April 10, 1970.
63. Wiederholt IC, et al: Recurrent episodes of hypoglycemia induced by propoxyphene. Neurology 17:703, 1967.
64. Hansten PD: Personal observations, 1968–1969.
65. Smith RM, et al: Succinylcholine-pantothenyl alcohol: a reappraisal. Anesth Analg 48:205, 1969.
66. Ilopan®. Product Information. Dublin, Ohio, Adria Laboratories, 1984.
67. Worton AG: Personal communication, December 12, 1968.
68. Ghoneim MM, Long JP: The interaction between magnesium and other neuromuscular blocking agents. Anesthesiology 32:23, 1970.
69. Giesecke AH Jr, et al: Of magnesium, muscle relaxants, toxemic parturients, and cats. Anesth Analg 47:689, 1968.
70. Morris R, Giesecke AH Jr: Potentiation of muscle relaxants by mag-

References (CONT.)

nesium sulfate therapy in toxemia of pregnancy. South Med J 61:25, 1968.

71. USUBIAGA JE, et al: Interaction of intravenously administered procaine, lidocaine, and succinylcholine in anesthetized subjects. Anesth Analg 46:39, 1967.

72. BELLVILLE JW, et al: The interaction of morphine and D-tubocurarine on respiration and grip strength in man. Clin Pharmacol Ther 5:35, 1964.

73. Tubocurarine Chloride Injection. Product Information. Abbott Laboratories, 1969.

74. CHASAPAKIS G, DIMAS C: Possible interaction between muscle relaxants and the kallikrein-trypsin inactivator "Trasylol." Br J Anaesth 38:838, 1966.

75. SPHIRE RD: Gallamine: a second look. Anesth Analg 43:690, 1964.

76. GOODWIN CS, SPARELL G: Inhibition of dapsone excretion by probenecid. Lancet 2:884, 1969.

77. SCHROEDER ET: Alkalosis resulting from combined administration of a "nonsystemic" antacid and a cation-exchange resin. Gastroenterology 56:868, 1969.

78. VIEWEG WVR, et al: Complications of intravenous administration of heparin in elderly women. JAMA 213:1303, 1970.

79. PEREL JM, et al: Studies of interactions among drugs in man at the renal level: probenecid and sulfinpyrazone. Clin Pharmacol Ther 10:834, 1969.

80. DIETZE F, BRUSCHKE G: Inhibition of iron absorption by pancreatic extracts (Letter). Lancet 1:424, 1970.

81. BLEIWEISS H: Salt supplements with lithium (Letter). Lancet 1:416, 1970.

82. THOMAS FB, et al: Inhibition of the intestinal absorption of inorganic and hemoglobin iron by cholestyramine. J Lab Clin Med 78:70, 1971.

83. DRETCHEN K, et al: The interaction of diazepam with myoneural blocking agents. Anesthesiology 34:463, 1971.

84. WEBB SN, BRADSHAW EG: Diazepam and neuromuscular blocking drugs (Letter). Br Med J 3:640, 1971.

85. FERNANDEZ PC, KOVNAT PJ: Metabolic acidosis reversed by the combination of magnesium hydroxide and a cation exchange resin. N Engl J Med 286:23, 1972.

86. LEON AS, et al: Pyridoxine antagonism of levodopa in Parkinsonism. JAMA 218:1924, 1971.

87. PAPAVASILIOU PS, et al: Levodopa in Parkinsonism: potentiation of central effects with a peripheral inhibitor. N Engl J Med 286:8, 1972.

88. COTZIAS GC, PAPAVASILIOU PS: Blocking the negative effects of pyridoxine on patients receiving levodopa (Letter). JAMA 215:1504, 1971.

89. EMORI W, et al: The pharmacokinetics of indomethacin in serum (Abstract). Clin Pharmacol Ther 14:134, 1973.

90. FLEMENBAUM A: Does lithium block the effects of amphetamine? A report of three cases. Am J Psychiatry 131:820, 1974.

91. ANGRIST B, et al: The antagonism of amphetamine-induced symptomatology by a neuroleptic. Am J Psychiatry 131:817, 1974.

92. LEON A, et al: The effect of antacid administration on the absorption and metabolism of levodopa. J Clin Pharmacol 12:263, 1972.

93. ZIESSMAN HA: Alkalosis and seizure due to a cation-exchange resin and magnesium hydroxide. South Med J 69:497, 1976.

References (CONT.)

94. MIMS RB, et al: Inhibition of L-dopa-induced growth hormone stimulation by pyridoxine and chlorpromazine. J Clin Endocrinol Metab 40:256, 1975.
95. SWEDBERG K, et al: Heart failure as complication of lithium treatment. Acta Med Scand 196:279, 1974.
96. LEVY ST, et al: Lithium-induced diabetes insipidus: manic symptoms, brain and electrolyte correlates, and chlorothiazide treatment. Am J Psychiatry 130:1014, 1973.
97. HANSSON O, SILLANPAA M: Pyridoxine and serum concentrations of phenytoin and phenobarbitone (Letter). Lancet 1:256, 1976.
98. VAN KAMMEN DP, MURPHY D: Attenuation of the euphoriant and activating effects of d- and l-amphetamine by lithium carbonate treatment. Psychopharmacologia 44:215, 1975.
99. GREENBLATT DJ, et al: Influence of magnesium and aluminum hydroxide mixture on chlordiazepoxide absorption. Clin Pharmacol Ther 19:234, 1976.
100. MENA I, COTZIAS GC: Protein treatment of Parkinson's disease with levodopa. N Engl J Med 292:181, 1975.
101. COHEN WJ, COHEN NH: Lithium carbonate, haloperidol and irreversible brain damage. JAMA 230:1283, 1974.
102. WEINBERGER M, et al: Interaction of ephedrine and theophylline. Clin Pharmacol Ther 17:586, 1975.
103. BIERMAN CW, et al: Exercise-induced asthma. Pharmacological assessment of single drugs and drug combinations. JAMA 234:295, 1975.
104. CHURCHILL D, et al: Toxic nephropathy after low-dose methoxyfluane anesthesia: drug interaction with secobarbital? Can Med Assoc J 114:326, 1976.
105. VESTAL RE, et al: Antipyrine metabolism in man: Influence of age, alcohol, caffeine, and smoking. Clin Pharmacol Ther 18:425, 1975.
106. ALGERI S, et al: Effect of anticholinergic drugs on gastrointestinal absorption of L-dopa in rats and man. Eur J Pharmacol 35:293, 1976.
107. SEGRE EJ, et al: Effects of antacids on naproxen absorption (Letter). N Engl J Med 291:582, 1974.
108. BASELT RC, CASARETT LJ: Urinary excretion of methadone in man. Clin Pharmacol Ther 13:64, 1972.
109. OLESEN OV: The influence of disulfiram and calcium carbimide on the serum diphenylhydantoin. Arch Neurol 16:642, 1967.
110. LUDIN HP, DUBACH K: Action of diazepam on muscular contraction in man. Z Neurol 199:30, 1971.
111. GREENBLATT DJ, et al: Clinical importance of the interaction of diazepam and cimetidine. N Engl J Med 310:1639, 1984.
112. D'ENCARNACAO PS, ANDERSON K: Effects of lithium pretreatment on amphetamine and DMI tetrabenazine produced psychomotor behavior. Dis Nerv Syst 31:494, 1970.
113. ALVARES AP, KAPPAS A: Influence of phenobarbital on the metabolism and analgesic effect of methadone in rats. J Lab Clin Med 79:439, 1972.
114. KAMPFFMEYER HG: Elimination of phenacetin and phenazone by man before and after treatment with phenobarbital. Eur J Clin Pharmacol 3:113, 1971.
115. DEMERS RG, HENINGER GR: Sodium intake and lithium treatment in mania. Am J Psychiatry 128:1, 1971.

References (CONT.)

116. WHITTAKER JA, EVANS DA: Genetic control of phenylbutazone metabolism in man. Br Med J 4:323, 1970.

117. AMBRUS JL, et al: Effect of the protease inhibitor trasylol on cholinesterase levels and on susceptibility to succinylcholine. Res Commun Chem Pathol Pharmacol 1:141, 1970.

118. ALDRETE JA, et al: Prevention of succinylcholine-induced hyperkalaemia by magnesium sulfate. Can Anaesth Soc J 17:477, 1970.

119. EMORI HW, et al: Indomethacin serum concentrations in man. Effects of dosage, food, and antacid. Ann Rheum Dis 35:333, 1976.

120. GEISLER A, KLYSNER R: Combined effect of lithium and flupenthixol on striatal adenylate cyclase. Lancet 1:430, 1977.

121. LOUDEN JB, WARING H: Toxic reactions to lithium and haloperidol. Lancet 2:1088, 1976.

122. BAASTRUP P, et al: Adverse reactions in treatment with lithium carbonate and haloperidol. JAMA 236:2645, 1976.

123. TINKELMAN DG, AVNER SE: Ephedrine therapy in asthmatic children. JAMA 237:553, 1977.

124. ALVARES AP, et al: Interactions between nutritional factors and drug biotransformations in man. Proc Nat Acad Sci 73:2501, 1976.

125. MELANDER A, et al: Bioavailability of propylthiouracil: interindividual variation and influence of food intake. Acta Med Scand 201:41, 1977.

126. LYLE WH: Penicillamine and iron (Letter). Lancet 2:420, 1976.

127. VESELL ES, PAGE JG: Genetic control of the phenobarbital-induced shortening of plasma antipyrine half-lives in man. J. Clin Invest 48:2202, 1969.

128. STAMBAUGH JE, et al: A potentially toxic drug interaction between pethidine (meperidine) and phenobarbitone. Lancet 1:398, 1977.

129. FANN WE, et al: Effects of lithium on adrenergic function in man. Clin Pharmacol Ther 13:71, 1973.

130. KOTHARY SP, et al: Plasma cholinesterase activity in relation to the safe use of succinylcholine in myasthenic patients on chronic anticholinesterase treatment (Abstract). Clin Pharmacol Ther 21:108, 1977.

131. GARNHAM JC, et al: Different effects of sodium bicarbonate and aluminum hydroxide on absorption of indomethacin in man. Postgrad Med J 53:126, 1977.

132. NAYLOR GJ, MCHARG A: Profound hypothermia on combined lithium carbonate and diazepam treatment. Br Med J 3:22, 1977.

133. BELLWARD GD, et al: Methadone maintenance: effect of urinary pH on renal clearance in chronic high and low doses. Clin Pharmacol Ther 22:92, 1977.

134. HILDICK-SMITH M: Pyridoxine in parkinsonism (Letter). Lancet 2:1029, 1973.

135. JONES CJ: Pyridoxine in parkinsonism (Letter). Lancet 2:1030, 1973.

136. STITT FW, et al: A clinical study of naproxen-diazepam drug interaction on tests of mood and attention. Curr Ther Res 21:149, 1977.

137. HILL GE, et al: Lithium carbonate and neuromuscular blocking agents. Anesthesiology 46:122, 1977.

138. BELLVILLE JW, et al: The hypnotic effects of codeine and secobarbital and their interaction in man. Clin Pharmacol Ther 12:607, 1971.

139. CAVANAUGH JH, et al: Effect of amphetamine on the pressor response to tyramine: formation of p-hydroxynorephedrine from amphetamine in man. Clin Pharmacol Ther 11:656, 1970.

References (CONT.)

140. KUNTZMAN RG, et al: The influence of urinary pH on the plasma half-life of pseudoephedrine in man and dog and a sensitive assay for its determination in human plasma. Clin Pharmacol Ther 12:62, 1971.
141. WIENER JD: Lithium carbonate-induced myxedema (Letter). JAMA 220:587, 1972.
142. YAHR MD, DUVOISIN RC: Pyridoxine and levodopa in the treatment of parkinsonism (Letter). JAMA 220:861, 1972.
143. JORGENSEN JV, et al: Possible synergism between iodine and lithium carbonate (Letter). JAMA 223:192, 1973.
144. JENKINS R, LAMID S: Gastric acidity and levodopa in parkinsonism (Letter). JAMA 223:81, 1973.
145. MORGAN JP, et al: Metabolism of levodopa in patients with Parkinson's disease. Arch Neurol 25:39, 1971.
146. GILLESPIE NG, et al: Diets affecting treatment of parkinsonism with levodopa. J Am Diet Assoc 62:525, 1973.
147. LINNOILA M, et al: Effect of food and repeated injections on serum diazepam levels. Acta Pharmacol Toxicol 36:181, 1975.
148. KORTTILA K, et al: Prolonged recovery after sedation: the influence of food, charcoal ingestion and injection rate on the effects of intravenous diazepam. Br J Anaesth 48:333, 1976.
149. KLOTZ U, et al: Food intake and plasma binding of diazepam (Letter). Br J Clin Pharmacol 4:85, 1977.
150. HOWARD LA, COLEMAN M: The effect of food or previous medication upon the action of an oral bronchodilator. J Asthma Res 8:197, 1971.
151. KAPPAS A, et al: Influence of dietary protein and carbohydrate on antipyrine and theophylline metabolism in man. Clin Pharmacol Ther 20:643, 1976.
152. CONNEY AH, et al: Enhanced phenacetin metabolism in human subjects fed charcoal-broiled beef. Clin Pharmacol Ther 20:633, 1976.
153. PECOUD A: Effect of foodstuffs on the absorption of zinc sulfate. Clin Pharmacol Ther 17:469, 1975.
154. ABDULLA M: Effect of food on zinc absorption (Letter). Lancet 1:217, 1974.
155. SCHELLING JL: Effect of food on zinc absorption (Letter). Lancet 2:968, 1973.
156. RHEINHOLD JG: Effects of purified phytate and phytate-rich bread upon metabolism of zinc, calcium, phosphorous, and nitrogen in man. Lancet 1:283, 1973.
157. ODELL BL: Effect of dietary components upon zinc availability. Am J Clin Nutr 22:1315, 1969.
158. WELLING PG, et al: Influence of diet and fluid on bioavailability of theophylline. Clin Pharmacol Ther 14:475, 1975.
159. STAMBAUGH JE, et al: The effect of phenobarbital on the metabolism of meperidine in normal volunteers. J Clin Pharmacol 18:482, 1978.
160. PALADINO JA, et al: Effect of secobarbital on theophylline clearance. Ther Drug Monit 5:135, 1983.
161. GRYGIEL JJ, et al: Differential effects of cimetidine on theophylline metabolic pathways. Eur J Clin Pharmacol 26:335, 1984.
162. MUSA MN, LYONS LL: Effect of food on the pharmacokinetics of propoxyphene. Curr Ther Res 19:669, 1976.
163. ALSOP WR, et al: The effects of five potassium chloride preparations on the upper gastrointestinal mucosa in healthy subjects receiving glycopyrrolate. J Clin Pharmacol 24:235, 1984.

References (CONT.)

164. McGilveray IJ, Mattok GL: Some factors affecting the absorption of paracetamol. J Pharm Pharmacol 24:615, 1972.

165. Mattok GL, McGilveray IJ: The effect of food intake and sleep on the absorption of acetaminophen. Rev Can Biol 32(s):77, 1973.

166. Jaffe JM, et al: Effects of dietary components on GI absorption of acetaminophen tablets in man. J Pharm Sci 60:1646, 1971.

167. Emori HW, et al: Indomethacin pharmacokinetics. Aust NZ Med J 4:212, 1974.

168. Indocin®. Physicians' Desk Reference. 31st Ed. Oradell, New Jersey, Medical Economics Company, 1977.

169. Coste JF, et al: In-vitro interactions of oral hematinics and antacid suspensions. Curr Ther Res 22:205, 1977.

170. Horwitz D, et al: The influence of allopurinol and size of dose on the metabolism of phenylbutazone in patients with gout. Eur J Clin Pharmacol 12:133, 1977.

171. Barbiturates and barbiturate-like drugs. JAMA 230:1440, 1974.

172. Goode DL, et al: Effect of antacid on the bioavailability of lithium carbonate. Clin Pharm 3:284, 1984.

173. Cousins MJ, Mazze RI: Methoxyflurane nephrotoxicity: a study of dose response in man. JAMA 225:1611, 1973.

174. Anderson KE, et al: Oxidative drug metabolism and inducibility by phenobarbital in sickle cell anemia. Clin Pharamcol Ther 22:580, 1977.

175. Buchanan N, et al: Symmetrical gangrene of the extremities associated with the use of dopamine subsequent to ergometrine administration. Intensive Care Med 3:55, 1977.

176. Pearce LA, Waterbury LD: L-methionine: a possible levodopa antagonist. Neurology 24:640, 1974.

177. Duvoisin RC: Antagonism of levodopa by papaverine. JAMA 231:845, 1975.

178. Gardos G, Cole J: Papaverine for tardive dyskinesia? (Letter). N Engl J Med 292:1355, 1975.

179. Posner DM: Antagonism of levodopa by papaverine (Letter). JAMA 233:768, 1975.

180. Juhl RP, et al: Concomitant administration of haloperidol and lithium carbonate in acute mania. Dis Nerv Syst 38:675, 1977.

181. Borden H, et al: The use of pancuronium bromide in patients receiving lithium carbonate. Can Anaesth Soc J 21:79, 1974.

182. Hill GE, et al: Potentiation of succinylcholine neuromuscular blockade by lithium carbonate. Anesthesiology 44:439, 1976.

183. Eilderton TE, et al: Reduction in plasma cholinesterase levels after prolonged administration of echothiophate iodide eyedrops. Can Anaesth Soc J 15:291, 1968.

184. Piafsky KM, et al: Effect of phenobarbital on the disposition of intravenous theophylline. Clin Pharmacol Ther 22:336, 1977.

185. Galeazzi RL: The effect of an antacid on the bioavailability of indomethacin. Eur J Clin Pharmacol 12:65, 1977.

186. Landay RA, et al: Effect of phenobarbital on theophylline disposition. J Allergy Clin Immunol 62:27, 1978.

187. McMahon FG, et al: Upper gastrointestinal lesions after potassium chloride supplements: a controlled clinical trial. Lancet 2:1059, 1982.

188. Advertisement for Slow-K. JAMA 250:281, 1983.

References (CONT.)

189. STEINBERG WM, et al: Antacids inhibit absorption of cimetidine. N Engl J Med 307:400, 1982.
190. MIHALY GW, et al: High dose of antacid (Mylanta II) reduces bioavailability of ranitidine. Br Med J 285:998, 1982.
191. FRISLID K, BERSTAD A: High dose of antacid reduces bioavailability of ranitidine. Br Med J 286:1358, 1983.
192. MAY DC, JARBOE CH: Effect of probenecid on dyphylline elimination. Clin Pharmacol Ther 33:822, 1983.
193. CHEN TWD, PATTON TF: Effect of probenecid on the pharmacokinetics of aminophylline. Drug Intell Clin Pharm 17:465, 1983.
194. KERRY RJ, et al: Possible toxic interaction between lithium piroxicam. Lancet 1:418, 1983.
195. HENDY MS, et al: Mazindol-induced lithium toxicity. Br Med J 280:684, 1980.
196. NIMMO J, et al: Pharmacological modification of gastric emptying: effects of propantheline and metoclopromide on paracetamol absorption. Br Med J 1:587, 1973.
197. NIMMO J: The influence of metoclopramide on drug absorption. Postgrad Med J 49 (July Supplement):25, 1973.
198. DAVID BO, YOEL G: Calcium and calciferol antagonise effect of verapamil in atrial fibrillation. Br Med J 282:1585, 1981.
199. PERKINS CM: Serious verapamil poisoning treatment with intravenous calcium gluconate. Br Med J 2:1127, 1978.
200. WOIE L, STORSTEIN L: Successful treatment of suicidal verapamil poisoning with calcium gluconate. Eur Heart J 2:239, 1981.
201. CHIMIENTI M, et al: Acute verapamil poisoning: successful treatment with epinephrine. Clin Cardiol 5:219, 1982.
202. LEVY G, HOUSTON JB: Effect of activated charcoal on acetaminophen absorption. Pediatrics 58:432, 1976.
203. DORDONI B, et al: Reduction of absorption of paracetamol by activated charcoal and cholestyramine: a possible therapeutic measure. Br Med J 3:86, 1973.
204. PERUCCA E, RICHENS A. Paracetamol disposition in normal subjects treated with antiepileptic drugs. Br J Clin Pharmacol 7:201, 1979.
205. PESSAYRE E, et al: Additive effects of inducers and fasting on acetaminophen hepatotoxicity. Biochem Pharmacol 29:2219, 1980.
206. McLEAN AEM, et al: Dietary factors in renal & hepatic toxicity of paracetamol. J Int Med Res 4(Supplement 4):79, 1976.
207. WILSON JT, et al: Death in an adolescent following an overdose of acetaminophen and phenobarbital. Am J Dis Child 132:466, 1978.
208. BOYER TD, ROUFF SL: Acetaminophen-induced hepatic necrosis and renal failure. JAMA 218:440, 1971.
209. NEUVONEN PJ, et al: Antipyretic analgesics in patients on antiepileptic drug therapy. Eur J Clin Pharmacol 15:263, 1979.
210. GANNON R, et al: Possible interaction between vidarabine and theophylline. Ann Intern Med 101:148, 1984.
211. HENDELES L, WEINBERGER M: Theophylline: a "state of the art" review. Pharmacotherapy 3:2, 1983.
212. Mulley BA et al: Interactions between diazepam and paracetamol. J Clin Pharm 3:25, 1978.
213. BOSTON COLLABORATIVE DRUG SURVEILLANCE PROGRAM: Clinical depres-

References (CONT.)

sion of the central nervous system due to diazepam and chlordiaze-poxide in relation to cigarette smoking and age. N Engl J Med 288:277, 1973.

214. KLOTZ U, et al: The effects of age and liver disease on the disposition and elimination of diazepam in adult man. J Clin Invest 55:347, 1975.

215. DESMOND PV, et al: No effect of smoking on metabolism of chlordiaze-poxide. N Engl J Med 300:199, 1979.

216. GREENBLATT DJ, et al: Diazepam disposition determinants. Clin Pharmacol Ther 27:301, 1980.

217. GREENBLATT DJ, et al: Lorazepam kinetics in the elderly. Clin Pharmacol Ther 26:103, 1979.

218. CROW JW, et al: Glutethimide and 4-OH glutethimide: pharmacokinetics and effect on performance in man. Clin Pharmacol Ther 22:458, 1978.

219. CIPOLLE RJ, et al: Heparin kinetics: variables related to disposition and dosage. Clin Pharmacol Ther 29:387, 1981.

220. KEERI-SZANTO M, POMEROY JR: Atmosphere pollution and pentazocine metabolism. Lancet 1:947, 1971.

221. VAUGHAN DP, et al: The influence of smoking on the intersubject variation in pentazocine elimination. Br J Clin Pharmacol 3:279, 1976.

222. JENNE J, et al: Decreased theophylline half-life in cigarette smokers. Life Sci 17:195, 1975.

223. JUSKO WJ, et al: Enhanced biotransformation of theophylline in marihuana and tobacco smokers. Clin Pharmacol Ther 24:406, 1978.

224. PFEIFER HJ, GREENBLATT DJ: Clinical toxicity of theophylline in relation to cigarette smoking. A report from the Boston Collaborative Drug Surveillance. Chest 73:455, 1978.

225. HUNT SN, et al: Effect of smoking on theophylline disposition. Clin Pharmacol Ther 19:546, 1976.

226. POWELL JR, et al: The influence of cigarette smoking and sex on theophylline disposition. Am Rev Respir Dis 116:17, 1977.

227. HADLER AJ: Phenmetrazine vs. phenmetrazine with amobarbital for weight reduction: double-blind study. Curr Ther Res 11:750, 1969.

228. KAUKINEN S, et al: Prolongation of thiopentone anaesthesia by probenecid. Br J Anaesth 52:603, 1980.

229. SOMOGYI A, et al: Influence of phenobarbital treatment of cimetidine kinetics. Eur J Clin Pharmacol 19:343, 1981.

230. MacLEOD SM, et al: Interaction of disulfiram with benzodiazepines. Clin Pharmacol Ther 24:583, 1978.

231. SELLERS EM, et al: Differential effects of benzodiazepine disposition by disulfiram and ethanol. Arzneimmittelforsch 30:882, 1980.

232. TOBERT JA, et al: Effect of antacids on the bioavailability of diflunisal in the fasting and postprandial states. Clin Pharmacol Ther 30:385, 1981.

233. VERBEECK R, et al: Effect of aluminum hydroxide on diflunisal absorption. Br J Clin Pharmacol 7:519, 1979.

234. HOLMES GI, et al: Effects of maalox on the bioavailability of diflunisal. Clin Pharmacol Ther 25:229, 1979.

235. WILKINSON GR, BECKETT AH: Absorption, metabolism and excretion of the ephedrines in man. I. The influence of urinary pH and urine volume output. J Pharmacol Exp Ther 162:139, 1968.

References (CONT.)

236. LEE KY, et al: Severe hypertension after ingestion of an appetite suppressant (phenylpropanolamine) with indomethacin. Lancet 1:1110, 1979.
237. TI TY, et al: Probable interaction of loperamide and cholestyramine. Can Med Assoc J 119:607, 1978.
238. RUNKEL R, et al: Naproxen-probenecid interaction. Clin Pharmacol Ther 24:706, 1978.
239. FROLICH JC, et al: Indomethacin increases plasma lithium. Br Med J 1:1115, 1978.
240. RAGHEB M, et al: Interaction of indomethacin and ibuprofen with lithium in manic patients under a steady-state lithium level. J Clin Psychiatry 41:397, 1980.
241. OSMAN MA, et al: Reduction in oral penicillamine absorption by food, antacid, and ferrous sulfate. Clin Pharmacol Ther 33:465, 1983.
242. HANSEN BS, et al: Influence of dextropropoxyphene on steady state serum levels and protein binding of three anti-epileptic drugs in man. Acta Neurol Scand 61:357, 1980.
243. ROSENBERRY KR, et al: Reduced theophylline half-life induced by carbamazepine therapy. J Pediatr 102:472, 1983.
244. YOSSELSON-SUPERSTINE S, LIPMAN AG: Chlordiazepoxide interaction with levodopa. Ann Intern Med 96:259, 1982.
245. SPRING G, FRANKEL M: New data on lithium and haloperidol incompatibility. Am J Psychiatry 138:818, 1981.
246. KAMLANA SH, et al: Lithium: some drug interactions. Practitioner 224:1291, 1980.
247. STRAYHORN JM, NASH JL: Severe neurotoxicity despite "therapeutic" serum lithium levels. Dis Nerv Syst 38:107, 1977.
248. THOMAS C, et al: Lithium/haloperidol combinations and brain damage. Lancet 1:626, 1982.
249. TURNER TH: Lithium/haloperidol combinations and brain damage. Lancet 1:856, 1982.
250. SILVERMAN G: Lithium/haloperidol combinations and brain damage. Lancet 1:856, 1982.
251. CARMAN JS, et al: Lithium combined with neuroleptics in chronic schizophrenic and schizoaffective patients. J Clin Psychiatry 42:124, 1981.
252. BIEDERMAN J, et al: Combination of lithium carbonate and haloperidol in schizo-affective disorder. Arch Gen Psychiatry 36:327, 1979.
253. TUPIN JP, SCHULLER AB: Lithium and haloperidol incompatibility reviewed. Psychiat J Univ Ottawa 3:245, 1978.
254. FETZER J, et al: Lithium encephalopathy: a clinical, psychiatric, and EEG evaluation. Am J Psychiatry 138:1622, 1981.
255. THOMAS CJ: Brain damage with lithium/haloperidol. Br J Psychiatry 134:552, 1979.
256. THORNTON WE, PRAY BJ: Lithium intoxication: a report of two cases. Can Psychiatr Assoc J 20:281, 1975.
257. BABER N, et al: The interaction between indomethacin and probenecid: a clinical and pharmacokinetic study. Clin Pharmacol Ther 24:298, 1978.
258. OSMAN MA, et al: Reduction in oral penicillamine absorption by food, antacid, and ferrous sulfate. Clin Pharmacol Ther 33:465, 1983.
259. MARTIN BA, KRAMER PM: Clinical significance of the interaction be-

References (CONT.)

tween lithium and a neuromuscular blocker. Am J Psychiatry 139:1326, 1982.

260. SIERLES FS, OSSOWSKI MG: Concurrent use of theophylline and lithium in a patient with chronic obstructive lung disease and bipolar disorder. Am J Psychiatry 139:117, 1982.
261. MILLER RR: Effects of smoking on drug action. Clin Pharmacol Ther 22:749, 1977.
262. BOSTON COLLABORATIVE DRUG SURVEILLANCE PROGRAM: Decreased clinical efficacy of propoxyphene in cigarette smokers. Clin Pharmacol Ther 14:259, 1973.
263. JACKSON JE, et al: Cimetidine decreases theophylline clearance. Am Rev Respir Dis 23:615, 1981.
264. REITBERG DP, et al: Alteration of theophylline clearance and half-life by cimetidine in normal volunteers. Ann Intern Med 95:582, 1981.
265. ROBERTS RK, et al: Cimetidine impairs the elimination of theophylline and antipyrine. Gastroenterology 81:19, 1981.
266. SCHWARTZ JI, et al: Impact of cimetidine on the pharmacokinetics of theophylline. Clin Pharm 1:534, 1982.
267. LALONDE RL, et al: The effects of cimetidine on theophylline pharmacokinetics at steady state. Chest 2:221, 1983.
268. KELLY JF, et al: The effect of cimetidine on theophylline metabolism in the elderly. Clin Pharmacol Ther 31:238, 1982.
269. FENJE PC, et al: Interaction of cimetidine and theophylline in two infants. Can Med Assoc J 126:1178, 1982.
270. CLUXTON RJ, et al: Cimetidine-theophylline interaction. Ann Intern Med 96:684, 1982.
271. JACKSON JE, PLACHETKA JR: More on cimetidine-theophylline interaction. Drug Intell Clin Pharm 15:809, 1981.
272. HENDELES L, et al: The interaction of cimetidine and theophylline. Drug Intell Clin Pharm 15:808, 1981.
273. WEINBERGER MM, et al: Decreased theophylline clearance due to cimetidine. N Engl J Med 304:672, 1981.
274. CAMPBELL MA, et al: Cimetidine decreases theophylline clearance. Ann Intern Med 95:68, 1981.
275. LOFGREN RP, GILBERTSON RA: Cimetidine and theophylline. Ann Intern Med 96:378, 1982.
276. BAUMAN JH, et al: Cimetidine-theophylline interaction: report of four patients. Ann Allergy 48:100, 1982.
277. ANDERSON JR, et al: A fatal case of theophylline intoxication. Arch Intern Med 143:559, 1983.
278. KLOTZ U, REIMANN I: Delayed clearance of diazepam due to cimetidine. N Engl J Med 302:1012, 1980.
279. DESMOND PV, et al: Cimetidine impairs elimination of chloridiazepoxide (Librium) in man. Ann Intern Med 93:266, 1980.
280. KLOTZ U, REIMANN I: Elevation of steady-state diazepam levels by cimetidine. Clin Pharmacol Ther 30:513, 1981.
281. PATWARDHAN RV, et al: Lack of tolerance and rapid recovery of cimetidine-inhibited chlordiazepoxide (Librium) elimination. Gastroenterology 81:547, 1981.
282. RUFFALO RL, et al: Cimetidine-benzodiazepine drug interaction. Am J Hosp Pharm 38:1365, 1981.
283. GOUGH PA, et al: Influence of cimetidine on oral diazepam elimina-

References (CONT.)

tion with measurement of subsequent cognitive change. Br J Clin Pharmacol 14:739, 1982.

284. Hiss J, et al: Fatal bradycardia after intentional overdose of cimetidine and diazepam. Lancet 1:982, 1982.
285. Greenblatt DJ, et al: The diazepam-cimetidine interaction: is it clinically important? Clin Pharmacol Ther 35:245, 1984.
286. Divoll M, et al: Cimetidine impairs drug oxidizing capacity in the elderly. Clin Pharmacol Ther 31:218, 1982.
287. Greenblatt DJ, et al: Old age, cimetidine, and disposition of alprazolam and triazolam. Clin Pharmacol Ther 33:253, 1983.
288. Greenblatt DJ, et al: Halazepam, another precursor of desmethyldiazepam. Lancet 1:1358, 1982.
289. Klotz U, Reimann I: Influence of cimetidine on the pharmacokinetics of desmethyldiazepam and oxazepam. Eur J Clin Pharmacol 18:517, 1980.
290. Patwardhan RV, et al: Cimetidine spares the glucuronidation of lorazepam and oxazepam. Gastroenterology 79:912, 1970.
291. Fernandes E, Melewicz FM: Ranitidine and theophylline. Ann Intern Med 100:459, 1984.
292. Dobbs JH, Smith RN: Ranitidine and theophylline. Ann Intern Med 100:769, 1984.
293. Breen KJ, et al: Effects of cimetidine and ranitidine and hepatic drug metabolism. Clin Pharmacol Ther 31:297, 1982.
294. Rogers JF, et al: The influence of cimetidine vs ranitidine on theophylline pharmacokinetics. Clin Pharmacol Ther 31:261, 1982.
295. Ruff E: Interferences medicamenteuses de la theophylline—Absence d'interaction theophylline-ranitidine. Nouvelle Presse Med 11:3512, 1982.
296. Ost L: Effects of cyclosporin on prednisolone metabolism. Lancet 1:451, 1984.
297. Klintmalm G, Sawe J: High dose methylprednisolone increases plasma cyclosporin levels in renal transplant recipients. Lancet 1:731, 1984.
298. Ferguson RM, et al: Ketoconazole, cyclosporin metabolism, and renal transplantation. Lancet 2:882, 1982.
299. Cunningham C, et al: Ketoconazole, cyclosporin, and the kidney. Lancet 2:1464, 1982.
300. Morgenstern GR, et al: Cyclosporin interaction with ketoconazole and melphalan. Lancet 2:1342, 1982.
301. Ringden O, et al: Nephrotoxicity by co-trimoxazole and cyclosporin in transplanted patients. Lancet 1:1016, 1984.
302. Fine A, Churchill DN: Potentially lethal interaction of cimetidine and morphine. Can Med Assoc J 124:1434, 1981.
303. Lam AM, Parkin JA: Cimetidine and prolonged post-operative somnolence. Can Anaesth Soc J 28:450, 1981.
304. Knodell RG, et al: Drug metabolism by rat and human hepatic microsomes in response to interaction with H_2-receptor antagonists. Gastroenterology 82:84, 1982.
305. Lee HR, et al: Effect of histamine H_2-receptors fentanyl metabolism. Pharmacologist 24:145, 1982.
306. Mojaverian P, et al: Cimetidine does not alter morphine disposition in man. Br J Clin Pharmacol 14:309, 1982.

References (CONT.)

307. PHILBIN DM, et al: The use of H_1 and H_2 histamine antagonists with morphine anesthesia: a double-blind study. Anesthesiology 55:292, 1981.
308. GRUND VR, HUNNINGHAKE DB: Inhibition of histamine-stimulated increases in heart rate in man with the H_2-histamine receptor antagonist cimetidine. J Clin Pharmacol 21:87, 1981.
309. LOI CM, et al: The effect of multiple-dose cimetidine on the pharmacokinetics of verapamil. Drug Intell Clin Pharm 18:494, 1984.
310. KIRCH W, et al: Influence of the two histamine H_2-receptor antagonists cimetidine and ranitidine on plasma levels and clinical effect of nifedipine and metoprolol (Abstract). 14th Congress, European Society of Toxicologists, 28–30th March 1983 in Rome, p. 46.
311. HETZEL DJ, et al: Cimetidine interaction with phenytoin. Br Med J 228:1512, 1981.
312. ALGOZZINE GJ, et al: Decreased clearance of phenytoin with cimetidine. Ann Intern Med 95:244, 1981.
313. NEUVONEN PJ, et al: Cimetidine-phenytoin interaction: effect on serum phenytoin concentration and antipyrine test. Eur J Clin Pharmacol 21:215, 1981.
314. SALEM RB, et al: Effect of cimetidine on phenytoin serum levels. Epilepsia 24:284, 1983.
315. ITEOGU MO, et al: Effect of cimetidine on single-dose phenytoin kinetics. Clin Pharm 2:302, 1983.
316. BARTLE WR, et al: Dose-dependent effect of cimetidine on phenytoin kinetics. Clin Pharmacol Ther 33:649, 1983.
317. WATTS RW, et al: Lack of interaction between ranitidine and phenytoin. Br J Clin Pharmacol 15:499, 1983.
318. BELZ GG, et al: Digoxin plasma concentrations and nifedipine. Lancet 1:844, 1981.
319. PEDERSEN KE, et al: Digoxin-verapamil interaction. Clin Pharmacol Ther 30:311, 1981.
320. KLEIN HO, et al: Verapamil and digoxin: their respective effects on atrial fibrillation and their interaction. Am J Cardiol 50:894, 1982.
321. BELZ GG, et al: Interaction between digoxin and calcium antagonists and antiarrhythmic drugs. Clin Pharmacol Ther 33:410, 1983.
322. KLEIN HO, et al: The influence of verapamil on serum digoxin concentration. Circulation 65:998, 1982.
323. KOUNIS N: Asystole after verapamil and digoxin. Br J Clin Pract 34:57, 1980.

INDEX

In the following index, the drug interactions are divided into three categories of clinical significance which are designated by differing type faces.

Bold type—Major Clinical Significance: includes those interactions which are relatively well documented and which have the potential of being harmful to the patient.

Italic   —Moderate Clinical Significance: includes those interactions for which more documentation is needed and/or the potential harm to the patient is less.

Roman   —Minor Clinical Significance: includes those interactions which may occur but are least significant because of one or more of the following factors.

   1) documentation is poor.
   2) potential harm to the patient is slight.
   3) incidence of the interaction is quite low.

See Instructions to Users, page ix, for a discussion of the criteria used in assigning interactions to these three categories.

439

445

447

Dopamine *(continued)*
  phenytoin, 126
Dopar. See levodopa.
Dopram. See doxapram.
Doriden. See glutethimide.
Doxapram
  beta-adrenergic blockers, 31
  monoamine oxidase inhibitors, 335
Doxepin. See also antidepressants,
    tricyclic.
  bethanidine, 170
  guanethidine, 177
Doxinate. See docusate.
Doxorubicin
  barbiturates, 264
Dymelor. See antidiabetics.
Dyphylline
  probenecid, 402
Dyrenium. See triamterene.

E

Echothiophate iodide
  procaine, 402
  succinylcholine, 403
Edecrin. See ethacrynic acid.
Edrophonium. See also cholinergic
    agents.
  digitalis glycosides, 277
Ephedrine
  acetazolamide, 286
  ammonium chloride, 381
  bethanidine, 171
  corticosteroids, 320
  guanethidine, 178
  methyldopa, 183
  monoamine oxidase inhibitors, 335
  reserpine, 187
  sodium bicarbonate, 403
  theophylline, 404
Epinephrine
  antidepressants, tricyclic, 370
  antidiabetics, 155
  beta-adrenergic blockers, 32
  monoamine oxidase inhibitors, 335
Equanil. See meprobamate.
Ergot alkaloids
  beta-adrenergic blockers, 33
  dopamine, 402
  nitroglycerin, 47
Erythromycin
  anticoagulants, oral, 80
  beta-adrenergic blockers, 33
  carbamazepine, 117
  clindamycin, 208
  digitalis glycosides, 209
  lincomycin, 210
  penicillins, 210
  theophylline, 211
Eskalith. See lithium carbonate.
Estrogens. See contraceptives, oral.

Ethacrynic acid
  aminoglycosides, 197
  anticoagulants, oral, 81
  cisplatin, 262
  corticosteroids, 289
  lithium carbonate, 289
Ethanol (alcohol)
  acetaminophen, 303
  aminosalicyclic acid, 200
  anticoagulants, oral, 66
  antidepressants, tricyclic, 304
  antidiabetics, 155
  antipyrine, 304
  ascorbic acid, 304
  barbiturates, 305
  benzodiazepines, 305
  beta-adrenergic blockers, 33
  bromocriptine, 306
  caffeine, 306
  cephalosporins, 204
  chloral hydrate, 306
  chloramphenicol, 206
  chloroform, 307
  cimetidine, 307
  cromolyn, 308
  disulfiram, 308
  ethionamide, 212
  food, 309
  furazolidone, 212
  glutethimide, 309
  guanethidine, 178
  isoniazid, 216
  meprobamate, 309
  methotrexate, 265
  metoclopramide, 309
  metronidazole, 221
  milk, 309
  monoamine oxidase inhibitors, 336
  narcotic analgesics, 310
  nitroglycerin, 47
  paraldehyde, 310
  penicillin, 225
  phenothiazines, 310
  phenytoin, 127
  procainamide, 15
  procarbazine, 268
  quinacrine, 229
  salicylates, 311
  sulfonamide, 236
  tetrachloroethylene, 312
  tetracycline, 240
  tolazoline, 312
  trichloroethylene, 312
  vitamin C, 304
Ethclorvynol
  anticoagulants, oral, 81
  antidepressants, tricyclic, 370
Ethionamide
  ethanol (alcohol), 212
Extended spectrum penicillins.
  aminoglycosides, 194

Kaolin-pectin *(continued)*
lincomycin, 219
pseudoephedrine, 409
Kaopectate. See kaolin-pectin.
Kayexalate. See sodium polystyrine
sulfonate resin.
Ketamine
thyroid hormones, 327
Ketoconazole
antacids, 218
cimetidine, 218
cyclosporine, 400

L

Lanoxin. See digitalis glycosides.
Larodopa. See levodopa.
Lasix. See furosemide.
Laxatives
anticoagulants, oral, 86, 89, 93
contraceptives, oral, 326
isoniazid, 216
quinidine, 20
sulfonamide, 236, 237
vitamin A, 415
L-DOPA. See levodopa.
Levarterenol. See norepinephrine.
Levodopa
antacids, 385
anticholinergics, 387
antidepressants, tricyclic, 371
benzodiazepines, 394
beta-adrenergic blockers, 37
clonidine, 173
food, 409
guanethidine, 179
methionine, 410
methyldopa, 184
monoamine oxidase inhibitors, 337
papaverine, 410
phenothiazines, 349
phenylbutazone, 410
phenylephrine, 410
phenytoin, 130
pyridoxine, 411
reserpine, 187
Levophed. See norepinephrine.
Levoprome. See methotrimeprazine.
Librium. See benzodiazepines.
Lidocaine
ajmaline, 7
aminoglycosides, 7
amiodarone, 3
barbiturates, 8
beta-adrenergic blockers, 8
cephalosporins, 9
cimetidine, 9
diazepam, 10
digitalis glycosides, 10

Lidocaine *(continued)*
diphenhydramine, 10
disopyramide, 5
isoproterenol, 10
levarterenol, 11
neuromuscular blocking agents,
11
phenytoin, 11
polymixin B, 7
procainamide, 12
ranitidine, 12
smoking, 12
Lignocaine. See lidocaine.
Lincocin. See lincomycin.
Lincomycin
erythromycin, 210
food, 218
kaolin-pectin, 219
Liquamar. See anticoagulants, oral.
Lithane. See lithium carbonate.
Lithium carbonate
acetazolamide, 287
amphetamine, 383
antacids, 386
antidepressants, tricyclic, 371
benzodiazepines, 395
carbamazepine, 118
ethacrynic acid, 289
furosemide, 291
haloperidol, 404
indomethacin, 406
levarterenol, 411
mazindol, 411
methyldopa, 184
neuromuscular blocking agents,
412
norepinephrine, 411
phenothiazines, 350
phenytoin, 130
piroxicam, 412
potassium iodide, 412
spironolactone, 293
sodium bicarbonate, 413
sodium chloride, 413
tetracycline, 242
theophylline, 413
thiazide diuretics, 296
urea, 414
Lithonate. See lithium carbonate.
Loperamide
cholestyramine, 397
Lopressor. See beta-adrenergic
blockers.
Lorazepam. See benzodiazepines.
Loxapine
phenytoin, 130
Loxitane. See loxapine.
Ludiomil. See antidepressants,
tricyclic.
Lufyllin. See dyphylline.

Placidyl. See ethchlorvynol.
Platinol. See cisplatin.
Polymyxin
  lidocaine, 7
  neuromuscular blockers, 228
Pondamin. See fenfluramine.
Ponstel. See mefenamic acid.
Potassium salts
  anticholinergics, 388
  antidiabetics, 159
  disopyramide, 6
  spironolactone, 294
  triamterene, 298
Prazepam. See benzodiazepines.
Prazosin
  beta-adrenergic blockers, 43
  indomethacin, 186
Primidone
  acetazolamide, 138
  barbiturates, 139
  clonazepam, 120
  clorazepate, 139
  isoniazid, 139
  phenytoin, 134
  valproic acid, 140
Pro-banthine. See propantheline.
Probenecid
  allopurinol, 381
  aminosalicylic acid, 201
  antidiabetics, 159
  barbiturates, 392
  bumetanide, 288
  captopril, 172
  cephalosporin, 205
  dapsone, 401
  dyphylline, 402
  furosemide, 292
  indomethacin, 407
  methotrexate, 267
  nalidixic acid, 222
  naproxen, 415
  rifampin, 233
  salicylate, 361
  sulfinpyrazone, 419
Procainamide
  acetazolamide, 13
  ammonium chloride, 13
  antacids, 13
  beta-adrenergic blockers, 14
  cholinergic agents, 14
  cimetidine, 14
  ethanol (alcohol), 15
  isoniazid, 15
  lidocaine, 12
  neuromuscular blocking agent, 15
  sodium bicarbonate, 16
Procaine. See also anesthetics, local.
  echothiophate iodide, 402
  neuromuscular blockers, 417

Procarbazine
  central nervous system depressants, 268
  ethanol (alcohol), 268
  sympathomimetics, 269
Procardia. See nifedipine.
Pronestyl. See procainamide.
Propadrine. See phenylpropanolamine.
Propantheline. See also anticholinergics.
  acetaminophen, 380
  digitalis glycosides, 280
Propoxyphene
  anticoagulants, oral, 93
  antidepressants, tricyclic, 373
  barbiturates, 392
  beta-adrenergic blockers, 43
  carbamazepine, 119
  food, 419
  orphenadrine, 418
  smoking, 420
  spironolactone, 294
Propranolol. See beta-adrenergic blockers.
Propylthiouracil
  food, 420
Protriptyline. See antidepressants, tricyclic.
Pseudoephedrine
  ammonium chloride, 382
  kaolin, 409
  monoamine oxidase inhibitors, 340
  sodium bicarbonate, 420
Psyllium
  anticoagulants, oral, 93
Purinethol. See mercaptopurine.
Pyopen. See extended spectrum penicillins.
Pyrazinamide
  aminosalicylic acid, 201
  isoniazid, 217
Pyridostigmine. See also cholinergic agents.
  methocarbamol, 414
Pyridoxine
  barbiturates, 392
  levodopa, 411
  phenytoin, 134
Pyrimethamine
  folic acid, 229
  quinine, 229

Q

Quaalude. See methaqualone.
Questran. See cholestyramine.
Quinacrine
  ethanol, 229